ELECTROENCEPHALOGRAPHY

Hans O. Lüders
Staff, Epilepsy Center, University Hospitals, Cleveland

Soheyl Noachtar
Staff, Epilepsy Center Munich, Department of Neurology,
LMU University Hospital, Ludwig Maximilian University Munich

Jan Rémi
Head of the Epilepsy Center Munich, Vice Chair, Department of Neurology,
LMU University Hospital, Ludwig Maximilian University Munich

ELECTROENCEPHALOGRAPHY

Textbook and Atlas

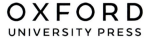

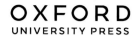

OXFORD
UNIVERSITY PRESS

Oxford University Press is a department of the University of Oxford. It furthers the University's objective of excellence in research, scholarship, and education by publishing worldwide. Oxford is a registered trade mark of Oxford University Press in the UK and certain other countries.

Published in the United States of America by Oxford University Press
198 Madison Avenue, New York, NY 10016, United States of America.

Library of Congress Cataloging-in-Publication Data
Names: Lüders, Hans, author. | Noachtar, Soheyl, author. | Rémi, Jan, 1977– author.
Title: Electroencephalography : textbook and atlas / Hans O. Lüders, Soheyl Noachtar, Jan Rémi.
Description: New York, NY : Oxford University Press, [2024] |
Includes bibliographical references and index. |
Identifiers: LCCN 2023049388 (print) | LCCN 2023049389 (ebook) |
ISBN 9780197502334 (hardback) | ISBN 9780197502358 (epub) |
ISBN 9780197502365 (electronic)
Subjects: MESH: Electroencephalography—methods
Classification: LCC RC386.6.E43 (print) | LCC RC386.6.E43 (ebook) |
NLM WL 150 | DDC 616.8/047547—dc23/eng/20231204
LC record available at https://lccn.loc.gov/2023049388
LC ebook record available at https://lccn.loc.gov/2023049389

DOI: 10.1093/med/9780197502334.001.0001

Printed by Integrated Books International, United States of America

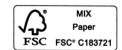

Contents

Contents

1 Introduction

Electroencephalogram (EEG) technology has changed significantly since its discovery in 1924 by Hans Berger (Berger, 1929). Digital EEG devices with an adequate number of amplifiers are available at relatively low cost. Digital recording allows us to change the montage, the filters, and the amplification of the EEG channels after the actual recording session has been completed. This allows us to display and analyze the EEG optimally after the recording. In addition, the ability to store a large amount of digital data and advances in computer analysis of EEG data are being used most effectively in the analysis of continuous EEG/video recordings. All these developments call for an innovative, new approach to electroencephalography.

The introduction of clinical EEG approximately 70 years ago was followed by the identification of different EEG patterns related to more or less specific clinical scenarios. Some of these EEG patterns, such as ictal and interictal epileptiform discharges, are still powerful diagnostic tools. Other patterns, such as focal EEG slow, are of limited practical value because more accurate and more sensitive different diagnostic methods such as magnetic resonance imaging are now used preferentially for the diagnosis of these conditions.

This book systematically describes abnormal EEG findings and their differentiation from normal variants, which may imitate the abnormal EEG patterns. The framework of the book is a structured classification of EEG findings, with the description of more or less specific EEG patterns that have a typical frequency, amplitude, distribution, and/or waveform evolution of EEG potentials over time (Lüders & Noachtar, 2000a). Such a rigid classification does not reflect the fluid transitions of nature but, rather, defines relatively objective rules for EEG interpretation, which traditionally has been very subjective (Goldensohn & Koehle, 1975). This leads to a weak interrater reliability that negatively affects the reliability of the EEG (Grant et al., 2014; Williams et al., 1985) and can result in diagnostic errors and subsequent incorrect treatments (Benbadis, 2013; Kaplan & Benbadis, 2013).

This book approaches EEG use from a direct clinical reading and interpretation perspective, i.e. reading of pages of curves in certain montages. EEG has a host of possibilities for further interpretation and application, like quantitative analysis, coherence analysis and more recently deep-learning approaches to the whole richness of the EEG (Tveit et al., 2023). These other applications will certainly be used more and more and add much value to the general method. This book focuses on the analysis of the actual EEG for a structured approach to the clinical EEG. A thorough understanding of the EEG should be the ground to the abstractions of the other analysis methods.

This book illustrates all essential abnormal EEG patterns that can be recorded with scalp electrode and physiological EEG patterns ("normal variants") that can be confused with these abnormities. For example, frontal slow activity can only be reliably classified if one is able to distinguish it from eye movements that can cause EEG potentials of similar frequency, distribution, and waveform.

The EEG examples in this book come from the EEG laboratory and the EEG video monitoring unit of the Epilepsy Center of the Department of Neurology and the Department of Neuropediatrics of the University Hospital of Munich (Ludwig-Maximilians-University Munich). The montages were designed following the guidelines of the American Clinical Neurophysiology Society (Acharya et al., 2016; see **Appendix 1**). Some illustrations show clearly defined EEG patterns with a minimum of underlying artifacts ("clean recordings"). Other illustrations show less clearly defined EEG patterns partially obscured by other EEG potentials and/or artifacts. These "not so clean" illustrations were selected purposefully to reflect more accurately "everyday life" of an EEG lab. In addition, efforts were made to also illustrate as many normal EEG patterns as possible that may simulate abnormal EEG patterns. Most of the illustrations are shown in high-resolution vector graphics. However, a few lower resolution screen shots are also included because the original EEG recordings were no longer available. We thank Dr. Christian Vollmar for his efforts to improve the resolution and to "clean up" some of the more poorly defined EEG traces. In addition, we appreciate that Prof. Ingo Borggräfe allowed us to include some of the EEG samples recorded in the Neuropediatric Section of our Epilepsy Center. We appreciate Nicholas Fearns' valuable assistance in the preparation of the figures and the manuscript.

Most EEG examples are between 15 and 18 s long, but in selected cases, shorter or longer EEG sections are shown to better illustrate a given EEG pattern. Moreover, some illustrations are excerpts from 24 to 128 channel recordings. For most EEG examples, additional images in various reformatted montages are available online on the server of Oxford University Press. This makes it possible to appreciate and evaluate the EEG sections shown in the book in different montages. The reformatting of EEG during the reading process is an important tool to optimally assess and interpret EEG recordings. For optimal display of the online figures, we recommend a screen with full high-definition resolution (1920 × 1080) or better.

The electrode designation follows the international recommendation of the 10/20 (▶ **Figure 1.1**) or 10/10 system (▶ **Figure 1.2**) (Klem et al., 1999). The nomenclature of the 10/20 system is identical to the nomenclature of the 10/10 system except for electrodes T7/T8 and P7/P8 in the 10/10 system that correspond to the designations T3/T4 and T5/T6, respectively, in the 10/20 system. The EEG terminology follows the international recommendation (Kane et al., 2017; Noachtar et al., 1999). The abbreviation EEG refers equally to electroencephalography and electroencephalogram.

In the book, mostly bipolar longitudinal montages are shown (▶ **Figures 1.3 and 1.4**). Occasionally, reference derivations (▶ **Figures 1.5–1.7**) and, more rarely, bipolar transverse rows (▶ **Figure 1.8**) are shown. In the routine EEG, ear electrodes are applied and labeled as A1 and A2 in the different montages. In prolonged recordings, however, ear electrodes are not well tolerated by most patients and are relatively susceptible to electrode artifacts. Therefore, in long-term recordings, ear electrodes are usually replaced by electrodes applied to the mastoid processes labeled as TP9/TP10.

Electrode nomenclature in the 10/20 system

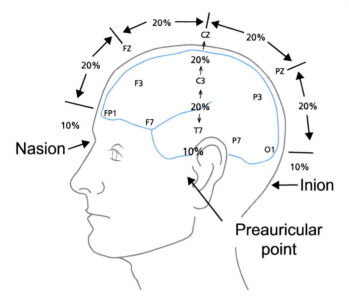

Electrode positions in the 10/10 system

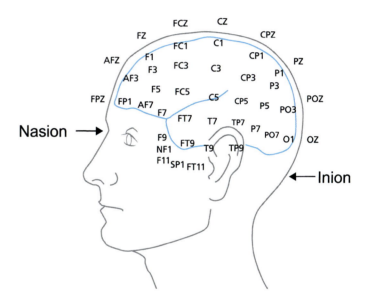

▶ **Figure 1.1** **Electrode nomenclature in the 10/20 system.** The head convexity is divided lengthwise and crosswise in steps of 10% and 20%. In the side view, the nasion, inion, and preauricular point represent reference points. Electrodes located over the left hemisphere are identified by odd numbers, and electrodes located over the right hemisphere are identified by even numbers. Electrodes over the midline are identified by a Z. The capital letters FP, F, C, P, T, and O identify electrodes placed approximately over the frontopolar, frontal, central, parietal, and occipital regions. The electrodes T7/T8 and P7/P8 correspond to the electrodes T3/T4 and T5/T6 of the old nomenclature (Klem et al., 1999).

▶ **Figure 1.2** **Electrode positions in the 10/10 system.** The head convexity is divided into steps of 10%—that is, electrode points are inserted at half the distance between the electrodes of the 10/20 system, and the nomenclature used to label the electrodes follows the same principles outlined in **Figure 1.1** (e.g., FT9/10 = frontotemporal, CP3/4 = centroparietal, and PO7/8 = parieto-occipital). The numbers 1 and 2 indicate that the electrode is 10% from the midline, the numbers 3 and 4 indicate that the electrode is 20% from the midline, and the numbers 7 and 8 specify that the electrode is 40% from the midline. Additional electrodes, such as the sphenoidal electrodes (SP1/2), are also listed. Here, too, the left-side electrodes are labeled with odd numbers and the right-side electrodes with even numbers.

Bipolar longitudinal montage

FP1-F7
F7-T7
T7-P7
P7-O1
FP2-F8
F8-T8
T8-P8
P8-O2
FP1-F3
F3-C3
C3-P3
P3-O1
FP2-F4
F4-C4
C4-P4
P4-O2
FZ-CZ
CZ-PZ

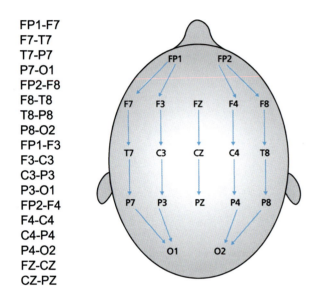

▶ **Figure 1.3** **Bipolar longitudinal montage.** Bipolar connection of the electrodes following the American convention from rostral to caudal and from left to right. Each arrow symbolizes one channel of the EEG montage. The base of the arrow is at input 1 and the tip of the arrow is at input 2 of the amplifier.

Bipolar longitudinal montage with an anterior temporal electrode (FT9)

FP1-F7
F7-FT9
FT9-T7
T7-P7
P7-O1
FP2-F8
F8-FT10
FT10-T8
T8-P8
P8-O2
FP1-F3
F3-C3
C3-P3
P3-O1
FP2-F4
F4-C4
C4-P4
P4-O2
FZ-CZ
CZ-PZ

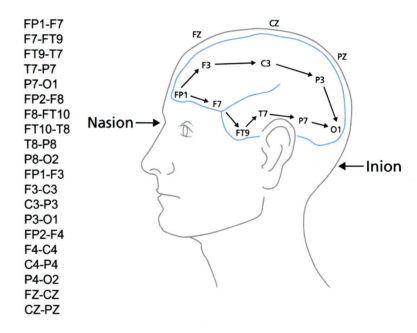

▶ **Figure 1.4** **Bipolar longitudinal montage with an anterior temporal electrode (FT9).** Bipolar longitudinal montage with an additional electrode of the 10/10 system (FT9) inserted. Each arrow symbolizes a channel of the EEG montage. The base of the arrow is at input 1 and the tip of the arrow is at input 2 of the amplifier. Only the left sided electrodes of this montage are shown here.

Vertex reference montage

FP1-CZ
FP2-CZ
F7-CZ
F8-CZ
T7-CZ
T8-CZ
P7-CZ
P8-CZ
F3-CZ
F4-CZ
C3-CZ
C4-CZ
P3-CZ
P4-CZ
O1-CZ
O2-CZ
FZ-CZ
PZ-CZ

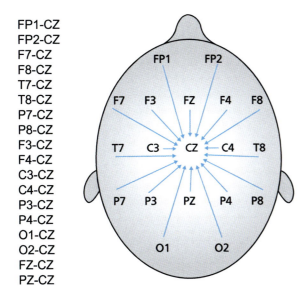

▶ **Figure 1.5**   **Vertex reference montage.** Referential montage of all electrodes to the vertex electrode CZ. Each arrow symbolizes one channel of the EEG montage. The base of the arrow is at input 1 and the tip of the arrow is at input 2 of the amplifier.

Ipsilateral ear reference montage

FP1-A1
F7-A1
T7-A1
P7-A1
FP2-A2
F8-A2
T8-A2
P8-A2
F3-A1
C3-A1
P3-A1
O1-A1
F4-A2
C4-A2
P4-A2
O2-A2
FZ-A1
CZ-A2
PZ-A1

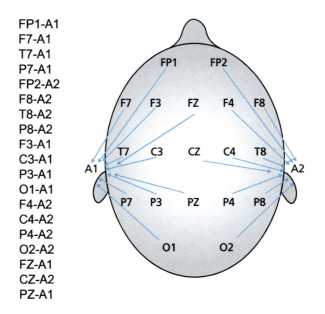

▶ **Figure 1.6**   **Ipsilateral ear reference montage.** Referential wiring of the left- and right-sided electrodes against the ipsilateral ear electrodes A1 and A2. Each arrow symbolizes one channel of the EEG montage. The base of the arrow is at input 1 and the tip of the arrow is at input 2 of the amplifier.

Unilateral ear reference montage

FP1-A2
F7-A2
T7-A2
P7-A2
FP2-A2
F8-A2
T8-A2
P8-A2
F3-A2
C3-A2
P3-A2
O1-A2
F4-A2
C4-A2
P4-A2
O2-A2
FZ-A2
CZ-A2
PZ-A2

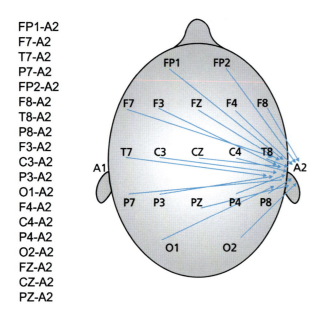

▶ **Figure 1.7** **Unilateral ear reference montage.** Referential connection of all electrodes to an ear electrode (A2). Each arrow symbolizes one channel of the EEG montage. The base of the arrow is at input 1 and the tip of the arrow is at input 2 of the amplifier.

Bipolar transverse montage

F7-FP1
FP1-FP2
FP2-F8
F7-F3
F3-FZ
FZ-F4
F4-F8
A1-T7
T7-C3
C3-CZ
CZ-C4
C4-T8
T8-A2
P7-P3
P3-PZ
PZ-P4
P4-P8
P7-O1
O1-O2
O2-P8

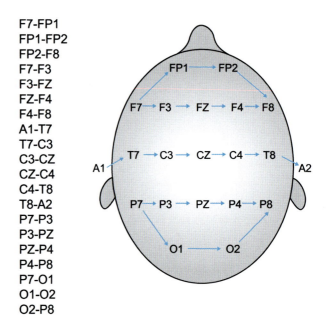

▶ **Figure 1.8** **Bipolar transverse montage.** Bipolar wiring of the electrodes from left to right. Each arrow symbolizes one channel of the EEG montage. The base of the arrow is at input 1 and the tip of the arrow is at input 2 of the amplifier.

2

FUNDAMENTALS OF ELECTROENCEPHALOGRAPHY

2.1 Biological Basis of Electroencephalography

The electroencephalogram (EEG) reflects electrical potentials generated by brain activity as well as other potentials (biological and external "artifacts") in high temporal resolution. The brain potentials represent the summed field potential of millions of neurons and glial cells. Neurons generate action potentials and synaptic potentials. Action potentials are rapid changes of the membrane potential, which in turn represents a difference in the electric potential between compartments that hold a certain electric charge (e.g., intra- vs. extracellular). The synaptic transfer occurs chemically but is accompanied by chemo-electric changes. The result of the propagation of the associated electromagnetic waves is the field potential, where the electrical events at the membrane are a typical source of these electromagnetic waves.

2.1.1 Source of EEG Signal

2.1.1.1 Action Potentials

Action potentials, due to their short duration, contribute little to the field potential derived in the EEG. However, their function and effect on the field potential should first be explained because other electrical events at the cell membrane are based on them. The membrane potential indicates the charge difference between intra- and extracellular space. Action potentials are rapid changes in this charge state and are largely caused by rapid sodium influxes into the intracellular space. The action potentials and the predominant membrane potential can be recorded by insertion of microelectrodes. The changing membrane potentials causes an electromagnetic field, which extends into the extracellular space. These field potentials can be recorded with extracellular and ultimately also with extracranial electrodes. However, there is a major difference in the contribution to the field potential, which is ultimately recorded by the EEG. Individual action potentials are typically too fast and are limited in their spatial spread by the electrochemical properties of the extracellular space (Humphrey, 1968). Typically, therefore, the field potentials of individual action potentials are not recorded by extracellular electrodes. Exceptions are (mostly hippocampal) synchronized action potentials (Buzsáki, 1986), which can be detected either with depth electrodes (Buzsáki, 2002) or with surface EEG as ultrafast frequencies (600 Hz) if appropriate sampling and filtering techniques are used (Curio, 2000).

2.1.1.2 Synaptic Potentials

In general, only electrical potentials that last long enough contribute significantly to the field potential recorded with scalp electrodes. In contrast to action potentials, the duration of synaptic potentials is 10–15 times longer. Depending on the neurotransmitter, synaptic activity causes an excitatory postsynaptic potential (EPSP) or an inhibitory postsynaptic potential (IPSP). They result in changes to the electric charge across the cell membrane, typically measured in the interstitial compartment because the intracellular changes do not contribute as much to the EEG signal. EPSPs are typically mediated by the inflow of sodium or calcium ions, resulting in a local increase of negative charge in the interstitium (loss of positive ions). IPSPs lead to a local interstitial positivity mediated by potassium outflow or chloride inflow. In order to eventually maintain a general charge equilibrium in the electrical spaces, as a result of the previous EPSP or IPSP, the same amount of charges will flow in a different direction elsewhere on the cell membrane or opposite charges flow in the same direction. The distribution of local interstitial negativities or positivities during an EPSP or IPSP at a neuron (▶ Figure 2.1) can therefore assume several states. For example, an apical dendritic EPSP leads to an active negativity, through the influx of cations, which is compensated by a passive positivity (e.g., at the cell body). On surface EEG, a negativity can therefore

Origin of the field potential

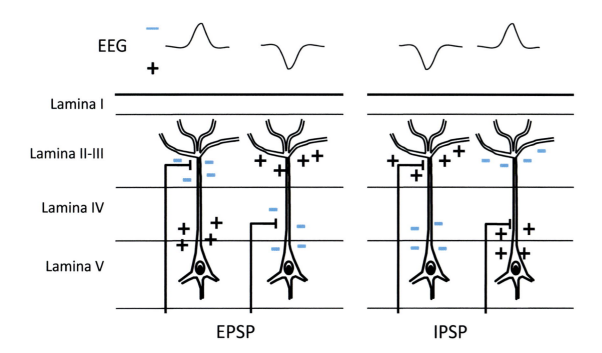

Figure 2.1 Origin of the field potential. The localization of the postsynaptic potentials (PSPs) at the neuron determines the expression of the field potential. An excitatory PSP (EPSP) close to the dendrite leads to a negativity at the scalp, and an EPSP close to the axon leads to a positivity at the scalp. With inhibitory PSPs (IPSPs), the orientation of the field potential is opposite to the EPSPs.

be determined by either an apical EPSP or a proximal IPSP (▶ **Figure 2.1**). Therefore, each neuron basically acts as an electrical dipole with negative and positive poles. For example, cortical somatosensory evoked potentials typically show a positivity at the posterior bank of the central sulcus (Brodmann's area 3) because the afferent somatosensory fibers synapse connects deep in the cortex in lamina IV and, therefore, an apically located EPSP is recorded as a positivity on the scalp surface (▶ **Figure 2.1**). However, an electrode placed caudally with respect to the central sulcus will record the negative pole of the dipole.

The different orientation of the local negativities and positivities, depending on the distribution of IPSP and EPSP at the neuron, also explains why the slow wave ("wave") is also negative after a cortical negative epileptiform discharge ("spike"), when recording from the cortical surface. The EPSP of the spike causes an active negativity at the apical dendritic tree, resulting in a passive positivity close to the soma (▶ **Figure 2.1**). The following slow wave of the spike and slow wave complex is most probably generated by an IPSP (Haglund & Schwartzkroin, 1990) located close to the soma as an active source with a more apical passive sink. The IPSP generating the slow wave of the spike and slow wave complex is most probably produced by outflow of potassium ions (Schwartzkroin & Stafstrom, 1980). Therefore, both events—the spike and the following slow wave—have similarly oriented field potentials, even though one is an EPSP and the other is an IPSP.

2.1.1.3 Spatial Arrangement of Electric Fields

The spatial arrangement of neurons is important when recording summation field potentials (▶ **Figure 2.2**) (Niedermeyer & da Silva, 2005).

Open versus closed field

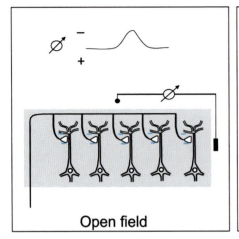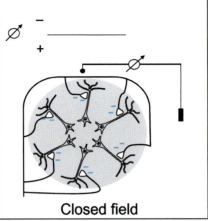

Open field	Closed field

▶ **Figure 2.2** **Open versus closed field.** The orientation of the neurons determines the field potential. With an open field, a relatively large field potential can be derived. With a closed field, no field potential can be recorded because the individual potentials cancel each other out.

Parallel-arranged large pyramidal cells of the cortex—an arrangement labeled as "open field"—generate the largest EEG potentials (▶ **Figure 2.2**). On the other hand, neurons arranged in all directions with a similar number of neurons in the opposite direction form what is called a "closed field." Synchronous excitation of approximately equal degree of all the neurons in a closed field will cancel the summation field (Timofeev et al., 2004) (▶ **Figure 2.2**). This must be taken into consideration when analyzing the EEG, because inhibitory synaptic connections are often arranged in a semi-closed field and, therefore, are represented poorly in scalp recordings. So, two waves of the same amplitude may not reflect the same neuronal activity, depending on the origin and orientation of that activity. On the other hand, the slow wave of spike-and-wave discharges, which is most likely an inhibitory potential, is usually clearly visible in scalp recordings, suggesting that it is, like the initial spike, due to synchronous discharges of neurons arranged in a semi-open field.

Solid angle concept

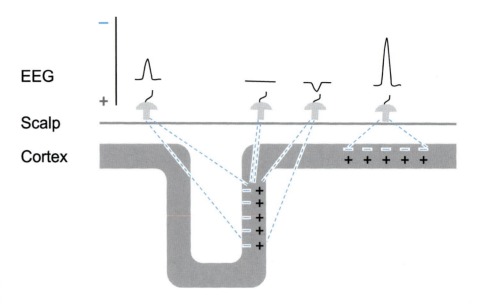

▶ **Figure 2.3** **Solid angle concept.** The orientation of the electrodes relative to the potential generator determines the amplitude of the potential recorded at the scalp (solid angle) (Gloor, 1985). Notice that a generator in a fissure is recorded as a dipole and is of relatively low amplitude. On the other side, a generator on the crown of a gyrus will behave as a monopole and will be of relatively large amplitude. In the diagram, the solid angle is represented by an active line. In reality, the solid angle is defined by the three-dimensional active surface "seen" by the recording electrode from different points of view.

In addition to the spatial arrangement of neurons, the summation field potential will be influenced by the angle between the activated cortex and the recording electrode (▶ **Figure 2.3**; Gloor, 1985). ▶ **Figure 2.3** illustrates the concept of the solid angle, which allows us to predict the polarity and the amplitude of a field potential when the recording is placed at different positions with respect to the activated cortex. It is important to remember, however, that the solid angle is a three-dimensional angle, not a two-dimensional angle as illustrated in ▶ **Figure 2.3** (Gloor, 1985).

How Is the EEG Generated?

The EEG represents mainly the sum of IPSP and EPSP occurring relatively synchronously in cortical neurons oriented perpendicularly with respect to the cortical surface. Action potentials usually do not contribute to the scalp EEG recordings.

2.1.2 Fundamentals of Rhythmic EEG Activity

A normal EEG usually includes typical rhythms of characteristic frequencies that can be recorded from different brain regions. One of the most typical examples is the occipital background rhythm, which usually has an alpha frequency. However, occasionally it may be in the beta range ("fast alpha variant") or in the theta range ("slow alpha" background rhythm). The "slow alpha variant" is frequently approximately half the normal background frequency (4–6 Hz).

The thalamus is the relay station for almost all sensory afferents (except the sense of smell), and it also receives reciprocal corticothalamic connections, not only from sensory areas but also as afferents from frontal lobe motor areas (Steriade, 2006). The different EEG rhythms generated by a normal brain are, therefore, in great part determined by the characteristics of thalamocortical and corticothalamic interconnections. The influence of the thalamus on the cortex is determined not just by its function as a relay station; the thalamic neurons also have electrophysiological properties that actively modify afferences and control states of vigilance (Llinás & Steriade, 2006). Not infrequently, the rhythmic cortical activity shows spindle-like modulations. These phenomena can be generated when two rhythms of similar frequencies occur simultaneously. The summation of these two rhythms of similar but clearly different frequency will generate a rhythm of spindle-like shape (▶ **Figure 2.4**). There is evidence that sleep spindles are generated by the interaction of thalamocortical rhythms of slightly different frequencies (Steriade, 2005). The generator of the occipital background rhythms is still poorly understood. It has been hypothesized that short bursts of efferent activity alternate with hyperpolarizations of approximately 100 ms, which would lead to a fundamental frequency of approximately 10 Hz. In addition, there is evidence that intracortical mechanisms may also

Origin of spindles

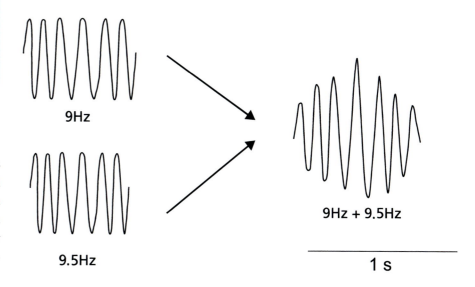

9Hz

9.5Hz

9Hz + 9.5Hz

1 s

▶ **Figure 2.4   Origin of spindles.** Spindles can be generated by combining oscillations of two generators with similar but clearly distinctive frequencies. At the vertex of the spindle (highest amplitude), the two oscillations are in phase. They then are progressively more out of phase until they are completely out of phase when the amplitude of the spindle is zero.

play a role in the generation of occipital rhythms (Lopes da Silva et al., 1980; Steriade, 2006).

The mechanism of generation of delta rhythms in the routine EEG is also still poorly understood. We know, however, that resection of the thalamus or its cortical projections in different animals (Gloor et al., 1977; Nakamura & Ohye, 1964) will not prevent the generation of cortical slow waves. We know also that during the generation of delta activity of sleep, there are rhythmic intracortical oscillations between activity and silence, leading to modulation of thalamic afferent activity from the reticular formation (Csercsa et al., 2010).

It is important to realize that cortical rhythms that have similar morphological characteristics may be generated by different neurophysiological mechanisms and therefore have very different clinical implications. For example, the delta-range slow activity seen during normal sleep frequently is morphologically very similar to the delta activity seen in patients in coma. However, these two rhythms are most likely generated by completely different mechanisms, thus explaining why the two delta rhythms have completely different clinical implications.

In summary, we may conclude that the generating mechanisms of the different physiological and pathological EEG rhythms are only partially understood and that their interpretation is based primarily on empirical electroclinical correlations. In part, this is due to the fact that the rhythms we record in scalp EEG are the summation of different rhythms generated simultaneously by different neuronal networks of millions of cells each.

2.2 Physical and Technical Fundaments of the EEG

2.2.1 Technical Structure

An EEG consists of the recording, amplification, and display of very low amplitude potentials generated by the brain. The difference in electric potential of the EEG signal recorded at the two inputs to the differential preamplifier is fed to a second amplifier, and then the signal is filtered and displayed on a PC screen. ▶ **Figure** 2.5 illustrates the different hardware components used to record EEGs. Notice that the scalp recorded EEG consists mainly of potentials that usually have only an amplitude of 20–100 μV. Occasionally, normal individuals may even have EEG recordings that do not show any activity exceeding 10 μV. On the other hand, electrodes applied to the scalp will also record eye movement potentials, electromyography (EMG) potentials, and glossokinetic potentials, which are usually of higher amplitude than brain activity. This makes EEG recording and interpretation particularly challenging.

2.2.1.1 Electrodes and Skin Contact

To get an adequate brain activity recording, it is essential to establish a stable contact of low electrical resistance between the scalp and the corresponding recording electrodes. This is achieved by applying an electrolyte paste and using relatively flat electrodes measuring a few millimeters. Flat electrodes increase the contact between scalp and the electrode, leading to a lower resistance between electrode and scalp.

Unfortunately, poorly cleaned human skin, with keratinized and sebaceous layers, frequently results in a high resistance between the scalp and the electrode. Therefore, the skin must be cleaned well—that is, the hair may have to be washed and a cleansing paste must be applied—before attempting any EEG recordings. The cleansing paste usually contains a slightly abrasive material (e.g., pumice stone) with which excess keratin layers and sebum can be removed.

At the same time, the cleansing paste contains electrolytes that also decrease the resistance between head surface and electrodes. The total resistance between scalp and electrode is called the contact resistance or electrode impedance (*resistance* refers to a direct current and *impedance* refers to alternating current). In general, for adequate scalp EEG recordings, the electrode impedance should be less than 10 kΩ (see **Appendix** 1). An increase of electrode impedance causes a slight reduction of EEG signal amplitude. This is of little importance given the capacity for amplification of modern amplifiers. On the other hand, differential amplifiers that are used in routine EEG do not amplify potentials that involve equally both inputs of the amplifier. However, if the electrode impedance between two recording electrodes is too large, the 60 Hz main signal may be amplified, obscuring the underlying brain activity. In this case, the amplitude of the artifact will be a function of the relative difference in impedance between the two electrodes. The most outstanding setting occurs when one electrode is loose (not touching the scalp), producing an infinite electrode impedance difference. Under these circumstances, the EEG usually shows a high-amplitude 60 Hz artifact produced by the electrical main and making evaluation of the brain activity impossible. Modern differential amplifiers, however, have extremely high common mode rejection ratios of up to 100,000, allowing recordings of brain activity even when there are major differences in electrode impedance between the different electrodes. However, good EEG technology requires recordings with uniformly low electrode impedance. To achieve relatively low electrode impedances, we can use an abrasive paste as also selectively light "scratching" of the skin below electrodes with relatively high impedance. In some patients, however, such as newborns and patients with severe renal insufficiency, the skin tends to be very sensitive, and care must be taken to avoid skin injuries. In these patients, we may also opt to record the EEG with relatively higher electrode impedance if the impedance is similar in all electrodes. In addition, the 60 Hz artifact from the main may also be essentially eliminated by using a notch filter (see below).

Components of an EEG system

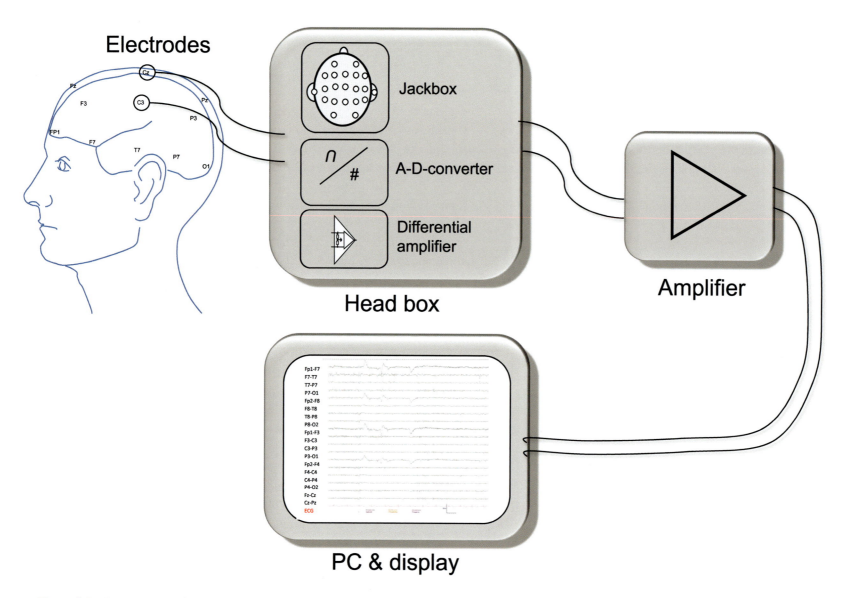

2.2.1.2 Electrodes

Metal electrodes are typically used for contact between the skin and the EEG device. For technical reasons, different materials are used. Some of these materials differ significantly in their electrical properties (▶ Figure 2.6). When metals (e.g., EEG electrodes) come into contact with a salt solution (e.g., the electrode paste), the ions of the metal strive to dissolve, depending on its electronegativity. The less noble a metal, the more likely it is that metal ions will enter the solution. When two different metals meet a saline solution and are connected outside of the solution, a half-cell battery is formed—a classic Volta element. The strength of the electrical potential produced depends on the metals and the salt solution (Cooper, 1963). For example, the combination of silver/silver chloride electrodes with gold electrodes has a potential of up to 1.28 V. This DC voltage can lead to very slow fluctuations (<<1 Hz) in the EEG, which

can be eliminated by using low-frequency filters. The different properties of the metals are relevant not only because of the combination of different metals but also because the metals influence the representation of the electrical signals (▶ Figure 2.6). Individual electrodes have a metal-dependent resistance and act like a capacitor due to its finite surface. Therefore, the electrodes themselves can act like frequency filters (see the section titled "EEG Filters"). The influence of different metals on the EEG signal is depicted in ▶ Figure 2.6 (Cooper, 1963). It is easy to see that silver/silver chloride electrodes represent the DC square wave signal well. Copper also has good conducting properties, but it is too toxic for use on the scalp.

In routine EEG, silver/silver chloride electrodes (▶ Figure 2.7) are usually used. Pure silver electrodes are not useful because of a polarization effect. However, pure silver electrodes can be chloridized by placing them in a sodium chloride solution and connecting the electrodes to a battery (e.g., 9 V block battery). A physiological sodium chloride solution for infusion therapy can be used to chloridize the silver electrodes. The silver electrodes are connected to the anode of the battery, producing an accumulation of chloride ions. This results in the characteristic gray–black coating of the electrodes. This coating chips off over time from usage in EEG recordings. Therefore, the process outlined above must be repeated regularly. To avoid having to chloridize the electrodes regularly, sintered electrodes were introduced. These electrodes consist of a mixture of very small silver and silver chloride grains firmly pressed into one another at temperatures well below the melting point (metallurgically, this process is called "sintering"). In sintered electrodes, the mixture of silver and silver chloride is more or less uniformly distributed and not just in the outside of the electrode, as is the case of silver electrodes chloridized in a physiological sodium chloride solution. Sintered electrodes, however, may be the source of artifacts. When sintered electrodes are exposed to a strong force (e.g., falling onto the floor), microscopic, not necessarily visible, cracks may occur between the grains of silver and silver chloride. Electrolytes may now penetrate these cracks (e.g., the electrolyte paste for EEG derivation or skin sweat) and, as explained above, a half-cell battery is formed, leading to an active direct current. The DC potential generated at the broken electrode is consistently higher than the DC potential at intact electrodes. Therefore, even drift-free differential amplifiers will not be able to compensate for the artifact produced by cracked sintered electrodes. Chipping-off of the silver chloride layer is also possible when using silver/silver chloride electrodes, but in this case, the damage to the silver chloride layer

EEG electrodes conducting property

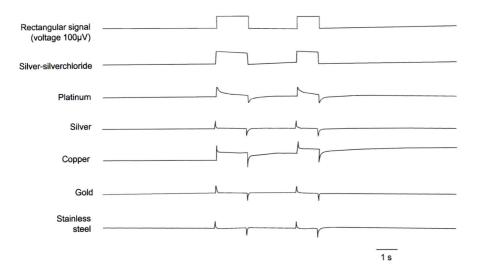

▶ **Figure 2.6** **EEG electrodes conducting property.** The rectangular calibration signal (top track) is recorded in different ways by electrodes made of different metals. The silver–silver chloride electrodes commonly used in routine EEG most accurately records the square–wave signal.

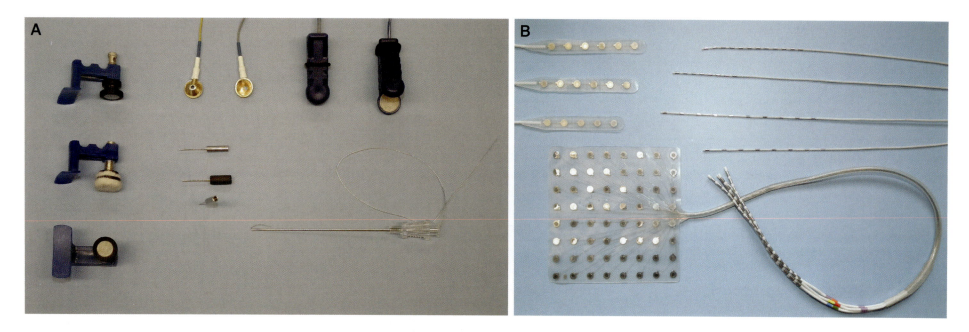

▶ **Figure 2.7** **EEG electrodes.** (A) Noninvasive EEG electrodes. Left: Stamp electrodes with chlorided silver layer (the middle electrode has the typical felt protection). Top middle: Gold-plated cup electrodes (attached with electrode adhesive, for use in EEG monitoring). Top right: Clamping electrodes used for recording potentials from the ears. Middle: Needle electrodes. Bottom right: Sphenoidal electrode consisting of a Teflon-coated steel wire that is pierced with a hollow needle. (B) Invasive electrodes. Left: Subdural strip and plate electrodes (the latter with connection tree) for use on the cortex. Right: Depth electrodes that are inserted stereotactically into the brain. The contacts of depth electrodes are usually made of platinum (steel electrodes should be avoided because they have poorer conductivity properties for slow waves; see ▶ **Figure 2.6**).

is macroscopically visible. It is hoped that further progress will be made in the manufacturing process of the electrodes to prevent these artifact sources outlined above. Currently in clinical practice, silver/silver chloride electrodes chloridized in physiological sodium chloride solutions are preferred to sintered silver/silver chloride electrodes. Unfortunately, ear electrodes that are attached to the ear with clips are only available in sintered form.

Silver/silver chloride electrodes can cause skin irritation when used for a prolonged period of time. For this reason, gold-plated silver cup electrodes filled with electrolyte paste are used for long-term EEG recordings, as for example in EEG video monitoring or in sleep laboratories (▶ **Figure 2.7**).

However, gold plating of another metal implies that cracks or scratches in the electrodes in combination with an electrolyte may again result in a half-cell battery and, therefore, electrode artifacts. To prevent cracks, the EEG electrodes must be handled carefully, and the integrity of the gold layer should be checked regularly.

In intensive care units or during surgical anesthesia, needle electrodes made of steel alloys are occasionally used. The needles are inserted subcutaneously and have the advantage that the skin resistance is roughly the same for all electrodes without the need to use electrolyte paste or to abrase the skin. As explained above, having relatively similar impedances at all electrodes minimizes the generation of artifacts produced by external sources that affect all electrodes more or less equally. When needle electrodes are used in intensive care units, it must be considered that the conductive properties for slow waves are worse for steel than for silver/silver chloride and that therefore slow waves have a relatively lower amplitude. However, because needle electrodes are more susceptible to infections, they are not used when surface electrodes can be applied. Sphenoidal electrodes (SP1 and SP2) are also made of steel. They are used mainly in the epilepsy monitoring units when a temporal lobe epilepsy is suspected (Kanner et al., 2002; D. King et al., 1986). Mesial temporal epileptiform discharges are far better represented in sphenoidal electrodes than in the routine 10/20 system (▶ Figure 2.8). The better representation of mesial temporal lobe discharges at the sphenoidal electrode is determined (a) by the position of the sphenoidal electrode immediately in front of the foramen ovale, in proximity of the uncus and adjacent mesial temporal structures; and (b) by the electrical properties of steel, which displays epileptiform discharges "more pointed" due to a faster electric decay of the potential (▶ Figure 2.6). In clinical practice, anterior temporal electrodes (FT9 and FT10) not infrequently may show mesial temporal discharges significantly better than standard 10/20 electrodes (▶ Figure 2.9) (Kanner et al., 2002). The literature on sphenoidal and FT9/FT10 electrodes emphasizes the advantage of being able to record epileptiform discharges that were not visible when using standard 10/20 or 10/10 electrodes alone. This approach, however, is misleading. The main advantage of sphenoidal electrodes is in using them together with 10/10 electrodes and then mapping the potential field distribution of epileptiform or actual ictal discharges more precisely. Under this condition, the field distribution will then allow us to determine if the discharge arises from the neocortical temporal convexity (maximum at T7/T8), the temporal pole (F7/F8), or the mesial temporal region (maximum at SP1/SP2) (▶ Figure 2.8).

So-called dry electrodes, a completely different type of electrodes, have been developed in recent years. These electrodes consist of steel coated with a ceramic layer (e.g., titanium oxide or barium oxide) (Fonseca et al., 2007; Matsuo et al., 1973). They are called dry electrodes because no electrolyte paste is used. However, in clinical practice, electrode paste is applied when recording from dry electrodes. The derived signals using dry electrodes are very similar to the signals derived from silver/silver chloride electrodes (Fonseca et al., 2007). The dry electrodes typically have a low-frequency filter on the order of 0.2 Hz, which is sufficient for clinical conditions. Their use is not yet widespread.

2.2.1.3   Differential Amplifier

The field potentials of brain activity derived from the scalp are of very low amplitude, ranging from 10 to a few hundred microvolts. These potentials must be amplified by a factor of approximately 100,000 to adequately visualize them. In addition to the field potentials of brain activity, the electrodes also record interference activities (like the mains current of electrical devices). The field strength of these interference potentials can exceed the strength of the brain potentials by several orders of magnitude. These interference potentials obscure the presence of brain activity field potentials unless differential amplifiers are used. With differential amplifiers, two input signals (electrodes A and B) are amplified individually, but mainly the difference of potential between the two input signals is displayed (▶ Figure 2.10).

The ability of the differential amplifier to reject signals that affect both inputs equally is expressed as the common mode rejection ratio (CMRR). This ratio compares the ability of the amplifier to amplify unequal signals compared to equal signals. Typical values of CMRR for modern EEG devices are 1:100,000 or higher. A CMRR of 1:100,000 implies that unequal signals are amplified 100,000 times more than equal signals.

The following example illustrates the advantages of using differential amplifiers of a high CMRR. Let's assume we are recording a 60 Hz interference signal of 100 mV that with a gain of 70 μV/cm would result in a deflection of 1,428 cm. With a CMRR of 10,000:1, this signal would only have an amplitude of 1.43 mm, and with a CMRR of 100,000:1, it would only produce a deflection of 0.143 mm.

2.2.1.4   Analog-to-Digital Conversion

In older EEG devices, the voltage difference between two electrodes was amplified and was used to deflect a lever with a pen attached to it. The change of

Advantage of sphenoidal electrodes

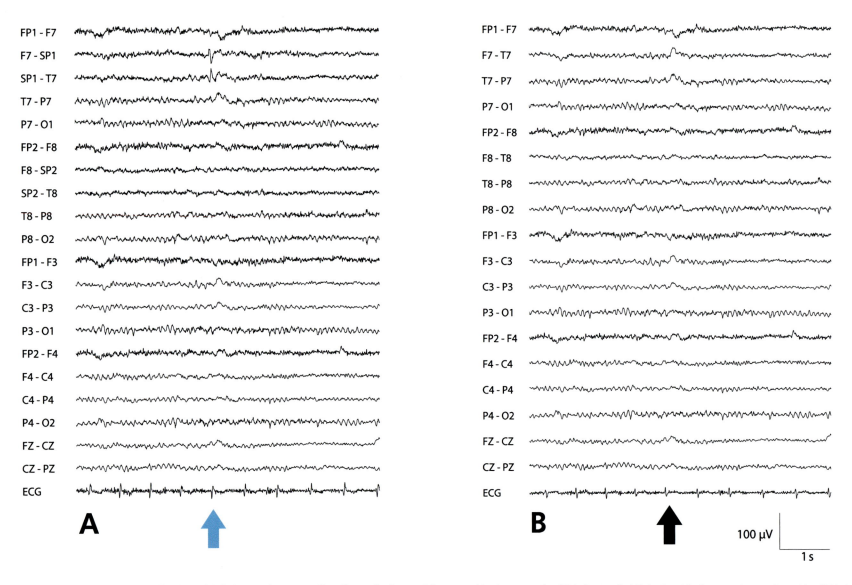

▶ **Figure 2.8** **Advantage of sphenoidal electrodes.** An epileptiform discharge (blue arrow) is shown at the SP1 electrode (A), but not in the montage where the SP1 electrode is missing (B). In **Figure 2.8B** only left temporal slow can be seen (black arrow). Recording spikes only in sphenoidal electrodes is rare. The real advantage of the sphenoidal electrodes is, however, that in mesial temporal epilepsies sphenoidal electrodes tends to be of highest amplitude, whereas in lateral extra-mesial temporal lobe epilepsies, the sphenoidal electrodes tend to be of relatively low amplitude compared to T7 or other more posterior temporal lobe electrodes.

Advantage of anterior temporal electrodes

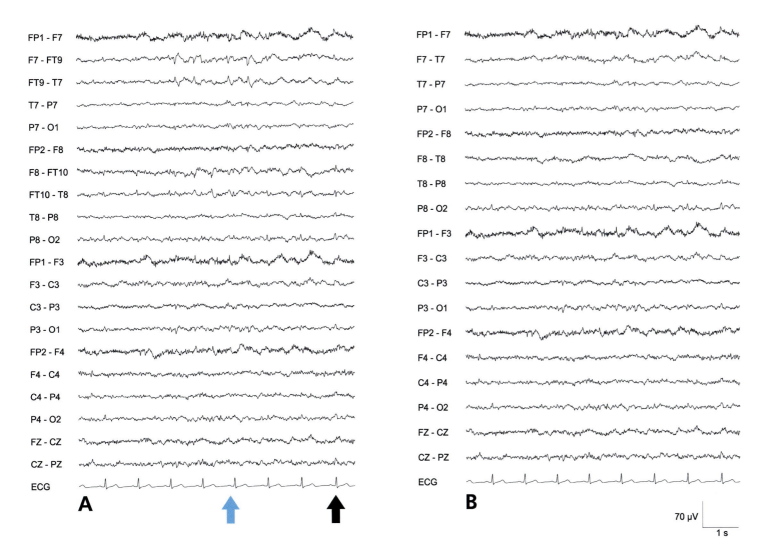

▶ **Figure 2.9** **Advantage of anterior temporal electrodes.** (A) Several spikes localized at FT9 (blue arrow). (B) The same EEG recording, but it does not include the FT9 electrode. No spikes can be detected in panel B. Note the ECG artifacts most conspicuous at P8–O2 (black arrow), which can easily be mistaken for right temporal spikes. An analysis of the relative amplitude of spikes at FT9/FT10 electrodes, sphenoidal electrodes, and other temporal lobe electrodes is very helpful in the differential diagnosis between mesial temporal and extra-mesial temporal lobe epilepsy.

Differential amplifiers, as the name implies, mainly amplify differences of voltage between input 1 and input 2

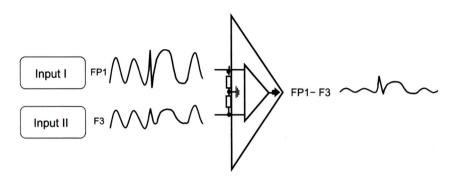

▶ **Figure 2.10** **Differential amplifiers, as the name implies, mainly amplify differences of voltage between input 1 and input 2.** Potentials that are equally affecting inputs 1 and 2 are only minimally amplified. Modern amplifiers with a common mode rejection of 100,000 will amplify voltage differences 100,000 times more than signals that affect both inputs equally.

voltage over time was then displayed graphically on a continuous paper writing system. The signal reproduction was continuous—that is, each change of the signal was transferred almost immediately to a corresponding change in the recording.

In modern EEG devices, the analog EEG signal is first converted into a digital signal by means of an analog-to-digital (AD) converter. Digital EEG devices always first record the EEG in a referential montage. The electrode used as reference in this montage should be a special reference electrode not included in the clinically used 10/10 electrode system. Only in this way will all clinically used 10/10 electrodes be available for reformatting. Only electrodes that are connected to amplifier input 1 of the different amplifiers can be used for reformatting. In our lab, we use CPZ, an electrode from the 10/10 electrode system located between CZ and PZ, as a reference (Klem et al., 1999).

▶ **Figure 2.11** illustrates how digitalization of a signal transforms a continuous curve into a sequence of discrete steps. The horizontal resolution of the curve depends on the sampling rate. The more samples over unit of time that

are taken, the higher the time resolution. Typical sampling rates in a standard EEG are 200–500 Hz. A sampling rate of 200 Hz implies that a digital sampling of the amplitude of the EEG signal is obtained every 5 ms. A sampling rate of 500 Hz calls for a measurement of the amplitude of the EEG signal every 2 ms. In invasive EEG video monitoring, sampling rates of 1000 Hz or more are used to optimally display even higher frequency signals. It is frequently argued that the minimum sampling rate for EEG technology should be at least twice as high as the highest frequency to be displayed (Nyquist–Shannon sampling theorem; Shannon, 1998). This is certainly true if our aim is just to detect the presence of these high-frequency signals. In clinical EEG, however, we are looking for an actual display of the waveform of all the frequencies we are interested in analyzing. To give a good display of the details of the waveform of the highest frequency we are interested in, we need at least 10–15 points per wave.

A sampling rate that is too low can also lead to "aliasing." This means that with a too low sampling rate of a signal, slow frequencies that do not exist in the original signal will be displayed (▶ **Figure 2.11**). One can reduce the aliasing effect by using a sufficiently high sampling rate and applying anti-aliasing filters to limit the width of the recorded frequency band.

The vertical resolution of a digital EEG trace depends on the sampling width (▶ **Table 2.1**). Currently, the signal is sampled with a width of 12–16 bits. A sampling width of 12 bits corresponds to a resolution of 0.24 μV per single step, and a sampling width of 16 bits corresponds to a resolution of 0.015 μV, assuming that 1,000 μV of EEG signal is measured (▶ **Figure 2.12**). Only with a sampling width of at least 12 bits (2^{12}) is the amplitude resolution sufficient to keep the EEG amplitude below the amplitude of the noise of EEG devices (<2 μV) and below the image system display capability. A lower resolution is unsuitable for EEG recordings (▶ **Figure 2.13**). Otherwise, fast frequencies cannot be reliably distinguished from artifacts.

2.2.1.5 Video

Currently, most EEG manufacturers offer the option of recording video image synchronized to the EEG signal (▶ **Figure 2.14**). This option offers, at relatively low additional cost, the possibility to correlate patients' behavior and their response to actions of the technicians. EEG video recordings are

Aliasing

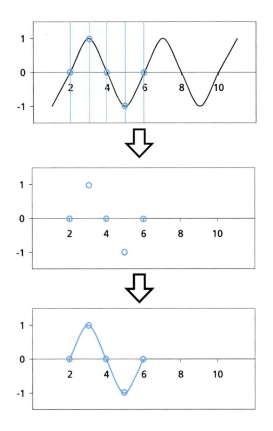

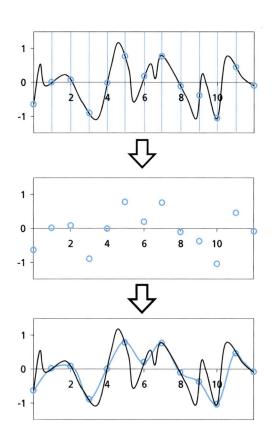

▶ **Figure 2.11** **Aliasing.** On the left are the sampling steps for digitizing an EEG signal. If a signal is acquired with poor horizontal resolution (i.e., temporal sampling steps), a wrong representation may result (see the example on the right side). On the right side of this example, fast waves that were part of the original signal (shown in black on the right side) are not displayed (blue curve). In the upper right corner, the original signal is shown as a curve; in the middle, the sampled values are shown; and at the bottom, the original curve (black) as well as the curve (blue) distorted by insufficient sampling are shown.

particularly useful in the evaluation of patients with seizures or other paroxysmal abnormalities. Usually, only clinically significant video segments of EEG video recordings are archived because of the large amount of data generated (see **Appendix 1**).

2.2.1.6   Electrical Safety

Electroencephalogram devices typically use the mains current for operation. However, other power sources, such as battery-power devices, are used, for

example, in functional magnetic resonance imaging (MRI). Alternating mains current is potentially dangerous for patients and technicians. Therefore, several precautions have been taken in the design of EEG devices to avoid electrical accidents. The coupling between the preamplifier and the second amplifier is usually not electrical, but the signals are converted into light signals and transmitted to the second amplifier via (short) optical fibers so that the part of the EEG device that has direct galvanic contact with the patient is disconnected from the mains voltage. In addition, special connectors of a unique shape are used on the preamplifier (headbox) to ensure that only proper devices are connected to the preamplifiers. EEG devices should only

Bits	Sampling Steps	Single Voltage Steps for Span of 1,000 µV (µV)
1	2^1	500
2	2^2	250
3	2^3	150
4	2^4	62.5
8	2^8	3.9
12	2^{12}	0.24
16	2^{16}	0.015

Vertical resolution

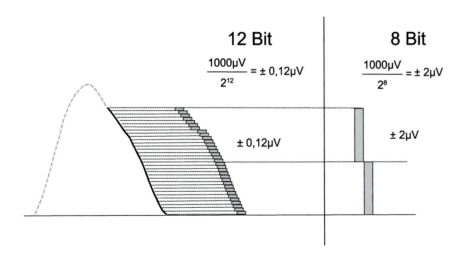

12 Bit

$$\frac{1000\mu V}{2^{12}} = \pm 0{,}12\mu V$$

± 0,12µV

8 Bit

$$\frac{1000\mu V}{2^8} = \pm 2\mu V$$

± 2µV

▶ **Figure 2.12** **Vertical resolution.** In the digital EEG, the EEG signal is also divided into discrete steps in the vertical direction. The vertical resolution is defined by the bit rate of the sampling. A low bit rate of 8 bits (right) results in coarse steps compared to a high bit rate of 12 bits (left).

Differences in vertical resolution

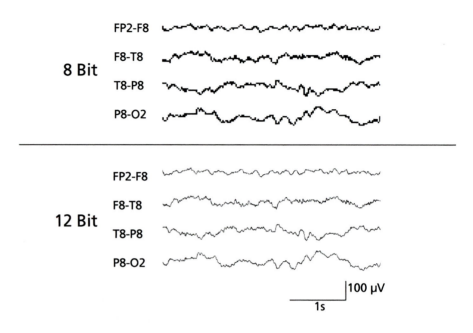

8 Bit
FP2-F8
F8-T8
T8-P8
P8-O2

12 Bit
FP2-F8
F8-T8
T8-P8
P8-O2

100 µV
1s

▶ **Figure 2.13** **Differences in vertical resolution: The same four-channel EEG signal recorded with a lower (8 bit) and higher (12 bit) resolution.** The low-resolution leads to a reduction of points in the EEG line, leading to reduced visibility of high frequencies.

be used if they display a technical approval mark indicating that they have been tested for safety. It is technically possible to create a functioning EEG device from parts supplied by EEG manufacturers (e.g., preamplifier and second amplifier) and commercially available PCs. However, this is strongly discouraged because there is no guarantee that the assembled system is safe to use.

The patient always should only have one connection to ground. In our institution, the ground electrode is usually placed between FP1 and FP2 (10/20 system; see **Figure 1.2**) at FPZ. Two earth electrodes should never be attached to a patient because current will flow through the patient between the two earth electrodes in the event of a short circuit.

Simultaneous EEG video recording

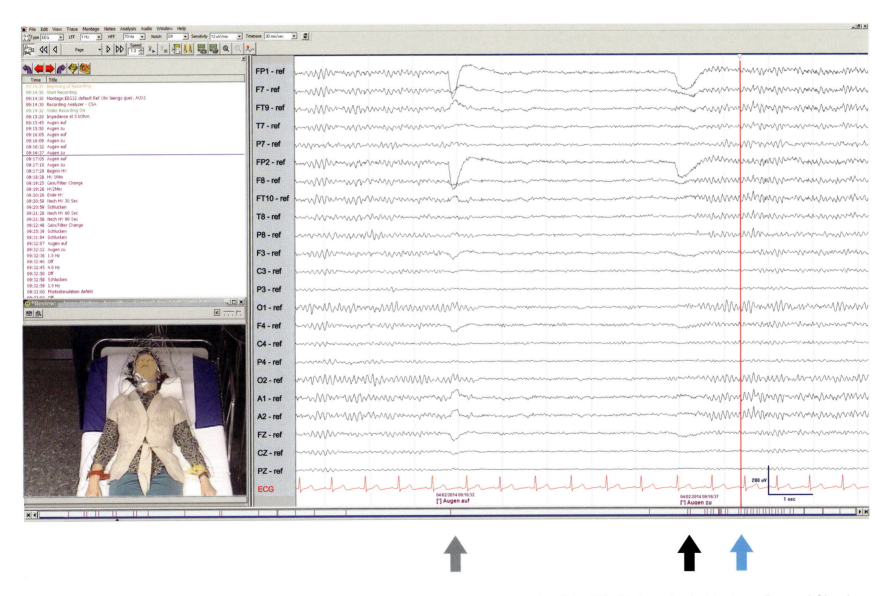

▶ **Figure 2.14** **Simultaneous EEG video recording.** In modern EEG systems, simultaneous registration of the EEG with the patient's video image (bottom left) and comments from the EEG technician (top left) is possible (split screen). The EEG is referenced to the electrode CPZ (ref). The video image is synchronized with the time of the red line in the EEG (blue arrow). The gray arrow marks the eye opening, and the black arrow marks the eye closure.

2.2.2 Technical Characteristics of EEG Recording

2.2.2.1 EEG Filters

EEG filters permit selective display of specific EEG frequencies, facilitating the interpretation of the EEG.

2.2.2.1.1 Electrotechnical Basis of Filters

▶ **Figure 2.15** explains the basic circuitry of a filter. A filter usually consists of a combination of resistors and capacitors. A capacitor consists of two spatially separated plates of an electrical conductor. The electrical properties of a capacitor result from the material and size of the plates as well as from the distance between the plates. If current is applied to a capacitor, it takes a certain amount of time until its plates are fully charged or fully discharged. The time it takes for the plates of a capacitor to be fully charged varies depending on the design of the capacitor. Depending on the arrangement of the circuit components, slow or fast frequencies of the EEG signal may only be displayed partially or not at all.

Considering the circuitry of a filter, it is obvious that, for example, a high-frequency filter does not filter out 100% of all frequencies above its specified cutoff frequency and that, on the other hand, it will not let all frequencies below the cutoff frequency pass through. Instead, the cutoff frequency is typically referred to as the frequency at which the amplitude of the input signal is reduced to approximately 80% (▶ **Figure 2.16**). Filtering of high frequencies at, for example, 30 Hz leads to a "rounding off" of the peak component of the calibration signal and of spikes (▶ **Figure 2.17**). In addition, in patients with an EEG with abundant EMG artifact, the filtering of frequencies higher than 15

Function of filters

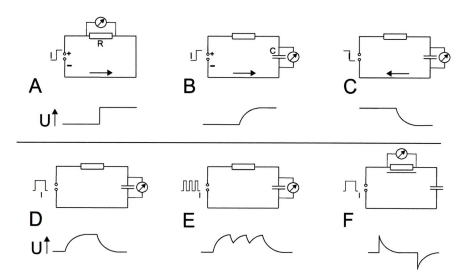

A

B

C

D

E

F

U↑

▶ **Figure 2.15** **Function of filters.** (A) If a current I is applied in a circuit with a resistor R, a voltage U can be measured, which follows the applied current in its time course. (B) If a capacitor C is installed in the circuit, it needs a finite time until it is charged, the voltage U rises slowly. (C) When the current flow is reversed, the capacitor discharges over time. (D) If the current is switched on and then off again, charging and discharging result via the capacitor. (E) If the switching on and off takes place too quickly for full discharge, the voltage curve shown in this panel results. Thus, a high-frequency filter is simulated—for example, with too fast changes of voltage, the changes can no longer be fully represented. High frequencies are therefore not fully represented. (F) If the voltage is measured across the resistance, the result simulates a low-frequency filter.

Frequency response of a filter

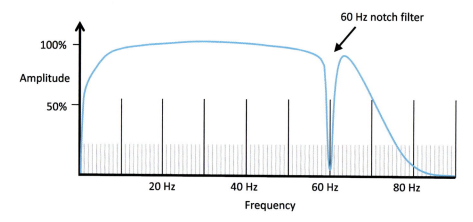

▶ **Figure 2.16** **Frequency response of a filter.** An EEG filter causes a gradual filtering of the desired frequencies and, thus, a gradual reduction of the amplitude above or below the filter frequency. The notch filter at 50 Hz reduces more or less selectively the 50 Hz main signal. The main current is at 60 Hz in the United States.

Influence of filters

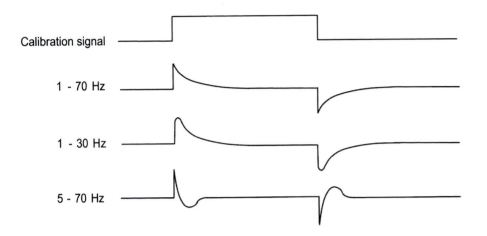

Calibration signal

1 - 70 Hz

1 - 30 Hz

5 - 70 Hz

▶ **Figure 2.17** **Influence of filters.** EEG filters significantly change the appearance of the original signal. The top trace shows the actual input. The second montage illustrates the changes in wave form when using the standard high- and low-frequency filters applied in routine EEG recordings. The lower two traces illustrate the changes of waveform when additional filtering is done.

Hz may be misleading and, by rounding off the peaks of the EMG artifact, an EMG artifact may be confused with pathological epileptiform discharges or seizure rhythms (see ▶ **Figures 3.138–3.140**). When analyzing slow frequencies, we must understand the concept of time constant. The time constant defines the time it takes for an EEG signal to drop to approximately 37% of the maximum amplitude. The lower the low-frequency filter that is selected, the longer it takes the signal to decay (▶ **Figure 2.17**). There is a reciprocal relationship between time constant and the specific lower cutoff frequency:

$$f u = 1/2 \, \pi \times \tau$$

where τ is the time constant, and $f u$ is the specific low-frequency cutoff. Using this formula, a time constant of 0.3 s corresponds approximately to a lower cutoff frequency of 0.5 Hz, and a time constant of 0.1 s corresponds to a lower cutoff frequency of approximately 1.6 Hz. Most EEG machines now permit adjustments of the low-pass frequency filters. Modern EEG machines allow adjustments of the high-pass as well as the low-pass filter settings. The option for the high-pass filter is expressed directly in frequencies that will be recorded with an amplitude of >20%. For high-pass filters, however, the unit of the dial of frequencies to be filtered out is expressed in time constants. We believe that the function of low-pass frequency filters should also be expressed by the frequency at which the amplitude of any slower rhythms is reduced by more than 80%.

2.2.2.1.2   Phase Shift due to Filters

Filters not only change the amplitude of the input signal but also shift the input signal in time. This effect of the phase shift is schematically illustrated in ▶ **Figure 2.18**. A high-frequency filter (▶ **Figure 2.18A**) reduces the amplitude of the higher frequency components and shifts the corresponding signal to the right—that is, the peak of those components is delayed. A low-frequency filter (▶ **Figure 2.18B**) reduces the amplitude of the low-frequency components and shifts the signal to the left—that is, the peak of those components occurs earlier. In addition to the filter setting, the frequency of the input signal determines the phase shift. The slower the frequency, the clearer the phase shift. The phase shift due to the low-frequency filters tends to affect the EEG significantly, whereas the phase shift due to high-frequency filters is so small that it is not relevant in daily practice (▶ **Figure 2.18**). ▶ **Figure 2.19** shows the effect of different filter settings on the amplitude and phase shift of EEG waves.

2.2.2.1.3   Recommended Filter Settings

Digital EEG allows adapting the filters after the recording is finished. However, the range of frequencies that can be displayed will depend on the frequencies originally recorded. Therefore, the original EEG recordings should be obtained using the broadest frequency range the amplifiers allow. The American Clinical Neurophysiology Society (ACNS) recommends 0.5 Hz as the low-frequency filter and 70 Hz as the high-frequency filter. A 60 Hz notch filter can be used if there is significant electrical interference from the mains.

Notch filters should only be used if necessary, such as in intensive care units, in which it is frequently not possible to avoid interference from the mains. Notch filters tend to trigger dampened oscillations called "ringing" (▶ **Figure 2.20**). Notch filter ringing is usually not a problem in routine EEG readings. However, in invasive recordings, notch filter ringing can be difficult to differentiate from high-frequency oscillations, particularly when the high-frequency oscillations

Phase shift produced by different filters

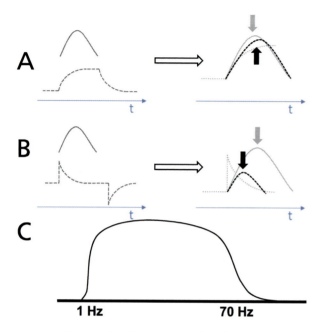

filter reduction results in signal delay

filter increase results in signal advance

▶ **Figure 2.18** **Phase shift produced by different filters.** (A) The combination of a high-frequency filter (dashed gray line) and the original signal (solid gray line) results in a new filtered signal (black) that is smaller and later in time. (B) The combination of a low-frequency filter (dotted gray line) and the original signal (solid gray line) results in a new filtered signal (black) that is smaller and earlier in time. C) Summary of the phase shift. A reduction of the high- and low-frequency filters leads to a delay of the potential and an increase to an advance of the EEG signal relative to a filter setting of 1–70 Hz.

are superimposed on high-amplitude spikes (Kirac et al., 2016). Ringing occurs most often when there are abrupt high-amplitude changes of the EEG signal.

As mentioned above, the EEG signal of digitally recorded EEGs can be filtered using high-frequency, low-frequency, or notch filters. These filters are used to either minimize artifacts (e.g., applying low-frequency filters to minimize the effect of sweating on the EEG) or better visualize EEG abnormalities

Phase shift due to low-frequency filter (LFF)

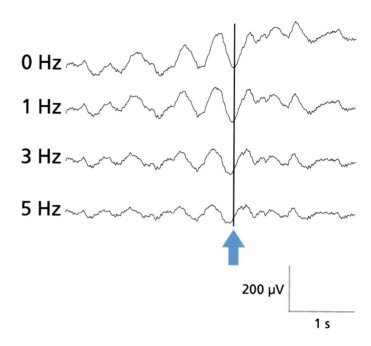

▶ **Figure 2.19** **Phase shift due to low-frequency filter (LFF).** Example of an actual EEG trace. By increasing the LFF, the amplitude of the slow waves is lowered and shifted in time earlier (see orientation line; blue arrow). The high-frequency filter is at 70 Hz in all four tracings.

(e.g., applying a high-frequency filter to better visualize sharp waves or paroxysmal theta activity that is obscured by EMG artifact). EEG filtering should be used very carefully because filtering can significantly alter the recorded EEG signals. For example, filtering from 70 to 30 or 15 Hz may make it impossible to distinguish polyspikes from EMG artifacts (see **Figures 3.138–3.140**).

2.2.2.2   Editing the Digital EEG

Digitally recorded EEGs can be processed in many ways, including reformatting (displaying the EEG in different montages to optimally map the potential in question), filtering, source analysis, and automated analysis of EEG patterns.

Filter artifact

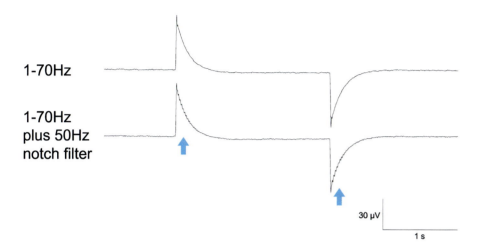

1-70Hz

1-70Hz
plus 50Hz
notch filter

30 µV

1 s

▶ **Figure 2.20** **Filter artifact.** In comparison to the original curve (top), a notched filter (here 50 Hz; bottom) causes a low-amplitude oscillation (blue arrows) on a calibration signal. This artifact is called ringing.

Digital EEG

Digital EEG is first referentially recorded against an electrode that is not in the 10/20 system (e.g., CPZ). Silver/silver chloride electrodes are placed on the scalp according to the 10/20 or 10/10 system. The filter and amplifier settings, as well as the reformatting in different montages, should follow the guidelines of the ACNS (see **Appendix 1**).

2.2.2.2.1   Reformatting

The original referential recording can be displayed in different EEG montages (reformatting). This allows analyzing the same EEG signal of interest in different montages. This has advantages when trying to localize the EEG potential or when trying to differentiate between artifacts and actual brain activity.

There are two types of EEG montages: referential and bipolar. Referential montages are sometimes called monopolar montages. **Appendix 1** contains a summary of useful montages as recommended by the ACNS. In some EEG

laboratories, selected montages that do not follow the general guidelines of the ACNS are still used for historical reasons or as an expression of loyalty to earlier EEG instructors who may not permit meaningful changes. This is strongly discouraged.

2.2.2.2.2   Referential Montages

As mentioned above, digital devices always record potential differences with respect to a so-called referential lead that is an electrode placed on the scalp but should not be part of the 10/20 electrode system. We use CPZ of the 10/10 system as the reference electrode (see Figure 1.2). In referential montages, the desired recording electrodes are each connected to input 1 of the amplifier and the common electrode (reference electrode) is connected to amplifier input 2 (see Figure 1.5). According to an international convention, the reference electrode is always connected to amplifier input 2. An exception to this rule is the ipsilateral ear reference montage, in which the electrodes on one side are connected to the ear on the same side (see Figure 1.6). In other words, in that montage, there are two referential electrodes. Although we show some examples of this traditionally established montage, we discourage the use of two reference electrodes. With two references, it is not possible to compare electrodes with one another.

The following electrodes typically serve as reference electrodes in routine EEG:

- Vertex (CZ)
- Ear (A1 or A2)
- Mastoid (TP9 or TP10)

In clinical practice, any electrode can be used as a reference. However, when choosing a reference electrode, the following criteria should apply:

1. Ideally, the reference electrode should not contain any artifacts. That makes the frontopolar electrodes FP1 and FP2, for example, less than ideal reference electrodes in awake (or rapid eye movement sleep) patients because of the possible large eye movement artifacts.
2. The signal of interest should ideally not be reflected in the reference electrode or at least be of low amplitude in that electrode. When the reference electrode is less affected than all the other electrodes, all the deflections will point in the same

direction (see Section 2.2.3), making analysis of the EEG easier. The presence of deflections in opposite directions between the different channels (phase reversal) implies that the reference is active with some electrodes more negative and others more positive than the reference electrode. This is also called a "contaminated reference."

For example, temporal potentials can be best analyzed (i.e., without phase reversal) in a vertex reference (▶ **Figure 2.21**). The same potential, however, when using an ear reference will be difficult to analyze because it will show a phase reversal (▶ **Figure 2.21**). Placing (i.e., selecting) a reference electrode as physically distant as possible from the generator (e.g., on the contralateral hemisphere) seems like a simple first approach to using an uncontaminated reference. However, not infrequently, the electrode physically most distant from the potential of interest may also be recording relatively high-amplitude noise or other physiological or pathological rhythms (vertex waves, eye movement potentials, EMG activity, glossokinetic artifacts, high-amplitude alpha activity, etc.). In that circumstance, it is best to use a reference that is partially contaminated but is as artifact-free as possible. Low-amplitude deflections of opposite polarity to the main potential will be seen but can easily be ignored (see Section 2.2.3.3).

2.2.2.2.3 Bipolar Montages

In bipolar montages, adjacent EEG channels each have a common electrode. The electrode in amplifier input 2 of one channel is switched to amplifier input 1 in the next channel. This arrangement is applied to either longitudinal or transverse rows. Following the recommendations of the ACNS, bipolar montages should always be arranged in straight rows or columns running respectively from left to right and from front to back (see **Figures 1.3** and **1.8**).

In bipolar montages, it is best to connect the ends of columns or rows. For example, in the montage illustrated in **Figure 1.3**, both ends (FP1/FP2 and O1/O2) form the beginning and end of both the temporal and parasagittal longitudinal rows. When two bipolar chains of electrodes are connected, the relative amplitude of the potential of interest at all the electrodes of these two chains can be calculated. This would not be possible with unconnected rows of electrodes. Therefore, the ACNS does not recommend unconnected longitudinal rows (see **Appendix 1**).

Localization rules of potentials displayed with referential or bipolar montages are discussed in detail in Section 2.2.3.

2.2.2.2.4 Source Analysis and Mapping

Many attempts have been made to display the EEG signal in a more universally understandable way. "Brain mapping" illustrates the electric field distribution over the head. The hope was that such displays would help the novice EEG reader localize potentials without having to go through the trouble of polarity localization theory. Brain mapping, however, has numerous methodological problems. The EEG does not provide absolute potential values but only potential differences between electrodes. Thus, to display the distribution of the potentials, an assumption must be made regarding the polarity of the generator and if the generator is a monopole or a dipole. This conflict (inverse problem) can only be alleviated, but not resolved, by complex plausibility assumptions. Necessary assumptions about skull shapes and conductivities of the individual layers as well as assumptions about the number and spatial extent of the generators greatly complicate the calculations. Another difficulty is that the artifacts contained in the EEG cannot be identified reliably. Therefore, mapping cannot replace visual analysis of the EEG; it can only complement it. In other words, it is always necessary to analyze the original EEG curve before performing mapping. Thus, according to the ACNS, prospective evaluation of EEG discriminant analysis has not yet demonstrated its practical use in clinical differential diagnosis (see https://www.acns.org/practice/guidelines).

Modern structural and functional imaging methods, such as MRI and positron emission tomography/single-photon emission computed tomography, are much more reliable than EEG for lesion detection and localization. Thus, the clinical relevance of EEG mapping in such cases is low. On the other hand, EEG is still the most powerful tool in the evaluation of epileptiform discharges as well as EEG seizure patterns.

The localization of ictal and interictal epileptiform discharges is important in the localization of the epileptogenic zone. Suitable computer programs can support the analysis of potentials, for example, for localization determination. In combination with the raw signal, such programs can facilitate the work of the inexperienced EEG evaluator. In these patients, surface electrodes in the 19 basic positions of the 10/20 system may not yield enough spatial resolution to be sufficient for an exact localization. Therefore, in patients who are surgical candidates, epileptiform discharges are usually distributed using the 10/10 system

Advantages and disadvantages of different reference montages

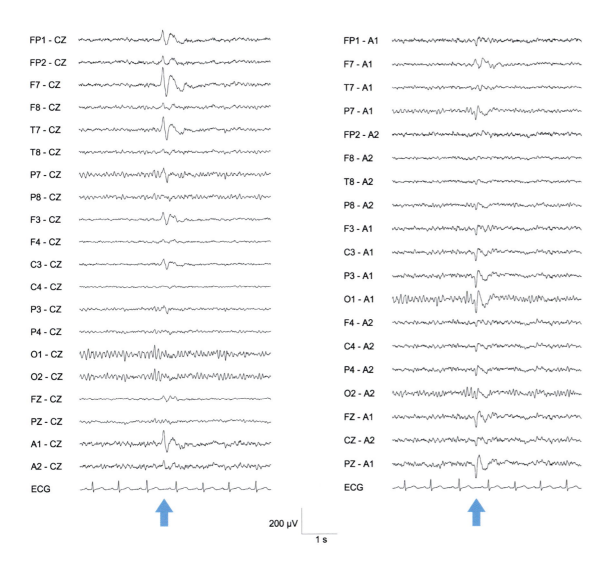

200 µV

1 s

▶ **Figure 2.21 Advantages and disadvantages of different reference montages.** The left temporal spike (blue arrows) is easily recognizable in the vertex reference montage because no phase reversal occurs. Absence of a phase reversal indicates that the reference is either more active or less active than all the other electrodes connected to the same reference. The same EEG signal is difficult to locate in an ipsilateral ear reference montage because the ear reference is located in the field of the negative spike ("contaminated reference"). A phase reversal in a reference montage implies that some electrodes are more negative and others more positive than the reference electrode ("contaminated reference").

with electrodes spaced approximately 2.5 cm apart. Experience shows, however, that most likely due to volume conduction, it does not make sense to place the electrodes on the skull surface closer than 2.5 cm from each other. Software can display distribution maps of potentials of interest (Ebersole, 1994; Scherg et al., 2012). These programs contribute little to the distribution maps that can be deduced from direct visual analysis of the potentials of interest in a 10/10 system. These computer programs can also display the propagation of potentials of interest. However, the propagation of distribution maps of epileptiform discharges is of little practical use.

Paradoxical lateralization of epileptiform discharges due to parasagittal epileptogenic zones has been described and further complicates localization matters in EEG (Adelman et al., 1982; Catarino et al., 2012; Cruse et al., 1982). Some source localization algorithms may wrongly lateralize EEG potentials located close to the midline (Jayakar et al., 1991).

2.2.2.2.5 Automatic Spike Detection/AI implementation

Several automatic spike detection programs have been developed, and are commercially available. In recent years, AI-applications further support EEG analysis (Tveit et al., 2023). In many of these programs, the sensitivity of the spike detection program can be adjusted. Obviously, an increase in spike detection sensitivity goes along with a decrease of spike detection specificity. The development of spike detection programs is greatly limited by the lack of an objective golden standard—that is, the golden standard is the subjective assessment of an experienced electroencephalographer. We know, however, that even between experienced electroencephalographers, there is no absolute agreement on which EEG potentials are actually epileptiform. In addition, automatic spike detection programs not infrequently have difficulties differentiating between spikes and artifacts of similar distribution and/or similar waveform. Despite these limitations, spike detection programs can be very helpful in the analysis of prolonged EEG/video recordings. Sometimes spike detection programs may accurately identify a given epileptiform discharge. In those cases, the spike detection program can be used to assess the frequency of occurrence of those discharges because these algorithms can reliably reproduce the marking of closely similar potentials. At other times, the spike detection program may identify an epileptiform discharge that was missed by the electroencephalographer because they may have been overwhelmed by the large amount of data.

The technological advances of recent years make it easier to continuously record EEG signals over many hours and days. In combination with video recordings, these long-term EEG/video recordings are important for the diagnosis of epilepsies and essentially indispensable for assessment of surgical treatment options. In epilepsy surgery diagnostics, recordings from 128 and even more channels are frequently used. Storing of this information with the synchronized video recordings frequently exceeds even the current storage capability. In most long-term EEG/video recordings, more than 95% of the information is redundant. At this point, the neurophysiologist reviewing the EEG/video usually decides what parts of the recording will be clipped for long-term storage.

Automatic spike recognition, as mentioned above, can be of significant assistance to the electroencephalographer (Jing et al., 2020). Spike detection can identify epileptiform discharges that the electroencephalographer missed because large amounts of data cannot be reviewed with the same precision as short EEG recordings. In addition, as mentioned above, spike detection in selected cases can give a very precise, automatic assessment of spike frequency over time. This may be of some help when assessing the effect of a given anti-seizure treatment. It has been suggested that automatic spike and seizure detection is currently precise enough to allow the electroencephalographer to limit the review of prolonged recordings to careful analysis of EEG segments selected by the spike or seizure detection program (Scherg et al., 2012). This is certainly not the case because automatic spike and seizure detection programs not infrequently still miss essential EEG potentials and lastly, the electroenephalographer needs to be the last instance in judging the discharge, making an analytical EEG-training necessary.

2.2.2.2.6 Automatic Seizure Detection

Automatic seizure detection programs have the same limitations as spike detection programs (Baumgartner et al., 2018). In some cases, the program is extremely accurate in detecting essentially all EEG seizures and, therefore, can be used to quantify the occurrence of EEG seizures. EEG seizure quantification is useful when evaluating the effect of treatment on seizure count. It also may be useful if one is trying to assess the relative frequency of seizures arising, for example, from the left versus right temporal lobe. This may be important if one is considering a unilateral lobectomy in a patient with seizures arising from both temporal lobes. In addition, the electroencephalographer may miss epileptic seizures, particularly if large amounts of EEG/video data must be reviewed. Moreover, the patient may not notice seizure symptoms or may be amnestic of the seizure symptoms. In some cases, even observers may not be aware that a seizure occurred. In selected situations, a seizure detection program may be useful to detect changes in the EEG that the electroencephalographer missed. Therefore, both spike and seizure detection programs are useful adjuncts to the visual analysis of the EEG, but they certainly do not replace the direct visual analysis of the EEG, especially when using automated detection systems, because then the EEG reader must be the last instance of judgment for many collected patterns. Investigators have been trying to design reliable EEG seizure detection programs for more than 40 years. Previous attempts at seizure and spike detection used algorithms that were derived from what was believed to be a typical spike. New approaches such as artificial intelligence in general and deep learning methods in particular are being developed and implemented as an approach to automate EEG analysis (Tveit et al., 2023). In the future, highly precise automated spike and seizure detection will be implemented, but, again, the electroencephalographer will still need to be well-trained and experienced to judge the findings on their relevance and the clinical impact. Therefore we believe a structured and analytical approach to EEG reading is paramount.

2.2.2.2.7 Long-Term EEG Monitoring

In the past 5–10 years, there has been an increased demand for long-term continuous EEG monitoring. It has been demonstrated to have a positive impact on clinical outcome (Hill et al., 2019). The objectives of long-term monitoring vary but frequently include the following:

- Assess precisely the frequency of interictal epileptiform discharges or of EEG seizures. This information is then used to manage the seizure medication.
- Assess the fluctuations of the degree of encephalopathy over time.
- Alert of a sudden change of the EEG pattern suggesting a neurological complication.

Simple quantification of the EEG is of great help in the long-term evaluation of the EEG. The most useful parameters include the following:

- Continuous evaluation of the predominant EEG frequencies in the two hemispheres.
- Continuous evaluation of the degree of asymmetry of the predominant EEG frequency bands between the two hemispheres.
- EEG seizures tend to modify the characteristics of the different EEG frequency bands in a very specific way that is typical for each

individual. Once these patterns have been recognized, they can usually be easily identified and, therefore, quantified.

- The long-term EEG quantification may also assist in defining more precisely the degree of encephalopathy. Patients in deep coma show EEG frequency bands that do not change over time and also reveal no change when stimulating the patient. On the other hand, less severely encephalopathy patients tend to show at least two distinctive EEG patterns, namely an awake-like pattern and an asleep-like pattern. In addition, the EEG frequency analysis shows significant changes when stimulating the patient.

It is outside the scope of this book to discuss in detail the advances being made in quantification of long-term EEG recordings. The objective of this section is to advise the reader that EEG quantification is an indispensable tool in the routine evaluation of long-term EEGs.

2.2.3 Localization of EEG Potentials

The localization and definition of the polarity of EEG potentials over the scalp are important criteria for the identification of physiological and abnormal EEG patterns and thus essential for accurate EEG evaluation. Vertex waves, for example, are negative and—as the name suggests—show highest amplitude at the vertex. Positive occipital sharp transients of sleep (POSTS) are of positive polarity and located occipitally. In the case of epileptiform discharges, the localization at which they have the highest amplitude usually also points to the approximate location of the epileptogenic zone or, in the case of circumscribed slow, to the localization of a structural lesion. Artifacts also tend to have a characteristic field distribution that may be useful when distinguishing them from brain activity—for example, to distinguish between eye movements and frontal slow (see Section 2.3.2.1).

2.2.3.1 Polarity Convention

In electroencephalography, differential amplifiers with two inputs are used. The following convention is applied in clinical neurophysiology, with the first

Polarity convention

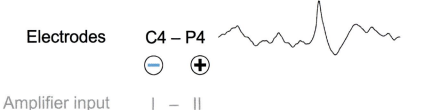

Electrodes C4 – P4

Amplifier input I – II

▶ **Figure 2.22** **Polarity convention.** Following an international convention, all EEG devices are connected as follows: A preponderance of negativity at amplifier input 1 or a preponderance of positivity at amplifier input 2 causes a deflection upwards.

electrode mentioned in the channel label being amplifier input 1 and the second amplifier input 2: An upward deflection means that amplifier input 1 is more negative than amplifier input 2 or that amplifier input 2 is more positive than amplifier input 1 (▶ **Figure 2.22**). Conversely, a downward deflection results from either a predominance of positivity at amplifier input 1 or a predominance of negativity at amplifier input 2 (▶ **Figure 2.23**). When the targeted waves face toward each other, they produce a negative phase reversal at the targeted electrode C4. When the targeted waves face in opposite directions, they produce a positive phase reversal (▶ **Figure 2.24**).

It is important to recognize that EEG potentials are generated within a volume conductor and, therefore, always both amplifier inputs are "active" to a certain degree. For any given EEG potential, however, amplifier input 1 or 2 will be relatively more positive or relatively more negative, leading to EEG deflections following the convention outlined above. Notice that the "differential amplifiers" used for amplification of the EEG signal only amplify voltage difference but do not measure absolute voltages. In the following paragraphs, we assume that the potential recorded with scalp electrodes is a monopole. We know that all brain potentials recorded with scalp electrodes are dipoles in principle. However, these dipoles usually are oriented perpendicularly with respect to the brain surface. Therefore, one of the poles of the dipole tends to point to the center of gravity of the brain, making it invisible to scalp electrodes. That is obviously not the case when we record brain activity with (deep) invasive electrodes.

Phase reversal

Channel 1 F4 – C4

Channel 2 C4 – P4

Amplifier input I – II

▶ **Figure 2.23** **Phase reversal.** In a bipolar longitudinal montage, the electrode C4 in channel 1 is connected to amplifier input 2 and in channel 2 to amplifier input 1. The sharp wave at C4 is of relatively negative polarity, producing a downward deflection at channel 1 and an upward deflection at channel 2. This is called a negative phase reversal at C4.

Negative and positive phase reversal

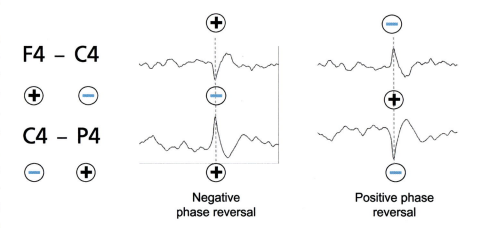

F4 – C4

C4 – P4

Negative phase reversal

Positive phase reversal

▶ **Figure 2.24** **Negative and positive phase reversal.** When the targeted waves face toward each other, they produce a negative phase reversal at the targeted electrode C4. When the targeted waves face in opposite directions, they produce a positive phase reversal.

For the analysis of the localization of EEG potentials, knowledge of the polarity and localization of typical EEG patterns is a prerequisite. For example, the peak component of vertex waves and epileptiform discharges (with rare exceptions) is negative, whereas the peak component of POSTS or 14 and 6 Hz positive spikes is positive.

2.2.3.2 Systematic Approach to Localization of EEG Potentials

The potential voltage that we can derive from such potential sources depends on the spatial arrangement of the electrodes to the surface of the generator and is illustrated by the concept of the "spatial angle" (Gloor, 1985). In order to localize EEG potentials, we have to follow systematic rules that we discuss in detail in the following sections. The rules of localization apply only if we assume a unipolar potential source. However, these models are crude simplifications, and we have to assume that most potentials derived in clinical EEG are probably caused by much more complex generators aligning in multiple layers and different spatial orientations of dipoles (Speckmann et al., 1993). Even highly complex mathematical models cannot currently offer a satisfactory solution to this issue (Scherg et al., 2019). This simplification is justifiable from a practical standpoint. A large part of these dipoles lies perpendicular to the skull surface, which has the consequence that with electrodes fixed to the scalp, we only detect one pole, while the other pole remains hidden in the depth of the sulci (Jayakar et al., 1991). However, an accurate analysis sometimes allows the representation of both poles. When analyzing a potential field distribution, the possibility of a dipole should always be considered. The easiest way to display this graphically is to move the zero line up or down in an electrode-potential field distribution. It should be borne in mind that the displacement of the zero line also changes the orientation of the dipole. Typical examples of dipoles that can be derived from the skull surface are lateral eye movements (▶ **Figure 2.25**), electrocardiogram (ECG) artifact (▶ **Figure 2.26**), benign epileptiform discharges (▶ **Figure 2.27**), and epileptiform discharges in patients who had a skull defect and brain resection (▶ **Figure 2.28**) (Franco et al., 2018).

The localization rules discussed below apply exclusively to brain potentials that reflect on the scalp as apparent unipoles. They cannot be used to localize dipoles. However, all brain generators are dipoles, and usually thousands of generators participate in the generation of any given EEG potential. We certainly cannot localize each one of those generators. We just localize one pole of the equivalent dipole. As discussed below, when we apply the localization rules, we will always get two possible solutions. The reason for this is that identical deflections can be generated by a positive discharge or a negative discharge, depending on whether the affected electrode is in amplifier input 1 or 2. However, if we define either (a) the location of the discharge or (b) the polarity of the discharge, we are left with a unique solution. For example, the discharge in ▶ **Figure 2.22** can be generated by a positive discharge at P4 or a negative discharge at C4. If we now specify that the discharge is of negative polarity, there will be only one solution left, namely a negative discharge at C4.

The steps outlined below should always be followed when localizing EEG potentials:

STEP 1: Determine if the EEG montage is referential or bipolar or a mixture of both. For example, the montage shown in **Figure 1.3** is a bipolar montage, and that shown in **Figure 1.5** is a referential montage.

STEP 2: Determine how many chains are in the montage. A chain in a referential montage includes all the electrodes connected to a specific reference. For example, the montage shown in **Figure 1.5** consists of a single chain. A chain in a bipolar montage includes all the channels in which the electrode connected to input 2 in one channel is the same electrode that is connected to input 1 in the next channel. For example, the montage shown in **Figure 1.3** consists of five chains. In this case, some chains are interconnected.

STEP 3: Decide the chain in which you will localize the potential of interest.

STEP 4: Decide the exact point in time you would like to localize the EEG potential of interest.

STEP 5: Decide if the potential of interest shows a phase reversal or not (see below).

STEP 6: Skip this step if there is no phase reversal. If there is a phase reversal, decide if there is a positive or a negative phase reversal (see below).

STEP 7: Apply the appropriate localization rule (see below).

Phase reversal is an important concept when localizing scalp potentials. Phase reversal is a simple electric concept, stating different deflections (negative

Slow horizontal eye movements

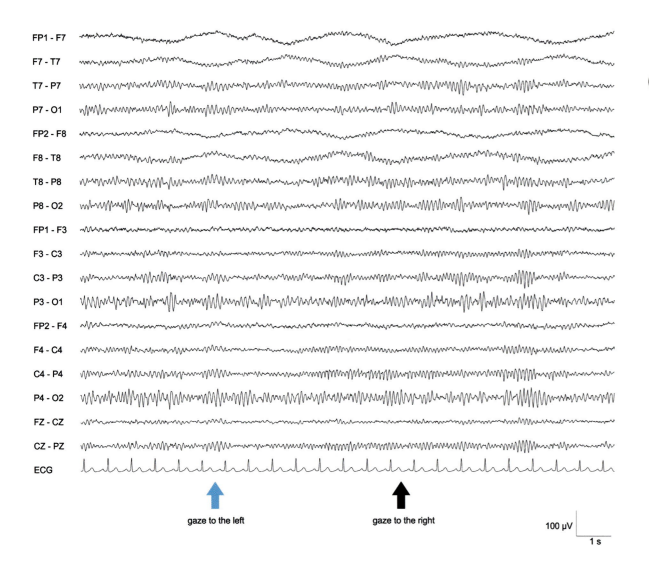

FP1 - F7

F7 - T7

T7 - P7

P7 - O1

FP2 - F8

F8 - T8

T8 - P8

P8 - O2

FP1 - F3

F3 - C3

C3 - P3

P3 - O1

FP2 - F4

F4 - C4

C4 - P4

P4 - O2

FZ - CZ

CZ - PZ

ECG

gaze to the left   gaze to the right

100 µV

1 s

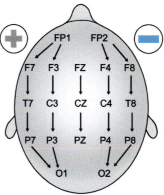

▶ **Figure 2.25 Slow horizontal eye movements.** Slow horizontal eye movements are an early sign of drowsiness. Gaze to the left (blue arrow) leads to positivity at electrode F7 and negativity at electrode F8 (head view). The opposite is true when looking to the right (black arrow).

ECG artifact

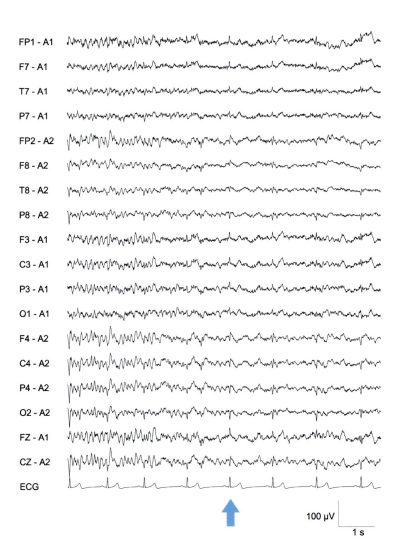

FP1 - A1

F7 - A1

T7 - A1

P7 - A1

FP2 - A2

F8 - A2

T8 - A2

P8 - A2

F3 - A1

C3 - A1

P3 - A1

O1 - A1

F4 - A2

C4 - A2

P4 - A2

O2 - A2

FZ - A1

CZ - A2

ECG

100 µV

1 s

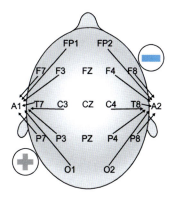

▶ **Figure 2.26** **ECG artifact.** ECG artifact in an ipsilateral ear reference montage. The ear electrodes are closest to the heart and are therefore particularly susceptible to ECG artifacts (blue arrow). Due to the electrical heart vector, there is a typical potential distribution with positivity of the QRS complex on the left posterior temporal/parietal region and negativity on the right frontal region. As evident in this figure, the left ear electrode is relatively positive compared to left scalp electrodes, and the right ear electrode is relatively negative compared to right scalp electrodes. In addition, the left ear electrode is relatively positive compared to the right ear electrode.

Dipole of a benign focal epileptiform discharge of childhood

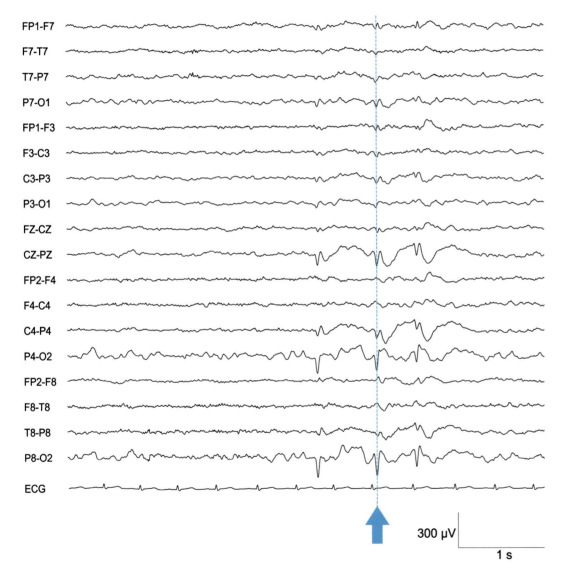

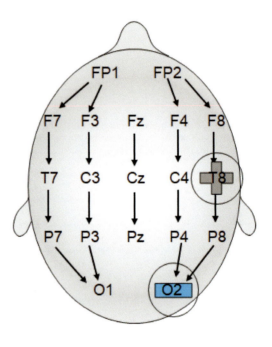

300 µV

1 s

▶ **Figure 2.27** **Dipole of a benign focal epileptiform discharge of childhood.** Bipolar longitudinal montage. This benign focal epileptiform discharge of childhood (blue arrow) shows a dipole with negative right occipital spike and corresponding right temporal positivity.

Positive left temporal spike

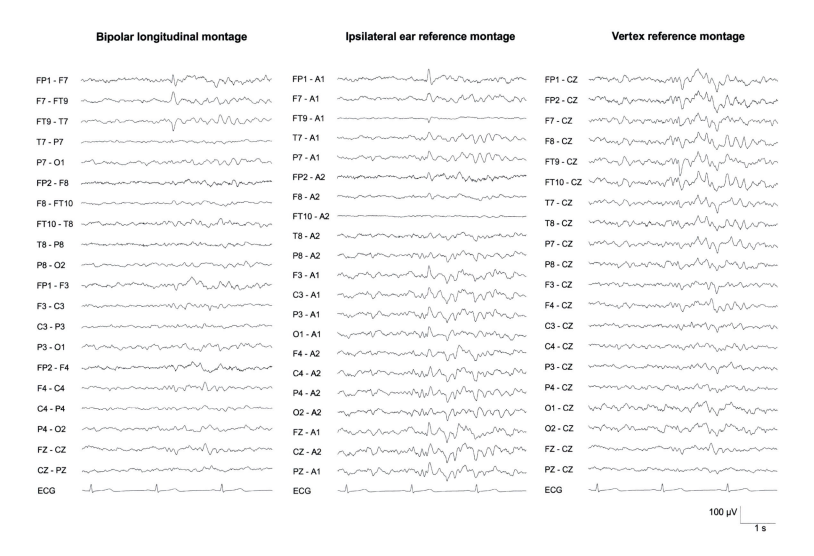

Bipolar longitudinal montage	Ipsilateral ear reference montage	Vertex reference montage
FP1 - F7	FP1 - A1	FP1 - CZ
F7 - FT9	F7 - A1	FP2 - CZ
FT9 - T7	FT9 - A1	F7 - CZ
T7 - P7	T7 - A1	F8 - CZ
P7 - O1	P7 - A1	FT9 - CZ
FP2 - F8	FP2 - A2	FT10 - CZ
F8 - FT10	F8 - A2	T7 - CZ
FT10 - T8	FT10 - A2	T8 - CZ
T8 - P8	T8 - A2	P7 - CZ
P8 - O2	P8 - A2	P8 - CZ
FP1 - F3	F3 - A1	F3 - CZ
F3 - C3	C3 - A1	F4 - CZ
C3 - P3	P3 - A1	C3 - CZ
P3 - O1	O1 - A1	C4 - CZ
FP2 - F4	F4 - A2	P3 - CZ
F4 - C4	C4 - A2	P4 - CZ
C4 - P4	P4 - A2	O1 - CZ
P4 - O2	O2 - A2	O2 - CZ
FZ - CZ	FZ - A1	FZ - CZ
CZ - PZ	CZ - A2	PZ - CZ
ECG	PZ - A1	ECG
	ECG	

100 µV

1 s

▶ **Figure 2.28** **Positive left temporal spike.** Spikes recorded from the scalp almost always are of negative polarity. In reality, these spikes are generated by a dipole whose negative pole is oriented to the surface of the brain, and the positive pole is not visible because it usually points toward the brain center. In some cases, after surgery, the positive pole of the dipole may become visible on scalp electrodes. In this example, the positive spike is shown in three different montages: The bipolar longitudinal montage shows a positive phase reversal at electrode FT9; in the ear reference montage, only the electrode FT9 shows a downward deflection; and in the vertex reference montage, the spike in the electrode FT9 and in the ear electrodes (A1 more pronounced than A2) clearly shows a downward deflection. This indicates that the maximum of the positivity of the spike is at electrode FT9, followed by electrode A1.

and positive) of a potential. A phase reversal is present when, within a chain, the potential of interest shows deflections in opposite directions. On the other hand, there is no phase reversal if all deflections within a chain point in one direction. This applies to both referential and bipolar montages. However, the conclusions we draw from the presence or absence of a phase reversal in any given chain are different for bipolar and referential montages.

It is often mentioned in EEG reports that a phase reversal has been found at an electrode. This statement is meaningless unless we specify the chain in which this phase reversal occurred (Benbadis & Lin, 2008). In addition, the presence or not of a phase reversal has nothing to do with the nature of the brain potential. In other word, the presence or not of a phase reversal does not assist us in deciding if a potential is epileptiform or not. Summarizing, phase reversal is a concept that is essential when localizing EEG potentials in bipolar or referential chains but has nothing to do with the epileptogenicity of the potential of interest and also does not necessarily identify the maximum amplitude of a potential of interest. We label a phase reversal as a negative phase reversal when, in a bipolar chain, the deflections point toward each other, and we label it as a positive phase reversal when the deflections point away from each other (▶ **Figure** 2.24). Phase reversal applies to all wave forms (normal and abnormal) and is a useful concept that helps in the localization of any EEG potential.

A phase reversal in a reference montage should be interpreted as follows (▶ **Figure** 2.29):

Phase reversal in a reference montage: The reference electrode is neither maximum nor minimum ("contaminated reference"). In other words,

some electrodes are more positive and others more negative than the reference electrode.

Positive generator: The electrode in the channel with the largest downward deflection will be maximum. On the other hand, the largest upward deflection points to the least active electrode.

Negative generator: The electrode in the channel with the largest upward deflection will be maximum. On the other hand, the largest downward deflection points to the least active electrode.

No phase reversal in a reference montage: The reference is either maximum or minimum.

Positive generator: The channel with the largest downward deflection is maximum positivity. If all the deflections are downward, then the reference is minimum positivity. If all the deflections are upward, then the reference is maximum positivity.

Negative generator: The channel with the largest upward deflection is maximum. If all the deflections are downward, then the reference is maximum negativity. If all the deflections are upward, then the reference is minimum negativity.

A phase reversal in a bipolar montage should be interpreted as follows (▶ **Figure** 2.30):

Phase reversal in a bipolar montage: The electrode at the phase reversal is either maximum or minimum.

Polarity rule for referential montages

| Phase reversal | → | The referential electrode is neither maximum nor minimum |
| No phase reversal | → | The referential electrode is maximum or minimum |

▶ **Figure 2.29** Polarity rule for referential montages.

Polarity rule for bipolar montages

| Phase reversal | → | The maximum or minimum is at the electrode of phase reversal |
| No phase reversal | → | The maximum or minimum is at the end of the electrode montage |

▶ **Figure 2.30** Polarity rule for bipolar montages.

Positive generator: The electrode at the phase reversal is maximum if there is a positive phase reversal. The electrode at the phase reversal is minimum if there is a negative phase reversal.

Negative generator: The electrode at the phase reversal is maximum if there is a negative phase reversal. The electrode at the phase reversal is minimum if there is a positive phase reversal.

No phase reversal in a bipolar montage: The maximum and minimum potentials are at the end of the chain.

Positive generator: Assuming we have a chain from front to back: If all the deflections are downward, the maximum positive electrode is in the front; if all the deflections are upward, the maximum positivity is in the back.

Negative generator: Assuming we have a chain from front to back: If all the deflections are upward, the maximum negative electrode is in the front; if all the deflections are downward, the maximum negativity is in the back.

There are some additional localization rules. In some bipolar chains, a phase reversal occurs across two or more channels, as shown in ▶ **Figure 2.31**. This is called a "broad phase reversal." The same localization rules outlined above for phase reversals across one electrode apply in this circumstance. In this case, the electrode at the phase reversal is of the same potential (isoelectric) as the adjacent electrodes. Broad phase reversals produce isoelectric recordings (no deflections) at one or more channels.

If a phase reversal includes one or more channels without deflection, the number of electrodes indicating the maximum or minimum is calculated according to the following rule:

Number of electrodes for maximum or minimum = number of isoelectric channels + 1

For example, in ▶ **Figure 2.31**, there is one channel with electrodes isoelectric with the phase reversal electrode. Therefore, there are 1 + 1 isoelectric electrodes = 2 = F7 and FT9.

Broad phase reversal means that a phase reversal occurs in a bipolar montage, and one or more channels placed between the phase reversal show no deflection (channel F8–T8 in ▶ **Figure 2.32**). When amplifying the EEG signal with differential amplifiers, a channel without deflection means that there is no

Broad phase reversal

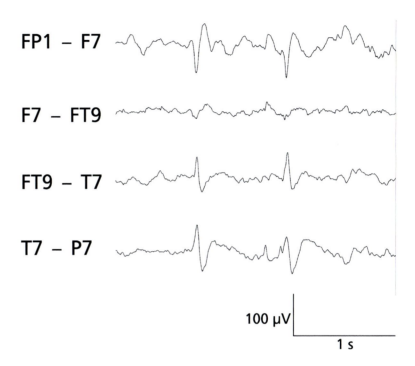

FP1 – F7

F7 – FT9

FT9 – T7

T7 – P7

100 µV

1 s

▶ **Figure 2.31** **Broad phase reversal.** The electrodes F7 and FT9 are almost equally negative for the spike, which is the reason the differential amplifier in channel F7–FT9 does not show a deflection for this spike. The adjacent channels show a phase reversal. Therefore, one speaks of a wide negative phase reversal at F7 and FT9—that is, there is a maximum negativity at electrodes F7 and FT9—and electrodes F7 and FT9 are of approximately equal negativity.

potential difference between the two connected electrodes. In this case, electrodes F8 and T8 have the same negative charge. The reference montage to the vertex (CZ) confirms this assumption: Electrodes F8 and T8 have similarly high upward deflections - that is, they are maximum and of almost equal negativity (▶ **Figure 2.33**). In such cases, additional closely placed electrodes (10/10 system) often show that the maximum lies between the two electrodes. In this case, for example, this could be the anterior temporal electrode FT10, which is not included in the 10/20 system (Morris et al., 1986). This example also illustrates that the temporal spike would be overlooked if only an 8-channel parasagittal

Right temporal spike in a bipolar longitudinal montage

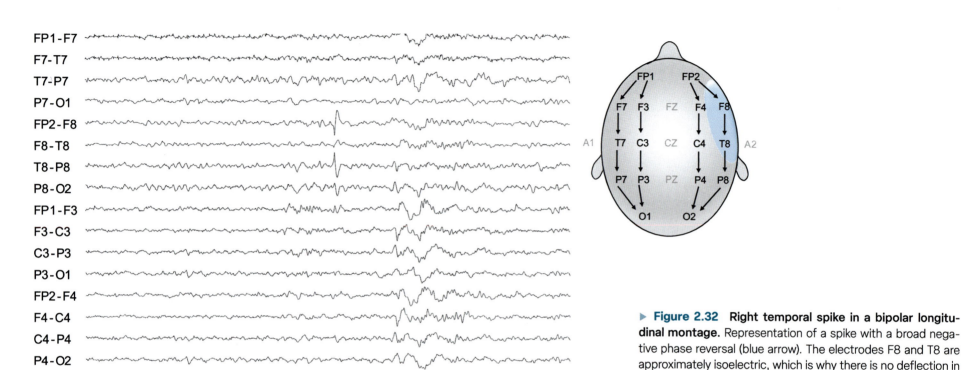

▶ **Figure 2.32** **Right temporal spike in a bipolar longitudinal montage.** Representation of a spike with a broad negative phase reversal (blue arrow). The electrodes F8 and T8 are approximately isoelectric, which is why there is no deflection in the channel F8–T8 higher than the background activity (broad phase reversal). The open arrow marks a vertex wave followed by a K-complex with sleep spindle (sleep stage 2).

longitudinal row were used. The lower 8 channels show nothing of the spike (▶ Figure 2.32).

In the vertex reference derivation of ▶ Figure 2.33, a vertex wave is also shown. The vertex wave shows a downward deflection because vertex waves are negative and usually, as the name implies, maximum at the vertex (CZ) (▶ Figure 2.33, open arrow). This is another example of a referential montage with no phase reversal in which the reference is highly "contaminated," namely

it reflects the maximum negativity. In the bipolar montage of ▶ Figure 2.32, the vertex wave is poorly defined because the vertex electrode is missing.

In the reformatted reference montage to ipsilateral ear electrodes (▶ Figure 2.34), the analysis of the EEG becomes more difficult. As can be seen, there is now a phase reversal implying that the reference electrode is "contaminated." This makes the analysis in an ear reference montage more complex (blue arrow; ▶ Figure 2.34). The electrodes F8 and T8 show

Right temporal spike in vertex reference montage

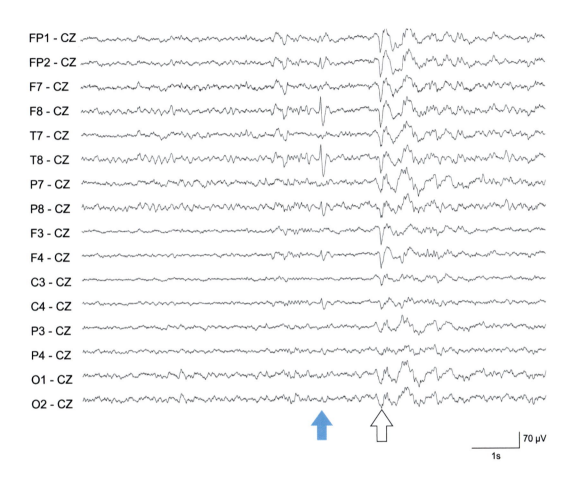

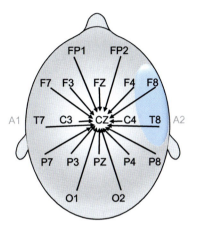

70 µV

1s

▶ **Figure 2.33** **Right temporal spike in vertex reference montage.** The same EEG section as in ▶ **Figure 2.32** in a reference montage to electrode CZ. The negative epileptiform discharge (blue arrow) shows a nearly equal deflection in electrodes F8 and T8. The vertex wave (open arrow) points downwards in all channels because the electrode in amplifier input 2 (electrode CZ) is more negative than all other electrodes.

similarly small upward deflections, while the largest deflections point downward. This means that in channels FP2–A2, P8–A2, F4–A2, C4–A2, P4–A2 and O2–A2, the right ear electrode A2 is more negative than the electrode in amplifier input I (▶ **Figure 2.34**). Therefore, the deflection is downward.

We can conclude from this that the right ear electrode is slightly less negatively charged than the electrodes F8 and T8. The right temporal spike is best displayed in the vertex reference (▶ **Figure 2.33**) and the left ear reference montages (▶ **Figure 2.35**).

Right temporal spike in reference montage to the ipsilateral ear

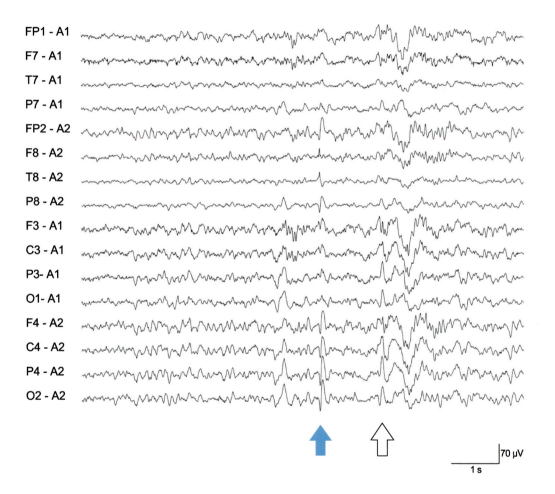

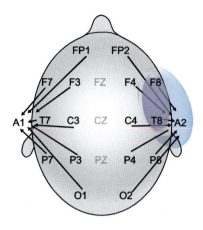

▶ **Figure 2.34** **Right temporal spike in reference montage to the ipsilateral ear.** The same EEG section as in ▶ **Figures 2.32** and **2.33** in a reference montage to the ipsilateral ear (A1 and A2). The right temporal spike (blue arrow) shows a phase reversal in the referential montage. This means that the reference electrode is neither maximum nor minimum. It lies in the field of the temporal spike, which means the reference electrode is "contaminated." This is understandable for a temporal spike in the same side as the ear reference. In a temporal spike, the left ear electrode A1 is always more negative than left parasagittal electrodes, all of which showed a downward deflection (F3–A1, C3–A1, P3–A1, and O1–A1). The open arrow marks the vertex wave.

Right temporal spike in a reference montage to the left ear

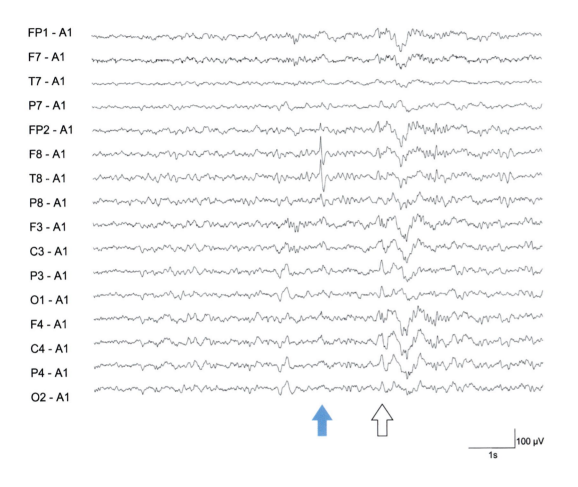

FP1 - A1
F7 - A1
T7 - A1
P7 - A1
FP2 - A1
F8 - A1
T8 - A1
P8 - A1
F3 - A1
C3 - A1
P3 - A1
O1 - A1
F4 - A1
C4 - A1
P4 - A1
O2 - A1

100 µV

1s

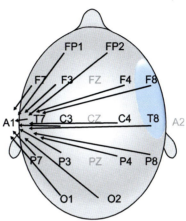

▶ **Figure 2.35   Right temporal spike in a reference montage to the left ear.** The same EEG section as in **Figures 2.32–2.35** in a reference montage to the left ear (A1). The right temporal spike (blue arrow) shows no phase reversal in this ear reference montage, indicating that the reference electrode is the least relative negative electrode. The open arrow marks the vertex wave.

Occasionally, more than one phase reversal occurs in a bipolar chain (▶ **Figure 2.36**). Let us here apply the rules of localization:

STEP 1:   ▶ **Figure 2.36** shows a bipolar montage with two additional isolated channels (FT9–FT10 and TP9–TP10).

STEP 2:   We analyze the four bipolar channels.

STEP 3:   We see a downward deflection in the first channel.

STEP 4:   We will analyze the time of the maximum deflection of the sharp wave.

STEP 5:   There are three phase reversals: Negative at F7, positive at FT9, and negative at T7.

Triple phase reversal

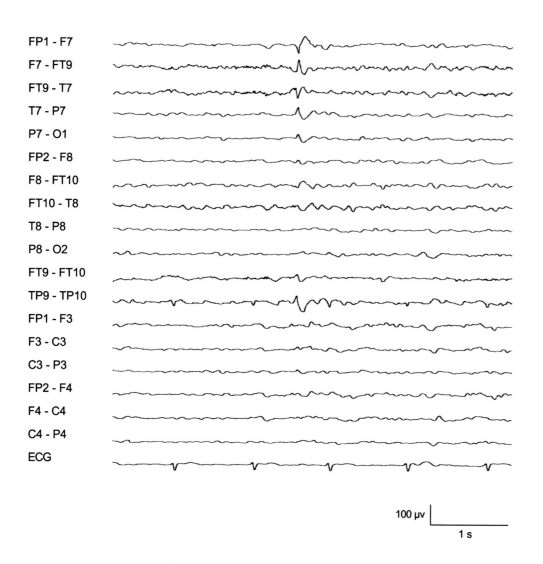

FP1 - F7
F7 - FT9
FT9 - T7
T7 - P7
P7 - O1
FP2 - F8
F8 - FT10
FT10 - T8
T8 - P8
P8 - O2
FT9 - FT10
TP9 - TP10
FP1 - F3
F3 - C3
C3 - P3
FP2 - F4
F4 - C4
C4 - P4
ECG

100 µv

1 s

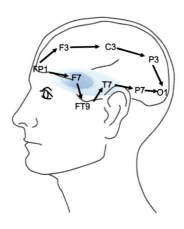

▶ **Figure 2.36 Triple phase reversal.** The maximum of the sharp wave lies in the electrodes F7 and T7. The FT9 electrode is less negative than F7 and T7. By connecting electrode F7 to electrode FT9, one moves away from the maximum negativity, and in channel FT9–T7 one returns to the maximum negativity again. This results in a triple phase reversal for this sharp wave—that is, the electrodes F7 and T7 are more negative than the electrode FT9.

If we assume the generator is negative, there are two maxima in the chain: F7 and T7.

If we assume that the discharge is positive, the maximum positivity is either at the positive phase reversal or in one of the extremes of the bipolar chain we are analyzing (FT9, FP1, or O1).

Finding more than one phase reversal in a bipolar chain is unusual, and we discuss later in this chapter how to decide on a localization in this case.

If a bipolar montage shows a threefold phase reversal (▶ Figure 2.36), this means the following:

Number of "phase reversals" = number of polarity reversals in the montage

In summary, the triple phase reversal is due to the bipolar montage, which includes anterior temporal electrodes that do not represent the maximum of the negative spike. The spike maximum is at electrode F7, and therefore electrode FT9 is more positive than electrode F7. This leads to the triple phase reversal.

Let us now apply the step-by-step localization rules in the analysis of the EEG illustrated in ▶ Figure 2.37:

STEP 1:   ▶ Figure 2.37 shows a bipolar montage.

STEP 2:   There are four bipolar channels.

STEP 3:   We will analyze the potentials in channels 2 and 3, which show the potential of interest best.

STEP 4:   We will analyze the time of the maximum deflection of the sharp wave.

STEP 5:   There is a negative phase reversal. Therefore, the two possible solutions are the following:

Solution 1: The potential of interest is negative and maximum at the electrode where the phase reversal is: C4.

Solution 2: The potential is of positive polarity and minimum at C4 (or, in other words, maximum at the end of the chain FP2 or O2). Notice that Solution 1 is the mirror image of Solution 2.

Which one of the two solutions is correct? The correct solution can be determined when we know other characteristics of the potential of interest:

Localization in bipolar longitudinal montage with phase reversal

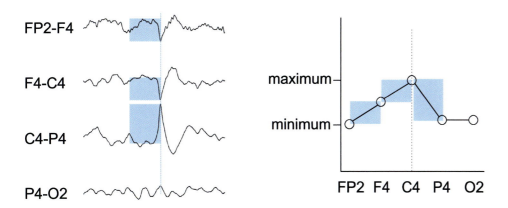

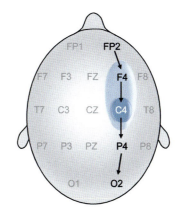

▶ **Figure 2.37** **Localization in bipolar longitudinal montage with phase reversal.** Right central spike (maximum negativity at electrode C4) in a bipolar longitudinal montage. Localization of the potential field by determining the amplitudes and transferring the potential field gradient to an electrode potential field graph (middle of ▶ **Figure 2.30**) and then to an isopotential head model (graph on the right side of ▶ **Figure 2.30**). The higher excursion in C4–P4 compared to channel F4–C4 indicates that electrode P4 is less negative than electrode F4.

A. The potential of interest is epileptiform, and epileptiform discharges usually are of negative polarity when recording with scalp electrodes. Therefore, Solution 1 is most probably the correct one.

B. In this chain, the highest potential difference occurs at C4–P4 and the lowest potential differences at P4–O2 and FP2–F4. Again, we conclude that Solution 1 is the correct one because in a volume conductor, the potentials fall off exponentially.

C. On the other hand, the shape of the generator of the potential of interest would be extremely unusual if we assume that the generator is of positive polarity—that is, the generator would be minimum at C4. This is highly unlikely. Therefore, we would again reach the conclusion that the generator is negative and maximum at C4.

STEP 6: Once we have defined the maximum of the potential of interest, we should proceed to determine the distribution of the potential of interest.

Therefore, the question arises as to which electrode is the next most active—that is, the most negatively charged one. The next most negatively charged electrode will show a smaller deflection compared to C4. If one considers that the potential of interest was recorded with differential amplifiers, in the example in ▶ Figure 2.37, the deflection in channel F4–C4 is smaller than the deflection in channel C4–P4, which means that electrode F4 is the next negatively charged electrode.

Potential fields of a potential of interest can be plotted in two ways:

1. A bar graph with all the electrodes of a chain plotted on the x-axis, and the y-axis showing the relative amplitude of the potential at any given electrode (the maximum potential equals 100%). The definition of the maximum, however, is arbitrary. It is essential to understand that we can only plot the "shape" of the distribution curve but do not know what the absolute values are. They can be negative or positive potentials—that is, because of the inverse problem, we do not know where along the y-axis they are actually located. The differential amplifier in EEG provides only current differences between electrodes. We do not have a zero baseline. Thus, we can only derive

information on the relative negativity or positivity. In this book, for the purpose of illustration, negative potentials are plotted above the y-axis and positive potential below the y-axis. As mentioned above, the localization rules only apply for monopoles. Therefore, in these plots, all the potentials are either above or below the y-axis.

▶ Figure 2.37 shows such a graph. The amplitude of the spike in channel F4–C4 (e.g., measured from the baseline to the maximum of the spike) is plotted in the graph as maximum, reflecting the maximum negativity in that chain. Then the relative amplitude drop of the spike in the adjacent channels can be plotted—that is, first C4–P4 and F4–C4 and then P4–O2 or FP2–F4 (▶ Figure 2.37). The voltage difference between the electrodes in this bipolar chain is plotted above the zero line, thus indicating a maximum negativity at electrode C4. If we would move the graph down, we would end up with two positive maxima at FP2 and P4/O2. Because epileptiform discharges are usually negative, it is more likely that this plot is correct than to assume two positive generators in the front and back of the head.

2. An isopotential line graph showing all the electrodes in its spatial relationship to the brain (▶ Figure 2.37). In this graph, the electrode with the maximum negative or positive potential is encircled first. The second circle includes all the electrodes with potential amplitudes of >90%. This can be followed by more circles that include all the electrodes with potential amplitudes of more than 80%, 70%, or 60%. However, in general, the area of brain involved in the generation of any scalp potential corresponds to approximately the area encircled by 80% of the isopotential lines.

Figures 2.32–2.42, 2.44, 2.45, and 2.47–2.49 show examples of different potentials localized following the localization rules with the corresponding distribution maps. ▶ Figure 2.38 shows the same spike illustrated in ▶ Figure 2.37 but now recorded in a transverse bipolar chain. The figure only shows one chain. Again, we analyze the distribution of the spike at its maximum amplitude. Notice that the higher amplitude of the spike at C4–CZ implies that T8 is more negative than CZ.

▶ Figure 2.39 shows a spike in a bipolar distribution. There are three chains, and the spike has only been distributed in two chains. The two chains are not

Localization analysis of a spike in a bipolar transverse montage with phase reversal

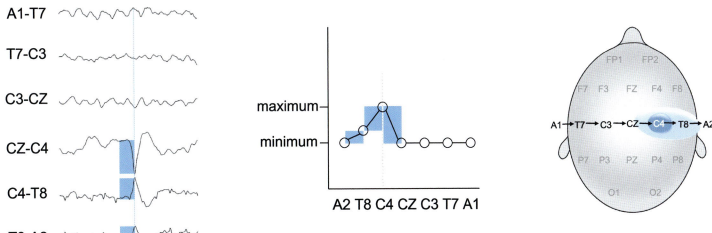

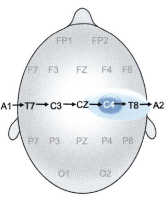

▶ **Figure 2.38**   **Localization analysis of a spike in a bipolar transverse montage with phase reversal.** The same right central spike (maximum negativity at electrode C4) of ▶ **Figure 2.30** in a bipolar transverse montage. Localization of the potential field by determining the amplitudes and transferring the potential field gradient to an electrode potential field graph and then to an isopotential head model. The higher excursion in C4–CZ compared to channel T8–C4 means that electrode CZ is less negative than electrode T8.

▶ **Figure 2.38**

linked; therefore, we must make some assumptions to distribute the spike over the two chains:

Assumption: O1 and O2 are very distant from the spike and, therefore, most probably not involved and equal.

Assumption: There is a low-amplitude downward deflection in channels 4, 7, 8, and 10. Therefore, if we assume a monopole, we obtain an unusual distribution with a maximum positivity at electrodes F3, C3, P3, F4, C4, and P4 and an abrupt falloff of positivity from F3 and F4 to FP1 and FP2, respectively. A better assumption would be to assume that the activity at O1 and O2 is generated by an independent generator at O1 and O2 that is independent of the frontal spikes (e.g., alpha rhythm) but happens to be synchronous with the frontal spikes. The other possibility is that we are dealing with a dipole with maximum negativity at FP1 and FP2, and a maximum positivity at O1 and O2. As previously mentioned, however, the localization

rules explained in this book only refer to monopoles. Therefore, we are only going to distribute the negative pole of the discharge and neglect the small occipital deflection, which is likely a reflection of intermixed occipital alpha activity. In other words, we are going to assume that all channels except channels 1 and 5 are flat. We can then see that channel 5 has a slightly higher amplitude than channel 1. That is also reflected in the attached distribution maps.

If we make the assumptions outlined above, ▶ **Figure 2.39** would be an example of two bipolar chains without a phase reversal. In that case, the maximum amplitude is at one of the extremes of the chain (▶ **Figure 2.30**). The following criteria can be used to localize the spike in these two chains:

1. Epileptiform discharges usually are of negative polarity.
2. The highest amplitude of spikes in a volume conductor occurs close to the generator.

Localization analysis in bipolar longitudinal montage without phase reversal

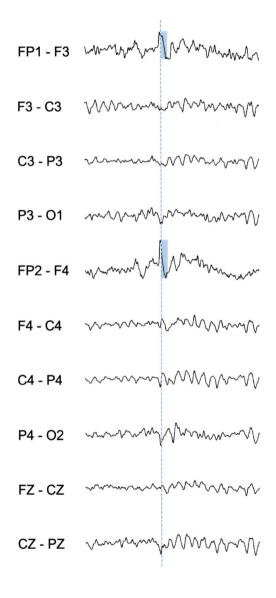

FP1 - F3

F3 - C3

C3 - P3

P3 - O1

FP2 - F4

F4 - C4

C4 - P4

P4 - O2

FZ - CZ

CZ - PZ

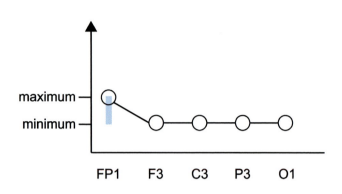

maximum —

minimum —

FP1   F3   C3   P3   O1

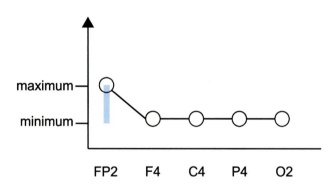

maximum —

minimum —

FP2   F4   C4   P4   O2

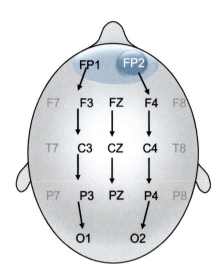

▶ **Figure 2.39 Localization analysis in bipolar longitudinal montage without phase reversal.** The deflections of the spike point upwards in all channels. There is no phase reversal. The maximum negativity is at electrodes FP1 and FP2, respectively, in the left and right hemisphere. Unfortunately, the two chains are not connected; therefore, we cannot directly compare the amplitudes. However, because there are no significant deflections in all channels except at FP1–F3 and FP2–F4, it is reasonable to assume that these are very focal discharges almost exclusively reflected at electrodes FP1 and FP2. The two graphs in the middle, and the isopotential map on the right make this assumption, and it is concluded that the discharge is maximum at FP2 and that FP1 is significantly smaller than FP2.

3. It is very unlikely that three or more channels are maximum and almost of equal amplitude unless they are inactive.

All these arguments support the conclusion that the maximum potential is at FP2 and FP1. In addition, it can be seen that the upward deflection is of higher amplitude at FP2–F4 compared to FP1–F3. This implies that the discharge is maximum at FP2.

In summary, the spike distribution in this 10-channel derivation would be typical for a right frontal lobe epilepsy. Generalized spikes typically show shifting maximum negativity around the midline (electrodes FZ, F3/F4, and FP1/FP2). However, only a 10-channel parasagittal longitudinal row is shown here.

▶ **Figure 2.40** shows the same spike illustrated in ▶ **Figure 2.39** in an 18-channel bipolar montage that includes all the scalp electrodes of the 10/20 system. Using the stepwise approach mentioned above, we should first analyze the right temporal chain. It shows a clear negative phase reversal at F8. In addition, FP2–F8 shows a downward deflection indicating that F8 is more negative than FP2, which was maximum in the more restricted chains of ▶ **Figure 2.39**. This example illustrates that 10-channel montages in certain instances (as shown in ▶ **Figures 2.39** and **2.40**) may be inadequate and may lead to misinterpretations of the EEG. Notice also that chains 1 and 2, as well as 3 and 4, in ▶ **Figure 2.40** are linked by FP1/FP2 and O1/O2. The corresponding amplitude/electrode position graphs reflect these linkages. An additional transverse chain, such as F3–FZ, FZ–F4, would link all five chains together and permit a precise potential localization.

▶ **Figure 2.41** shows the same potential as in ▶ **Figure 2.37** (bipolar longitudinal montage) and ▶ **Figure 2.38** (bipolar transverse montage) but in a referential derivation of five electrodes (parasagittal chain) connected to the ipsilateral ear (electrode A2). In this limited chain, the sharp transient shows no phase reversal. Therefore, we can apply the rule of a referential montage with no phase reversal (▶ **Figure 2.29**). This leads us to the conclusion that if we assume that the generator is negative, A2 is the least negative electrode and C4 is the highest negativity.

▶ **Figure 2.42** shows the same electrodes as in ▶ **Figures 2.37, 2.38** and **2.41** in a referential montage to CZ. Again, in this case, there is no phase reversal, indicating—if the generator is negative—that the reference is not contaminated. Notice that the electrode position/amplitude map and also the isopotential map of ▶ **Figures 2.37** and **2.38** are almost identical in the two figures. This is because A2 and CZ are essentially uninvolved and therefore approximately of equal potential (0 V). In the figures discussed above, only selected chains of electrodes are displayed and analyzed. However, in most laboratories, 18- to 20-channel recordings are obtained. In the following figures, 18 channels are displayed and analyzed.

▶ **Figure 2.43** shows a spike displayed in four 18-channel montages. Let us apply the stepwise approach to the first montage of ▶ **Figure 2.43**:

STEP 1: This is a bipolar longitudinal montage.
STEP 2: There are five bipolar chains.
STEP 3: We will first analyze the fourth chain.
STEP 4: We will analyze the time of the maximum deflection of the sharp wave.
STEP 5: There is a negative phase reversal at C4. That would imply that the C4 is the maximum if we assume that the generator is negative. Applying the same arguments discussed in the analysis of ▶ **Figure 2.37**, we can conclude that the discharge is negative and, therefore, maximum at C4. The deflection F4–C4 is smaller than the deflection C4–P4, indicating that F4 is the most negative electrode after C4. There are no other significant deflections in this montage. However, the EEG shows a well-developed alpha activity at P7–O1 that is almost absent at P8–O2, suggesting that the patient has a structural lesion on the right hemisphere.

Let us now analyze the EEG shown in ▶ **Figure 2.44**. Using the stepwise approach, we have the following:

STEP 1: This is a referential montage.
STEP 2: There is only one chain because all the electrodes are referred to CZ.
STEP 3: Therefore, there is only one chain to consider.
STEP 4: We will analyze the time of the maximum deflection of the sharp wave.
STEP 5: There is no phase reversal, implying that the reference is either maximum or minimum. If we now apply the criteria discussed in ▶ **Figure 2.37**, we can assume that the generator is negative and, therefore, that the reference electrode is minimum (or most probably inactive).

Localization analysis in a bipolar longitudinal montage with phase reversal

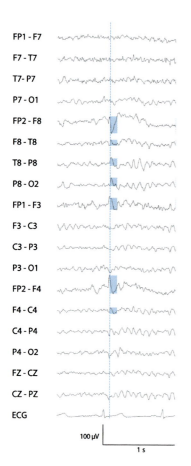

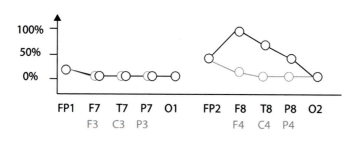

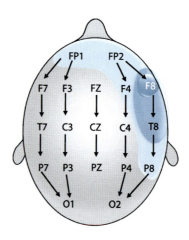

▶ **Figure 2.40** **Localization analysis in a bipolar longitudinal montage with phase reversal.** The same EEG signal as in ▶ **Figure** 2.39 in a bipolar 18-channel longitudinal montage. The additional temporal montage shows a negative phase reversal at electrodes F8 and T8 that was missing in the parasagittal longitudinal montage in ▶ **Figure** 2.39. This analysis shows that replacing an 18-channel recording by a 10-channel recording (▶ **Figure** 2.39) would falsely localize this right temporal spike.

We can now also conclude that the maximum negativity (deflection upwards due to negativity at amplifier input 1) is at electrode T8, followed by C4. The next negative electrodes—P8, P4, and FP2—show significantly lower upward deflections. Defining the potential distribution is relatively simple if there is no phase reversal in a referential montage and the reference is the minimum as in this case.

Let us now analyze the EEG shown in ▶ **Figure** 2.45, which shows the same spike analyzed in ▶ **Figure** 2.44 but using a different reference electrode, namely the ipsilateral ear:

STEP 1:   This is a referential montage.

STEP 2:   There are two chains (referenced to A1 or A2).

STEP 3:   We will analyze first chain 2 with reference to A2.

Localization analysis in an ear reference montage without phase reversal

FP2-A2

F4-A2

C4-A2

P4-A2

O2-A2

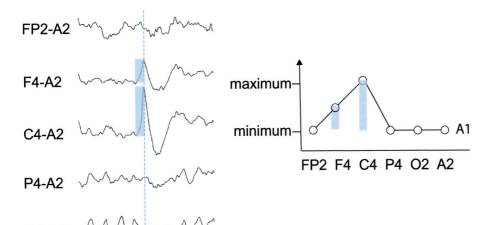

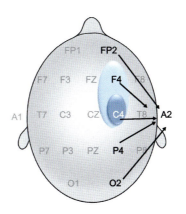

▶ **Figure 2.41** Localization analysis in an ear reference montage without phase reversal. The same EEG section as in ▶ **Figures 2.37** and 2.38 but now displayed in a reference montage to the ipsilateral ear. Electrode C4 shows the largest upward deflection, followed by electrode F4. Electrode C4 also shows the highest negativity, followed by electrode F4.

2 Fundamentals of EEG

Localization analysis in a vertex reference montage without phase reversal

FP2-CZ

F4-CZ

C4-CZ

P4-CZ

O2-CZ

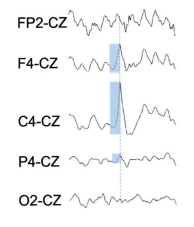

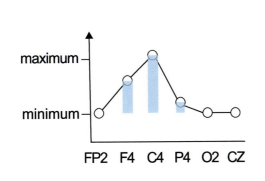

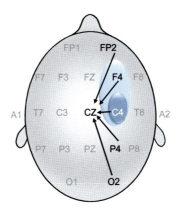

▶ **Figure 2.42** Localization analysis in a vertex reference montage without phase reversal. The same EEG section as in ▶ **Figures 2.37**, 2.38, and 2.41 in a reference montage to the vertex. The amplitude is the largest in C4, second largest at F4, and third largest at P4. There is a high-amplitude potential difference between C4 and CZ even though the electrode CZ is anatomically close to C4.

Right central spike in four different montages

Bipolar longitudinal montage	Vertex reference montage	Ipsilateral ear reference montage	Bipolar transverse montage
FP1 - F7	FP1 - CZ	FP1 - A1	F7 - F3
F7 - T7	F7 - CZ	F7 - A1	F3 - FZ
T7- P7	T7- CZ	T7- A1	FZ - F4
P7 - O1	P7 - CZ	P7 - A1	F4- F8
FP2 - F8	FP2 - CZ	FP2 - A2	A1 - T7
F8 - T8	F8 - CZ	F8 - A2	T7 - C3
T8 - P8	T8 - CZ	T8 - A2	C3 - CZ
P8 - O2	P8 - CZ	P8 - A2	CZ - C4
FP1 - F3	F3 - CZ	F3 - A1	C4 - T8
F3 - C3	C3 - CZ	C3 - A1	T8 - A2
C3 - P3	P3 - CZ	P3 - A1	P7 - P3
P3 - O1	O1 - CZ	O1 - A1	P3 - PZ
FP2 - F4	F4 - CZ	F4 - A2	PZ - P4
F4 - C4	C4 - CZ	C4 - A2	P4 - P8
C4 - P4	P4 - CZ	P4 - A2	FP1 - A1
P4 - O2	O2 - CZ	O2 - A2	FP2 - A2
FZ - CZ	FZ - CZ	FZ - A1	O1 - A1
CZ - PZ	PZ - CZ	CZ - A1	O2 - A2
ECG	ECG	ECG	ECG

200 µV

1 s

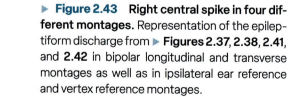

▶ **Figure 2.43** **Right central spike in four different montages.** Representation of the epileptiform discharge from ▶ **Figures 2.37**, **2.38**, **2.41**, and **2.42** in bipolar longitudinal and transverse montages as well as in ipsilateral ear reference and vertex reference montages.

Localization analysis in a vertex reference montage without phase reversal

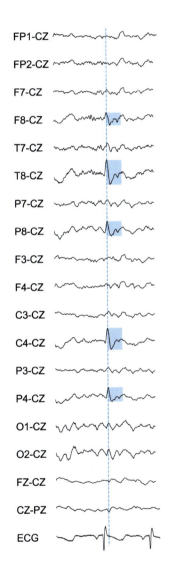

FP1-CZ

FP2-CZ

F7-CZ

F8-CZ

T7-CZ

T8-CZ

P7-CZ

P8-CZ

F3-CZ

F4-CZ

C3-CZ

C4-CZ

P3-CZ

P4-CZ

O1-CZ

O2-CZ

FZ-CZ

CZ-PZ

ECG

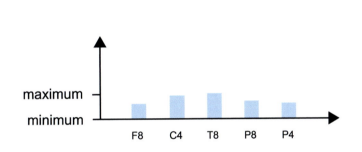

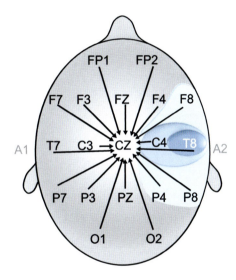

▶ **Figure 2.44** **Localization analysis in a vertex reference montage without phase reversal.** The epileptiform discharge in this montage shows only upward deflections—that is, no phase reversal. Thus, the maximum of the negativity of the potential in the electrode T8 (followed by C4) can be determined by the height of the upward deflections.

Localization analysis in an ipsilateral ear reference montage with phase reversal

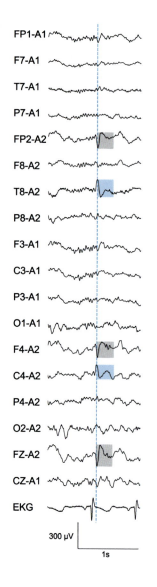

300 μV

1s

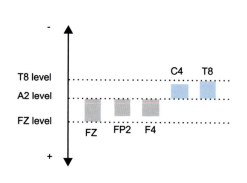

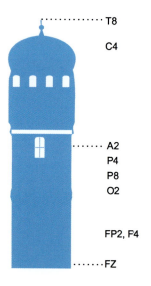

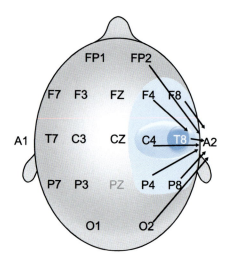

▶ **Figure 2.45 Localization analysis in an ipsilateral ear reference montage with phase reversal.** Same EEG section as in ▶ **Figure 2.44**. This referential montage shows a phase reversal. The reference thus lies in the potential field ("contaminated reference"). The upward deflections in the electrode T8 and slightly lower in electrode C4 are thus more negative than the reference electrode, and the electrodes pointing downward are more positive (FZ, FP2, and F4). The analogy of the potential field to the tower is explained in the text. In this example the amplitude has been measured from the maxmum negativity to the following maximum positivity of the spike.

STEP 4:   We will analyze the time of the maximum deflection of the sharp wave.

STEP 5:   There is a phase reversal with some deflections pointing upward and other deflections pointing downward. Specifically, at electrodes T8 and C4, there is an upward deflection, and at electrodes FZ, FP2, and F4, there is a downward deflection. At the other electrodes (F8, P8, P4, and O2), there is no deflection beyond the background activity.

This is a typical example of a "contaminated" reference. Applying the same arguments discussed in the analysis of ▶ Figure 2.37, we can conclude that the discharge is negative and, therefore, the highest amplitude negative discharge will be the highest upward deflection (C4 and T8). The least involved electrode will be the highest downward deflection. As this example shows, the analysis of the distribution of EEG potentials is much more complex when there is a "contaminated" reference. To illustrate the difference between contaminated and non-contaminated references, we place the reference electrode at different heights of a church tower. In this example, FZ is at the bottom of the tower, and T8 is at the peak of the tower. Therefore, if the generator is negative, all the electrodes are above FZ, and the degree of negativity will be an expression of the height of a given electrode. Assuming that the generator is negative, we can conclude that the highest electrode is also the most negative. On the other hand, if we choose the most negative electrode as a reference (T8), we will see no phase reversal because all the other electrodes are located under T8. In this case, the electrode that shows the highest amplitude is also the most different from the reference and, therefore, the least active electrode (FZ). Finally, if we choose an electrode as the reference placed in the middle of the tower (e.g., A2 at the window of the tower), there will be some electrodes above the window and others below the window. This implies that we will have a phase reversal, indicating that the reference is active. ▶ Figure 2.46 shows the spike in ▶ Figures 2.44 and 2.45 reformatted into four common montages. To assess the height of the tower, it is easier to look upward from the front door (level of FZ) or to look down from the top (level of T8). It is, however, more difficult to assess the height by looking out of the window (level of electrode A2) and adding the height difference down- and upward the window level. Therefore,

we always try to find a reference electrode that is not contaminated by the potential of interest.

2.2.3.3 Advantages and Disadvantages of Bipolar and Referential Montages

In clinical EEG, reference and bipolar montages are both used because each system has advantages and disadvantages. Bipolar montages display small steep potential fields very well. However, flat potential gradients are poorly shown. The ideal reference electrode should be completely inactive and free of any artifacts, such as EMG activity. However, there is no reference electrode that could never be contaminated. The reference electrode must therefore be selected in such a way that the potential of interest is optimally represented. This usually implies that the reference is inactive or the least active electrode, and the reference is not contaminated by artifacts or other EEG potentials, such as relatively high-amplitude background activity.

In the example in **Figures 2.33–2.35**, the temporal spike is better represented in a vertex reference (▶ **Figure 2.33**) and a contralateral ear reference (▶ **Figure 2.35**) than in an ipsilateral ear reference (▶ **Figure 2.34**). It is often said that in reference montages, the spatial distance between the reference electrode and electrodes placed on homologous areas of the two hemispheres should be approximately equal. It certainly is helpful to have the display of the potential in different channels follow some anatomical landmarks, but it is not necessary. Actually, the essential feature is a relatively less active reference with a minimum of interfering potentials (other EEG activity or artifacts). The example in ▶ **Figure 2.35** shows that a reference to the left (mutual) ear is excellently suited to optimally map the right temporal spike because the left ear is not affected by the potential field of the right temporal spike. As you can see, the different spatial distances between the different electrodes and the left ear are irrelevant.

The next example demonstrates the importance of the location of the reference electrode (▶ **Figure 2.47**). In this bipolar longitudinal row, there is no phase reversal for the small spike that in all channels is pointing downward. Following the rules of localization, the maximum or minimum of the spike lies at the beginning or end of the electrode row. Because we assume negativity for

Right temporocentral spike in four different montages

Bipolar longitudinal montage	Vertex reference montage	Ipsilateral ear reference montage	Bipolar transverse montage
FP1-F7	FP1-CZ	FP1-A1	F7-F3
F7-T7	FP2-CZ	F7-A1	F3-FZ
T7-P7	F7-CZ	T7-A1	FZ-F4
P7-O1	F8-CZ	P7-A1	F4-F8
FP2-F8	T7-CZ	FP2-A2	A1-T7
F8-T8	T8-CZ	F8-A2	T7-C3
T8-P8	P7-CZ	T8-A2	C3-CZ
P8-O2	P8-CZ	P8-A2	CZ-C4
FP1-F3	F3-CZ	F3-A1	C4-T8
F3-C3	F4-CZ	C3-A1	T8-A2
C3-P3	C3-CZ	P3-A1	P7-P3
P3-O1	C4-CZ	O1-A1	P3-PZ
FP2-F4	P3-CZ	F4-A2	PZ-P4
F4-C4	P4-CZ	C4-A2	P4-P8
C4-P4	O1-CZ	P4-A2	FP1-A1
P4-O2	O2-CZ	O2-A2	FP2-A2
FZ-CZ	FZ-CZ	FZ-A2	O1-A1
CZ-PZ	CZ-PZ	CZ-A1	O2-A2
ECG	ECG	ECG	ECG

300 µV | 1s

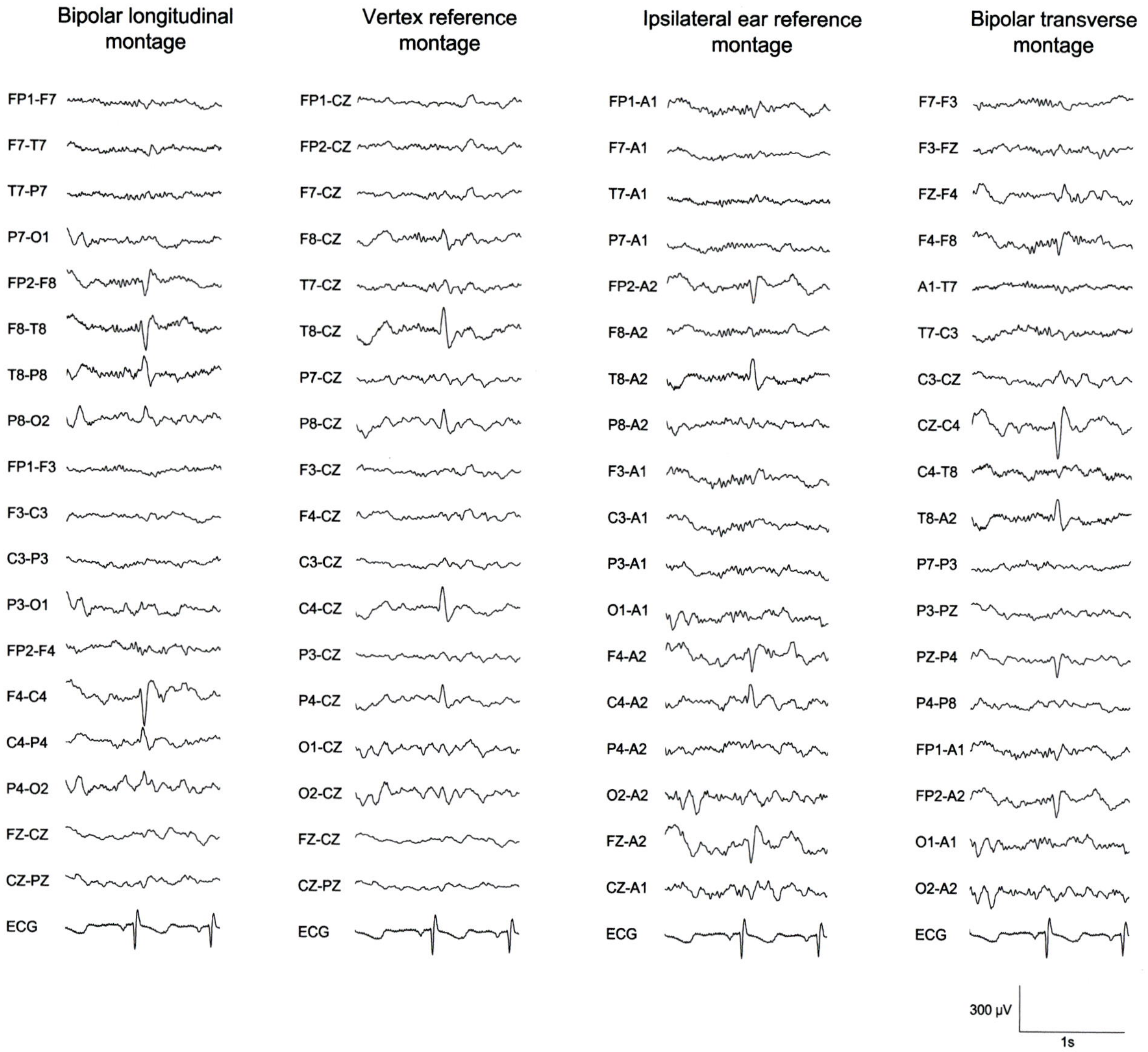

► **Figure 2.46** **Right temporocentral spike in four different montages.** Illustration of the spike from ► Figures 2.37 and 2.38 in bipolar longitudinal and transverse montages as well as in ipsilateral ear reference and vertex reference montages.

Occipital spike in a bipolar longitudinal montage

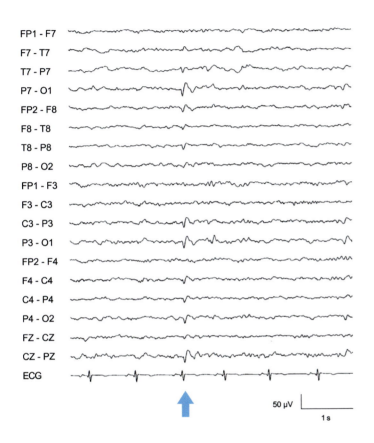

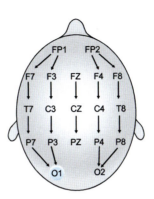

▶ **Figure 2.47** **Occipital spike in a bipolar longitudinal montage.** The spike points downwards in all channels. Thus, there is no phase reversal and, therefore, the maximum of the potential lies at the beginning or end of the electrode montage. The downward deflection means predominance of negativity at the amplifier input 2 and, thus, maximum negativity at O1 and O2. In this case, it is reasonable to assume that FP1 and FP2 are probably inactive (because they are located at a large distance from O1 and O2) and, therefore, of equal (inactive) potential. To calculate the voltage at O1 and O2, we must sum all the deflections of channels 9–12 and compare with the sum of the deflections at channels 13–16. The deflection at C3–P3 and P3–O1 is much larger then in homotopic right-sided electrodes. However, the spike on the right extends significantly more anterior than the spike on the left side (notice that there is no deflection at F3–C3). At this point, the best approach would be to get a referential montage with a single, inactive reference because of the imprecision of visual measurements and the possibility that the basic assumption is not correct (FP1 = FP2 = inactive) (see ▶ **Figure 2.49**).

epileptiform spikes and the deflection points downwards, we conclude that the negative spike originates from the electrodes O1 and/or O2. Unfortunately, the left and right parasagittal chains are not connected, and therefore we cannot simply compare amplitudes in P3–O1 and P4–O2. However, we know that in a volume conductor, the higher amplitudes occur in the immediate neighborhood of the generator. In this case, the higher amplitude deflections are in all the posterior leads. Therefore, it is most likely correct if we assume that FP1 and FP2 are either inactive or minimally involved. If we now assume that FP1 = FP2,

then we can compare the amplitudes at O1 and O2 by summing the amplitudes of the sharp wave in FP1–F7 + F7–T7 + T7–P7 + P7–O1 and compare it with the amplitudes at FP2–F8 + F8–T8 + T8–P8 + P8–O2. This clearly showed that the spike is of higher amplitude at O1 (▶ **Figure 2.47**). The same EEG recording reformatted to a referential montage with ipsilateral ear electrodes shows high-amplitude downward deflections in all electrodes except for O1 and O2, which show only relatively small upward deflections (▶ **Figure 2.48**). The interpretation of this recording is complicated for the following reasons:

1. Both references are active ("contaminated") because both chains included in this montage show phase reversals. As mentioned previously, EEG recordings with active references are in general more difficult to analyze than referential montages in which the reference is the least active electrode.
2. In this case, we are dealing with two referential chains in which the references most likely have different degrees of activity. In general, when making recordings with referential montages, we

should select a single reference. Only with a single reference we can deduce a distribution map covering all the recording electrodes.

▶ **Figure 2.49** shows the same potential of interest as ▶ **Figures 2.47** and 2.48, but now all the electrodes are connected to a single reference, namely CZ. Notice that now all the deflections of the spike point upward except electrodes F3, C3, and, to a lesser degree, FZ, indicating that either CZ, if the generator is negative, is an active electrode or F3 and C3 are more positive than CZ. In this

Occipital spike in a reference montage to the ipsilateral ear

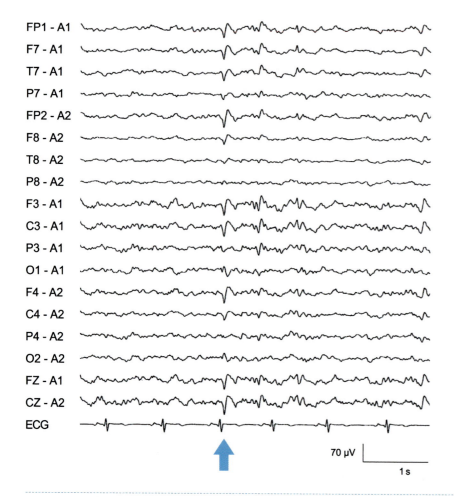

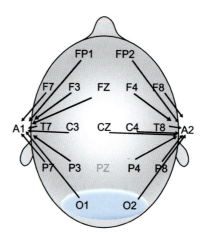

▶ **Figure 2.48 Occipital spike in a reference montage to the ipsilateral ear.** The same EEG section as in ▶ **Figure 2.47** in a reference montage to the ipsilateral ear (A1 and A2). There is a phase reversal for the spike (blue arrow). Only the electrodes O1 and O2 show small upward deflections. Therefore, the maximum of the negative spike lies in the electrodes O1 and O2.

example, we are dealing with a benign epileptiform discharge. These discharges are known to show dipoles, which in this case is likely a dipole with maximum negativity at O1 and a small positivity at F3 and C3.

As previously mentioned, in addition to brain activity, the EEG also records other physiological and nonphysiological potential fields that can disturb the recordings, such as ECG and EMG potentials. Such artifacts tend to occur preferentially in selected electrodes. For example, EMG artifacts are often found in the frontopolar (FP1 and FP2), inferior frontal (F7 and F8), and temporal electrodes (T7, T8, P7, and P8), whereas ECG artifacts usually have the highest amplitude in the ear electrodes (A1 and A2).

Although we list some typical montages for particular settings in ▶ **Table 2.2**, one should keep in mind that the EEG reader decides which reference to use by applying the principles mentioned above:

1. It should be an "indifferent" reference.
2. It should contain as little artifact and brain activity as possible.

Occipital spike in a reference montage to the vertex

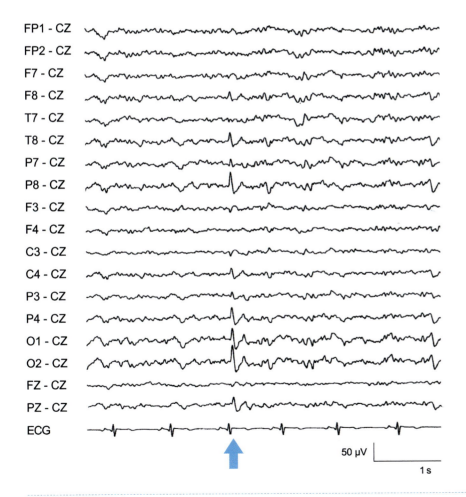

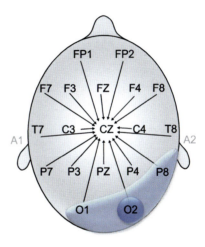

▶ **Figure 2.49   Occipital spike in a reference montage to the vertex.** The same EEG section as in ▶ **Figures 2.47** and **2.48** in a reference montage to the vertex (electrode CZ). When connected to the vertex, the amplitudes of the spike in electrodes O1 and O2 can be easily compared: The spike has the highest negative amplitude at electrode O2 (blue arrow). Notice also that the spike is a dipole (maximum negativity at O2 and small positivity at C3 and F3). As mentioned in the legend to ▶ **Figure 2.47**, the spike extended significantly more anteriorly on the right side given the wrong impression that the spike was possibly even higher amplitude at O1.

▶ Table 2.2   Potential Localization and Preferred EEG Montages

Localization	Montages
Temporal	Vertex reference, bipolar longitudinal row with inclusion of anterior temporal electrodes (FT9 and FT10)
Central	Ear reference, bipolar transverse, or longitudinal row
Frontal	Ear reference, bipolar transverse, or longitudinal row
Occipital	Vertex reference, bipolar longitudinal or transverse row
Generalized	Ear reference, bipolar transverse row

EEG, electroencephalogram.

For instance, one may decide to use an ipsilateral mastoid reference for a mesial temporal spike if it is indifferent and has no artifact (▶ **Figure 2.50**). The left temporal spike is best displayed in the longitudinal bipolar and ipsilateral mastoid reference montage but hardly identifiable in the vertex reference montage. In this case, CZ contains relatively high-amplitude background activity that obscures the left temporal spike.

The following examples (**Figures 2.51–2.54**) illustrate the advantages and disadvantages of the different montages. ▶ **Figure 2.51** is a bipolar run with longitudinal chains of electrodes. It shows two spikes in the right temporal region (blue and black arrows) that stand out from the background rhythms and from a continuous right temporal slow. By reformatting the same EEG section to a referential run with CZ as reference (▶ **Figure 2.52**), the first spike (blue arrow) is clearly identifiable and can be easily distributed. CZ is an inactive reference and at the time of the first spike shows no artifacts and only a negligible amount of background brain activity. For the second spike (black arrow), the reference CZ is highly "contaminated" with a K-complex, making analysis of the spike almost impossible (▶ **Figure 2.52**). K-complexes and V-waves tend to be of highest amplitude at the vertex and of relatively low amplitude in the temporal leads. Therefore, the difference of potentials of K-complexes when using temporal electrodes with a reference montage to CZ is very large. In other words, analysis of temporal spikes that occur at the time of a K-complex may be very difficult or almost impossible if a referential montage to the vertex is used

(▶ **Figure 2.52**) However, as shown for the first spike (blue arrow), a referential montage to the contralateral mastoid (TP9; ▶ **Figure 2.53**) may be an excellent reference for a temporal lobe spike if it happens to occur in between vertex waves or K-complexes.

▶ **Figure 2.53** shows the same section of the EEG as ▶ **Figures 2.51** and **2.52** but in a referential montage to the contralateral mastoid bone. The display of the first spike (blue arrow) is almost identical to the CZ reference (▶ **Figure 2.52**). This implies that both CZ and TP9 are inactive and excellent references for spike number 1. However, the use of a contralateral left mastoid reference does not really make the analysis of the second temporal spike any easier (▶ **Figure 2.53**). Spike number 2 (black arrow) is still "drowned" in the K-complex, which evidently extends all the way from the vertex down into the temporal region. Finally, when using an ipsilateral mastoid reference (▶ **Figure 2.54**), both spikes (blue and black arrows) are difficult to distribute because the reference is active for both spikes (notice that there is a phase reversal for both spikes) and, in addition, a significant amount of K-complex activity is still recorded and obscures even more the second spike (black arrow).

▶ **Figure 2.55** illustrates the fact that EEG analysis by waveform (EEG pattern) should always be complemented by a careful analysis of the distribution of the potential of interest applying the rules described above. This figure shows a sharp transient followed by a slower wave that clearly stands out from the background activity, and by pattern recognition alone it suggests primarily an epileptiform discharge. Let us now apply the stepwise approach to localization outlined above. We will first analyze the EEG on the left-hand side:

STEP 1:   This is a bipolar montage.

STEP 2:   There are five bipolar chains.

STEP 3:   We will first analyze chain 4, which shows the sharp transient best.

STEP 4:   We will analyze the time of the maximum deflection of the sharp wave.

STEP 5:   There is no phase reversal. Therefore, the potential is maximum or minimum at the end of the chain.

The following arguments can now be used to define the actual localization:

1. The maximum must be at O2 because the highest amplitude differences occur at O2, and in a generator in a volume conductor, the highest

Left temporal spike

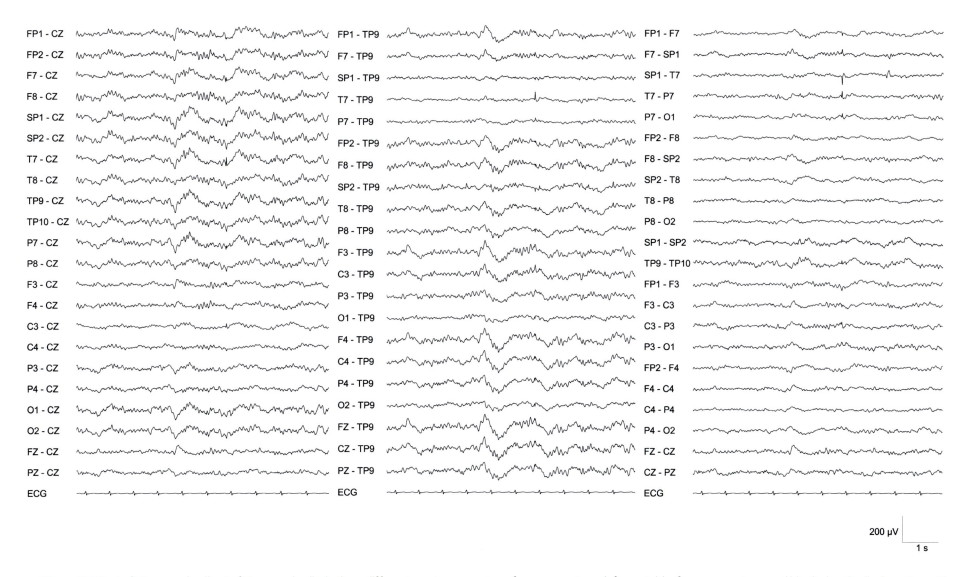

200 µV

1 s

▶ **Figure 2.50** **Left temporal spike.** Left temporal spike in three different montages: vertex reference montage, left mastoid reference montage, and bipolar longitudinal montage. The patient was suffering from left temporal lobe epilepsy. The left temporal spike is best displayed in the longitudinal bipolar and left mastoid reference montage but hardly identifiable in the vertex reference montage. In this case, CZ contains relatively high-amplitude background activity that obscures the left temporal spike.

Right temporal spike in a bipolar longitudinal montage

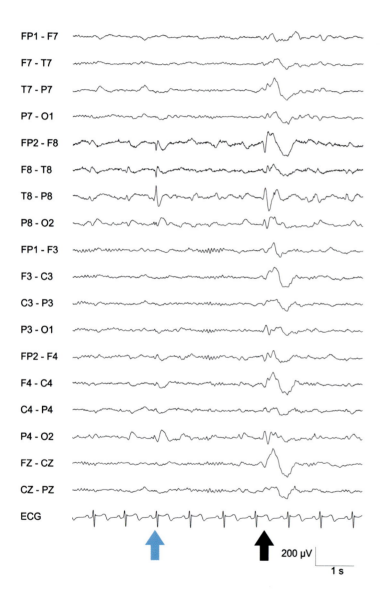

FP1 - F7

F7 - T7

T7 - P7

P7 - O1

FP2 - F8

F8 - T8

T8 - P8

P8 - O2

FP1 - F3

F3 - C3

C3 - P3

P3 - O1

FP2 - F4

F4 - C4

C4 - P4

P4 - O2

FZ - CZ

CZ - PZ

ECG

200 μV

1 s

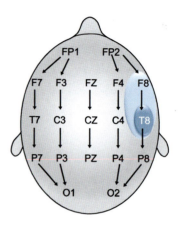

▶ **Figure 2.51** **Right temporal spike in a bipolar longitudinal montage.** There are two epileptiform discharges, one with maximum at electrode T8 (blue arrow) and one isoelectric at electrodes F8 and T8 and coinciding with a K-complex (black arrow).

Right temporal spike in a vertex reference montage

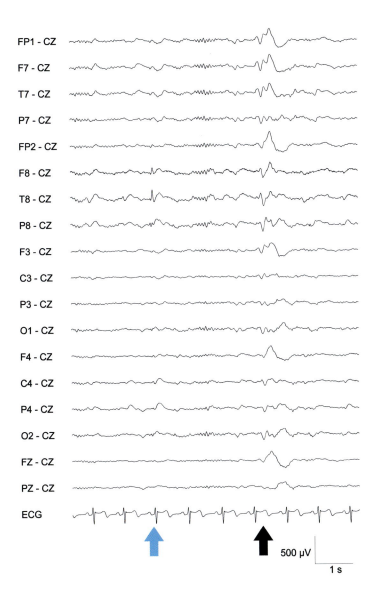

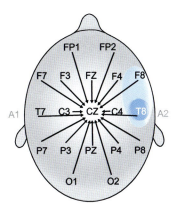

▶ **Figure 2.52** **Right temporal spike in a vertex reference montage.** The same EEG section as in ▶ **Figure 2.51** in a reference montage to the vertex. The first temporal spike (blue arrow) is still easily visible in the CZ reference. The second spike (black arrow) can hardly be identified because the vertex electrode CZ scatters the high-amplitude potential of the K-complex into all channels, obscuring the low-amplitude right temporal spike.

Right temporal spike in a contralateral mastoid reference montage

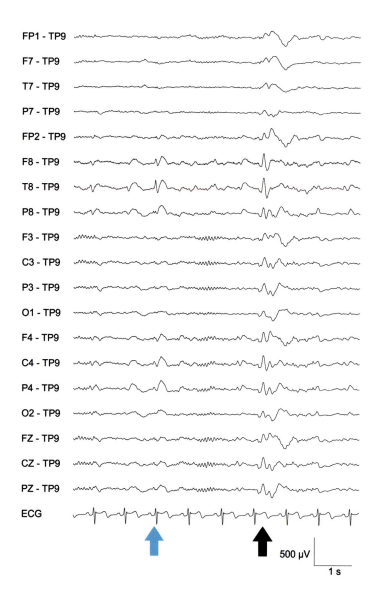

FP1 - TP9
F7 - TP9
T7 - TP9
P7 - TP9
FP2 - TP9
F8 - TP9
T8 - TP9
P8 - TP9
F3 - TP9
C3 - TP9
P3 - TP9
O1 - TP9
F4 - TP9
C4 - TP9
P4 - TP9
O2 - TP9
FZ - TP9
CZ - TP9
PZ - TP9
ECG

500 µV

1 s

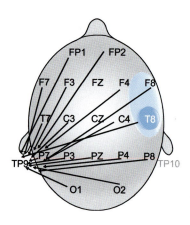

▶ **Figure 2.53** **Right temporal spike in a contralateral mastoid reference montage.** The same EEG section as in ▶ **Figures 2.51** and **2.52** in a reference montage to the contralateral left mastoid (TP9). The first spike (blue arrow) is still visible. The second spike (black arrow) is now more clearly visible than in **Figure 2.52** but still difficult to distinguish from the K-complex.

Right temporal spike in a right mastoid reference montage

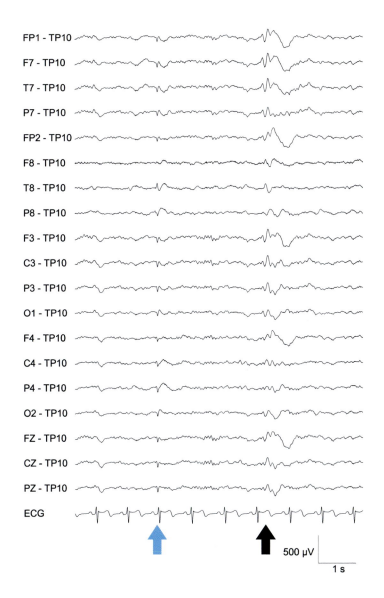

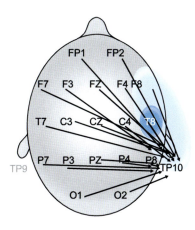

▶ **Figure 2.54** **Right temporal spike in a right mastoid reference montage.** The same EEG section as in ▶ **Figures 2.51–2.53** in a reference montage to the right mastoid (TP10). In the right mastoid reference montage, the first spike (blue arrow) shows a small upward deflection only in electrode T8, whereas all other electrodes show downward deflections due to the contaminated right mastoid reference. The second spike (black arrow) is hardly distinguishable from the K-complex.

Pattern recognition: Spike versus POSTS

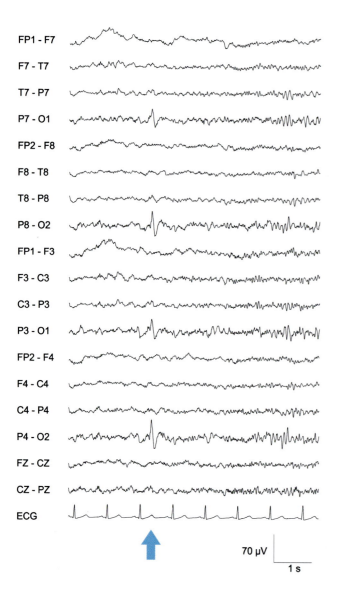

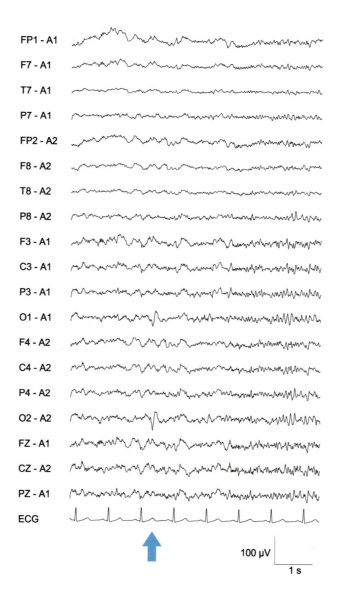

▶ **Figure 2.55 Pattern recognition: Spike versus POSTS.** The peak of the potential (blue arrow) points upwards in the bipolar longitudinal montage (left) and is followed by a slow wave. Only analyzing the waveform of the discharge ("pattern recognition") suggests that the potential represents an epileptiform discharge (spike). However, the transient has a positive polarity, as illustrated in an ear reference montage (right) that shows a downward deflection at O1 and O2. This finding indicates that the transient is a positivity (blue arrow) at electrodes O1 and O2 and, therefore, is a POSTS.

amplitude differences occur at electrodes placed in proximity of the generator. If the potential is maximum at O2, then the transient is positive (and not negative, as we would expect for an epileptiform discharge).

2. On the other hand, if we assume the generator is maximum at FP2, we would also conclude that all the electrodes in the right temporal chain except O2 are maximum and of identical voltage. That is extremely unlikely. Therefore, this argument also supports the hypothesis that the potential seen in chain 4 is extremely localized to O2 and of positive polarity.

3. We know also that there are occipital transients of positive polarity in normal stage N1 sleep: the POSTS (Positive Occipital Sharp Transients of Sleep).

The above analysis shows that the sharp transient, which by waveform looks like an epileptiform discharge, when carefully distributed is most likely a physiological occipital transient, namely POSTS. The referential montage shown in the right side of ▶ **Figure 2.55** confirms the analysis we made of the sharp transient using a bipolar chain.

Figures 2.56–2.58 show the advantages and disadvantages of bipolar and referential derivations in another example. The bipolar montage (▶ **Figure 2.56**) displays an occipital (O1; blue arrow) and temporo-occipital spikes (P7 > O1; gray arrow) and vertex waves (black arrows). The occipital spike (blue arrow) points downward and shows no phase reversal. Thus, the maximum negativity is in electrode O1. The temporo-occipital spike (gray arrow) has a phase reversal at electrode P7 and no phase reversal in the parasagittal row. Thus, the maximum negativity is higher at electrode P7 than O1. The vertex waves (black arrows) have a phase reversal at the vertex and the central electrodes bilaterally. This localization is confirmed by the vertex reference showing upward pointing spikes (blue and gray arrows) at O1 and P7/O1, respectively (▶ **Figure 2.57**). In the ipsilateral ear reference montage (▶ **Figure 2.58**), the vertex waves (black arrows) are well displayed but the occipital (blue arrow) and temporo-occipital spikes wave (gray arrow) are hardly identifiable from the sleep-related diffuse slow. Thus, in an ipsilateral ear reference montage, the occipital and temporo-occipital spikes may be easily missed. The vertex reference and the longitudinal bipolar montage were more appropriate to display the abnormality in this case.

The advantage of a referential montage can be illustrated in the analogy of isopotential lines shown in ▶ **Figure 2.59**. The contour map of isopotential lines gives a good overview from a distant perspective (▶ **Figure 2.59**) if the reference is not "contaminated," which is the case if the view is from the top of the mountain. However, the cyclist in the mountains will appreciate the information of the respective gradient on certain stretches of road as provided by the bipolar derivation (▶ **Figure 2.60**). The experienced electroencephalographer will make sensible use of the advantages and disadvantages of the different montages to present the potentials as optimally as possible.

Choice of Montage

The display of EEG potentials is greatly influenced by the choice of montages (bipolar montages vs. referential montages). In addition, when using referential montages, the choice of the reference electrode influences greatly the display of the EEG potentials. Montages must be chosen carefully to optimally represent the different EEG potentials: With inappropriate montages, EEG patterns can be concealed or misjudged.

In the report of the location (maximum amplitude) of an EEG abnormality, the corresponding brain location (and not the EEG electrode that shows highest amplitude) is mentioned. This facilitates communication with clinicians less familiar with EEG terminology. ▶ **Table 2.3** presents some examples of this rule.

The designation of these terms should use the electrode position with care. Electrodes F7/F8 are anatomically located over the most anterior part of the Sylvian fissure. It would be tempting to localize discharges with an F7/F8 maximum as "frontotemporal." Frontotemporal epilepsies—that is, epilepsies that originate from both the frontal and the temporal lobe ("temporal[+] epilepsy")—are extremely rare. Therefore, the localizing term "sharp waves, left or right frontotemporal" should be avoided except in very special situations. To decide if an epileptiform discharge points to a frontal epilepsy or a temporal epilepsy, we must analyze the complete distribution of the epileptiform potential. If the second highest electrode after F7 is a temporal electrode (FT9 or T7), a temporal generator is most likely (in this case, "sharp waves, left temporal"). On the other hand, if the second highest amplitude is at a frontal electrode (F3 or FP1), the generator is most likely frontal ("sharp waves, left frontal").

Left occipital spikes and vertex wave

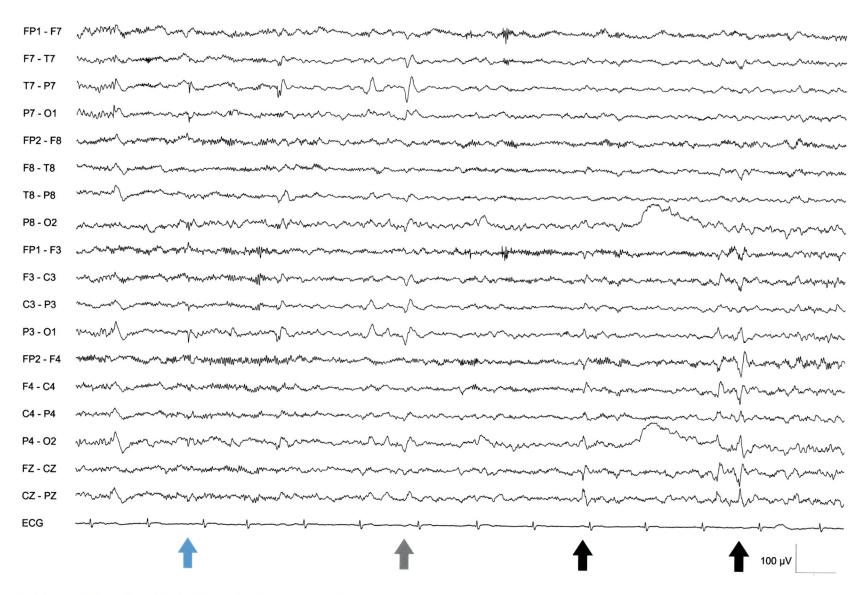

Left occipital spikes and vertex wave. An 18-year-old patient with bilateral occipital lobe epilepsy due to bilateral occipital heterotopias. Bipolar longitudinal montage showing left occipital (O1; blue arrow) and temporo-occipital (P7 > O1; gray arrow) spikes and sharply contoured vertex waves (black arrows). The advantages of the different montages are addressed in the text.

Same EEG section as in Figure 2.56 in a vertex reference montage

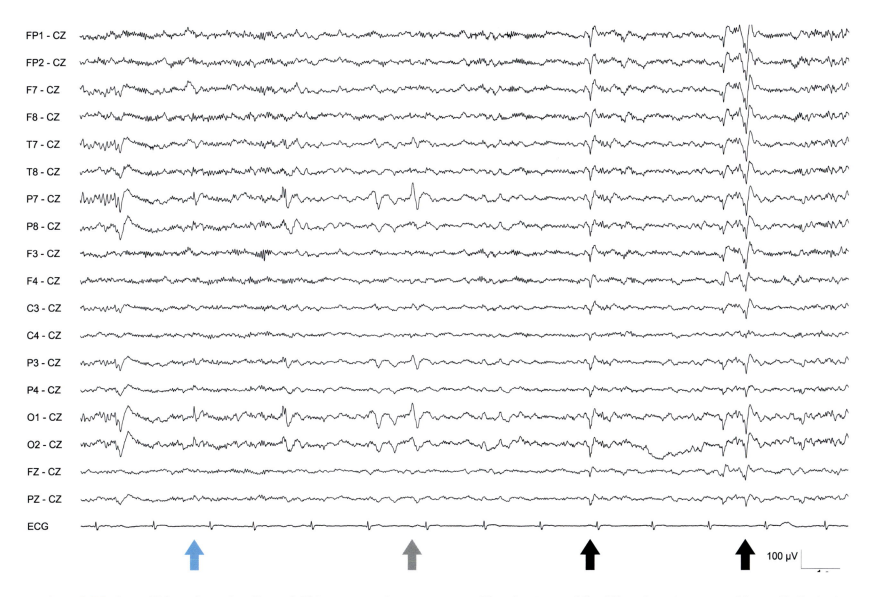

FP1 - CZ

FP2 - CZ

F7 - CZ

F8 - CZ

T7 - CZ

T8 - CZ

P7 - CZ

P8 - CZ

F3 - CZ

F4 - CZ

C3 - CZ

C4 - CZ

P3 - CZ

P4 - CZ

O1 - CZ

O2 - CZ

FZ - CZ

PZ - CZ

ECG

100 µV

▶ **Figure 2.57**   Same EEG section as in ▶ Figure 2.56 in a vertex reference montage. The advantages of the different montages are addressed in the text.

Same EEG section as in Figures 2.56 and 2.57 in an ipsilateral ear reference montage

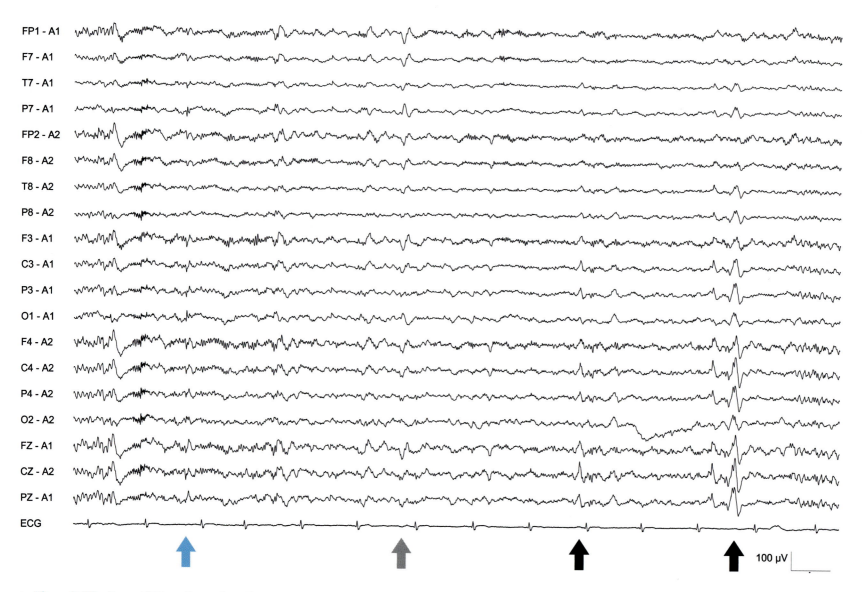

Analogy for reference montages

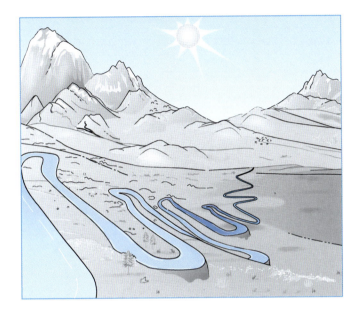

▶ **Figure 2.59** **Analogy for reference montages.** The reference montage gives a good overview as with contour lines on a mountain map but hardly allows an estimation of the gradient in individual curves.

Some essential principles must be considered when determining the localization of a potential of interest. In clinical practice as also in EEG interpretation, we frequently use the expression "generalized," implying that the whole brain is epileptogenic. It is well known that in the strict sense, bilaterally synchronous, generalized EEG discharges do not exist. Interconnecting homologous brain regions should not show any potentials if indeed bilateral bisynchronous discharges exist. We know that so-called bilateral synchronous discharges have a latency difference of approximately 10–20 ms between the two hemispheres. Spikes as an expression of a generalized epilepsy are usually relatively generalized with maximum amplitude bifrontally. Furthermore, patients with genetic, generalized epilepsy may have areas of the brain that are relatively more epileptogenic. That explains the frequent occurrence of lateralizing signs in patients with generalized epilepsy. The typical examples are patients with juvenile myoclonic epilepsy who may show consistent versive

Analogy for bipolar montages

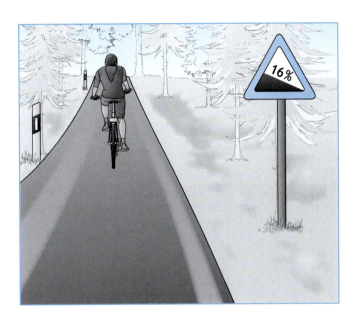

▶ **Figure 2.60** **Analogy for bipolar montages.** The bipolar montage allows a very accurate estimation of the slope of a mountain curve, like a cyclist's mountain map.

seizures at the beginning of the seizure (Usui et al., 2005). Not infrequently, the EEG of these patients may also show differences in amplitude and/or of latency between the two hemispheres. This asymmetry or asynchrony should be documented in the EEG report by specifying the asymmetry or asynchrony

▶ **Table 2.3** **Electrode Localization**

Epileptiform Discharge with Maximum Amplitude At	Report
T7	Sharp waves, left lateral temporal
FT9	Sharp waves, left mesial temporal
P7 = P3	Sharp waves, left temporoparietal

Secondary bilateral synchrony

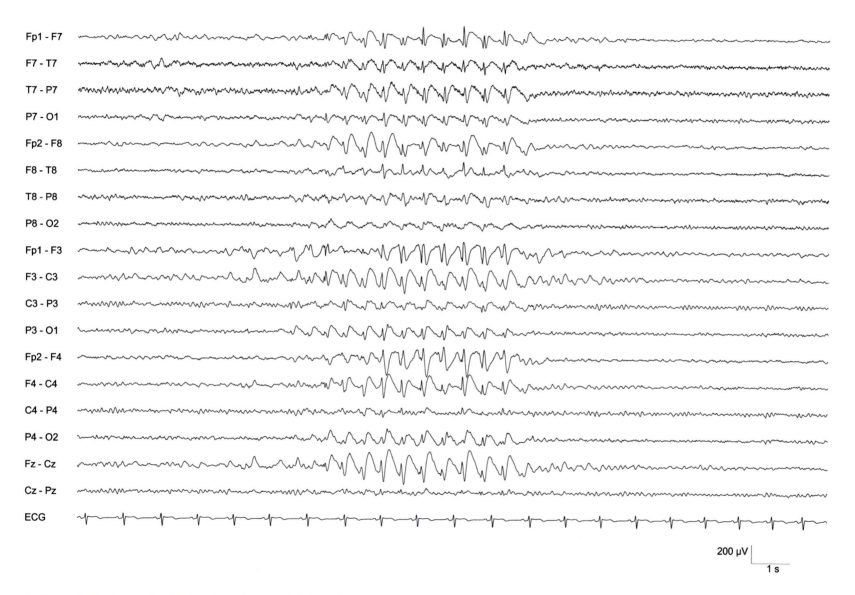

Fp1 - F7

F7 - T7

T7 - P7

P7 - O1

Fp2 - F8

F8 - T8

T8 - P8

P8 - O2

Fp1 - F3

F3 - C3

C3 - P3

P3 - O1

Fp2 - F4

F4 - C4

C4 - P4

P4 - O2

Fz - Cz

Cz - Pz

ECG

200 µV

1 s

▶ **Figure 2.61 Secondary bilateral synchrony.** A left frontal slow and spike in electrode F3 is followed by generalized spike–waves. This phenomenon has been described for patients with parasagittal lesions (Tükel & Jasper, 1952). This patient had a left frontal epilepsy secondary to a glioma in the left medial frontal gyrus.

as follows: Spike–wave, generalized maximum left frontal. By classifying the EEG abnormality as generalized, even if the maximum is in a region of one hemisphere, we still indicate that we think the patient has a generalized epilepsy. On the other hand, a classification as "spikes, left frontal" would imply a focal left frontal epilepsy. A special constellation results from the so-called secondary bilateral synchrony, in which initially regional epileptiform discharges generalize in the further course (▶ **Figure 2.61**). The concept of bilateral secondary synchrony, however, refers to patients with parasagittal lesions, in whom the interictal EEG shows both generalized spikes–waves and generalized discharges that were shortly preceded by regional epileptiform discharges (Tükel & Jasper, 1952).

The localization terms "focal" and "lateralized" do not need to be specified prior to localization. It is sufficient to specify the localization—for example, left temporal or left hemisphere—and the terms focal and lateralized would be redundant. An exception is the term "multifocal," which is used in the classification with reference to the hemisphere. ▶ **Table 2.4** summarizes the localization terms.

Most EEG abnormalities require a localization for their correct designation. However, there are EEG abnormalities that are diffuse and have no localization. In case of invasive EEG recordings, the term focal is used for localization of invasively detected epileptiform discharges in one or two electrodes, whereas "regional" is the term for noninvasive localization (▶ **Tables 2.5** and **2.6**).

▶ **Table 2.4** **Explanation of Localization Terms**

Localization	Term Explanation
Focal	EEG changes that are limited to a lobe or part of a lobe. With scalp electrodes, the highest localization level is regional.
Multifocal	Three or more regional foci (epileptiform discharges) exist. When there are only two distinctive regional foci, we classify both specifying the two regions. When there are spike foci arising from three or more regions, we use the following nomenclature: Spikes, multiregional left (or right) hemisphere *or* spikes, multiregional, bihemispheric.
Lateralized	EEG changes that are limited to one hemisphere but not to one lobe or region of the hemisphere.
Generalized	EEG abnormalities that occur bilaterally and relatively diffusely. They usually have a frontal maximum. When a discharge is generalized, the term "generalized, maximum . . ." can be used to indicate where the maximum of the change is, such as "continuous slow, generalized, maximum frontal." If it occurs regionally, the exact localization should be given—for example, "continuous slow, right frontal." "Generalized maximum . . ." and "Generalized and regional . . ." or "Generalized and lateralized . . ." are not identical. For example, "continuous slow, generalized maximum right frontal" points to a diffuse dysfunction with a relative maximum in the right frontal region. In contrast, "continuous slow, generalized and right frontal" expresses that in addition to a diffuse brain dysfunction, there is also a right frontal lesion (e.g., a tumor). In such a case, the diffuse brain dysfunction could be caused both by the frontal lesion and by another cause (e.g., medication).
Non-lateralized	This is only used for the localization of EEG seizure patterns. This term is used when the onset of the seizure pattern does not allow lateralization but there is no clear EEG or clinical evidence that the seizure was generalized.
Localization artifact obscured	This is only used when classifying an EEG seizure pattern whose onset cannot be adequately localized due to artifacts by excessive motion, EMG artifacts, or other artifacts.

EEG, electroencephalogram.
Sources: Lüders and Noachtar (2000a).

▶ **Table 2.5** **Pathological EEG Changes for Which a Localization Must Always Be Specified**

EEG Classification	Figure Examples
Intermittent slow (IS)	3.71, 3.72, 3.75
Continuous slow (CS)	3.101–3.104
Asymmetry (ASY)	3.274–3.282
Spikes (SP)	3.118–3.123
Polyspikes (PSP)	3.132, 3.133, 3.138–3.140
Benign focal epileptiform discharges (BFED)	2.27, 3.141–3.144
Spike–waves (SW)	3.145–3.148, 3.150, 3.151, 3.153
Polyspike–waves (PSPW)	3.127
3 Hz spike–waves (3SW)	3.149, 3.152
Slow spike–waves (SSW)	3.154–3.156
Hypsarrhythmia (HYP)	3.157–3.159
Photoparoxysmal response (PR)	3.12–3.14, 3.160, 3.161, 3.166
Seizure pattern (SEP)	3.167–3.197
Status pattern (STP)	3.198–3.231
Periodic discharges (PD)	3.246–3.252
Periodic epileptiform discharges (PED)	3.253, 3.255–3.259
Burst attenuation (BUA)	3.271, 3.272
Burst suppression (BUS)	3.267–3.270
Background attenuation (BA)	3.111, 3.112
Background suppression (BSU)	3.113, 3.114
Electrocerebral silence (ECS)	3.115

EEG, electroencephalogram.

▶ **Table 2.6** **Abnormal EEG Changes That Are Nonlocalized/Generalized**

EEG Classification	Figure Examples
Background slow (BS)	3.64, 3.68, 3.69
Excessive beta (EB)	3.273
Sleep-onset REM (SOREM)	3.283
Alpha coma (AC)	3.284, 3.287–3.289
Spindle coma (SC)	3.290, 3.291
Beta coma (BC)	3.292
Theta coma (TC)	3.293
Delta coma (DC)	3.294, 3.295

EEG, electroencephalogram.

2.2.3.4 Localization of Asymmetries

Asymmetry is the only EEG abnormality that requires specification of three parameters. It is important to realize that the three parameters refer always to an activity that can be visualized in the more normal hemisphere but is asymmetrically distributed. The following three parameters should be specified:

- Is the amplitude of the activity increased or decreased?
- What activity is increased or decreased?
- Where is the activity increased or decreased?

Examples

Asymmetry, increased beta right frontal (see **Figure 3.46**)

Asymmetry, decreased background left hemisphere (see **Figure 3.109**)

Frequently when reading an EEG, we can only determine that an activity is of higher or lower amplitude on one hemisphere or region. We need to consider the clinical history to decide what hemisphere is the more normal one, and then we can decide if the activity is increased or decreased on the more abnormal hemisphere.

2.3 Artifacts

All potentials recorded in the EEG that do not originate from the brain are considered disturbances and are called artifacts (▶ **Table 2.7**). It is not surprising that EEGs recorded from the scalp are very susceptible to artifacts because of the relatively low amplitude of brain waves. ECG potentials, for example, are measured in millivolts and are almost 1,000 times higher amplitude than brain potentials, which are usually measured in microvolts. Although the principle of the differential amplifier has considerably reduced the EEG's susceptibility to artifacts (see Section 2.2.1.3), there are still typical artifacts that need to be identified and—as far as possible—eliminated. Some artifacts can be used for diagnostic purposes, such as nystagmus, myoclonia, or cardiac arrhythmia. Artifacts can be divided into two groups according to their origin: biological and nonbiological (▶ **Table 2.7**).

▶ **Table 2.7   Typical Artifacts in the EEG**

Artifacts	Figure Examples
Nonbiological Artifacts	
60 Hz mains interference	2.73
Electrostatic	2.76
Electrodes short-circuit	2.67
Electrode pop	2.63–2.66
Pulse (ballistic artifact)	2.68–2.70
Tremor	2.71
Ventilation machine	2.75
Infusion pump	2.74
Aliasing	2.11
Open channel (open grid)	2.72
Electrode wobbling	2.77–2.78
Biological Artifacts	
Eye movements	2.79–2.88
Blinking	2.89
ECG	2.26, 2.69, 2.112–2.116
Eye muscles	2.109–2.111
EMG	2.96–2.104
Swallowing, chewing, lip smacking	2.99, 2.101–2.102
Tongue movement (glossokinetic artifact)	2.107–2.108
Nystagmus	2.94–2.95
Photomyoclonic response	3.10–3.11

ECG, electrocardiogram; EEG, electroencephalogram; EMG, electromyogram.

Recognition of artifacts and their differentiation from brain activity is essential for accurate analysis of EEG tracings. Many artifacts have a relatively unique field distribution and/or polarity. Having a detailed understanding of the field of distribution, the polarity, and also the shape of the different artifacts that may be seen in EEG tracings is of great help for an accurate interpretation of the EEGs.

As previously mentioned, artifacts can be classified as biological and nonbiological artifacts. Exact knowledge of the polarity, distribution, and waveform of different eye movements permits confident differentiation of eye movements from frontal dominant brain waves or other frontally located artifacts (▶ **Figure 2.25**). Slow eye movements are easily misjudged as so-called sweat artifacts (▶ **Figure 2.25** and **2.66**). Detailed examples of eye movements in different directions are presented in Section 2.3.2.1 (see **Figures 2.81–2.88**).

Precise analysis of the potential field distribution of EEG potentials provides important clues as to whether it is a biological or nonbiological artifact or a potential generated by the brain. For example, an artifact produced by shaking of EEG wires (wobble artifact) will not reveal a logical distribution (nonbiological artifact) (▶ **Figure 2.62**).

Many artifacts are produced by movement of electrodes or movement of the wires carrying the EEG potential from its input to the amplifier. The movement of an electrode produces an abrupt change in the resistance between the electrode and the scalp and/or a change in the stray capacitance between the EEG input wires.

The different names for these artifacts reflect the phenomenon that produced the movement of the electrode (pulse, shaking, etc.). Nonbiological (technical) artifacts are frequently caused by relatively high-intensity voltage fields that cannot be eliminated by the CMRR of the differential amplifiers. Relatively high-intensity voltage fields stem frequently from 60 Hz (or 50 Hz in Europe) AC current, electrostatic artifacts, or infusion pumps in intensive care units. Random movements of the wires, because the patient moves or an observer is moving the wires, also cause artifacts. These movements lead to sudden changes of the electrode resistance and, therefore, an abrupt change in the voltage recorded in a channel. After the abrupt change in potential at the electrode of interest, the recording returns to the baseline. The time it takes for the recording to return to the baseline depends on the settings of the time constant (low-frequency filter). The movement can be the result of pulse artifact (artery pulsation moves the electrode), tremor artifact (tremor moves the electrode[s]), electrode pop (random movement of one electrode that may be loose), and electrode shaking. The extreme case of a loose electrode is called open grid (**Figure 2.72**).

Power supply interference of 60 Hz (United States) or 50 Hz (Europe) can occur ubiquitously, but it is usually not a major problem, except in situations such as recoding an EEG in the intensive care unit, where it can hardly be avoided because ventilators, infusion pumps, and so on cannot be switched off easily. Often, 60 (50) Hz current interference is caused by poor electrode contact or high electrical resistance to the scalp (see Section 2.2.1.1; see also **Figure 2.73**). This can be prevented by using contact resistances of less than 10 kΩ and of similar value in each electrode. The grounding of the patient must also be checked in such cases. Earth loops must be avoided. An essential rule is that only one earth electrode may be connected to the patient (typically FPZ).

2.3.1 Nonbiological Artifacts

2.3.1.1 Electrode Artifacts ("Electrode Pop")

An electrode "pop" usually affects only one electrode. In the recording, it will appear at all the channels we are recording from the affected electrode (▶ **Figure 2.63**). The polarity can be negative or positive, and the shape is very similar to the calibration potential generated by an abrupt injection of a given potential (triangular shape) (▶ **Figures 2.63** and **2.64**). Depending on the cause, the artifact can occur in a stereotypical manner, but it can also change its shape (▶ **Figures 2.65** and **2.66**). In clear contrast to brain-generated potential fields, neighboring electrodes frequently are not affected even when this artifact is of relatively very large amplitude. Electrode pops have different causes, but ultimately, they all lead to more or less rapid current changes of potentials at an electrode. The reasons often lie in poor fixation of the electrode, high resistance at the electrode, cable breakage, or wobbling at the electrode or electrode cable. Sometimes, small bubbles in the electrolyte gel can also lead to electrode pops. ▶ **Figure 2.64** shows a so-called electrode pop at electrode FT9 and a wobble artifact at electrode FT10. Electrode pops may also occur when sintered electrodes that have developed small fractures between the silver and silver chloride layers due to accidental falling are used (see Section 2.2.1.1). It is often necessary to replace the electrode or electrode cable to eliminate an electrode pop artifact.

If too much electrolyte gel is used, an electrolyte bridge (short circuit) between two adjacent electrodes may be established (▶ **Figure 2.67**). The channel that records between the two shorted inputs will be silent (no voltage difference recorded because of the bridge).

Wobble artifact

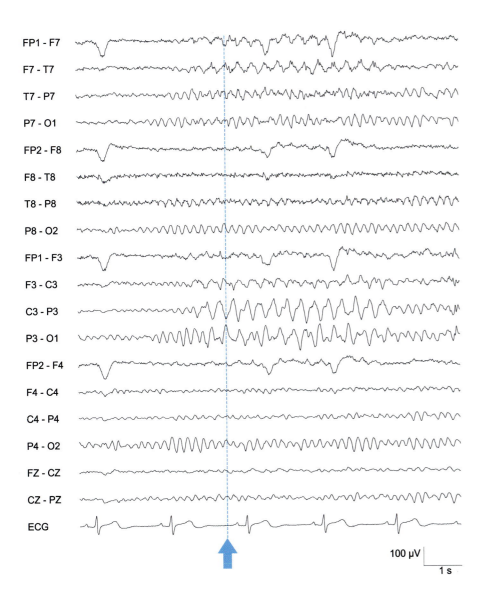

FP1 - F7
F7 - T7
T7 - P7
P7 - O1
FP2 - F8
F8 - T8
T8 - P8
P8 - O2
FP1 - F3
F3 - C3
C3 - P3
P3 - O1
FP2 - F4
F4 - C4
C4 - P4
P4 - O2
FZ - CZ
CZ - PZ
ECG

100 µV

1 s

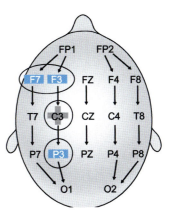

▶ **Figure 2.62** **Wobble artifact.** The wobble artifact can be easily identified by analyzing the potential field distribution at a given point in time (blue arrow). Potentials generated by wobbly artifacts do not follow biological potential field distributions and show unphysiological dipoles as in this case (F7, F3, and P3 negative; C3 positive).

Electrode artifacts

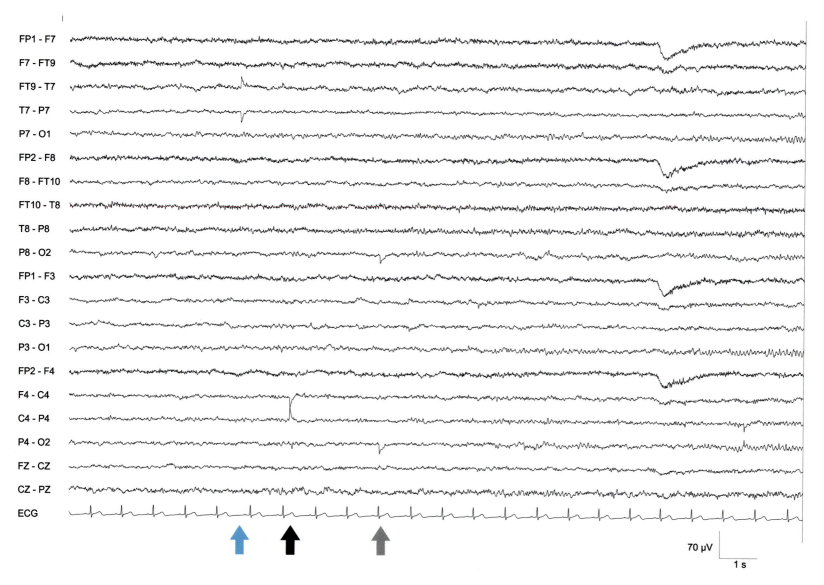

▶ **Figure 2.63** **Electrode artifacts.** In this bipolar longitudinal montage, electrode artifacts occur at electrodes T7 (blue arrow), C4 (black arrow), and O2 (gray arrow). A fast upward deflection is followed by a slower return to baseline. The artifact is of positive polarity at electrode T7 and of negative polarity at electrodes C4 and O2. This electrode artifact is produced by a sudden shift of DC potential, followed by a drop of potential as a function of the time constant. These artifacts are also called "pop" artifacts.

Electrode artifacts

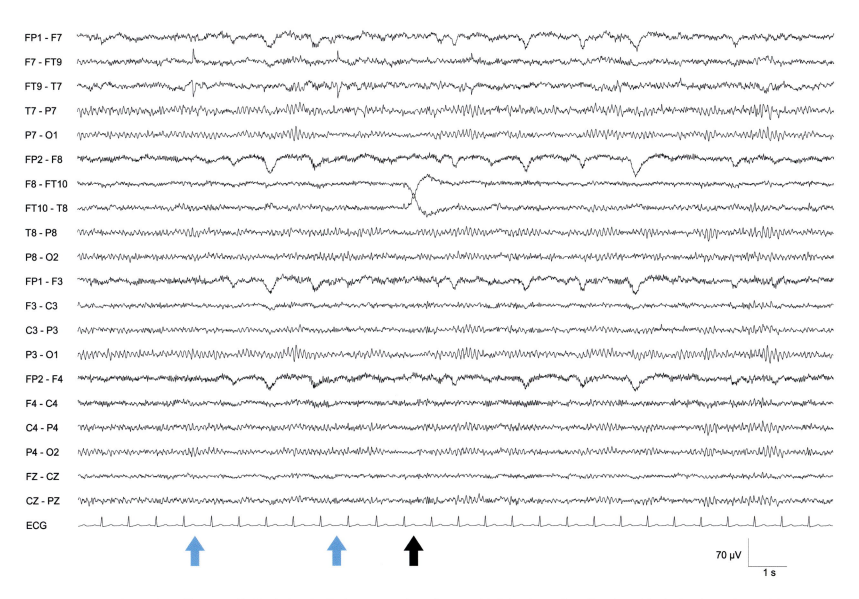

FP1 - F7
F7 - FT9
FT9 - T7
T7 - P7
P7 - O1
FP2 - F8
F8 - FT10
FT10 - T8
T8 - P8
P8 - O2
FP1 - F3
F3 - C3
C3 - P3
P3 - O1
FP2 - F4
F4 - C4
C4 - P4
P4 - O2
FZ - CZ
CZ - PZ
ECG

70 µV
1 s

▶ **Figure 2.64**　**Electrode artifacts.** In this bipolar longitudinal montage, the main potential of the electrode artifact is positive in the electrode FT9 (blue arrows) and negative in the electrode FT10 (black arrow).

Electrode artifact

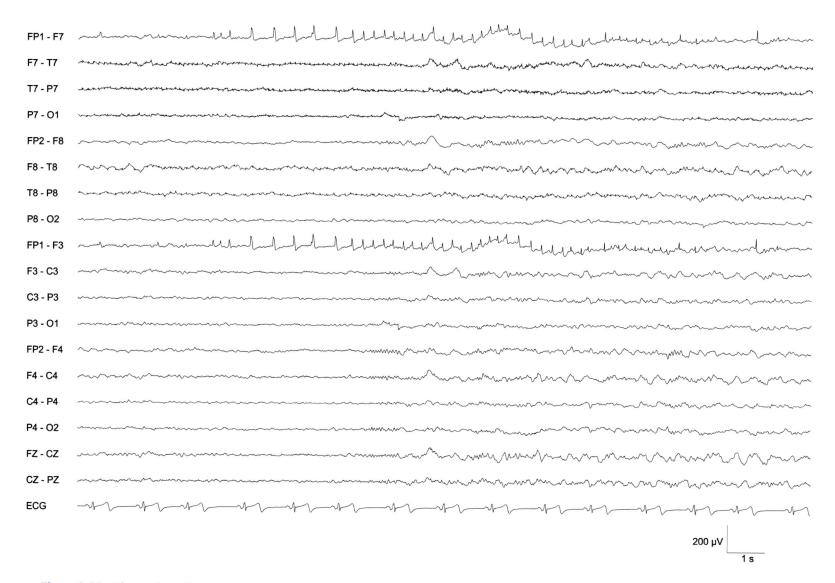

FP1 - F7

F7 - T7

T7 - P7

P7 - O1

FP2 - F8

F8 - T8

T8 - P8

P8 - O2

FP1 - F3

F3 - C3

C3 - P3

P3 - O1

FP2 - F4

F4 - C4

C4 - P4

P4 - O2

FZ - CZ

CZ - PZ

ECG

200 µV

1 s

▶ **Figure 2.65** **Electrode artifact.** Bipolar longitudinal montage. A stereotypical electrode artifact occurs at the FP1 electrode likely related to movements of the electrode FP1 with sudden changes of conductivity. The main component of the artifact is negative and returns repetitively at different intervals. A very slow wave is added after a few seconds.

Electrode artifact

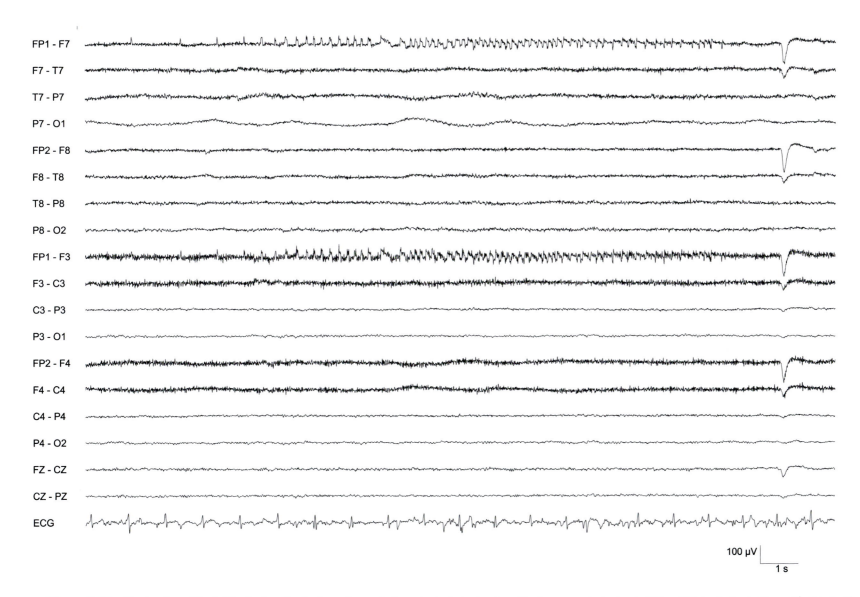

100 µV

1 s

▶ **Figure 2.66** **Electrode artifact.** Bipolar longitudinal montage. A stereotypical electrode artifact occurs at electrode FP1, which is similar to the artifact in ▶ **Figure 2.65** and is likely related to movements of the electrode with sudden changes of conductivity. The main component of the FP1 artifact is negative, and it recurs repetitively at different intervals. The small negative peaks at the beginning are not followed by slow waves, as would be the case with interictal epileptiform discharges. In addition, an EEG seizure pattern would not be limited to one electrode. Notice also the slow waves limited to P7 and F4, which most likely reflect sweating artifacts. A blink artifact occurs at the end of the EEG sample.

Short-circuit electrode artifact

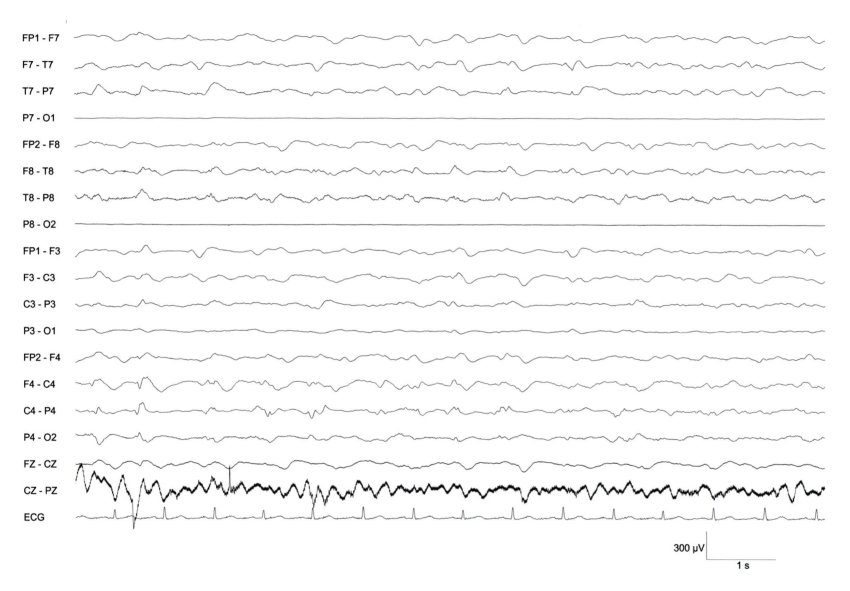

300 µV

1 s

▶ **Figure 2.67** **Short-circuit electrode artifact.** Bipolar longitudinal montage. The channels P8–O2 and P7–O1 are flat. This is most likely produced by an electrolyte bridge between electrodes P8 and O2 and also between electrodes P7 and O1. The patient most likely lies on their back, and a mixture of sweat and electrolyte paste produces the short circuit. This is a comatose patient with an EEG that reveals a periodic epileptiform discharge maximum at C4–P4 and a diffuse continuous slow. In addition, there is a 50 Hz main artifact (European power system), and there are pop artifacts at PZ.

2.3.1.2   Ballistic Artifacts

Movements at the electrode wires lead to so-called ballistic artifacts. Such movements occur due to various causes, such as tremor or pulse movements. The pulse artifact can be recognized because it synchronizes with the pulse and occurs approximately 300 ms after the QRS complex (▶ **Figures 2.68** and **2.69**). Arrhythmias can impair the regular recurrence of the pulse artifact, complicating its recognition. Pulse artifacts occur most frequently at temporal electrodes (F7/8, T7/8, and P7/8). In patients with background rhythm suppression or electrocerebral inactivity, blood flow through the internal carotid artery is frequently impaired, leading to an increased blood flow via the external carotid artery. This, together with the greater amplification we tend to use to analyze these recordings, explains why we frequently have pulse artifacts in these recordings (▶ **Figure 2.70**). Tremor leads to rhythmic shaking of electrodes and electrode wires, which is characteristically reflected in the EEG, for example, in Parkinson's disease (▶ **Figure 2.71**).

2.3.1.3   Open Channel

If an electrode connected to an amplifier input loses contact with the scalp—for example, because it falls off—the differential amplifier uses the ground electrode as the reference electrode instead. In such a case, the earth electrode records the potential differences against the reference electrode. In our lab, the earth electrode is placed at FPZ and, therefore, the channel with the loose electrode will record prominent eye blinks and eye movements (▶ **Figure 2.72**). This makes it easy to detect loose electrodes and is one of the reasons the earth electrode is placed at FPZ.

2.3.1.4   External Artifacts

A frequent artifact is the 50 Hz (Europe) or 60 Hz (United States) mains interference, which is most prominent if some electrodes have a poor impedance. Frequently, this artifact cannot be avoided because vital equipment cannot be switched off in the intensive care unit (▶ **Figure 2.73**). A notch filter can be applied in this setting to reduce 50/60 Hz artifact, and usually its use does not change significantly the EEG trace. EEGs in intensive care units are often disturbed by external artifacts such as infusion pumps (▶ **Figure 2.74**), ventilators (▶ **Figure 2.75**), or other electrical devices. Electrostatic artifacts show very short disturbances, which are like a line in the EEG (▶ **Figure 2.76**). Movements at the electrodes or cables lead to characteristic disturbances. Wobbling of the electrodes by tremor or other movements of the patient leads to artifacts whose electric field is erratic and certainly not consistent with a biological artifact or brain waves (▶ **Figures 2.77** and **2.78**).

2.3.2 Biological Artifacts

Biological artifacts are EEG interferences produces by biological generators located in the patient. Eye movements, ECG, EMG, and tongue movements (glossokinetic) are biological artifacts.

2.3.2.1   Bulb Movements

The eye forms a dipole with the retina negatively and the cornea positively charged (▶ **Figure 2.79**). The movements of the bulb lead to characteristic deflections in the EEG that correspond to changes in the location of the dipole of the eyes with respect to the scalp electrodes (▶ **Figure 2.80**). When using standard EEG montages, eye movements can be easily identified, making additional "eye leads" unnecessary. The eye bulb movement artifact shows characteristic deflections depending on the type of eye movement and the montage we use to record the eye movement. ▶ **Figures 2.81–2.88** summarize the different eye movements in 45° steps in all directions for four major EEG montages. Frequent blinking leads to artifacts that sometimes are difficult to differentiate from front-polar slow waves (▶ **Figure 2.89**).

Frequent eye blinking is seen in many seizures. It has been described mainly with occipital seizures, but its actual localizing or lateralizing value has not been elucidated. During a blink, the eyeball usually is moving very little. The artifact is due to the eyelid movement that when lowered decreases the impedance between the positivity of the cornea and the FP1 and FP2 electrodes. In addition, an upward eye movement produces a change in DC potential at FP1, FP2. Therefore, there is an abrupt downward deflection at FP1–F3 and

Pulse artifact

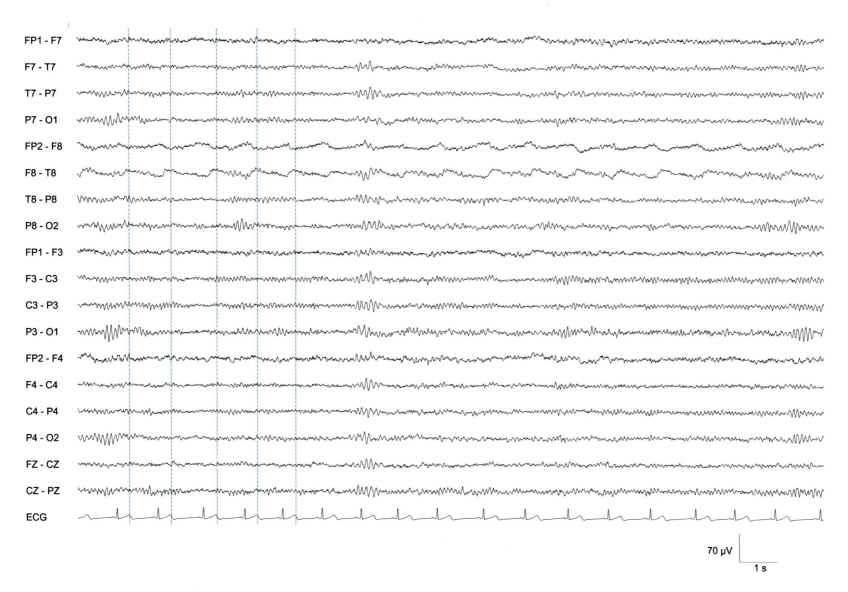

FP1 - F7

F7 - T7

T7 - P7

P7 - O1

FP2 - F8

F8 - T8

T8 - P8

P8 - O2

FP1 - F3

F3 - C3

C3 - P3

P3 - O1

FP2 - F4

F4 - C4

C4 - P4

P4 - O2

FZ - CZ

CZ - PZ

ECG

70 μV

1 s

▶ **Figure 2.68** **Pulse artifact.** Bipolar longitudinal montage. A ballistic pulse artifact at electrode F8 occurs with the same frequency as the ECG and a time delay that the pulse wave takes to reach the head. This time delay is typically one-third of the RR interval (200–300 ms) and corresponds approximately to the T-wave (markers). This example also shows a respiratory arrhythmia.

ECG and pulse artifact

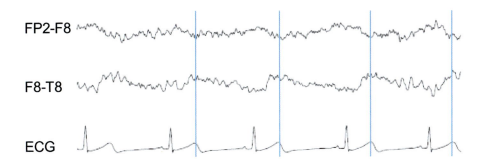

FP2-F8

F8-T8

ECG

▶ **Figure 2.69** **ECG and pulse artifact.** Enlargement of the pulse artifact at electrode F8 from ▶ **Figure 2.68**. After a fast negative deflection during the systole, the potential returns to baseline during the diastole. The vertical blue lines mark the transition from systole to diastole. The pulse artifact usually coincides with the T-wave.

FP2–F4, followed by a slow return to baseline according to the time constant (low-frequency filter) settings of the recording amplifier. The result is that the eye movement artifact will just return to baseline. There is no overshoot. On the other hand, during a blink, the lowering of the eyelid injects a positivity in FP1, FP2. Within 100 ms, however, the eyelid returns to the original position. This produces the characteristic overshoot of eyeblink (see typical waveform of a blink at approximately second 1 of ▶ **Figure 2.89**) (Iwasaki et al., 2005). On the other hand, forced eye closure is associated with an upward eye movement, the so-called Bell's phenomenon.

The rhythmic waves elicited by very fast eye flutter have been called kappa rhythm (▶ **Figures** 2.90 and 2.91). The differential diagnosis between eye movements and continuous frontal slow may be further complicated when there is additional pulse artifact (▶ **Figure 2.92**).

Slow, rhythmic, predominantly horizontal eye movements are an early indication of drowsiness, often before the occipital alpha activity abates (▶ **Figure 2.25**). The slow potential fluctuations observed during rowing, horizontal eye movements of drowsiness should be differentiated from sweat artifacts. However, the typical distribution of the horizontal, rowing eye movements (as opposed to the nonbiological distribution of sweat artifacts) allows reliable differentiation (▶ **Figure 2.80–2.88**).

Detailed knowledge of the artifact produced by eye movements in different directions is essential for differentiation of frontal slows from eye movement artifacts. In the bipolar longitudinal row, eye movements in any direction will almost always be of significantly higher amplitude in channels FP1–F3 and FP2–F4 compared to deflections in channels F3–C3 and F4–C4 (▶ **Figures** 2.81–2.91). This observation can be very helpful to distinguish frontal slow waves from eye movements.

In addition, it is important to remember that eye pathology may lead to total absence of the corneo-retinal potential and a unilateral or bilateral absence of eye movement or blink artifacts. This occurs in patients with unilaterally or bilateral blindness (▶ **Figure 2.93**) or retinopathies (Toljan et al., 2021).

A gaze evoked nystagmus in the EEG can be prevented by positioning the bulb in the resting position (▶ **Figure 2.94**), but a spontaneous nystagmus cannot be prevented. The downbeat nystagmus in ▶ **Figure 2.95** is blocked by fixation at eye opening and reappears after eye closure.

2.3.2.2 Muscle Artifacts

Muscle activity is often derived from the facial, head, and neck muscles in tense patients. Electrodes located in the forehead (FP1–2) and temporal region (F7-8 and T7-8) (▶ **Figure 2.96**) are particularly susceptible to record muscle potentials. EMG can be derived as the sum action potential of a motor unit (▶ **Figures 2.97** and **2.98**) or as a more or less dense pattern of different motor units such as seen during swallowing, typically associated with extensive scattering of EMG artifact into many electrodes (▶ **Figure 2.99**). Short phasic muscle activity may also occur during sleep and typically in the forehead region (▶ **Figure 2.100**). Three typical EMG artifacts are shown in ▶ **Figure 2.101**, namely swallowing (blue arrow), a short phasic muscle artifact in the forehead (gray arrow), and a tonic muscle artifact predominantly in the right forehead region (black arrow). Repetitive lip smacking is typical for seizures characterized by oral automatisms (oro-alimentary seizures) (E. Gibbs et al., 1948; Henkel et al., 2002; Lüders et al., 1998; Lüders & Noachtar, 2000a) and leads to characteristic artifacts in the EEG (▶ **Figure 2.102**). Tonic seizures lead to extensive EMG interferences (▶ **Figure 2.103**), which can occasionally completely mask the EEG. Nevertheless, as in this example, an EEG seizure pattern can often be detected shortly before the EMG artifact onset. Notice in the case

Pulse artifact

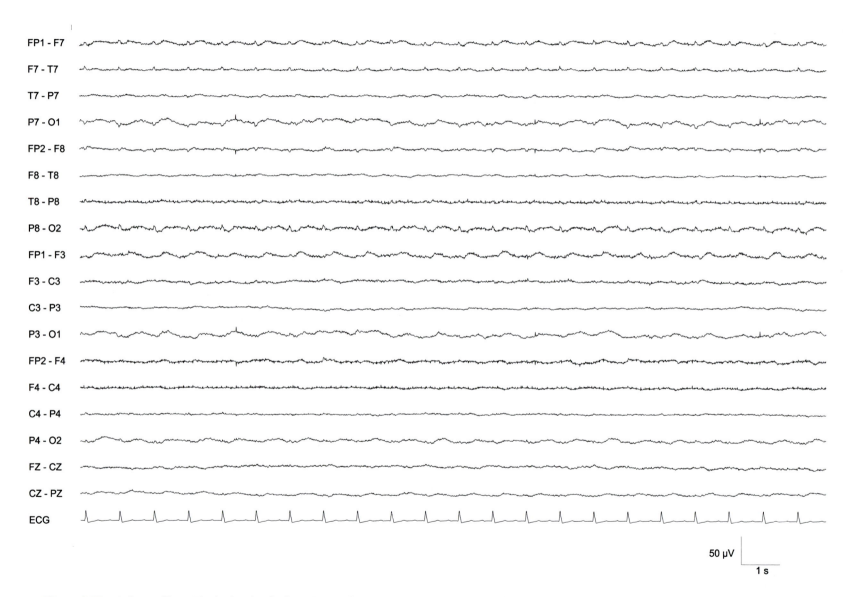

FP1 - F7

F7 - T7

T7 - P7

P7 - O1

FP2 - F8

F8 - T8

T8 - P8

P8 - O2

FP1 - F3

F3 - C3

C3 - P3

P3 - O1

FP2 - F4

F4 - C4

C4 - P4

P4 - O2

FZ - CZ

CZ - PZ

ECG

50 µV

1 s

▶ **Figure 2.70** **Pulse artifact.** Bipolar longitudinal montage. After severe brain damage, only low-amplitude brain activity can be recorded. The blood flow in the internal carotid artery is reduced and, thus, more blood flows into the external carotid artery, resulting in a pulse artifact that can be recorded on several electrodes on the head.

Tremor artifact

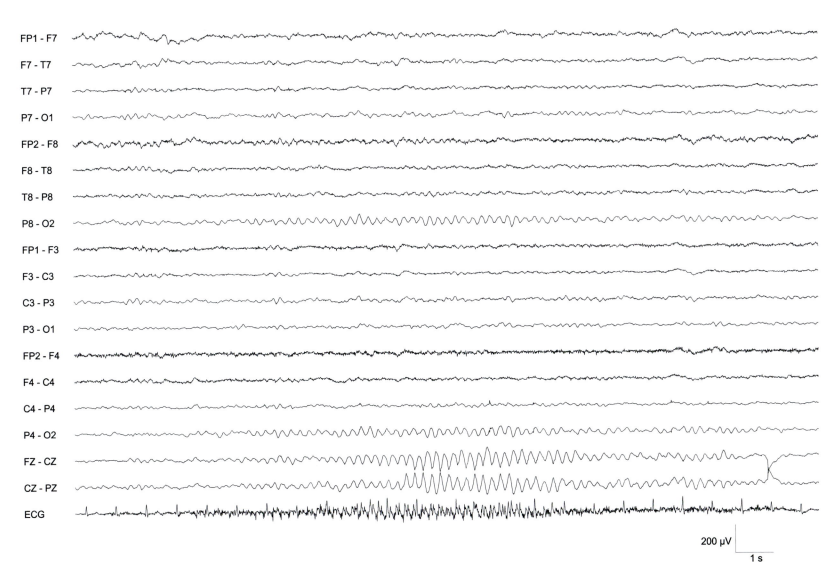

FP1 - F7

F7 - T7

T7 - P7

P7 - O1

FP2 - F8

F8 - T8

T8 - P8

P8 - O2

FP1 - F3

F3 - C3

C3 - P3

P3 - O1

FP2 - F4

F4 - C4

C4 - P4

P4 - O2

FZ - CZ

CZ - PZ

ECG

200 µV

1 s

▶ **Figure 2.71** **Tremor artifact.** Bipolar longitudinal montage. This typical artifact is caused by wobbling of several electrodes due to head tremor. The distribution of the wobble artifact is not logical (FZ = O2 > O1).

Loose electrode artifact

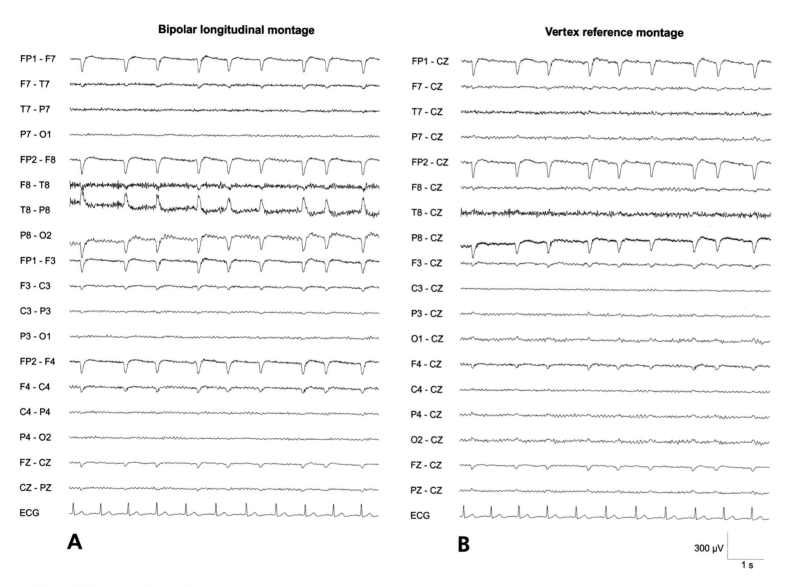

Bipolar longitudinal montage

FP1 - F7
F7 - T7
T7 - P7
P7 - O1
FP2 - F8
F8 - T8
T8 - P8
P8 - O2
FP1 - F3
F3 - C3
C3 - P3
P3 - O1
FP2 - F4
F4 - C4
C4 - P4
P4 - O2
FZ - CZ
CZ - PZ
ECG

A

Vertex reference montage

FP1 - CZ
F7 - CZ
T7 - CZ
P7 - CZ
FP2 - CZ
F8 - CZ
T8 - CZ
P8 - CZ
F3 - CZ
C3 - CZ
P3 - CZ
O1 - CZ
F4 - CZ
C4 - CZ
P4 - CZ
O2 - CZ
FZ - CZ
PZ - CZ
ECG

B

300 µV

1 s

▶ **Figure 2.72** **Loose electrode artifact.** Bipolar longitudinal montage (A) and vertex reference montage (B). The tracing shows a high-amplitude blink artifact at electrode P8. Blink artifacts always are of exponentially lower amplitude in relatively more posteriorly lying electrodes. In this case, electrode P8 has no contact with the scalp (e.g., it has fallen off), and the differential amplifier instead records from the ground electrode, which lies in the middle of the forehead (FPZ). This phenomenon is also called "open grid".

A 60 Hz artifact

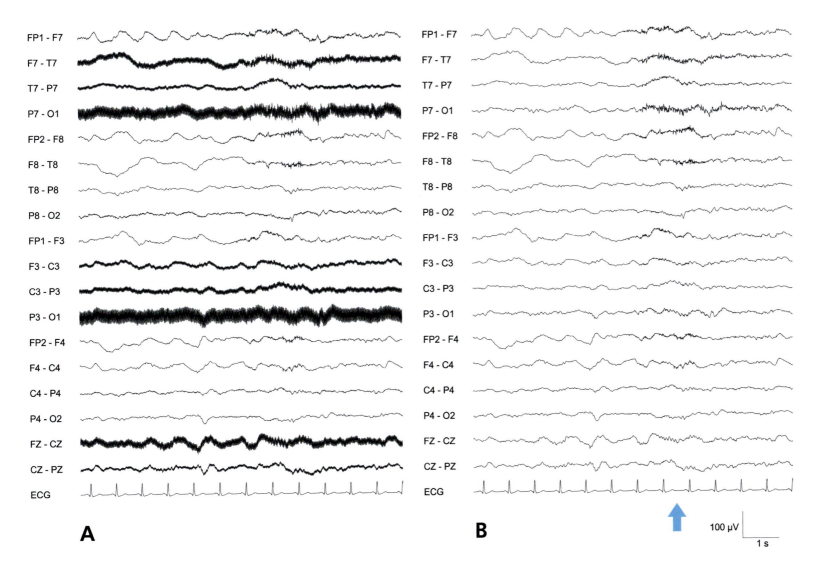

A   B

100 μV
1 s

▶ **Figure 2.73** **A 60 Hz artifact.** Bipolar longitudinal montage. The EEG shows a prominent 60 Hz artifact at electrodes O1, FZ, P7, and T7. By using a 60 Hz notch filter, the 60 Hz artifact (A) is almost completely eliminated. After filtering out the 60 Hz artifact (B), an EMG artifact (blue arrow) can now be distinguished.

Artifact caused by an infusion pump

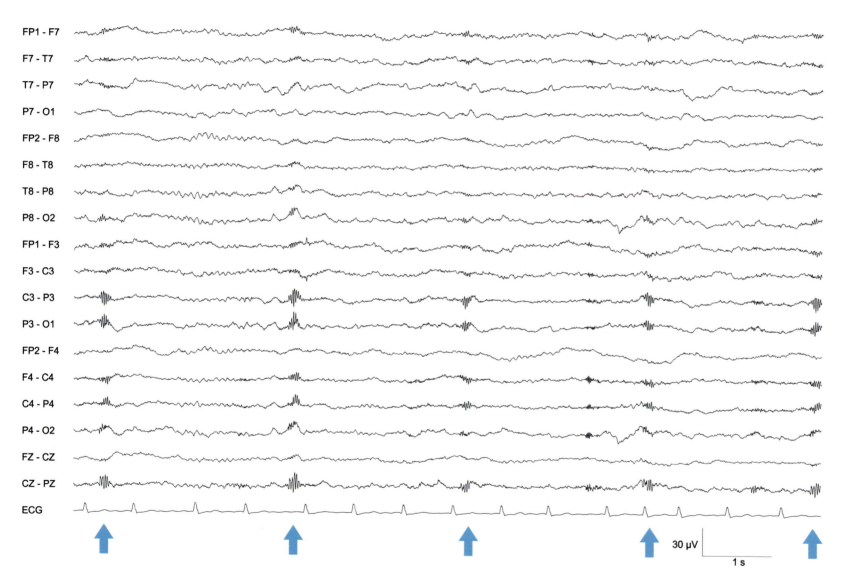

FP1 - F7
F7 - T7
T7 - P7
P7 - O1
FP2 - F8
F8 - T8
T8 - P8
P8 - O2
FP1 - F3
F3 - C3
C3 - P3
P3 - O1
FP2 - F4
F4 - C4
C4 - P4
P4 - O2
FZ - CZ
CZ - PZ
ECG

30 μV

1 s

▶ **Figure 2.74** **Artifact caused by an infusion pump.** Bipolar longitudinal montage. At relatively regular intervals (blue arrows), a short, high-frequency artifact occurs. Notice that the artifact occurs periodically but that the periods are not identical. In this patient, an infusion pump had been placed at the head end of the bed near some electrode cables. The infusion pump caused this artifact. It is also important to note that the artifact is only seen at selected electrodes, most likely those whose connecting cables were close to the infusion pump. Notice also that there is a small, positive pop artifact at F3, immediately after the second blue arrow.

Ventilator artifact

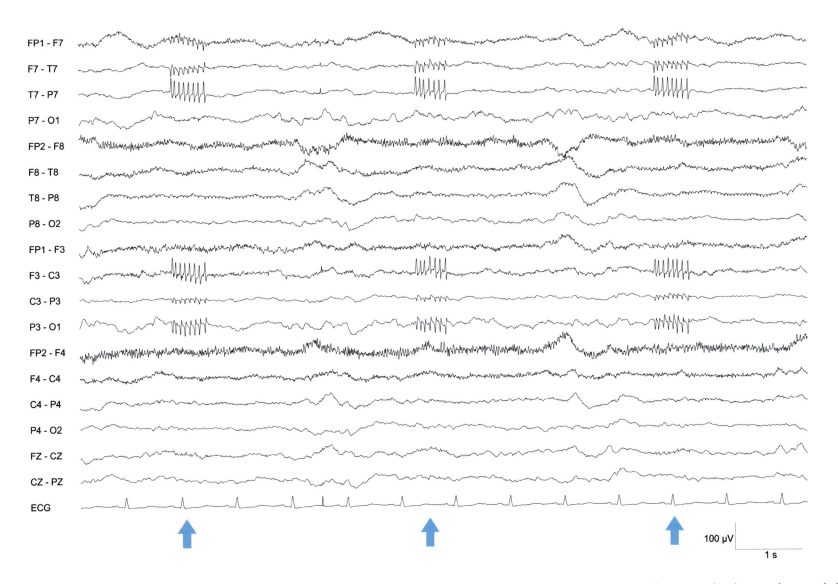

▶ **Figure 2.75** **Ventilator artifact.** Bipolar longitudinal montage. At regular intervals (blue arrows), a stereotypical high-frequency signal occurs in several electrodes. This EEG was recorded in a comatose patient in the intensive care unit. During this period of the recordings, the ventilator was very close to the left side of the patient's head. The polarity of the acute component of this artifact is negative at electrodes T7 > F7 and positive at electrodes C3 > P3. Notice that in this case the interburst period and also the waveform of each artifact are almost identical. Careful inspection reveals that the first and third artifacts contain eight "spikes," whereas the second burst contains seven "spikes." Moving the ventilator aside reduced the artifact.

Electrostatic artifact

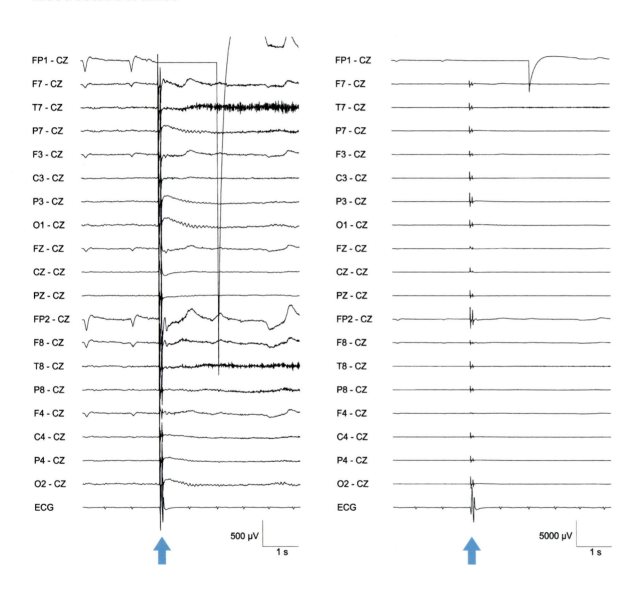

▶ **Figure 2.76 Electrostatic artifact.** Vertex reference montage. The electrostatic artifact is shown in two different amplifications. It caused a very short and high deflection involving all electrodes (blue arrows), including the thoraxic electrodes used for display of the ECG.

Wobble artifact

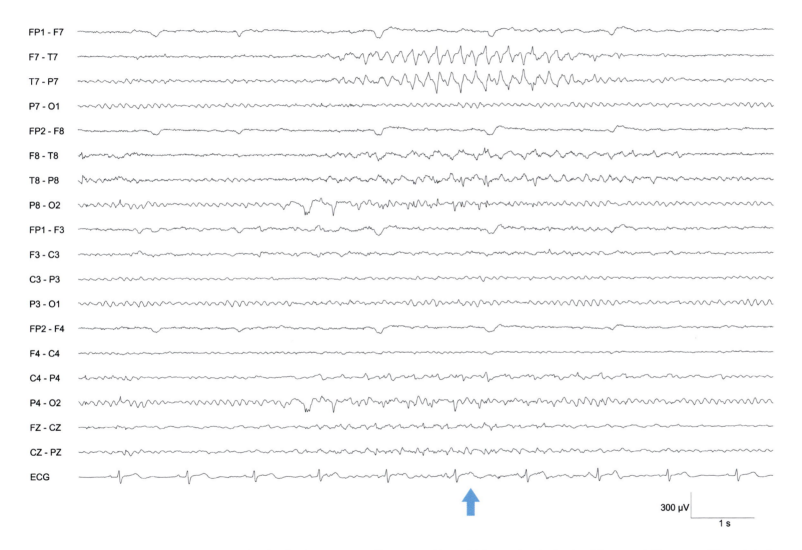

▶ **Figure 2.77** **Wobble artifact.** Bipolar longitudinal montage. Artifact caused by wobbling at the electrodes (blue arrow). There are different rhythms of different polarity and different waveforms affecting different electrodes. This produces a very complicated, nonphysiological distribution of potentials.

Wobble artifact: Bipolar longitudinal montage (A) and vertex reference montage (B)

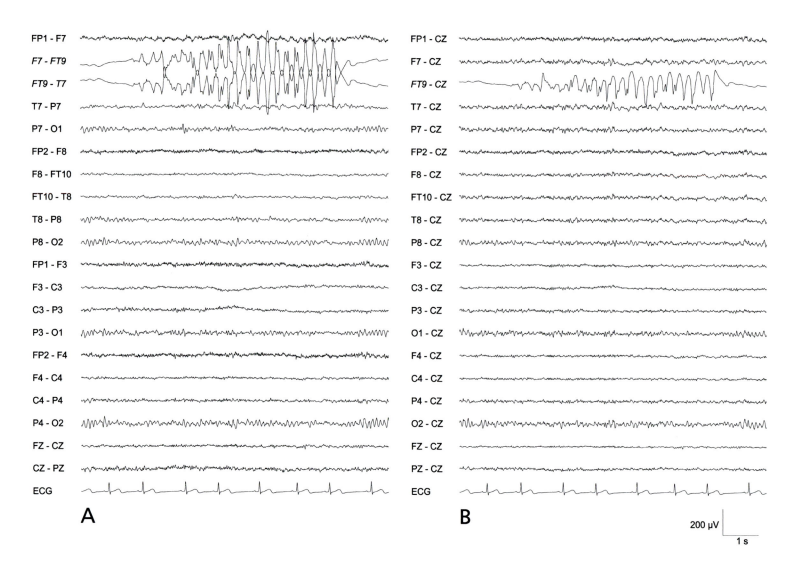

Figure 2.78 **Wobble artifact: Bipolar longitudinal montage (A) and vertex reference montage (B).** The scalp under electrode FT9 was rubbed with a cotton swab soaked in alcohol. This produced the wobble artifact shown in this sample. The amplification of the channels F7–FT9, FT9–T7, and FT9–CZ was reduced for better visualization of the artifact.

Dipole of the eye bulb

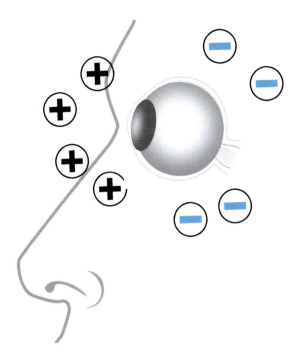

▶ **Figure 2.79** **Dipole of the eye bulb.** The retina is relatively negatively charged, and the cornea is relatively positively charged. This is because the retinal neurons produce a dipole that is perpendicular to the retina producing the effect shown in ▶ Figure 2.80. Most of the artifacts produced by eye movements can be explained by the anterior positive part of the eyeball moving away or closer to any given electrode. The potential change caused at scalp electrodes by movements of the posterior negative portion of the dipole is negligible because the posterior dipole is facing deep into the middle to the brain.

shown in ▶ **Figure 2.103** that a left mesial frontal EEG seizure pattern (paroxysmal fast) proceeds the EMG artifact by approximately 1.5 s. Generalized tonic–clonic seizures have a characteristic EMG artifact that usually obscures the entire EEG (▶ **Figure 2.104**). Myoclonic status in severe anoxic encephalopathy also shows typical muscle artifacts during twitching (▶ **Figure 2.105**). Palatal tremor leads to a fast, approximately 2 Hz, rhythmical EMG artifact of highest amplitude at the ear electrodes (▶ **Figure 2.106**).

A comfortable position in bed is essential to reduce EMG artifact, particularly in anxious patients. Hyperventilation also tends to relax patients and, therefore, preferentially should be done at the beginning of the EEG recoding. In general, use of 15 or 30 Hz filters to reduce EMG artifacts should be avoided because filtered EMG activity may erroneously appear as polyspikes or paroxysmal fast activity. However, sometimes it is helpful to aggressively filter out EMG activity temporarily when specifically trying to analyze EEG seizure patterns in the delta or theta range.

2.3.2.3   Glossokinetic Artifacts

The tongue is a dipole, with the tip of the tongue negatively charged and the base of the tongue positively charged. Movement of the tongue will produce an artifact that is named "glossokinetic artifact" (▶ **Figures 2.107** and **2.108**). Potentials caused by tongue movements decrease in amplitude from frontal to the vertex but increase again toward the occipital electrodes. This can be explained by the tip of the tongue moving toward the frontal electrodes but at the same time the positivity of the tongue base moving downwards, away from the occipital electrodes (▶ **Figure 2.108**). This would not be possible with a purely frontal generator, such as eye movements. In ▶ **Figure 2.108**, the difference between the potential fields of an eye blink and a tongue movement is illustrated.

2.3.2.4   Eye Muscle Artifacts

Eye muscle artifacts must be distinguished from eye bulb artifacts (▶ **Figure 2.109**). They are also referred to as rectus lateralis artifacts or rectus lateralis spikes. This, however, is misleading because all eye muscles, when contracted, produce muscle spicule artifacts at frontal electrodes (▶ **Figure 2.110**). The rectus lateralis artifact precedes horizontal eye movements ipsilaterally to the direction of eye movement. However, usually other eye muscle contractions also contribute to the artifact, with the respective contribution being difficult to assess. Vertical eye movements produce muscle spicules at FP1 and FP2 from contraction of the superior rectus muscles. If the pointed sum action potentials produced by contraction of eye muscles are followed by a slow wave, the erroneous impression of a spike with a following slow wave is created. ▶ **Figure 2.111**

Horizontal eye movements

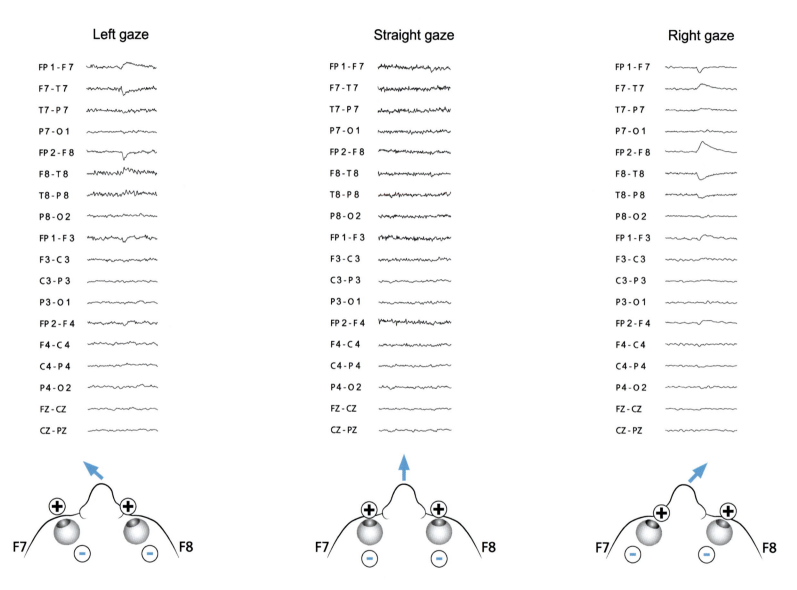

Left gaze

FP 1 - F 7	
F 7 - T 7	
T 7 - P 7	
P 7 - O 1	
FP 2 - F 8	
F 8 - T 8	
T 8 - P 8	
P 8 - O 2	
FP 1 - F 3	
F 3 - C 3	
C 3 - P 3	
P 3 - O 1	
FP 2 - F 4	
F 4 - C 4	
C 4 - P 4	
P 4 - O 2	
FZ - CZ	
CZ - PZ	

Straight gaze

Right gaze

F7 F8

▶ **Figure 2.80** **Horizontal eye movements.** Lateral eye movements have opposite effects on F7 and F8. Lateral movements to the left side produce a positivity at F7 and a simultaneous negativity at F8. Lateral movements to the right side produce just the opposite effect on F7 and F8. The effect of lateral movements on FP1 and FP2 is minimal because with lateral eye movements, the distance between the dipole and electrodes FP1 and FP2 changes very little.

Bulb movement when looking upwards

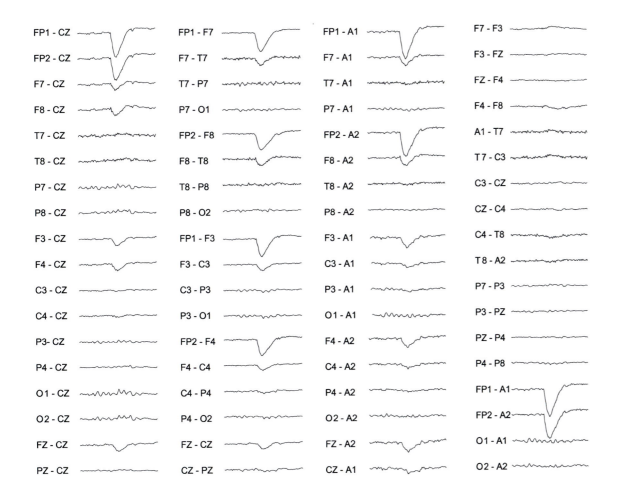

FP1 - CZ	FP1 - F7	FP1 - A1	F7 - F3
FP2 - CZ	F7 - T7	F7 - A1	F3 - FZ
F7 - CZ	T7 - P7	T7 - A1	FZ - F4
F8 - CZ	P7 - O1	P7 - A1	F4 - F8
T7 - CZ	FP2 - F8	FP2 - A2	A1 - T7
T8 - CZ	F8 - T8	F8 - A2	T7 - C3
P7 - CZ	T8 - P8	T8 - A2	C3 - CZ
P8 - CZ	P8 - O2	P8 - A2	CZ - C4
F3 - CZ	FP1 - F3	F3 - A1	C4 - T8
F4 - CZ	F3 - C3	C3 - A1	T 8 - A2
C3 - CZ	C3 - P3	P3 - A1	P7 - P3
C4 - CZ	P3 - O1	O1 - A1	P3 - PZ
P3- CZ	FP2 - F4	F4 - A2	PZ - P4
P4 - CZ	F4 - C4	C4 - A2	P4 - P8
O1 - CZ	C4 - P4	P4 - A2	FP1 - A1
O2 - CZ	P4 - O2	O2 - A2	FP2 - A2
FZ - CZ	FZ - CZ	FZ - A2	O1 - A1
PZ - CZ	CZ - PZ	CZ - A1	O2 - A2

200 µV

1 s

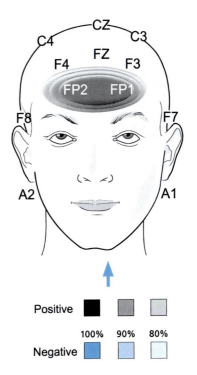

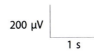

Positive — 100% 90% 80%

Negative

▶ **Figure 2.81 Bulb movement when looking upwards.** Representation of the movement of the bulb when looking upwards in referential and bipolar montages. When looking upwards, the artifact is mainly caused by the positively charged cornea getting closer to FP1 and FP2. The isopotential lines include the 80% gradient for the maps.

Bulb movement when looking up oblique to the left

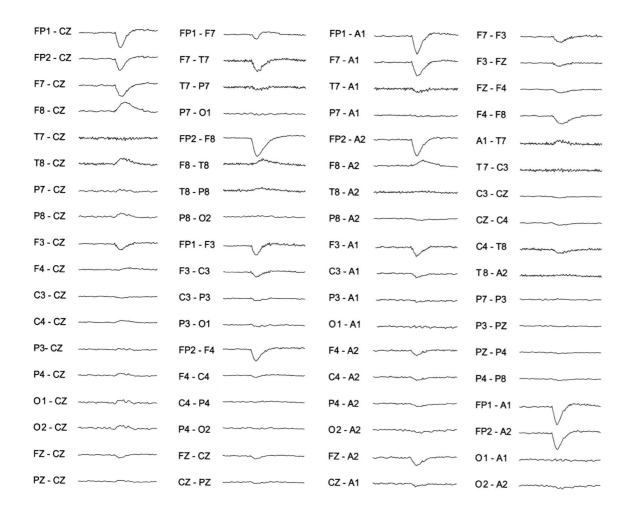

FP1 - CZ	FP1 - F7	FP1 - A1	F7 - F3
FP2 - CZ	F7 - T7	F7 - A1	F3 - FZ
F7 - CZ	T7 - P7	T7 - A1	FZ - F4
F8 - CZ	P7 - O1	P7 - A1	F4 - F8
T7 - CZ	FP2 - F8	FP2 - A2	A1 - T7
T8 - CZ	F8 - T8	F8 - A2	T7 - C3
P7 - CZ	T8 - P8	T8 - A2	C3 - CZ
P8 - CZ	P8 - O2	P8 - A2	CZ - C4
F3 - CZ	FP1 - F3	F3 - A1	C4 - T8
F4 - CZ	F3 - C3	C3 - A1	T8 - A2
C3 - CZ	C3 - P3	P3 - A1	P7 - P3
C4 - CZ	P3 - O1	O1 - A1	P3 - PZ
P3- CZ	FP2 - F4	F4 - A2	PZ - P4
P4 - CZ	F4 - C4	C4 - A2	P4 - P8
O1 - CZ	C4 - P4	P4 - A2	FP1 - A1
O2 - CZ	P4 - O2	O2 - A2	FP2 - A2
FZ - CZ	FZ - CZ	FZ - A2	O1 - A1
PZ - CZ	CZ - PZ	CZ - A1	O2 - A2

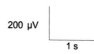

200 µV

1 s

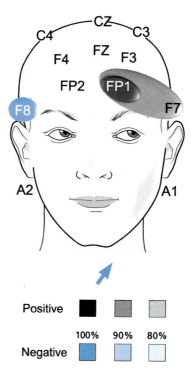

Positive ▪ ▪ ▪
100% 90% 80%
Negative ▪ ▪ ▪

▶ **Figure 2.82 Bulb movement when looking up oblique to the left.** Representation of the movement of the bulb when looking up to the left in referential and bipolar montage. The electrode F3 shows more of the positivity of the cornea than the electrode F4. The asymmetry of the deflections reflects the oblique eye movement.

Bulb movement when looking to the left

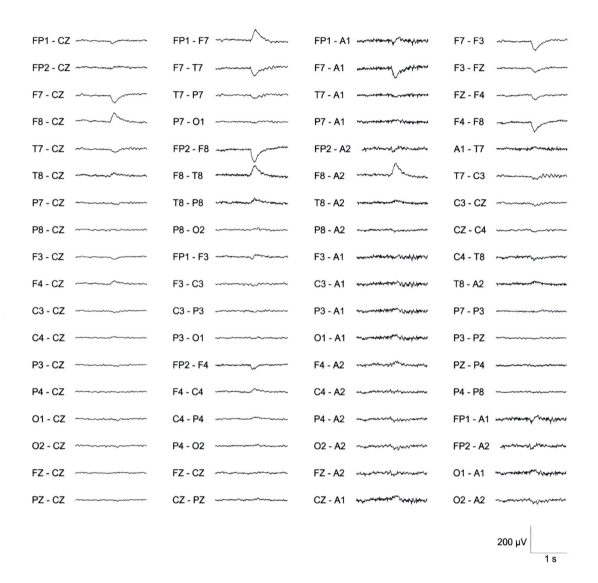

FP1 - CZ	FP1 - F7	FP1 - A1	F7 - F3
FP2 - CZ	F7 - T7	F7 - A1	F3 - FZ
F7 - CZ	T7 - P7	T7 - A1	FZ - F4
F8 - CZ	P7 - O1	P7 - A1	F4 - F8
T7 - CZ	FP2 - F8	FP2 - A2	A1 - T7
T8 - CZ	F8 - T8	F8 - A2	T7 - C3
P7 - CZ	T8 - P8	T8 - A2	C3 - CZ
P8 - CZ	P8 - O2	P8 - A2	CZ - C4
F3 - CZ	FP1 - F3	F3 - A1	C4 - T8
F4 - CZ	F3 - C3	C3 - A1	T8 - A2
C3 - CZ	C3 - P3	P3 - A1	P7 - P3
C4 - CZ	P3 - O1	O1 - A1	P3 - PZ
P3 - CZ	FP2 - F4	F4 - A2	PZ - P4
P4 - CZ	F4 - C4	C4 - A2	P4 - P8
O1 - CZ	C4 - P4	P4 - A2	FP1 - A1
O2 - CZ	P4 - O2	O2 - A2	FP2 - A2
FZ - CZ	FZ - CZ	FZ - A2	O1 - A1
PZ - CZ	CZ - PZ	CZ - A1	O2 - A2

200 µV
1 s

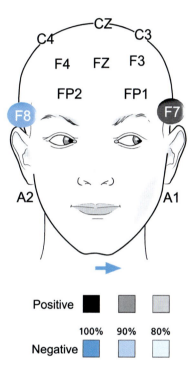

Positive 100% 90% 80%
Negative

▶ **Figure 2.83   Bulb movement when looking to the left.** Eye movement artifacts when looking to the left in referential and bipolar montages. The electrodes F7 and F8 show opposite deflections because the positivity of the cornea moves toward F7 and away from F8.

Bulb movement when looking oblique down to the left

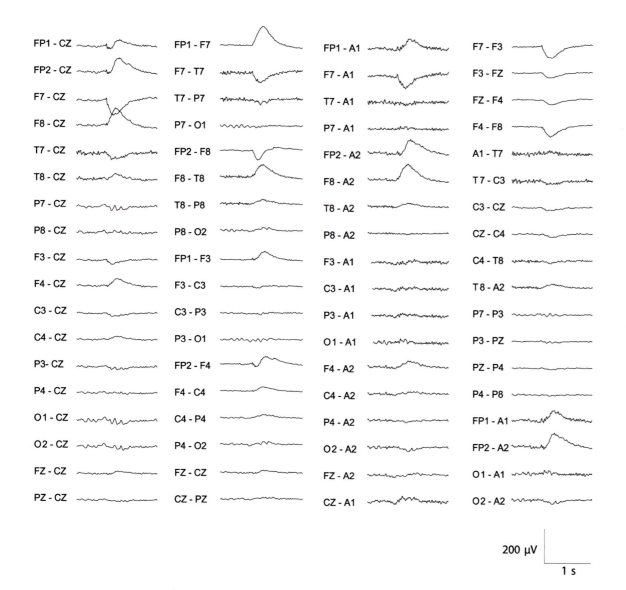

200 µV

1 s

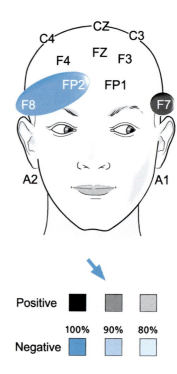

Positive: 100% 90% 80%

Negative

▶ **Figure 2.84** **Bulb movement when looking oblique down to the left**. Representation of the movement of the bulb when looking down to the left in referential and bipolar montage. The electrodes F7 and F8, as well as F3 and F4, show opposite deflections. All oblique eye movements show a characteristic artifact in the longitudinal bipolar montage, namely the waveform of the eye movement artifact in channel 1 is similar to the waveform in channel 6, and that in channel 2 is similar to that in channel 5.

Bulb movement when looking down

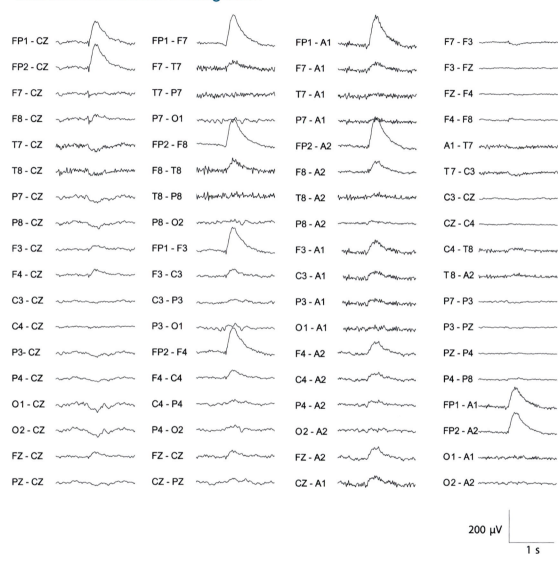

200 μV

1 s

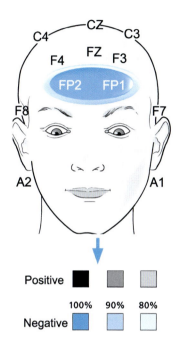

Positive

Negative

100%   90%   80%

▶ **Figure 2.85** **Bulb movement when looking down.** Illustration of the movement of the bulb when looking downwards in referential and bipolar montage. In all vertical eye movements, the artifact of the eye movement has a similar waveform in channel 1 and 5 and in channels 2 and 6 in a bipolar longitudinal montage.

Bulb movement when looking oblique down to the right

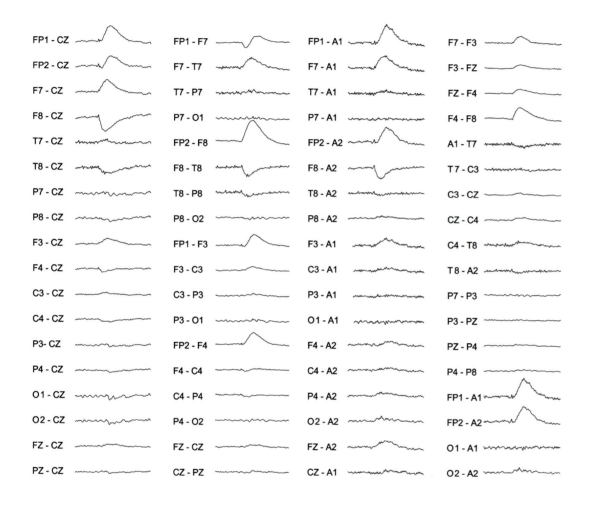

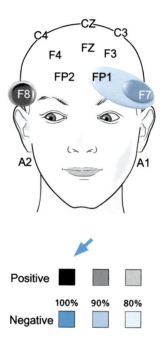

200 µV

1 s

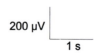

▶ **Figure 2.86 Bulb movement when looking oblique down to the right.** Illustration of the movement of the bulb when looking down to the right in referential and bipolar montage. The electrodes F7 and F8, as well as F3 and F4, show opposite deflections. Another example of the rule that in longitudinal bipolar montages, the eye movement artifact of all oblique eye movement is characterized by the waveform of the eye movement artifact being similar in channels 1 and 6 and also channels 2 and 5.

Bulb movement when looking to the right

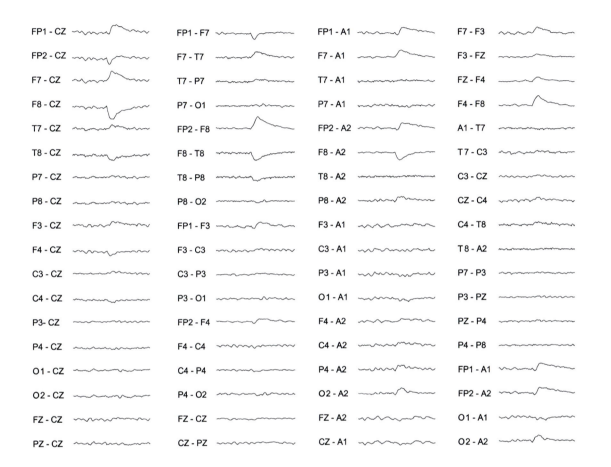

FP1 - CZ	FP1 - F7	FP1 - A1	F7 - F3
FP2 - CZ	F7 - T7	F7 - A1	F3 - FZ
F7 - CZ	T7 - P7	T7 - A1	FZ - F4
F8 - CZ	P7 - O1	P7 - A1	F4 - F8
T7 - CZ	FP2 - F8	FP2 - A2	A1 - T7
T8 - CZ	F8 - T8	F8 - A2	T7 - C3
P7 - CZ	T8 - P8	T8 - A2	C3 - CZ
P8 - CZ	P8 - O2	P8 - A2	CZ - C4
F3 - CZ	FP1 - F3	F3 - A1	C4 - T8
F4 - CZ	F3 - C3	C3 - A1	T8 - A2
C3 - CZ	C3 - P3	P3 - A1	P7 - P3
C4 - CZ	P3 - O1	O1 - A1	P3 - PZ
P3- CZ	FP2 - F4	F4 - A2	PZ - P4
P4 - CZ	F4 - C4	C4 - A2	P4 - P8
O1 - CZ	C4 - P4	P4 - A2	FP1 - A1
O2 - CZ	P4 - O2	O2 - A2	FP2 - A2
FZ - CZ	FZ - CZ	FZ - A2	O1 - A1
PZ - CZ	CZ - PZ	CZ - A1	O2 - A2

200 µV

1 s

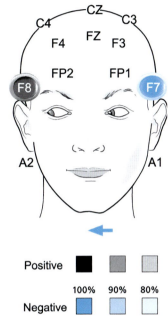

Positive

100% 90% 80%

Negative

► **Figure 2.87** **Bulb movement when looking to the right.** Representation of the eye movement when looking to the right in referential and bipolar montage. The corneal positivity moves away from F7, producing a relative negativity at F7, and rendering F8 relatively more positive.

Bulb movement when looking oblique up to the right

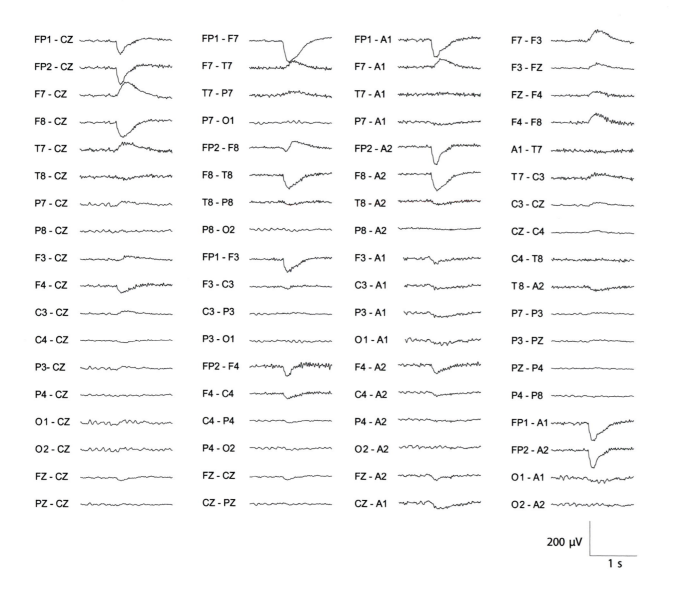

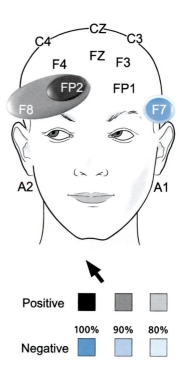

Positive ■ ■ ■
100% 90% 80%
Negative ■ ■ ■

200 µV

1 s

▶ **Figure 2.88 Bulb movement when looking oblique up to the right.** Representation of the movement of the bulb to the top right in referential and bipolar montage. The electrodes F7 and F8, as well as F3 and F4, show opposite deflections. Also in this case, the waveform of all oblique eye movements in the longitudinal bipolar montage reveals a similar waveform in channels 1 and 6 and also channels 2 and 5.

Frequent blinking

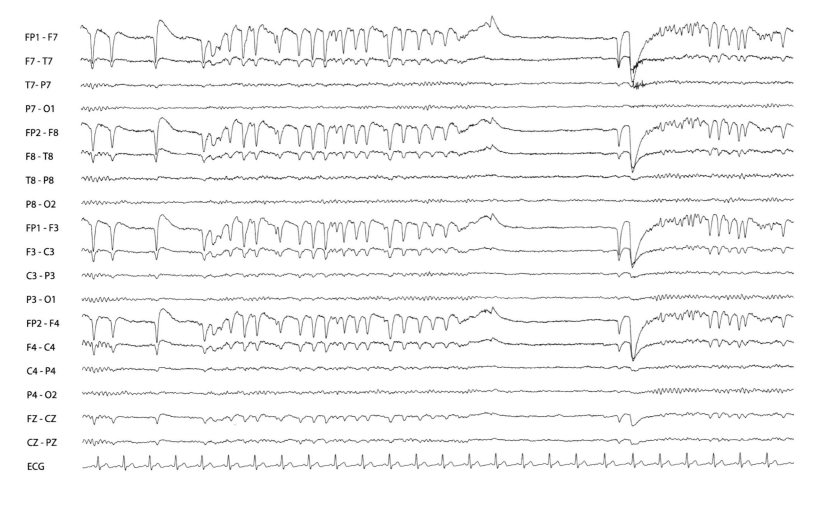

FP1 - F7
F7 - T7
T7- P7
P7 - O1
FP2 - F8
F8 - T8
T8 - P8
P8 - O2
FP1 - F3
F3 - C3
C3 - P3
P3 - O1
FP2 - F4
F4 - C4
C4 - P4
P4 - O2
FZ - CZ
CZ - PZ
ECG

100 µV

1 s

▶ **Figure 2.89**   **Frequent blinking.** Bipolar longitudinal montage. This EEG shows frequent eye blinking.

Kappa rhythm (fluttering of the eyelids)

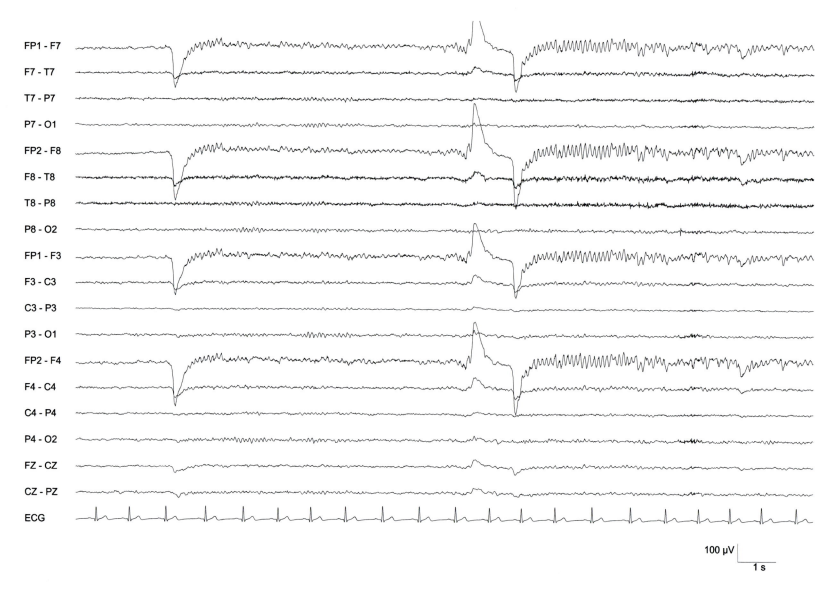

FP1 - F7
F7 - T7
T7 - P7
P7 - O1
FP2 - F8
F8 - T8
T8 - P8
P8 - O2
FP1 - F3
F3 - C3
C3 - P3
P3 - O1
FP2 - F4
F4 - C4
C4 - P4
P4 - O2
FZ - CZ
CZ - PZ
ECG

100 μV
1 s

▶ **Figure 2.90** **Kappa rhythm (fluttering of the eyelids).** Bipolar longitudinal montage. High-frequency eyelid movements lead to a typical eye movement artifact, which is also called kappa rhythm. It is an artifact caused by eyelid movements and does not reflect brain activity.

Kappa rhythm (fluttering of the eyelids)

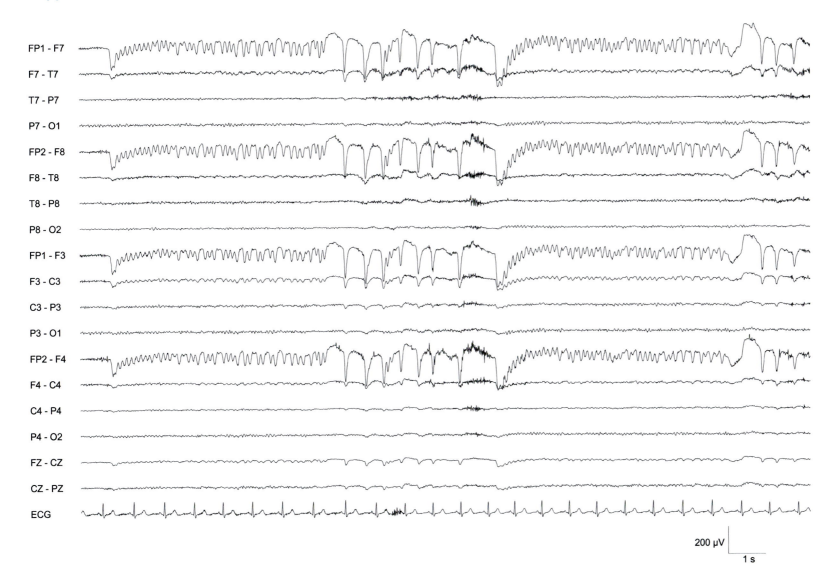

FP1 - F7
F7 - T7
T7 - P7
P7 - O1
FP2 - F8
F8 - T8
T8 - P8
P8 - O2
FP1 - F3
F3 - C3
C3 - P3
P3 - O1
FP2 - F4
F4 - C4
C4 - P4
P4 - O2
FZ - CZ
CZ - PZ
ECG

200 µV

1 s

▶ **Figure 2.91 Kappa rhythm (fluttering of the eyelids).** Bipolar longitudinal montage. Example of kappa rhythm by eyelid movements (eyelid flutter) of different frequency in an anxious patient.

Continuous slow, left frontopolar

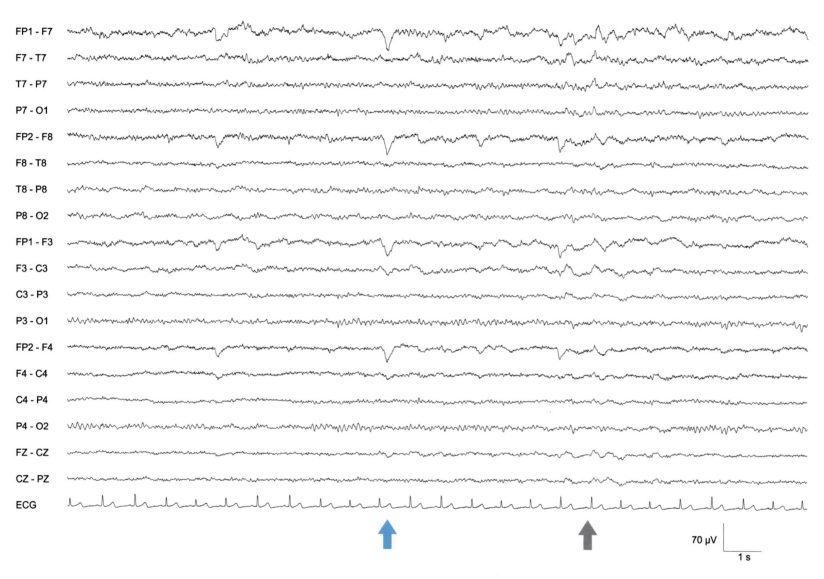

FP1 - F7

F7 - T7

T7 - P7

P7 - O1

FP2 - F8

F8 - T8

T8 - P8

P8 - O2

FP1 - F3

F3 - C3

C3 - P3

P3 - O1

FP2 - F4

F4 - C4

C4 - P4

P4 - O2

FZ - CZ

CZ - PZ

ECG

70 μV

1 s

▶ **Figure 2.92** **Continuous slow, left frontopolar.** Bipolar longitudinal montage. A 44-year-old patient with biopsy-proven left frontal glioblastoma. Status post left frontal seed implantation. Pulse artifact at the electrode P8. At the blue arrow, there is an artifact caused by either a blink or an upward eye movement (there is no clear overshoot). The blink or upward eyeball movement can be differentiated from pathological frontopolar slowing by analyzing in detail the distribution of the slow. Blinks or eyeball movement artifacts at a longitudinal bipolar montage will never be of higher amplitude at F3–C3 compared to FP1–F3 or F4–C4 compared to FP2–F4. In addition, blinks and eyeball movements are symmetrically distributed, whereas the continuous slow usually, as in this case, is lateralized. In this case, the slowing is clearly lateralized to the left hemisphere, and shortly before the gray arrow, there is another blink or eyeball movement artifact followed by slow activity that is of higher amplitude at F3–C3 than at FP1–F3.

Right eye amaurosis

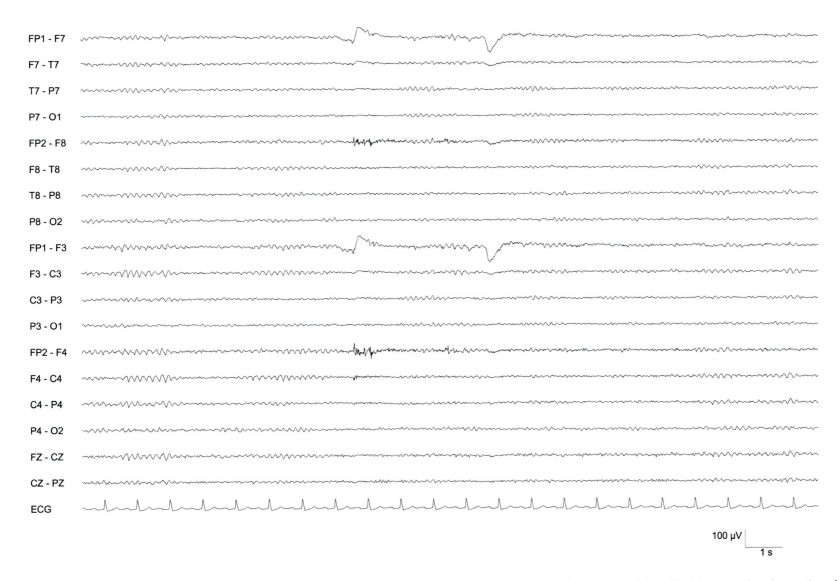

100 µV

1 s

▶ **Figure 2.93** **Right eye amaurosis.** Bipolar longitudinal montage. In this patient, eye movements are almost only visible at FP1. However, close inspection of the EEG shows that the eyeball movement artifact is of low amplitude but clearly visible at channels F3–C3, FP2–F4, and FP2–F8. This indicates that this is not an artifact at FP1. In addition, the amplitude at FP2 is similar to the amplitude at F3 because these two electrodes are at a similar distance from the left eye corneal potential. The abnormal eyeball artifact shown in this figure is due to a complete left retinal detachment producing a right eye amaurosis.

Gaze-induced nystagmus

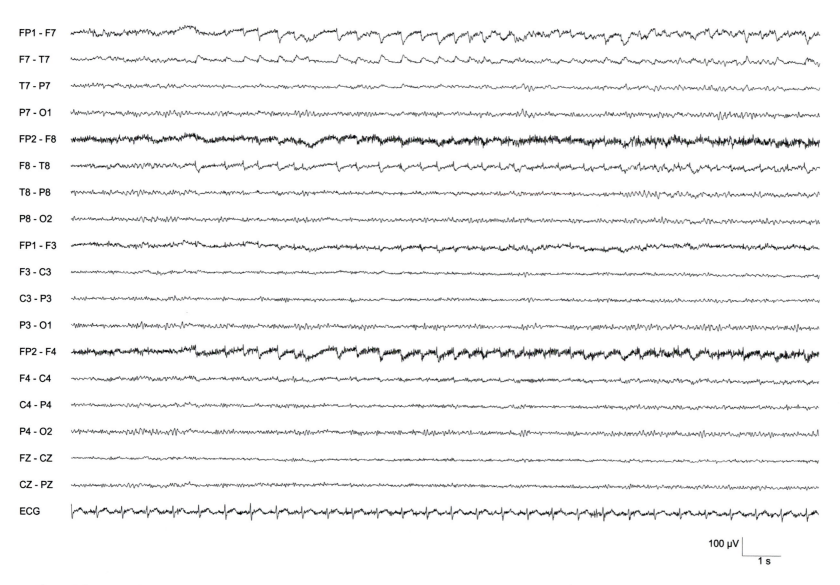

FP1 - F7

F7 - T7

T7 - P7

P7 - O1

FP2 - F8

F8 - T8

T8 - P8

P8 - O2

FP1 - F3

F3 - C3

C3 - P3

P3 - O1

FP2 - F4

F4 - C4

C4 - P4

P4 - O2

FZ - CZ

CZ - PZ

ECG

100 µV

1 s

▶ **Figure 2.94** **Gaze-induced nystagmus.** Bipolar longitudinal montage. This patient has a nystagmus with the fast component to the right and up. For the fast component of the nystagmus, electrode F7 is negative, whereas electrodes F8 and FP2 are positive. Notice also the muscle spicules at F8 and FP2 that most likely are caused by contraction of the right lateral rectus muscle and the right superior rectus muscle.

Downbeat nystagmus

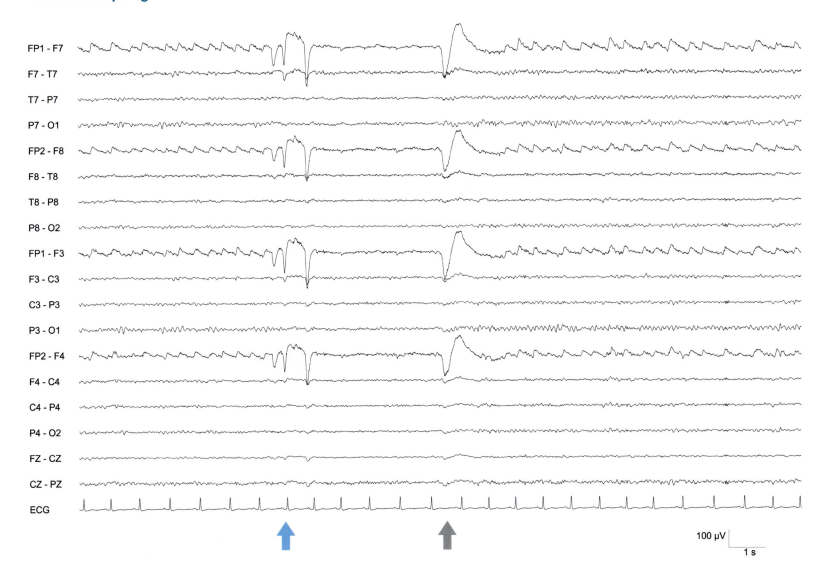

▶ **Figure 2.95** **Downbeat nystagmus.** Bipolar longitudinal montage. A downbeat nystagmus is reflected mainly at electrodes FP1 and FP2. The fast component of the nystagmus points upwards. During eye opening (blue arrow), the nystagmus was blocked and recurred with eye closure (gray arrow). The absence of muscle spicules at FP1 and FP2 is most likely related to the fact that blinking is associated with a relaxation of the superior rectus muscles and the levator palpebrae.

EMG artifact

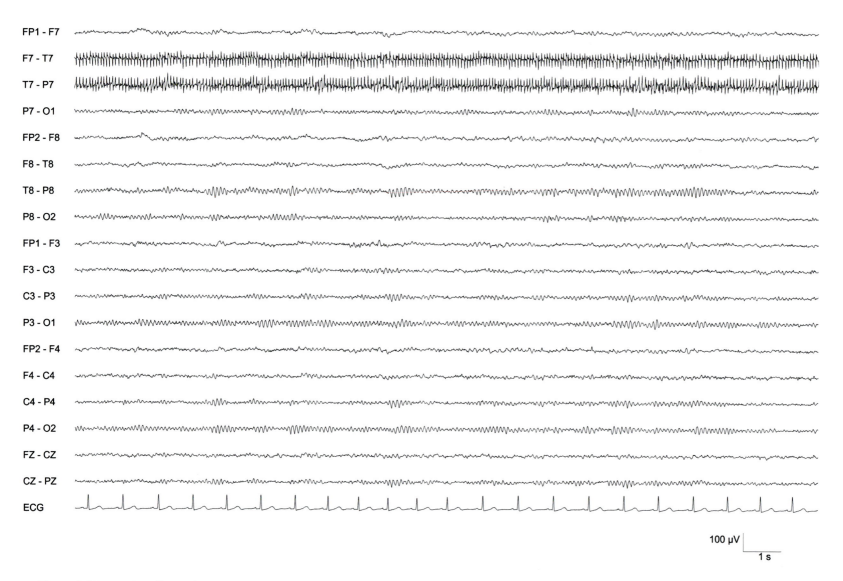

100 µV

1 s

▶ **Figure 2.96** **EMG artifact.** Bipolar longitudinal montage. The electrode T7 shows a continuous 11 or 12 Hz muscle artifact most likely reflecting a rhythmical firing of a muscle spicule. The artifact involves a single electrode; therefore, the possibility of an electrode artifact must also be considered. However, the following characteristics suggest that we are dealing with a muscle spicule: typical waveform with very short duration biphasic potentials, continuous changes in amplitude, and relative high repetition rate.

EMG artifact

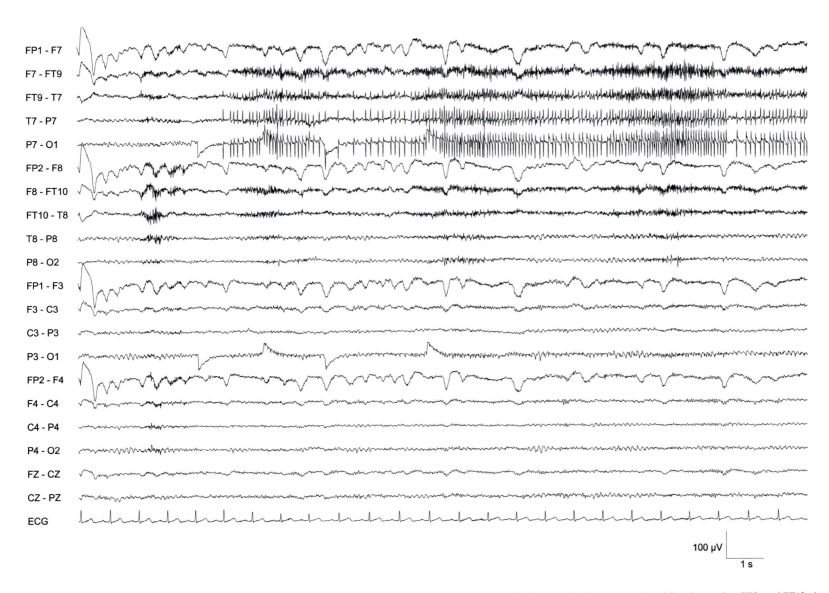

100 μV

1 s

▶ **Figure 2.97** **EMG artifact.** Bipolar longitudinal montage. Electrode P7 records a muscle artifact from a single motor unit, while electrodes FT9 and FT10 show a multiunit, denser EMG pattern. Notice the similarity of waveform and repetition rate between the artifacts of electrode T7 in ▶ **Figure 2.96** and P7 in this figure.

EMG artifact

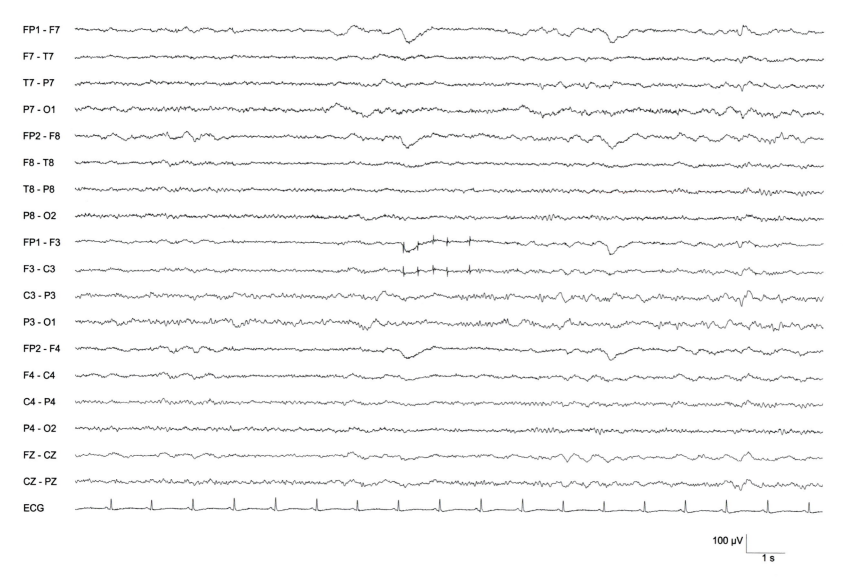

FP1 - F7
F7 - T7
T7 - P7
P7 - O1
FP2 - F8
F8 - T8
T8 - P8
P8 - O2
FP1 - F3
F3 - C3
C3 - P3
P3 - O1
FP2 - F4
F4 - C4
C4 - P4
P4 - O2
FZ - CZ
CZ - PZ
ECG

100 µV

1 s

▶ **Figure 2.98** **EMG artifact.** Bipolar longitudinal montage. Electrode F3 records five rhythmical single-unit muscle twitches. The discharges are reflected at a single electrode. Therefore, we must exclude an electrode artifact. However, the typical waveform and rhythmicity strongly suggest that the artifact is a muscle spicule discharge. This EEG also shows a continuous slow at P7, P3, and O1 as well as intermittent slow generalized and right frontopolar.

EMG artifact by swallowing

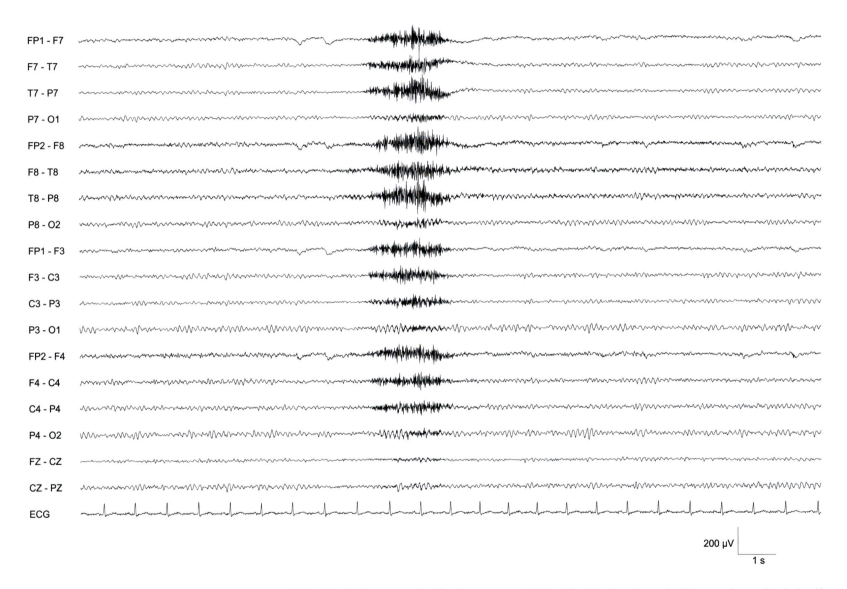

200 µV

1 s

▶ **Figure 2.99** **EMG artifact by swallowing.** Bipolar longitudinal montage. Swallowing causes an EMG artifact that, as shown in this example, can be derived in many EEG electrodes and lasts for 1 or 2 s. In addition, slow potentials produced by tongue movements (glossokinetic artifact) may typically occur together with the diffuse burst of EMG activity (see ▶ **Figures 2.102, 2.107**, and **2.108**). In this example, there appears to be a low-amplitude, approximately 1-s duration, negative potential at electrode T7.

Single muscle spicule artifact during sleep

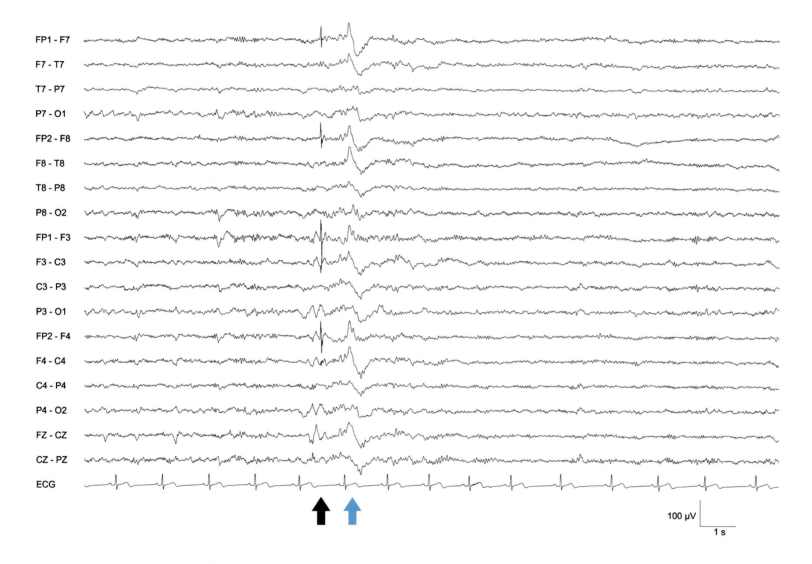

▶ **Figure 2.100** **Single muscle spicule artifact during sleep.** Bipolar longitudinal montage. A single muscle twitch occurs in the frontopolar electrodes FP1 and FP2 (black arrow) just before a K-complex (blue arrow).

Three different EMG artifacts

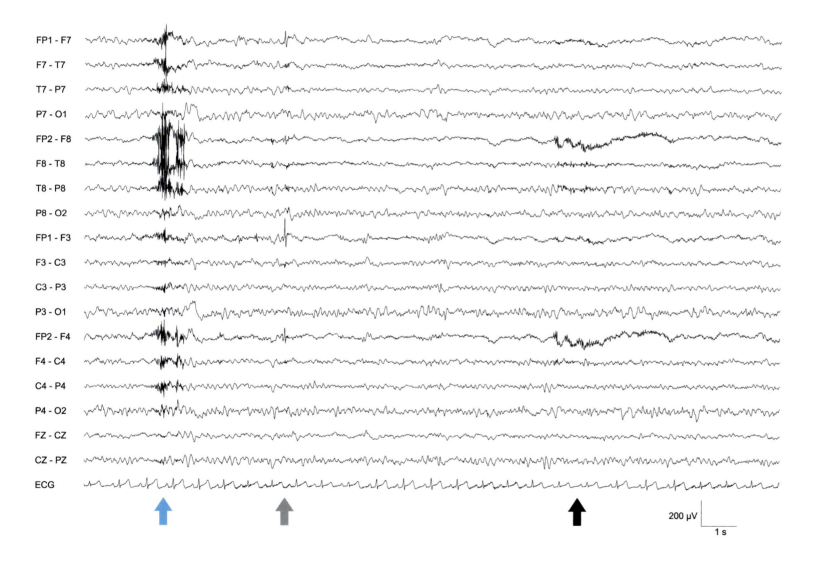

▶ **Figure 2.101** **Three different EMG artifacts.** Bipolar longitudinal montage. This example shows three different artifacts: (a) Swallowing (blue arrow), which also includes a slow positive potential at F8 and F7; (b) a very short single muscle spicule at FP1 > FP2 (gray arrow); and (c) a tonic muscle artifact at FP2 >> F8 > T8 > FP1 (black arrow).

Lip smacking artifacts

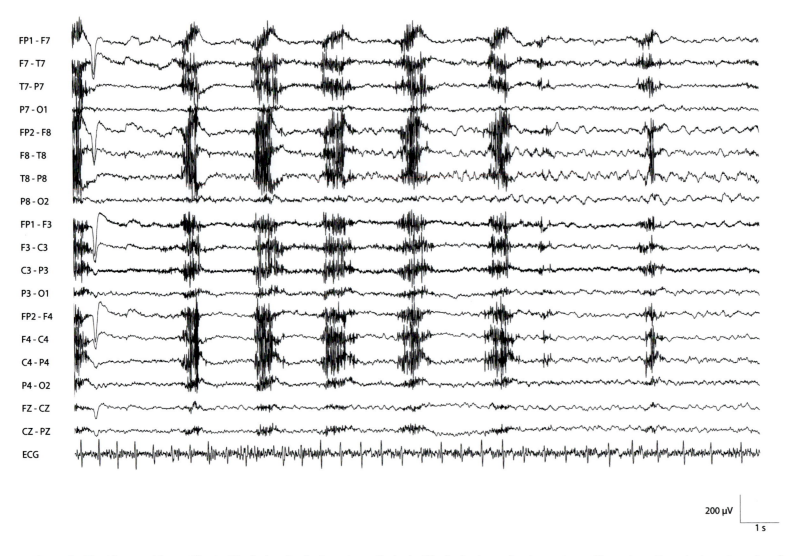

200 μV

1 s

▶ **Figure 2.102** **Lip smacking artifacts.** Bipolar longitudinal montage. Typical artifacts due to swallowing and smacking automatisms (automotor seizure) recorded during an epileptic seizure showing a right temporal EEG seizure pattern. The recording shows approximately 1-s bursts of dense EMG activity that recur every 2 s. Together with the bursts of EMG activity, there is a 1-s duration slow activity that is of relatively high amplitude and is of positive polarity at F7/F8 and less well-defined negative polarity at F3/F4. This slow potential is most likely generated by moving of the tip of the tongue (that is negatively charged) away from the right cheek and toward the left side of the mouth.

Muscle artifact and a left mesial frontal seizure pattern

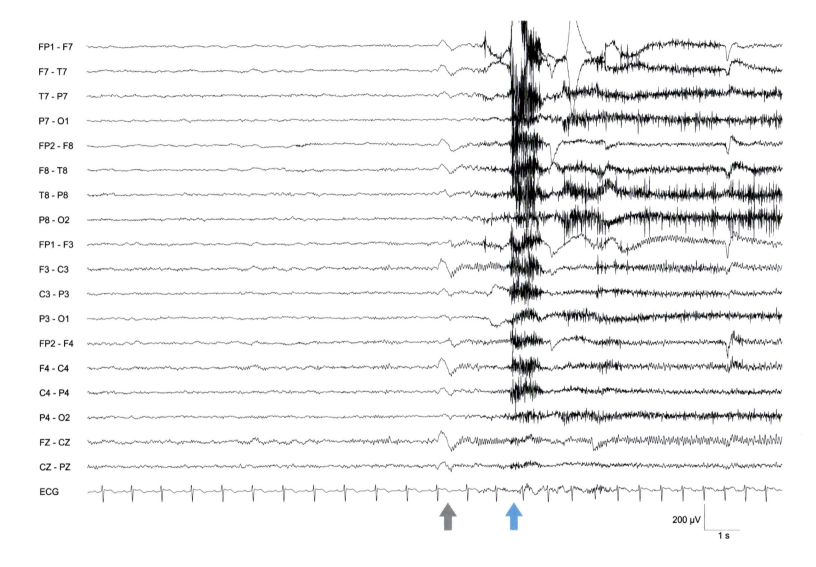

▶ **Figure 2.103** **Muscle artifact and a left mesial frontal seizure pattern.** Bipolar longitudinal montage. Soon after the beginning of a left mesial frontal EEG seizure, there is a prominent, generalized transient followed by paroxysmal fast activity localized to F3 and FZ (gray arrow). Approximately 2 s after the beginning of the paroxysmal fast activity, there is a typical muscle artifact associated (blue arrow) with a negative slow wave at the left and simultaneously a positive slow potential on the right side, suggesting that the patient deviated the tongue to the left side.

EMG artifact of a generalized tonic–clonic seizure

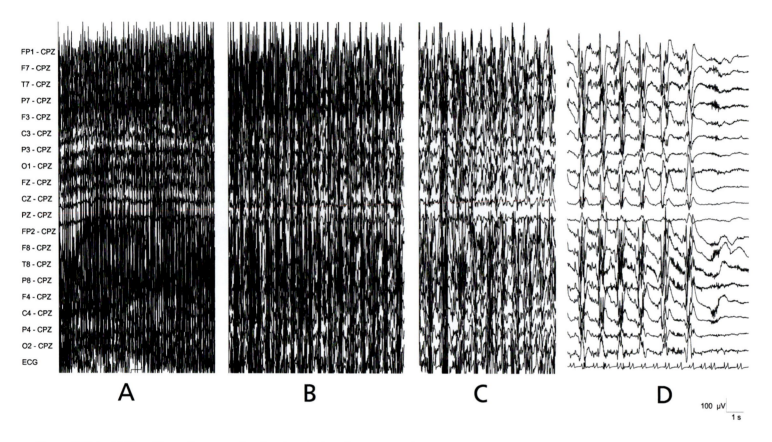

A   B   C   D

100 μV
1 s

▶ **Figure 2.104** **EMG artifact of a generalized tonic–clonic seizure.** CPZ reference montage. Generalized tonic–clonic seizures produce a characteristic EMG artifact that can be reliably used to diagnose that the patient indeed had a generalized tonic–clonic seizure. During the initial tonic phase, all electrodes, including the thoracic electrodes recording the ECG, record a dense muscle artifact that also obscures the ECG artifact (A). At this stage, the EMG activity may be interrupted by very short EMG free intervals (B). When the patient enters the "jittery phase," the EMG shows very brief pauses (C). Gradually, the jittery phase is replaced by clonic movements during which the agonist and antagonist muscle contract together. In the clonic phase, the interval between the muscle contractions becomes progressively longer (D). Eventually, the EMG artifacts disappear, and the EEG consists of relatively low-amplitude, diffuse slow activity.

illustrates a muscle spicule preceding a blink. In lateral eye movements, the muscle spicules are followed by a positive, slower wave at F7 and F8. Seldom are these artifacts confused with temporal lobe spike–waves because of the typical distribution and waveform of both, the initial muscle spicule, and the following slow artifact produced by the lateral eye movement.

2.3.2.5   ECG Artifacts

Electrocardiogram artifacts frequently are seen in patients with an increased neck circumference (▶ **Figure 2.112**). ECG artifacts are usually displayed more clearly if, with drowsiness, the background rhythms disappear, and the overall

EMG artifact in myoclonic status due to severe anoxic encephalopathy after cardiorespiratory arrest and resuscitation

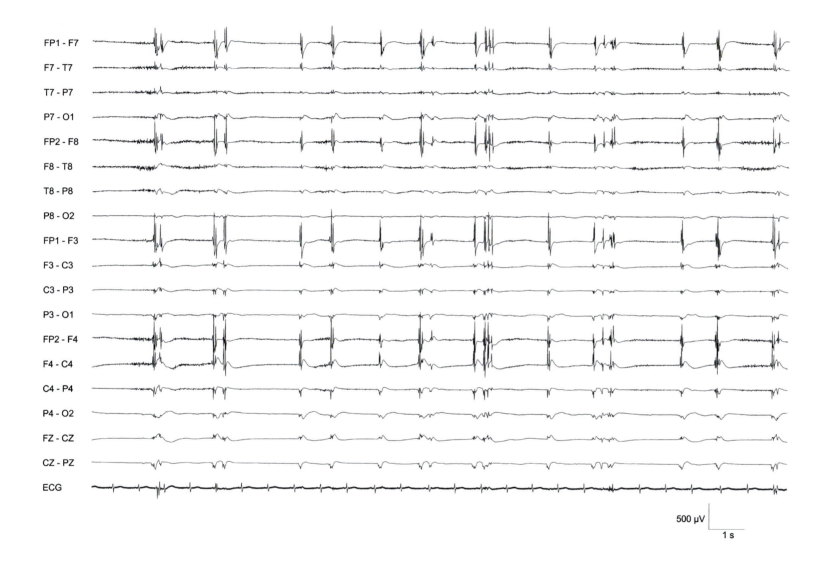

500 µV

1 s

▶ **Figure 2.105** **EMG artifact in myoclonic status due to severe anoxic encephalopathy after cardiorespiratory arrest and resuscitation.** Bipolar longitudinal montage. There is relatively high-amplitude EMG artifact affecting primarily the frontalis muscle. The EMG artifact only occasionally includes the ECG recording, suggesting that most of the myoclonic jerks were more or less limited to frontalis muscles. Due to the low sensitivity of the recordings (see calibration sign), it is not possible to assess the inter-myoclonic jerks EEG activity. Patients who show a generalized myoclonic status after an anoxic episode usually will not recover or will remain in a vegetative state. Most of these patients show background suppression (no brain activity exceeding 10 µV) in the inter-myoclonic jerks EEG recording. Patients who show only background attenuation (EEG activity between the bursts of more than 10 µV) between myoclonic jerks can potentially recover. This is the reason that in all these patients, the inter-myoclonic jerks EEG should be assessed using appropriate sensitivity settings.

Palatal tremor

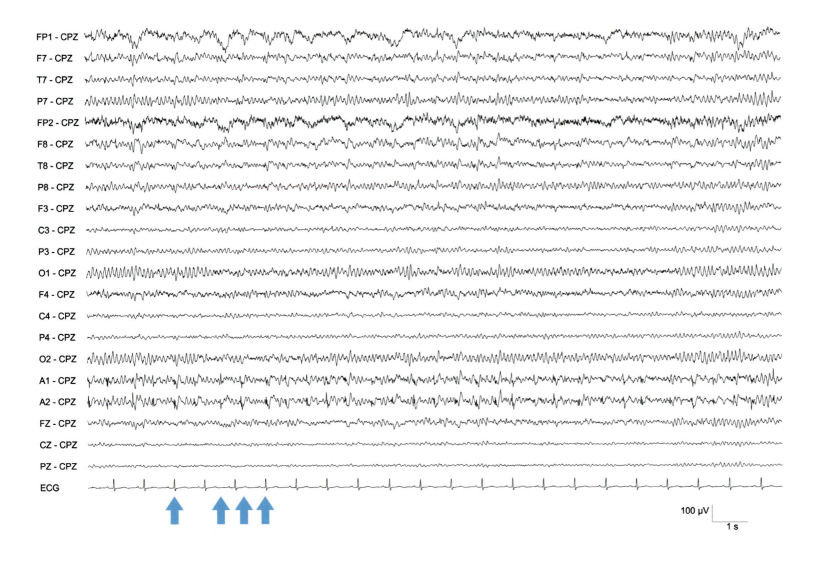

▶ **Figure 2.106** **Palatal tremor.** Vertex reference montage. The short EMG artifacts (blue arrows) caused by the palatal tremor are recorded mainly in the electrically close ear electrodes A1 and A2. The EMG artifact has a frequency of approximately 130 Hz. The high frequency of the contraction and its reflection mainly on ear electrodes is typical of palatal tremor (myoclonus).

Glossokinetic artifact

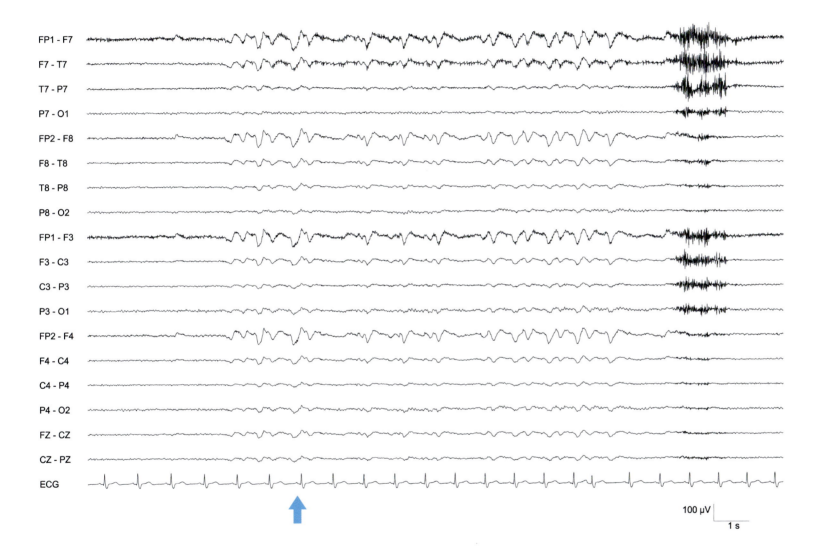

► **Figure 2.107   Glossokinetic artifact.** Bipolar longitudinal montage. The electric dipole of the tongue muscles causes a characteristic artifact of high-amplitude slow waves with frontal maximum when speaking. Note the nonlinear decrease of the potential gradient to occipital (blue arrow). The tip of the tongue is negatively charged, whereas the base of the tongue is relatively positively charged. In this example, the tip of the tongue moved away from electrodes FP1 and FP2. At the same time, the base of the tongue also moved away from O1 and O2. The deflection is higher in channels P4–O2 and P3–O1 compared to C4–P4 and C3–P3. Eye movement (blink) artifacts decay continuously, and there is either no potential visible at P3 or P3–O1 and P4–O2 or these channels are consistently of lower amplitude than C3–P3 and C4–P4, respectively (see ► **Figure 2.101**).

Glossokinetic artifact

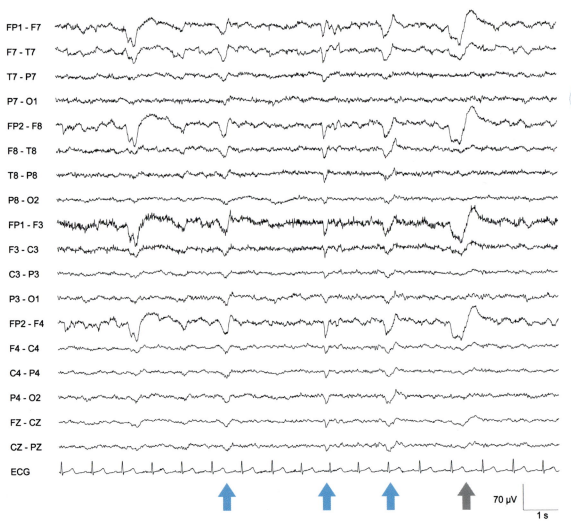

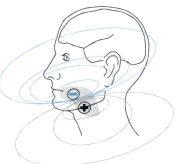

70 μV

1 s

▶ **Figure 2.108** **Glossokinetic artifact.** Bipolar longitudinal montage. See discussion of ▶ **Figure 2.106**. This EEG sample shows glossokinetic artifacts (blue arrows) and a prominent blink (gray arrow). Notice that the blink is not even reflected at the occipital leads. The glossokinetic artifacts, however, are of higher amplitude at the P3–O1 and P4–O2 channels compared with the C3–P3 and C4–P4 channels.

Eye muscle artifacts

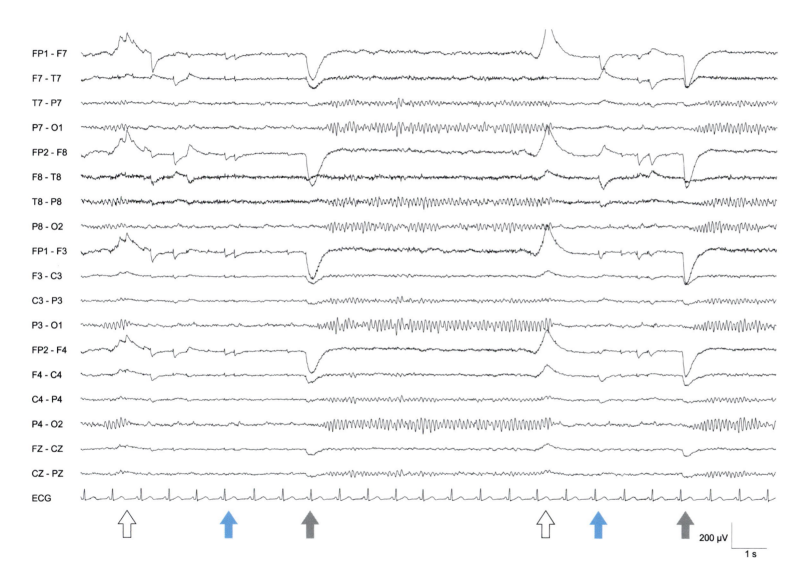

▶ **Figure 2.109** **Eye muscle artifacts.** Bipolar longitudinal montage. Between the eyes open (open arrows) and eyes closed (gray arrows), short-duration eye muscle artifacts (blue arrows) can be seen during horizontal and vertical eye movements. Notice, that the short-duration extraocular eye muscle artifacts always precede the eye movement, producing the characteristic picture of a muscle spicule followed by an acute DC shift with a slow return to baseline as a function of the time constant (low-frequency filter) of the amplifiers.

Eye muscle artifacts

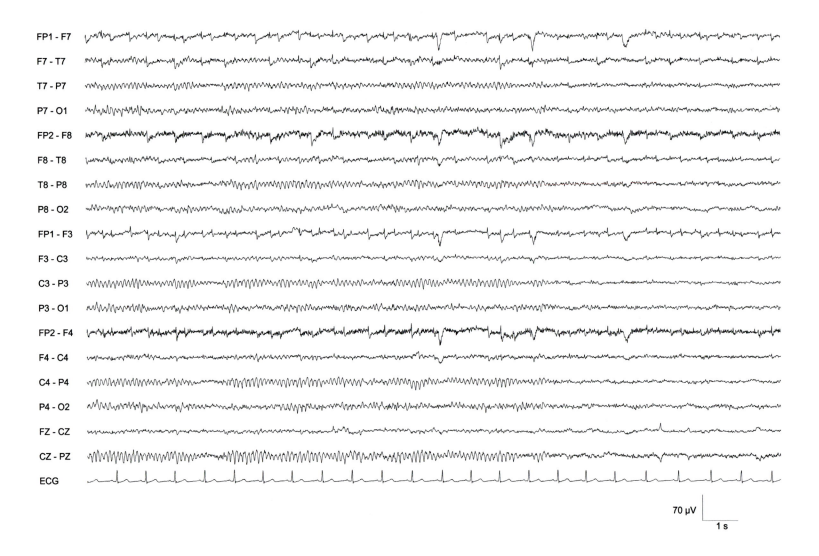

▶ Figure 2.110 **Eye muscle artifacts.** Bipolar longitudinal montage. Many short eye muscle artifacts are associated with small horizontal and vertical eye movements. The muscle spicules at FP1 and FP2 are most probably due to contraction of the superior rectus muscle, and the muscle spicules at F7 and are most probably due to contraction of the lateral rectus muscle.

Eye muscle artifacts

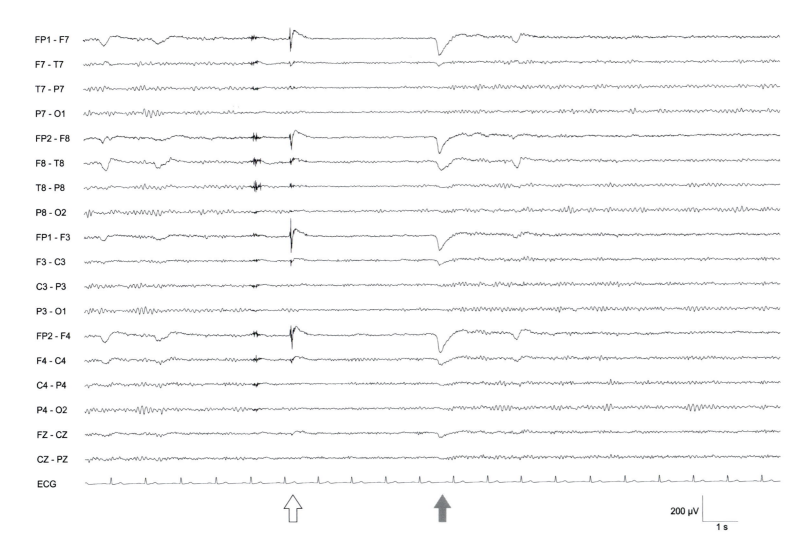

FP1 - F7

F7 - T7

T7 - P7

P7 - O1

FP2 - F8

F8 - T8

T8 - P8

P8 - O2

FP1 - F3

F3 - C3

C3 - P3

P3 - O1

FP2 - F4

F4 - C4

C4 - P4

P4 - O2

FZ - CZ

CZ - PZ

ECG

200 µV

1 s

▶ **Figure 2.111** **Eye muscle artifacts.** Bipolar longitudinal montage. At the beginning of the eye opening (open arrow), a short muscle artifact occurs, which in conjunction with following slow potential of the eyeball movement can be misinterpreted as spike–wave. The extremely short duration of the muscle spicule as also a small, polyphasic artifact of similar distribution as the muscle spicule preceding the eye opening suggests that this is not an epileptiform discharge. The gray arrow marks the eye closure.

ECG artifact

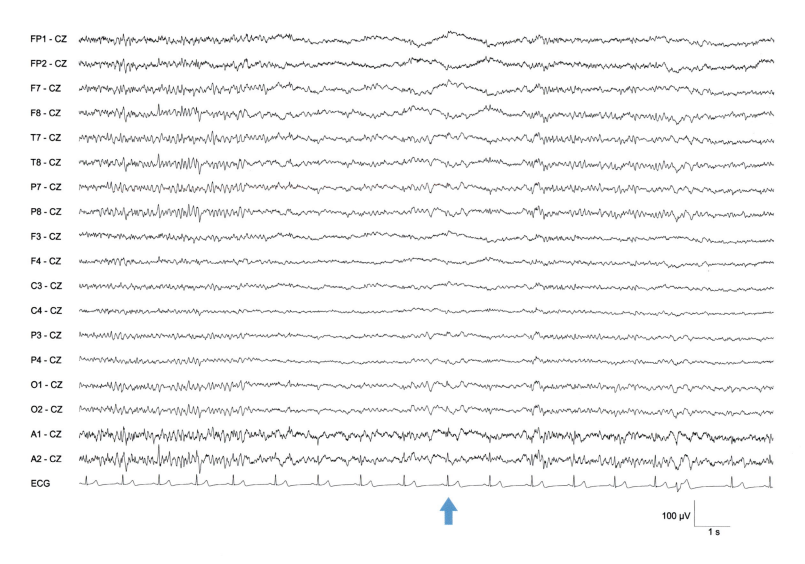

FP1 - CZ
FP2 - CZ
F7 - CZ
F8 - CZ
T7 - CZ
T8 - CZ
P7 - CZ
P8 - CZ
F3 - CZ
F4 - CZ
C3 - CZ
C4 - CZ
P3 - CZ
P4 - CZ
O1 - CZ
O2 - CZ
A1 - CZ
A2 - CZ
ECG

100 µV

1 s

▶ **Figure 2.112** **ECG artifact.** Vertex reference montage. An ECG artifact is of highest amplitude in the ear electrodes, most likely due to the proximity to the heart. The slow horizontal eye movements (blue arrow) reflect drowsiness. See also in ▶ **Figure 2.114**, the diagram of the distribution of the ECG potential over scalp electrodes.

ECG artifact

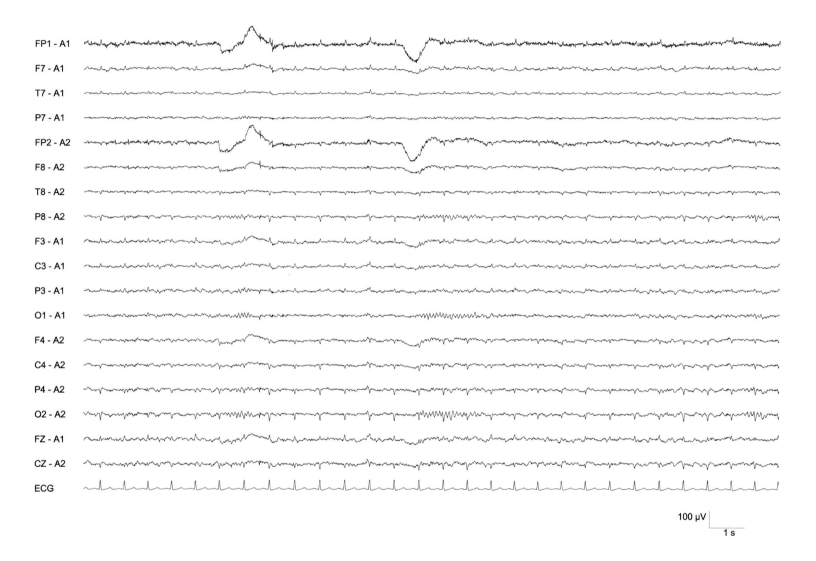

FP1 - A1

F7 - A1

T7 - A1

P7 - A1

FP2 - A2

F8 - A2

T8 - A2

P8 - A2

F3 - A1

C3 - A1

P3 - A1

O1 - A1

F4 - A2

C4 - A2

P4 - A2

O2 - A2

FZ - A1

CZ - A2

ECG

100 μV

1 s

▶ **Figure 2.113** **ECG artifact.** Ipsilateral ear reference montage. The ear electrodes record the ECG artifact in a characteristic manner: The ECG artifact deflections point upward in the left electrodes and downward in the right electrodes. This indicates that the right ear (A2) is negatively charged and the left ear is positively charged compared to the vertex reference (see ▶ **Figure 2.114**). The electrodes in the channels with the lowest deflections (P3 and O1) are electrically charged similar to the respective ears.

ECG artifact

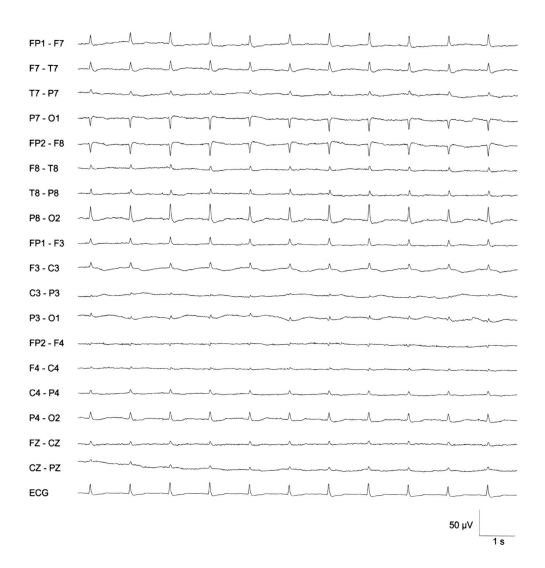

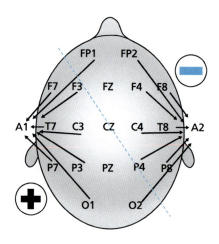

50 µV

1 s

▶ **Figure 2.114** **ECG artifact.** Bipolar longitudinal montage. In EEGs showing electrocerebral silence, the ECG is usually very large because there is no brain activity, and the sensitivity of the recording is increased to a maximum in an attempt to visualize lower amplitude brain activity. That is the case in this example, which corresponds to a patient who had electro-cerebral silence after a cardiopulmonary arrest. The electrical dipole of the heart is reflected on the scalp as a negativity in the left anterior temporal electrodes and as a positivity in the right posterior temporal electrodes. Interestingly, the distribution of the ECG artifact changes with the position of the head with respect to the heart—that is, when the patient moves the head, the ECG dipole vector remains constant at the thorax but its rela-tionship to the scalp electrodes changes.

ECG artifact

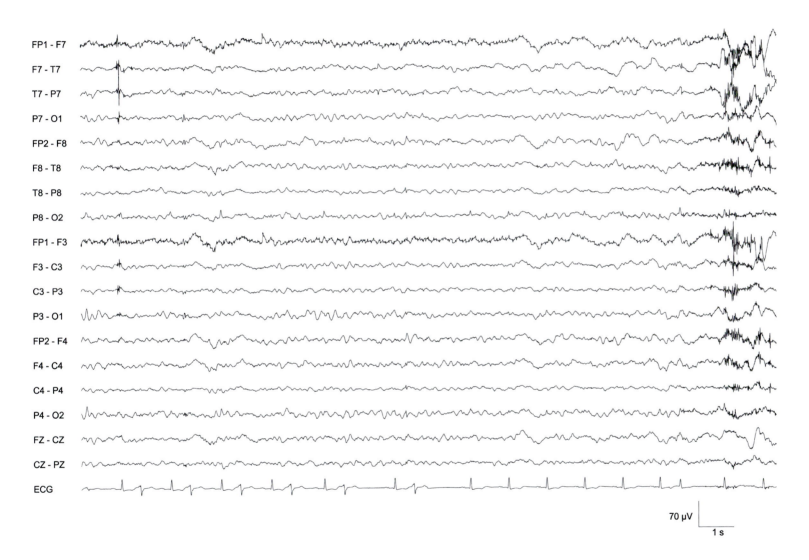

FP1 - F7
F7 - T7
T7 - P7
P7 - O1
FP2 - F8
F8 - T8
T8 - P8
P8 - O2
FP1 - F3
F3 - C3
C3 - P3
P3 - O1
FP2 - F4
F4 - C4
C4 - P4
P4 - O2
FZ - CZ
CZ - PZ
ECG

70 µV

1 s

▶ **Figure 2.115** **ECG artifact.** Bipolar longitudinal montage. In cardiac arrhythmias, the arrhythmia is also reflected in the ECG artifact (best seen at channel P8–O2).

ECG artifact of the mother in the EEG of the child

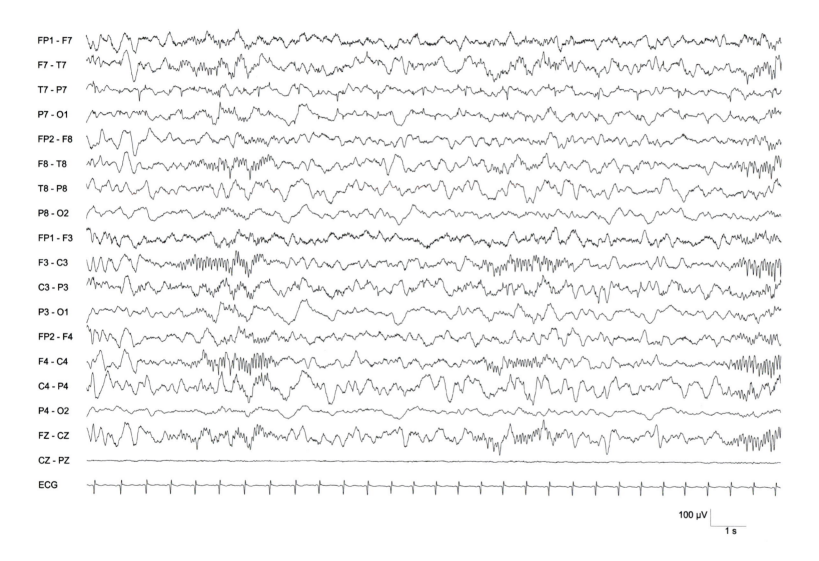

▶ **Figure 2.116** **ECG artifact of the mother in the EEG of the child.** Bipolar longitudinal montage. During this EEG, the sleeping infant is lying on the mother's chest. The infant's P7 electrode records the negative ECG artifact of the mother. The child's ECG artifact can also be seen in the same electrode with a positive polarity. The ECG of the child is recorded in the lowest channel.

amplitude of the EEG activity decreases (▶ **Figure 2.113**). The ECG artifact is consistently of higher amplitude at electrodes near the trunk on the ear or mastoid protuberance (▶ **Figure 2.113**). However, other electrodes may also show ECG artifacts. ECG artifacts are consistently seen in recordings showing electrocerebral silence because there is no brain activity, and those recordings are always reviewed using extremely high sensitivity (▶ **Figure 2.114**).

The ECG on the head is a dipole corresponding to the electrical axis of the heart (▶ **Figure 2.114**). The right ear is negative and the left ear positive, whereby the axis at the head is typically somewhat oblique. The regularity of the ECG artifact facilitates recognition. However, in patients with cardiac arrhythmias, the ECG can be confused with small temporal spikes (▶ **Figure 2.115**). The mother's ECG can be interspersed with the EEG of an infant who has been breastfed by the mother during the EEG (▶ **Figure 2.116**). The electrode P7 of the child touched the left breast of the mother and, thus, records the ECG of the mother (▶ **Figure 2.116**).

Artifacts

Artifacts must always be identified and, if possible, eliminated. However, some artifacts cannot be eliminated (EMG, movement artifacts, eye movement artifacts, etc.), and the EEG reader must be able to differentiate artifacts from other brain activity.

2 Fundamentals of EEG

3

CLINICAL ELECTROENCEPHALOGRAPHY

3.1 Recording of Electroencephalograms

The electroencephalogram (EEG) recording follows a standardized sequence. The electrodes (preferably silver/silver chloride) are placed according to the 10/20 system (see **Figure 1.1**). For long-term recordings, silver electrodes with gold coating are used to protect the skin (see **Figure 2.7**). The resistances of the electrodes are measured (ideal value: <5 kΩ), and a calibration of the device is carried out. Calibration consists of injecting a square wave signal of defined amplitude into the input of all channels. A standard recording lasts 20 min and should take place in a quiet room that can be darkened. There should be no distraction such as mobile phones or computer games. Restless young children should be accompanied by a familiar person. If necessary, the child could be breastfed. To promote rest and relaxation, we record all EEGs with patients lying in a comfortable bed. All electrodes of the 10/20 system and the two ear electrodes are recorded against a reference (CPZ; see **Figure 1.2**) that is not in the 10/20 system in digital EEG devices. The ECG is recorded simultaneously via electrodes on the wrists. For long-term EEG recordings, the ECG electrodes are placed on the chest. During the EEG, alertness and responsiveness (mental activation tests) must be tested. Simple cognitive tasks (e.g., counting) serve this purpose. When tongue movement artifacts (glossokinetic artifacts) occur during counting/speaking (see **Figures 2.107** and **2.108**), the patients should be asked to count silently. Responsiveness is tested during ictal events following a standardized protocol (Beniczky et al., 2016).

Additional electrodes (FT9 and FT10 and other 10/10 system electrodes) should be used (see Figure 1.2) if a patient is a surgical candidate. Recording from these additional electrodes improves the accuracy of the localization of interictal spikes or of EEG seizure patterns (▶ **Figure 3.1**). Without the anterior temporal electrodes FT9 and FT10, one might miss these spikes (▶ **Figure 3.2**). In mesial temporal lobe epilepsy, spikes tend to be of higher amplitude at FT9/FT10 than at T7/T8. The reverse is true for temporal lobe convexity epilepsy, namely spikes are of higher amplitude at T7/T8 compared to FT9/FT10.

Additional surface electromyogram (EMG) recordings can be used to document myoclonia (▶ **Figure 3.3**) or negative myoclonus (see ▶ **Figure 3.195** and Section 3.4.2.4.10).

At the beginning of the recording, the reactivity of the posterior background activity is checked several times by asking the patient to open and close the eyes. After that, the patient should remain relaxed with their eyes closed. The room in which the EEG is recorded should be quiet and comforting. After recording the EEG in a relaxed state for a few minutes, the patient should be asked to hyperventilate, which usually leads to (more) relaxation and drowsiness. This procedure also frequently helps reduce muscle and blinking artifacts. In restless patients, EMG artifacts should not be reduced by filters because filtered EMG activity not infrequently is difficult to differentiate from paroxysmal fast activity (see ▶ **Figures 3.138–3.140**). Photic stimulation is carried out soon after completing the hyperventilation test. Afterward, mental activation should be performed to assess fully awake EEG activity, and the blocking of the posterior background activity by eye opening and closing is tested again. A reaction test to acoustic or visual stimuli (the so-called "clicker test") is used to test and document responsiveness, for example, during generalized spike-waves or focal EEG patterns (▶ **Figures 3.145, 3.146** and **3.194**) (Browne et al., 1974).

3.1.1 Default Settings for EEG Recording

The default settings of gain and filters are listed in ▶ **Table 3.1**. These settings refer to conventional amplifiers. In general, the EEG should be recorded with maximum resolution and the least filtering possible.

The amplitude of EEG on the computer display should be set to optimally display the EEG potentials, but channel overlap should be avoided. Figures 2.15–2.20 show how filter changes influence the display of the calibration signal and ultimately of the EEG. An exception is the 50/60 Hz notch filter for EEG recordings in intensive care units (ICUs), where the surrounding equipment

Advantage of the anterior temporal electrode

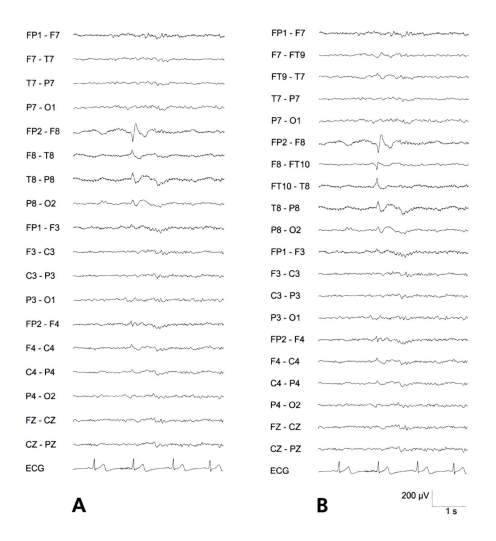

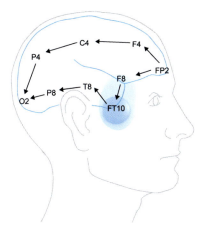

▶ **Figure 3.1** **Advantage of the anterior temporal electrode.** Bipolar longitudinal montage. A and B show the same EEG segment. With the anterior temporal electrode FT10, which is in the 10/10 system, the spike at F8 (A) can be better localized to the anterior mesial part of the temporal lobe (B).

can lead to this kind of interference. Frequently, this artifact cannot be avoided because vital equipment cannot be switched off in the ICU (see **Figure 2.73**). A notch filter can be applied to reduce 50/60 Hz artifact, and usually its use does not change the EEG trace significantly. On the other hand, filtering out of EEG activity should be avoided or done very cautiously because it may change the EEG significantly, and since filters can be applied when reviewing the EEG afterwards. The typical example is filtering out of EMG activity with the remaining activity appearing like paroxysmal fact activity (see ▶ **Figures 3.138–3.140**).

Advantage of the anterior temporal electrode

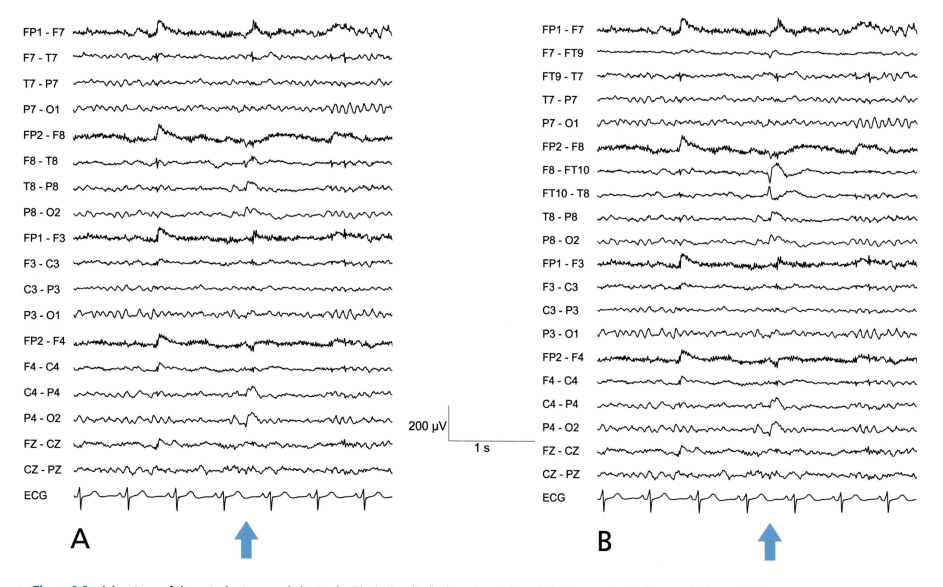

▶ **Figure 3.2** **Advantage of the anterior temporal electrode.** Bipolar longitudinal montage. The anterior temporal spike (blue arrow) in FT10 (B) is not visible in the montage without FT10 (A).

Myoclonic seizure

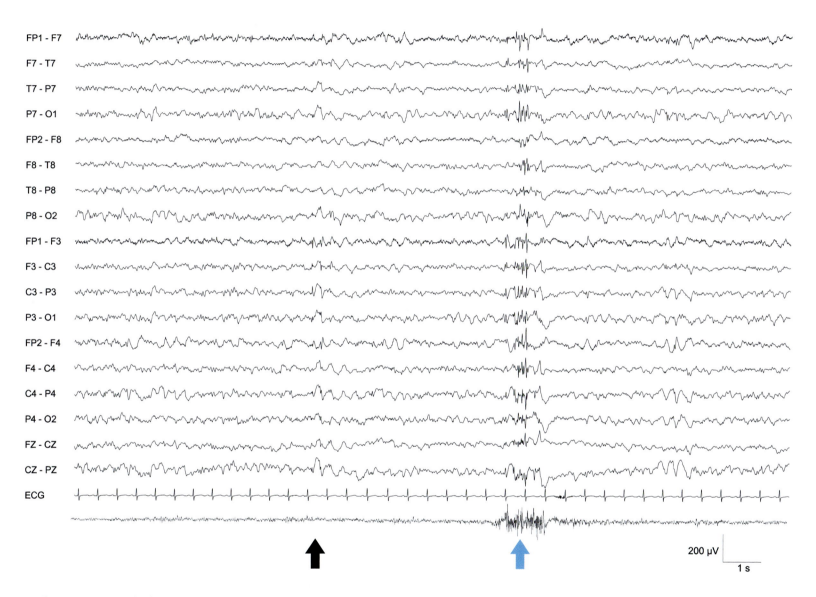

▶ **Figure 3.3** **Myoclonic seizure.** Bipolar longitudinal montage. This patient with mitochondropathy (myoclonic epilepsy with ragged red fibers [MERFF]) had bilateral myoclonic seizures of the legs (blue arrow). The myoclonic jerks were associated with a generalized muscle artifact, as can be seen in the ECG channel. The EEG shows the myogenic artifact presumably mixed with generalized polyspikes. The black arrow points at spike–waves most prominent at F3 and C3, followed by spike–waves at F4–C4 approximately 300 ms later. These spikes were not associated with any EMG or clinical manifestation.

> ▶ **Table 3.1 Default settings for EEG recording**

	Gain (µV/cm)[a]	Lower Cutoff Frequency (Hz)	Upper Cutoff Frequency (Hz)	Horizontal Sampling Rate	Vertical Resolution
EEG	70	0.5–1	70	>200 Hz	>12 bit
EOG	ca. 200	0.1	70		
ECG	500–1,000	0.5	70		
EMG	Individual	5–10	100		

[a]The gain in digital machines is set to optimally display the EEG according to the size and resolution of the screen.
ECG, electrocardiogram; EEG, electroencephalogram; EMG, electromyogram; EOG, electro-oculogram.

3.1.2 Recording of Newborn EEGs

The recording of EEGs in newborns differs significantly from the EEG recordings of adults or children. The head of newborns is very small, and the frontopolar electrodes show very little EEG activity. Therefore, the 10/20 frontopolar (FP1 and FP2) and superior frontal (F3 and F4) electrodes are replaced by electrodes at half the distance between FP2 and F4 or FP1 and F3 (Clancy et al., 2003). These electrodes are called AF4 and AF3 according to the 10/10 system nomenclature. ▶ **Table 3.2** illustrates one of the longitudinal montages with the reduced number of electrodes. In addition, in newborns it is essential to also record respiration, submental EMG activity, eye movements, and ECG. The polygraphic recordings obtained in this way are essential to assess if the newborn is awake or asleep and to determine the stage of sleep that is being recorded. In the interpretation of newborn recordings, it is very important to record a complete awake–sleep cycle. Therefore, the recordings should be more extensive to include all the different stages of awake and sleep. In addition, EEGs in newborns and premature infants are often derived under very difficult technical conditions, not infrequently with a patient in an incubator. This requires special technical abilities. Moreover, because the skin of newborns tends to be extremely sensitive, special care is required when applying the electrodes.

> ▶ **Table 3.2 Bipolar Neonatal Montage**

Channel	Electrodes/Device
1	AF3–C3
2	C3–O1
3	AF3–T7
4	T7–O1
5	AF4–C4
6	C4–O2
7	AF4–T8
8	T8–O2
9	FZ–CZ
10	CZ–PZ
11	Nasal air flow
12	Left inferior outer canthus–nasion
13	ECG
14	Submental EMG
15	Respiratory thoracic bands

ECG, electrocardiogram; EMG, electromyogram.

3.2 Activation Methods

The following activation methods (Fisch & So, 2003) can be used to increase the diagnostic yield of the EEG, mainly of interictal epileptiform discharges (IEDs):

- Hyperventilation
- Photic stimulation
- Sleep and sleep deprivation

3.2.1 Hyperventilation

Hyperventilation (HV) elicits in normal individuals medium- to high-amplitude rhythmical theta or delta waves frequently most prominent in the frontal region (frontal rhythmic delta activity [FIRDA]) (**Figures 3.4** and **3.5**). The HV-induced EEG slow disappears gradually 2 or 3 min after the patient breathes normally again. The magnitude of the HV-induced response depends on the HV effort made by the patient, the blood glucose level, and the age of the patient. Approximately 70% of children and 10% of adults show the typical physiological HV response in the EEG illustrated in ▶ **Figures 3.4** and **3.5** (Mendez & Brenner, 2006). HV-induced FIRDA is a physiological response of no diagnostic significance. On the other hand, HV is a potent activator of bursts of 3 Hz spike–waves and, therefore, a valuable diagnostic technique when absence epilepsy is suspected. In children with untreated absence epilepsy, HV triggers bursts of generalized spike–waves in approximately 80% of cases. Activation by HV of focal epileptiform discharges or actual focal seizures is significantly less frequent (4–9%) (Dalby, 1969). HV may also exaggerate EEG asymmetries with either a more pronounced slow or a relatively less clearly defined increase of slow on the pathological side or lobule. Clear asymmetries exaggerated by HV are usually an expression of a focal structural lesion.

HV is a very low-risk activation procedure. Relative contraindications include acute stroke; subacute cerebral hemorrhage, especially subarachnoid hemorrhage; critical stenosis of intra- or extracranial cerebral vessels, particularly moyamoya syndrome; severe cardiopulmonary disease; and sickle cell anemia.

HV helps most patients relax; the amplitude of posterior alpha activity tends to increase, and EMG activity also tends to become less prominent. That is the reason that in many laboratories, HV is performed relatively early during the EEG recording session. HV, if performed properly, induces an unpleasant dizziness and tingling of feet and hands. Most patients try to avoid these manifestations unless properly encouraged by the technologist. Obtaining a good HV effort is usually very difficult in children, particularly cognitively impaired children. Having the patient blow trying to activate a paper windmill may be helpful in these cases. On the other hand, a child who is crying usually will also hyperventilate. The crying-induced HV in turn will trigger different degrees of generalized slowing. Obviously, the HV-induced slow should not be considered abnormal.

It had been speculated that HV would produce hypocapnia, which secondarily produced vasoconstriction and a reduced supply of glucose and oxygen to the cortex. The reduced supply of glucose and oxygen to the cortex would be manifested by the typical EEG slow seen with HV. Later evidence demonstrated, though, that the direct effect of hypocapnia on the ascending reticular activating system in the brainstem and thalamus was responsible for the HV-induced EEG slow (Patel & Maulsby, 1987). It is also well established that hypoglycemia is related to a more pronounced HV slow (Drake, 1986).

3.2.2 Photic Stimulation

Photic stimulation (PS) activates epileptiform discharges in 20–30% of patients with generalized epilepsies but only in approximately 3% of patients with focal epilepsy (Binnie, 1999; Verrotti et al., 2004; Wolf & Goosses, 1986). PS is perceived as unpleasant by many patients and not infrequently associated with a significant increase of EMG and movement artifacts, making EEG

Frontal intermittent rhythmic delta activity (FIRDA)

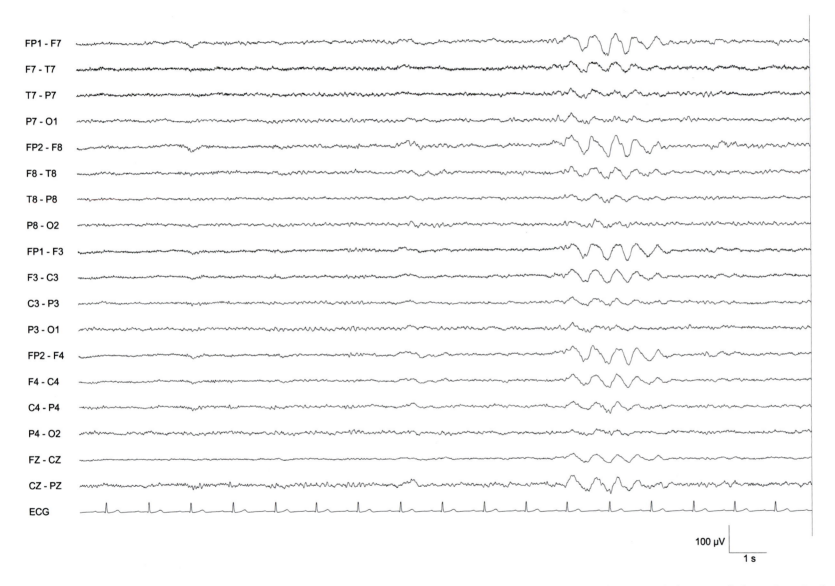

▶ **Figure 3.4** **Frontal intermittent rhythmic delta activity (FIRDA).** Bipolar longitudinal montage. After approximately 1-min hyperventilation, a 2- or 3-s burst of rhythmic, generalized maximum frontal delta waves interrupts the background activity. Burst of delta slowing during hyperventilation is seen mainly in children, but even in adults, it is a normal physiological response without clinical significance. FIRDA is a purely descriptive term.

Frontal intermittent rhythmic delta activity (FIRDA)

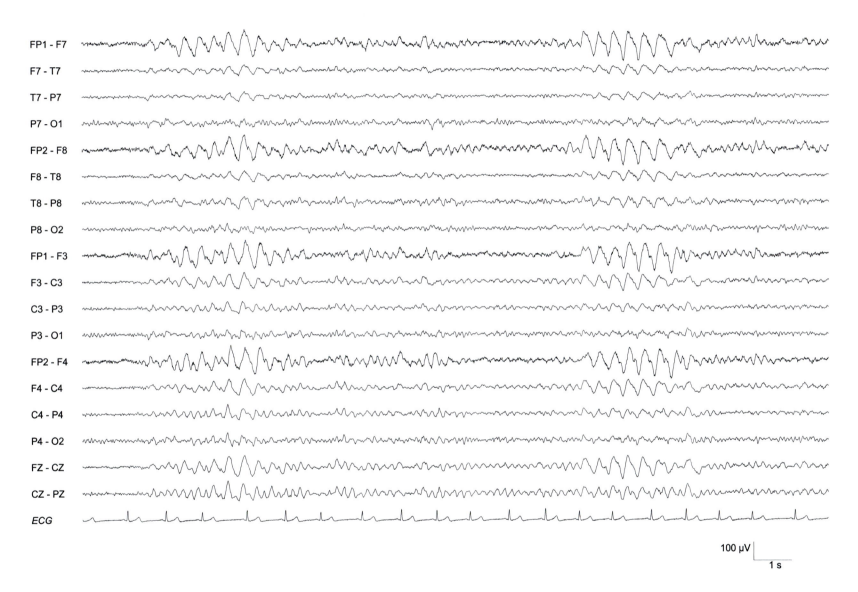

▶ **Figure 3.5** **Frontal intermittent rhythmic delta activity (FIRDA).** Bipolar longitudinal montage. Adult patient who had 3- or 4-s bursts of rhythmic, generalized maximum frontal delta waves interrupting the background activity after approximately 2-min hyperventilation. The same as ▶ **Figure 3.4**, this is a normal physiological response without clinical significance.

▶ **Table 3.3** **Parameters for Photic Stimulation**

Light intensity	Single flashes or flash series of constant intensity; >0.7 J per flash
Distance of the lamp	30 cm to the patient's nasion
Eyelids	Closed
Frequencies	1–60 Hz (first series: 1, 2, 3, 4, 6, 8, 10, 12, 14, 16, 18, and 20; second series: 60, 50, 40, 30, 25, and 20)
Duration of each stimulation frequency	4–10 s (up to 30 s)
Pause between different stimulations	7 s

Sources: Kasteleijn-Nolst Trenité et al. (1999, 2012).

interpretation difficult. That is the reason why in most laboratories, PS is performed at the end of EEG recordings. The parameters recommended for PS are listed in ▶ **Table 3.3.**

The stimulation lamp is positioned at a distance of 30 cm from the nasion. The eyes should be closed to minimize blink artifacts. With a light intensity of >0.7 J per flash, a good photic-induced response will be obtained even when the eyelids are closed. PS is performed in blocks of 4–10 s with a pause of more than 7 s between the blocks. In general, it is recommended that PS should be started manually for each frequency block and should end automatically after 10 s. In addition, to prevent PS from triggering epileptic seizures, PS must be switched off immediately if epileptiform activity is elicited by the stimulation.

Photic driving (▶ Figures 3.6–3.9) and photomyoclonic responses (▶ Figures 3.10 and 3.11) are physiological activations triggered by PS. Photic driving consists of synchronization of the posterior/occipital background rhythms to the photic stimulus. Typically, there is a 1:1 ratio between the light flash and the occipital rhythm, and the synchronized posterior/occipital rhythm occurs 70–150 ms after the flash ("photic driving"). Rarely, the synchronization ratio is 1:2 or higher. Photic driving occurs most frequently when PS is performed

at approximately ±1 or 2 Hz of the patient's background/occipital rhythm's frequency. Normal newborns and children frequently have high-amplitude visual evoked potentials. Therefore, when stimulating newborns or children at low frequency, each flash tends to be followed by a high-amplitude evoked potential localized to the occipital leads ("giant evoked potentials"). This is normal in newborn and infants, but in adults giant visual evoked potentials are frequently seen in patients with occipital cortex hyperexcitability, such as in Unverricht progressive myoclonus. Photic driving is not infrequently significantly asymmetric, most probably because it is mainly generated in the primary visual area of the occipital pole, which in normal individuals tends to have significant asymmetries in its orientation and also in its anatomy (▶ **Figure 3.9**). Therefore, EEGs that show only an asymmetric driving should not be classified as abnormal.

Photomyoclonic responses consist of muscle twitching in the facial and forehead areas that are strictly synchronized with the flash stimulus. They represent a muscular reflex that occurs in normal individuals and is not associated with epilepsy (▶ **Figures 3.10** and **3.11**) (Newmark & Penry, 1979).

Photoparoxysmal responses are epileptiform discharges triggered by PS (▶ **Figures 3.12–3.14**). The degree of epileptogenicity of a photoparoxysmal response depends on (a) the distribution of the epileptiform discharge, (b) whether the discharge is time-locked with the flash, and (c) the persistence of the epileptiform discharge after discontinuing the photic stimulus. According to these criteria, the following degrees of epileptogenicity are used:

Photoparoxysmal response I (EEG abnormal I)

Giant photic evoked responses that are limited mainly to the occipital leads, are strictly time-locked to the flash and disappear as soon as the photic stimulus is discontinued. As mentioned above, such giant evoked potentials are normal in newborns and infants but are indicative of slightly increased epileptogenicity of the occipital cortex when seen in adults (▶ **Figure 3.12** and **Figure 3.165**). Also notice that the photic driving in ▶ **Figure 3.9** is of constant amplitude and shape from one stimulus to the next at 1 Hz. In contrast, the photoparoxysmal response illustrated in ▶ **Figure 3.12** shows great variability in amplitude and only occurs after selected flash stimuli. The inconsistency of response also suggests a higher degree of epileptogenicity.

Photic driving

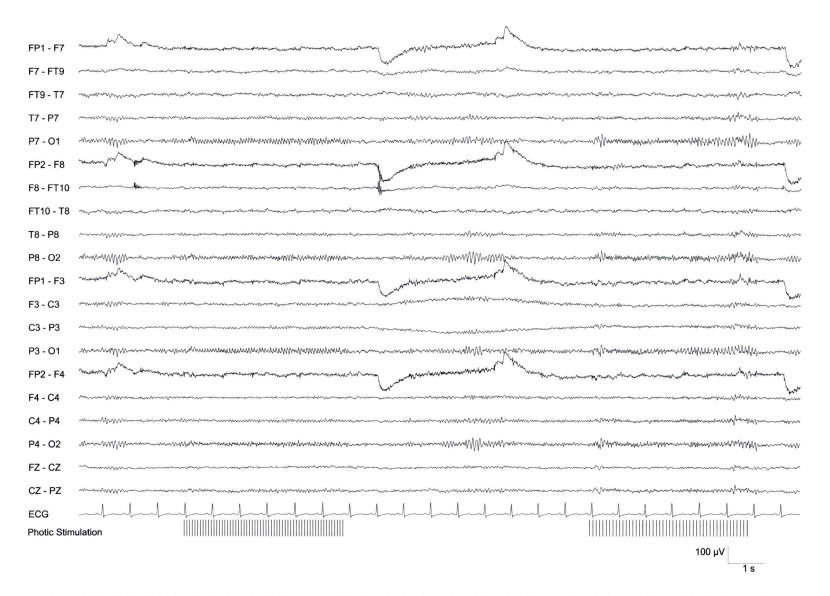

FP1 - F7
F7 - FT9
FT9 - T7
T7 - P7
P7 - O1
FP2 - F8
F8 - FT10
FT10 - T8
T8 - P8
P8 - O2
FP1 - F3
F3 - C3
C3 - P3
P3 - O1
FP2 - F4
F4 - C4
C4 - P4
P4 - O2
FZ - CZ
CZ - PZ
ECG
Photic Stimulation

100 µV

1 s

▶ **Figure 3.6** **Photic driving.** Bipolar longitudinal montage. Photic stimulation at 15 and 12 Hz leads to synchronization of the occipital background rhythm with the photic stimulus. At 15 Hz photic stimulation, the synchronization (1:1) occurs almost immediately and the amplitude of the derived response is more or less constant. At 12 Hz, initially there is a low-amplitude 1:2 synchronization. After a few seconds, the driving becomes 1:1 and the amplitude of the photic evoked potentials increases significantly. A spindle-like modulated occipital alpha background rhythm appears in the periods between photic stimulation. This is a normal response to photic stimulation.

Photic driving and mu rhythm

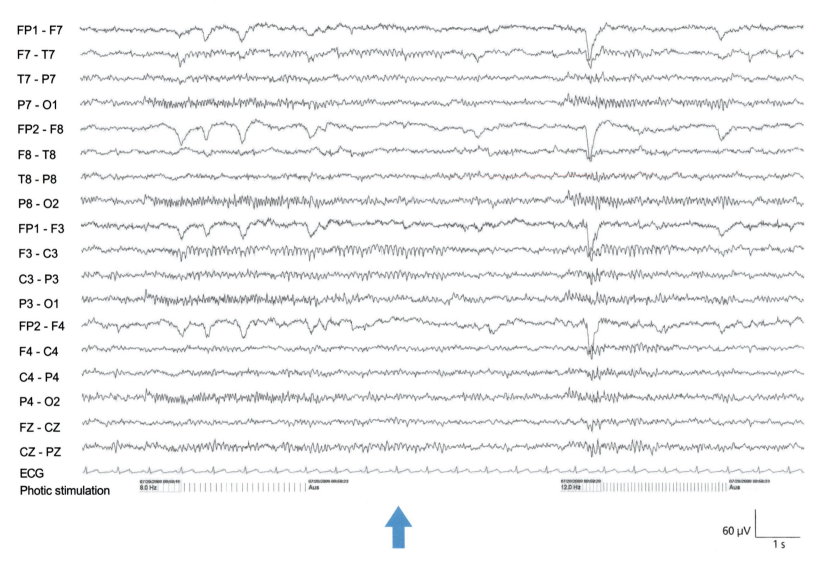

▶ **Figure 3.7**   **Photic driving and mu rhythm.** Bipolar longitudinal montage. Photic stimulation at 8 and 12 Hz leads to photic driving. There is a prominent mu rhythm at P4 and C4 (blue arrow) that is not driven by the photic stimulation.

Photic driving

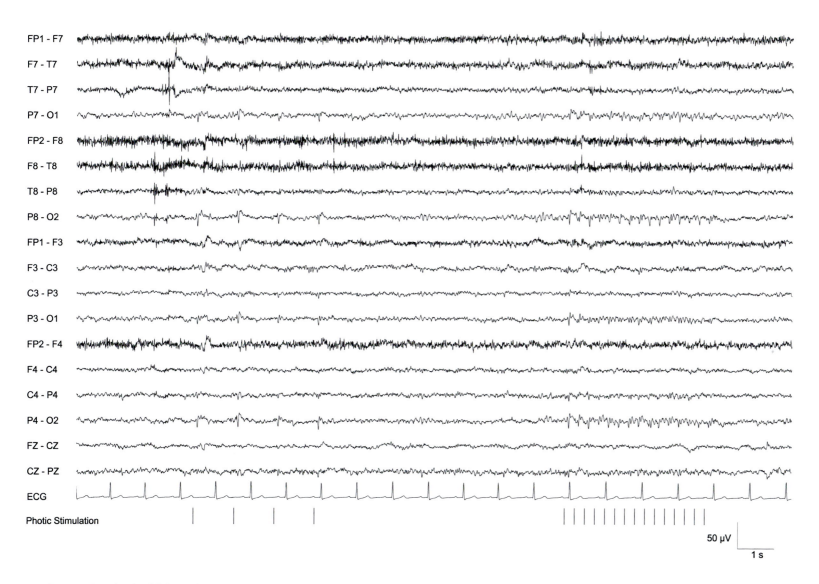

▶ **Figure 3.8** **Photic driving.** Bipolar longitudinal montage. Photic stimulation at 1 Hz elicits a clear photic evoked potential at O1 and O2. Stimulation at 6 Hz elicited a mixture of photic evoked responses and driving. The photic evoked response consisted of a small positivity followed by a relatively high-amplitude negative wave maximum at O1 and O2.

Photic driving, right occipital

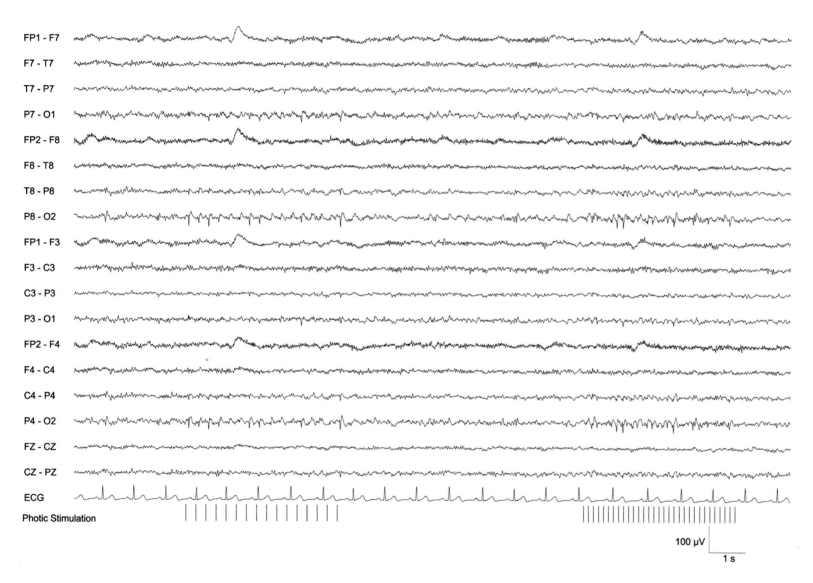

FP1 - F7	
F7 - T7	
T7 - P7	
P7 - O1	
FP2 - F8	
F8 - T8	
T8 - P8	
P8 - O2	
FP1 - F3	
F3 - C3	
C3 - P3	
P3 - O1	
FP2 - F4	
F4 - C4	
C4 - P4	
P4 - O2	
FZ - CZ	
CZ - PZ	
ECG	
Photic Stimulation	

100 μV

1 s

▶ **Figure 3.9** **Photic driving, right occipital.** Bipolar longitudinal montage. Photic evoked potentials and driving triggered by photic stimulation at 4 and 8 Hz. Photic evoked potentials and driving, even in normal individuals, frequently are asymmetric. This is most likely because the photic evoked potentials and the driving are generated in the occipital pole, and even small asymmetries of the anatomy will result in major asymmetries of the evoked potentials and also the driving.

Photic driving and photomyoclonic response

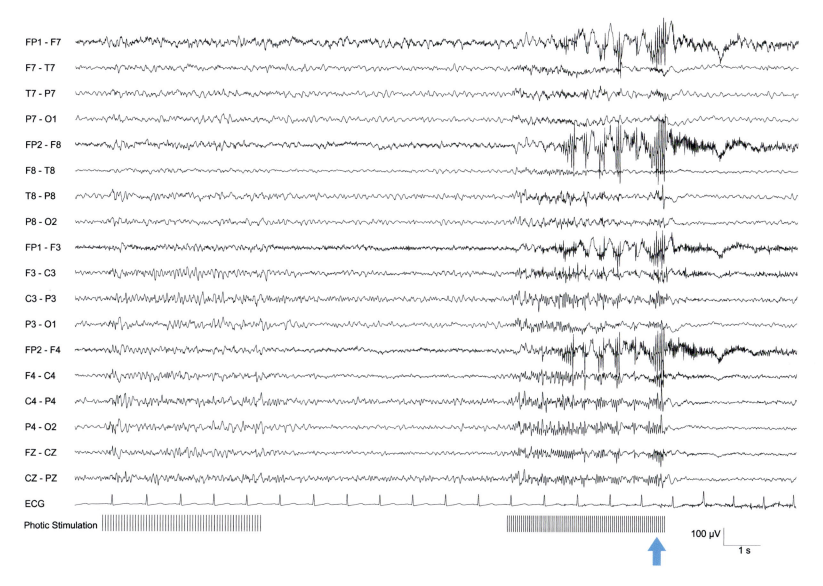

▶ **Figure 3.10** **Photic driving and photomyoclonic response.** Bipolar longitudinal montage. Photic stimulation at 15 Hz and more clearly at 20 Hz leads to photic driving. Stimulation at 20 Hz also leads to a photomyoclonic response (i.e., muscle twitching), most prominent at the frontalis muscle (blue arrow). Photomyoclonic response is an unusual but normal response to intermittent photic stimulation. The absence of photic-induced EMG artifact at the ECG indicates that the photomyoclonus is limited to cranial muscles. However, it is essentially impossible to differentiate the myoclonic response from the epileptiform discharge when both occur simultaneously.

Photomyoclonic response

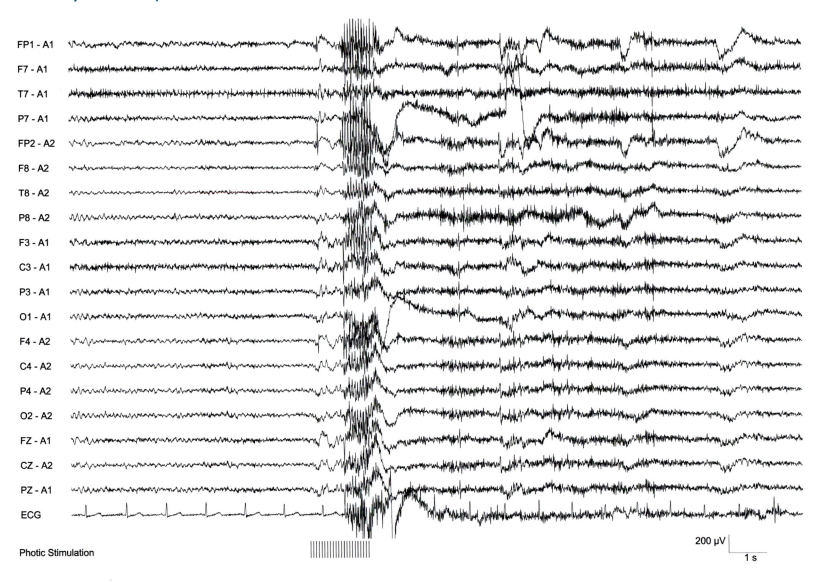

FP1 - A1

F7 - A1

T7 - A1

P7 - A1

FP2 - A2

F8 - A2

T8 - A2

P8 - A2

F3 - A1

C3 - A1

P3 - A1

O1 - A1

F4 - A2

C4 - A2

P4 - A2

O2 - A2

FZ - A1

CZ - A2

PZ - A1

ECG

Photic Stimulation

200 µV

1 s

▶ **Figure 3.11** **Photomyoclonic response.** Ipsilateral ear reference montage. Another example of photomyoclonus. See legend to ▶ **Figure 3.10**.

Photoparoxysmal response, occipital (EEG abnormal I)

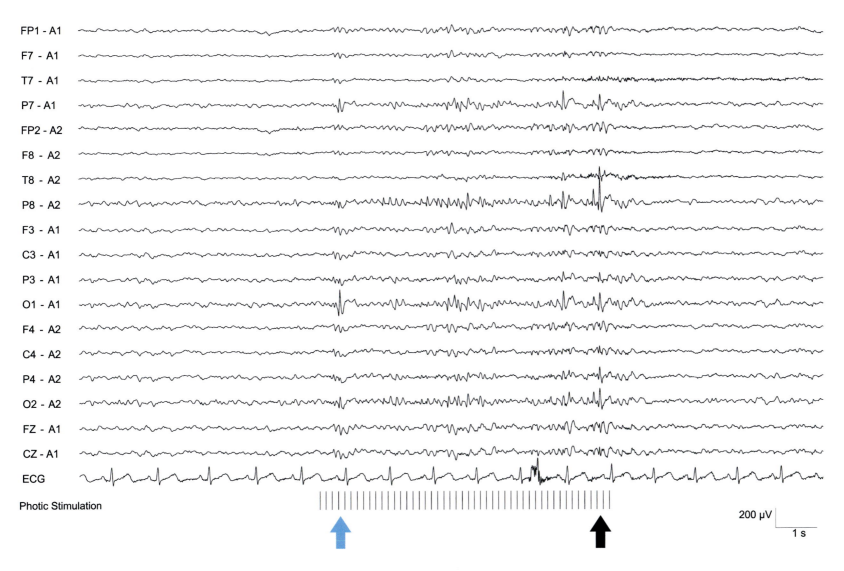

▶ **Figure 3.12** **Photoparoxysmal response, occipital (EEG abnormal I).** Ipsilateral ear reference montage. Photic stimulation at 8 Hz leads to left occipital (blue arrow) and later right posterior temporal (black arrow) spikes. Photic evoked spikes limited to the posterior leads are not indicative of abnormal epileptogenicity.

Photoparoxysmal response II (EEG abnormal II)

Generalized epileptiform discharges that are not time-locked to the stimulus. Included here are also photoparoxysmal responses that disappear despite continuous flash stimulation or that stop as soon as the flash stimulus is discontinued. These discharges are indicative of a moderately strong generalized epileptogenicity (▶ **Figure 3.13**).

Photoparoxysmal response III (EEG abnormal III)

Generalized epileptiform discharges that outlast the stimulus correlate strongly with the presence of generalized epilepsy (▶ **Figure 3.14**).

Note that patients with focal epileptogenic lesions of the occipital region only very infrequently have epileptiform discharges or epileptic seizures triggered by PS.

3.2.3 Sleep and Sleep Deprivation

Epileptiform discharges can be activated by sleep and sleep deprivation (Fountain et al., 1998; Gibbs & Gibbs, 1952). EEG derivation after sleep deprivation should include sleep because this increases the diagnostic yield compared to pure awake recordings (Fountain et al., 1998). Sleep is a potent activator of tonic seizures in patients with epileptic encephalopathies. Therefore, a sleep-deprived patient will sleep longer in the lab and have many more seizures compared to a patient who does not sleep during the recording.

Sleep deprivation can trigger epileptic seizures; therefore, patients should be warned of this possibility to ensure they take appropriate precautions. They should always be accompanied by family members or caregivers. Patients with juvenile myoclonic epilepsy are particularly prone to facilitation by sleep deprivation (Janz & Christian, 1957).

Protocols for sleep-deprived EEGs vary in the literature, and there is not sufficient objective evidence to determine which is the best protocol. We recommend the following procedure: Sleep-deprived EEGs are only ordered in patients in which epilepsy is suspected and the standard EEG shows no abnormality or at least no clearly defined epileptiform discharges.

In most cases, partial sleep deprivation is sufficient—that is, the bedtime on the day before the sleep-deprived EEG recording should be limited to less than half of the normal sleep duration (i.e. sleep only the second half of the typical night sleep (for example 3:00–7:00 a.m.). Stimulants (coffee, tea, energy drinks, etc.) should be avoided to facilitate sleep. The recording of the sleep-deprived EEG should be performed preferentially in the early afternoon after lunch to take additional advantage of postprandial sleepiness. The examination should take place in a comfortable bed in a darkened, quiet room to facilitate falling asleep. The duration of the examination should be set at 60 min.

3.2.4 Eye Closure

Eyelid closure may trigger either generalized or bilateral occipital epileptiform discharges in the EEG (▶ **Figure 3.15**). This phenomenon is called eyelid closure activity. It is a rare epileptiform abnormality and usually is seen in patients with idiopathic generalized and various occipital epilepsies (Sevgi et al., 2007; Tekin Güveli et al., 2013; Yang et al., 2008). Eyelid closure activity must be distinguished from rhythmic theta–delta wave bursts after eyelid closure, which are physiological phenomena, namely subharmonics of alpha activity ("alpha variants"; (▶ **Figure 3.16**) or occipital (posterior) slow waves of youth (see Section 3.4.1.1.1). Eyelid closure activity must also be distinguished from fixation-off sensitivity, in which generalized high-amplitude epileptiform discharges are triggered as soon as gaze fixation of central vision is lost—for example, during eye closure (▶ **Figure 3.17**) (Brigo et al., 2013). In this case, the EEG discharges disappear in complete darkness or when the eyes are opened. Epileptiform discharges can also be abolished if in complete darkness, the patient fixates vision on a very small, low-intensity red spot of light. An EEG with Frenzel glasses, which prevents fixation of the gaze, can also be obtained to distinguish between fixation-off sensitivity and inhibition of epileptiform discharges by eye opening. Fixation-off sensitivity is a rare EEG abnormality seen most frequently in patients with idiopathic epilepsy (syndrome of eyelid myoclonia with absences) and focal symptomatic epilepsies (Fattouch et al., 2013; Kaul et al., 2012). Occasionally, patients with benign occipital epileptiform discharges but no clinical seizures may also show fixation-off sensitivity (Brigo et al., 2013; Koutroumanidis et al., 2009).

Photoparoxysmal response, generalized (EEG abnormal II)

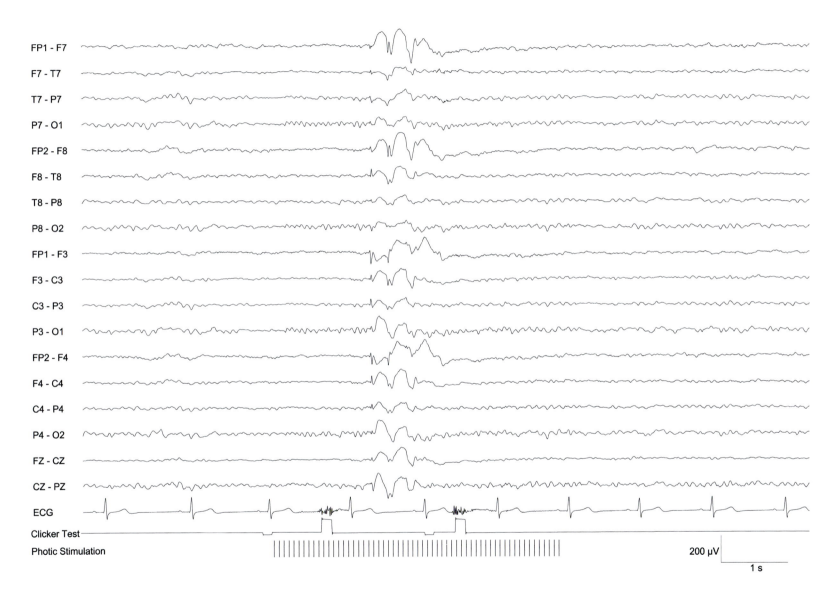

▶ **Figure 3.13** **Photoparoxysmal response, generalized (EEG abnormal II).** Bipolar longitudinal montage. Photic stimulation at 15 Hz leads to generalized spikes that end before photic stimulation is discontinued. This phenomenon (generalized spike–waves elicited by photic stimulation) is indicative of moderately increased, generalized epileptogenicity. However, in this case, it is unclear, from analyzing a single EEG page, if this burst of spike–waves was induced by photic stimulation or occurred spontaneously during photic stimulation. Spontaneously occurring spike–waves are classified as abnormal III, as are spike–waves that outlast the end of photic stimulation. This phenomenon has a high association with epilepsy (see ▶ **Figure 3.14**).

Photoparoxysmal response, generalized (EEG abnormal III)

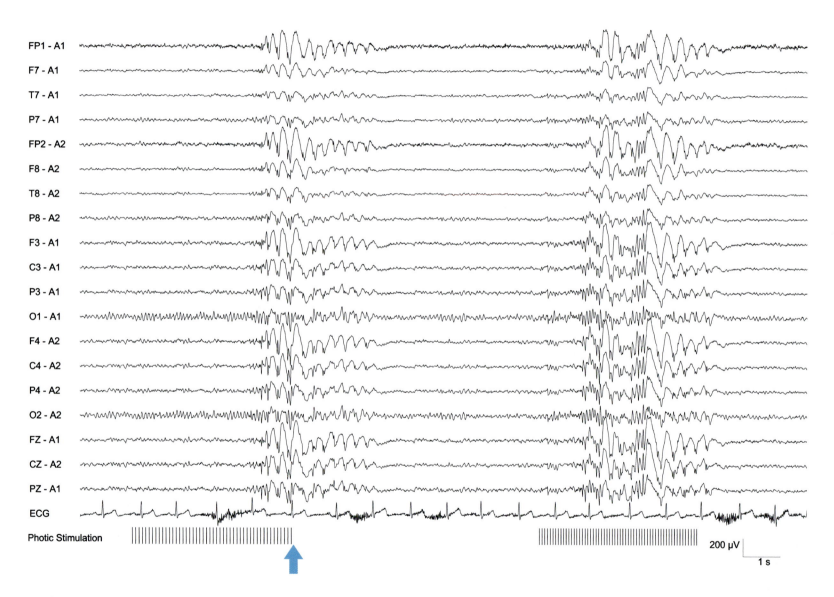

▶ **Figure 3.14** **Photoparoxysmal response, generalized (EEG abnormal III).** Bipolar longitudinal montage. During photic stimulation, generalized spike–waves outlast the end of photic stimulation, with stimulation at 12 Hz (blue arrow) more obvious than stimulation at 15 Hz. This phenomenon has a high association with epilepsy.

Eye closure triggered spikes

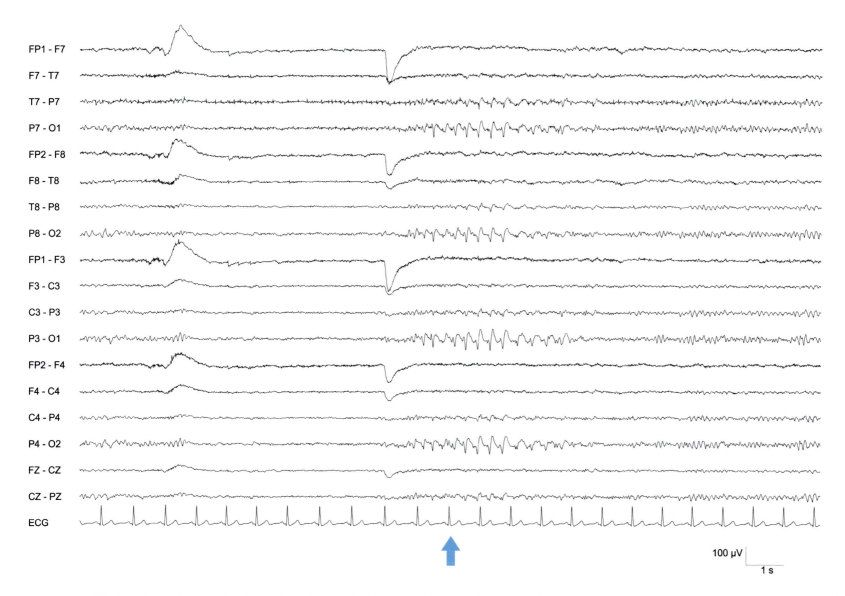

100 µV

1 s

▶ **Figure 3.15** **Eye closure triggered spikes.** Bipolar longitudinal montage. After eye closure, repetitive, bilateral occipital spikes occur for a few seconds (blue arrow). Eye closure triggered occipital spikes occur mainly in patients with idiopathic generalized epilepsies. Interestingly, focal occipital epilepsies only infrequently have an epileptogenic response to eye closure or photic stimulation.

Slow alpha variant background rhythm

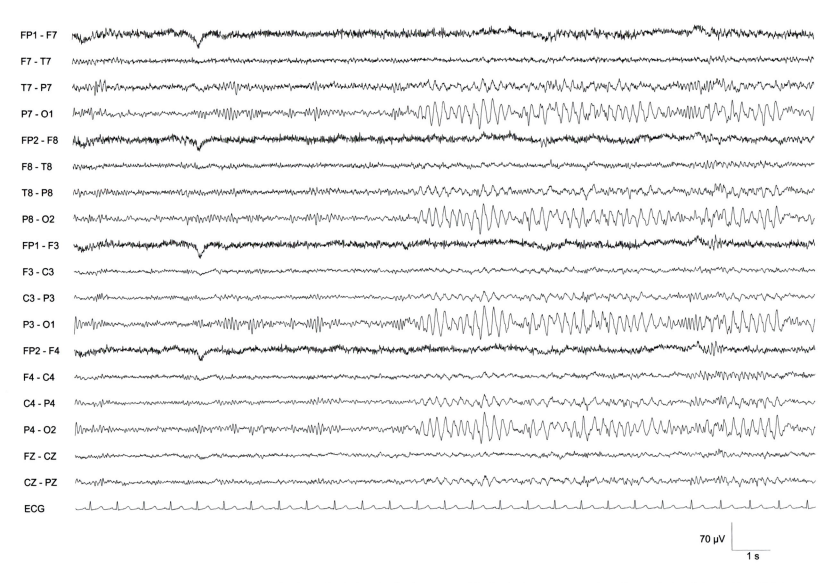

FP1 - F7
F7 - T7
T7 - P7
P7 - O1
FP2 - F8
F8 - T8
T8 - P8
P8 - O2
FP1 - F3
F3 - C3
C3 - P3
P3 - O1
FP2 - F4
F4 - C4
C4 - P4
P4 - O2
FZ - CZ
CZ - PZ
ECG

70 μV

1 s

▶ **Figure 3.16** **Slow alpha variant background rhythm**. Bipolar longitudinal montage. Rhythmic theta waves replace the posterior alpha rhythm. This is a normal phenomenon.

Fixation-off sensitivity

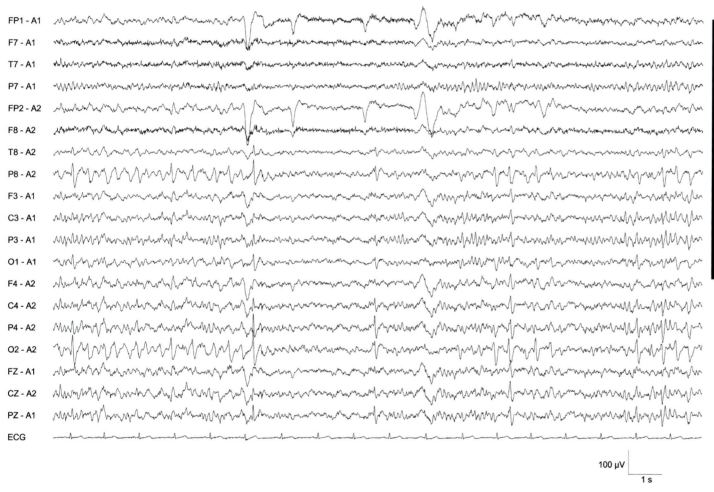
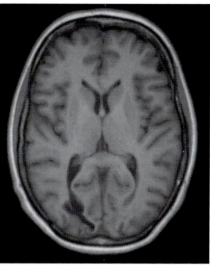

▶ **Figure 3.17** **Fixation-off sensitivity.** Ear reference montage. A 55-year-old female patient with right occipital lobe epilepsy due to an intracerebral hemorrhage caused by a skiing accident. Opening of the eyes ends the repetitive spikes. After eye closure, the spikes resume. Prevention of fixation by Frenzel glasses has the same effect as eye closure. This rare phenomenon indicates an increased epileptogenicity of the occipital lobe but also occurs in patients with generalized epilepsies. Magnetic resonance imaging (MRI) shows the right occipital post-hemorrhagic lesion.

3.3 EEG Reading

Clinical EEG evaluation consists of a mixture of objective and subjective criteria. For example, we define an epileptiform discharge as a sharp transient that stands out from the background activity, has a duration of less than 200 ms, is usually of negative polarity, and has a logical field distribution. However, there are usually many non–epileptiform transients that fulfill this definition (physiological vertex waves of sleep, etc.). Notice the highly subjective expression "that stands out from the background," which is very difficult to quantify. The difficulty in quantifying EEG abnormalities objectively is also the reason computer detection of epileptiform discharges is consistently less reliable than visual interpretation of EEGs and explains the poor agreement between different EEG evaluators (Williams et al., 1985).

The EEG report should provide a detailed description of the abnormal findings, taking into account the terminological recommendations of the International Federation of Clinical Neurophysiology (Kane et al., 2017; Noachtar et al., 1999). The description should also include the frequency of the background activity because it is an excellent index of the degree of encephalopathy if it is less than 8 Hz in adults.

Traditionally, it has been recommended that all EEG reports should include a detailed description (frequency, amplitude, polarity, etc.) of the different EEG patterns seen in normal individuals (e.g., posterior background alpha activity, sleep spindles, V-waves, photic driving, etc.). Over time, we have come to realize, however, that such a detailed description of normal patterns has no practical value. Therefore, we now limit the description of normal EEGs to specification of the frequency of the posterior background activity, the duration of the recording, and if awake and/or sleep has been recorded. The EEG interpreter certainly should be able to differentiate between normal and pathological findings, but the description of these normal EEG patterns (e.g., mu activity, positive occipital steep transients of sleep [POSTS], etc.) has no clinical value. A detailed description of these normal patterns will be of little help in allowing the recipient of the report to assess if indeed the EEG is normal or not. On the other hand, a sample of the EEG will give the recipient of the report, if they have been trained in EEG, an example of the activity that was reported as normal background activity. Therefore, the report of a normal EEG should always include a sample of the background activity. The sample that is included with the EEG report should not be just any EEG sample; rather, in the case of a normal EEG, it should be the best sample of the background activity. In the case of abnormalities, the samples should be the best examples of the abnormalities in the whole recording. The expression "a picture is worth a thousand words" certainly applies in this situation.

The pathological findings are classified according to the EEG classification described in this book. The abnormal classes described in this book all have clearly defined clinical correlates that help in determining the clinical implications of the EEG findings—for example, left frontal spikes supporting the diagnosis of left frontal epilepsy or sleep-onset rapid eye movement (REM) sleep suggesting that the patient has narcolepsy. After the classification of the EEG patterns, the evaluation of the EEG is carried out considering the clinical setting. Recommendations on reporting EEG have been published by the American Clinical Neurophysiology Society (ACNS; see **Appendix 1**).

3.3.1 Description of Abnormal EEG

The EEG description can be freely formulated or tabulated as shown in ▶ **Table 3.4** (Tatum et al., 2016; see **Appendix 1**).

In this book, pathological activity is divided into the following categories:

- Slow and suppression of background
- Epileptiform discharges
- Periodic discharges
- Special patterns
- EEG patterns in patients in stupor or coma

EEG Abnormality[b]	Background Rhythm	Spikes	Continuous Slow	Asymmetry
Sample No.	1	2	3	4
Frequency in Hertz or duration in milliseconds	11 Hz		Irregular 1.5–3 Hz	Beta
Amplitude (µV)		200	~220	<50
Localization of the maximum amplitude of the EEG abnormality	Occipital	FP1 > F7 > F3	Left frontopolar	Increased left frontotemporal
Amount		Four spikes in 20 min when awake	90%	
Triggering factors	Blocked by eye opening	Only seen when patient is awake		
Inhibitory factors		None	Awake	None

[a]See ▶ Figure 3.25.
[b]List one of the possible EEG abnormalities.
EEG, electroencephalogram.

Description of the abnormality in a tabulated form (▶ Table 3.4) has the advantage that it tends to be more concise and will include most of the essential parameters that characterize an EEG abnormality. A good description of an EEG abnormality should allow the reader to clearly visualize the abnormal EEG pattern and its evolution over time. In addition, even more or equally important as the detailed description, it is essential that for each EEG abnormality, the reader should include an actual EEG sample that illustrates best the EEG abnormality detected by the reader. That sample, which shows the most clearly defined abnormal EEG pattern, can then be reviewed by the recipient of the EEG report, and the recipient can then decide if they agree or not with the interpretation of the reader.

EEG abnormalities should be described in detail in addition to providing the best sample of them. The description is necessary because certain essential parameters of EEG abnormalities are not contained in the illustration. This includes mainly the amount, the variability of the pattern over time, and the influence of either triggering or inhibiting factors. More than one sample should be included if the "shape" of the abnormal EEG pattern varies significantly over time.

3.3.1.1   Frequency

Frequency is only specified for rhythms and is indicated as the number of waves per second (e.g., 8/s) or in Hertz (e.g., 8 Hz). If the frequency of a rhythmical abnormal EEG pattern varies greatly over time, the lower and upper limits of the respective frequency ranges should be specified. For non-rhythmical activity, the range of the maximum and minimum frequency is also given. Individual waves or complexes can occur repetitively in intervals of longer duration than their wavelength and are then called periodically, with the period being the time interval between them.

The frequencies of EEG rhythms are named according to the tradition of Hans Berger (1930) using Greek letters (▶ Figure 3.18). The measurement of frequency

Frequency ranges of the EEG

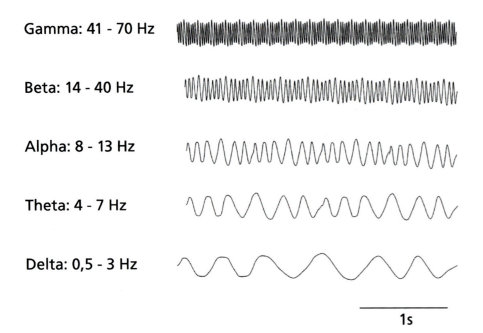

Gamma: 41 - 70 Hz

Beta: 14 - 40 Hz

Alpha: 8 - 13 Hz

Theta: 4 - 7 Hz

Delta: 0,5 - 3 Hz

1s

▶ **Figure 3.18   Frequency ranges of the EEG.** The frequency ranges of the clinical EEG are labeled with Greek letters.

and amplitude is illustrated in ▶ **Figure 3.19**. Alpha (8–13 Hz) and beta frequencies (14–40 Hz) in the occipital region were already described by Hans Berger in the 1930s. Later, slow frequencies were called delta waves (1–3 Hz) (Walter, 1936), with the letter "d" standing for "death," "degeneration," and "disease" because the usually unfavorable prognosis of these slow waves was recognized early on. Waves with frequencies between 4 and 7 Hz were first called intermediate waves in German but now are internationally labeled theta waves (Noachtar et al., 1999).

3.3.1.2   Amplitude

The amplitude and shape of any given EEG pattern depend on the montage used to record the EEG pattern because each channel is recording the difference

Measurement of amplitude and potential duration

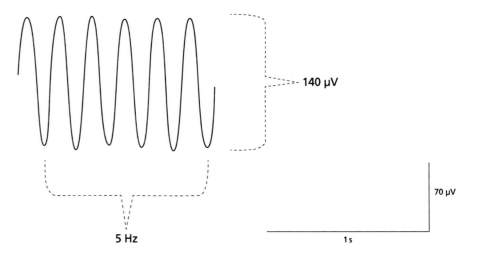

140 µV

5 Hz

70 µV

1s

▶ **Figure 3.19   Measurement of amplitude and potential duration.** Representation of the measurement of potential amplitude and frequency.

in voltage between the two inputs to the amplifier. In addition, the shape and amplitude of the potential of interest can be greatly influenced by application of EEG filters, and certainly the amplitude will vary depending on what brain region the EEG is recording. It is very difficult to precisely measure the amplitude of EEG potentials. On the other hand, amplitudes vary greatly from one individual to another without necessarily helping define an EEG abnormality. This is explained by the fact that amplitudes of normal and also pathological EEG patterns show a normal distribution. A good example is normal controls whose EEG may show extremely low-amplitude alpha waves of less than 10 µV even when measured in a montage referenced to an indifferent electrode and with all EEG filters disabled. In any given individual, however, EEG amplitudes tend to be relatively constant, and a major decrease or increase of amplitude over time is usually an index of a significant change. Exact measurement of amplitudes is extremely cumbersome and of very limited clinical value. On the other hand, as mentioned above, we recommend that all EEG reports should include samples of the background activity and also each EEG pathology. This allows the electroencephalographer to compare the amplitudes of the different

EEG findings and to determine if there was or was not any significant change of EEG amplitudes. Amplitude, however, is an extremely important variable when the patient is comatose or stuporous and we must decide if the patient has background suppression, background attenuation, burst suppression, or burst attenuation.

In general, measurements are made over the entire amplitude of the potential—that is, from maximum to minimum (▶ **Figure 3.19**). Qualitative amplitude expressions such as high, medium, or low should be avoided because they are meaningless. Whatever is high for one observer may be low for another.

3.3.1.3 Localization

Localization of EEG potentials can be very extensive across all brain regions or very limited to one brain area (see Chapter 2, Section 2.2.3). Generalized or diffuse activity occurs almost simultaneously everywhere on the surface of the scalp but may have a more circumscribed maximum. Lateralized activity is limited to one hemisphere. Regional or focal activity occurs only on a few electrodes. Each electrode position according to the 10/20 system reflects a topographical brain region. The more detailed EEG report (an example is shown in ▶ **Table 3.4**), which probably will only be reviewed by EEG-trained individuals, should specify for epileptiform discharges the electrode at which the epileptiform discharge showed the highest amplitude. In the interpretation, which is mainly addressed to neurologists or other nonspecialists, the corresponding brain region should be specified instead of the EEG electrode.

3.3.1.4 Shape and Temporal Behavior

EEG abnormalities may take an infinite number of shapes. That is the reason why the most accurate way to specify the shape is to use an actual picture of the EEG recording—in other words, the best EEG sample of the abnormality. Research and clinical experience (recording and analyzing EEGs in patients of different ages, with different degrees of encephalopathy, in different types of epilepsy, etc.) identified characteristic EEG patterns more or less specific for different ages and different pathologies. These patterns are the different classes

of the EEG classification, and the characteristics of each category are discussed in detail below.

In general, when discussing the shape of any given EEG pattern, we use the expressions specified here. The shape of an EEG pattern is determined by the change of voltage over time in any given channel of the potential of interest. For example, a spike consists of an acute increase of negative polarity of the potential of interest followed by an equally acute decrease of negativity. This acute increase/decrease of negative polarity produces the typical spike shape. Waves are called monophasic, biphasic, triphasic, or polyphasic depending on how often the EEG recording crosses the baseline (▶ **Figure 3.20**). If the waves are uniform—that is, have approximately the same frequency, amplitude, and shape—the activity is called regular, monomorphic, or rhythmic (special form: sinusoidal). Waves of different frequency, amplitude, and shape are called irregular or polymorphic. Different waveforms that form groups are referred to as complexes. They can be regular or irregular, but they also have changing configurations. Sharp or pointed waves are defined as transients that clearly stand out from the background activity. However, there is no objective definition of what "stand out" means. The polarity of an activity should always be defined (e.g., POSTS and 6 Hz positive spikes). EEG interpretation without considering the polarity of the potential of interested can lead to misinterpretation (▶ **Figures 3.21** and **3.22**). Modulation concerns the increase and decrease of amplitudes. Spindle-shaped waveforms occur when an EEG rhythm is the result of two generators that have frequencies close to each other (see **Figure 2.4** and Section 2.1.2).

Waveforms

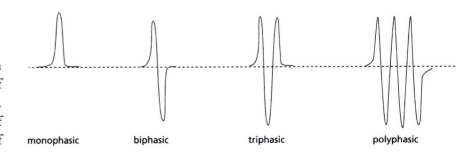

monophasic   biphasic   triphasic   polyphasic

▶ **Figure 3.20** **Waveforms.** Representation of mono-, bi-, tri-, and polyphasic potentials.

Photic evoked potentials versus spike

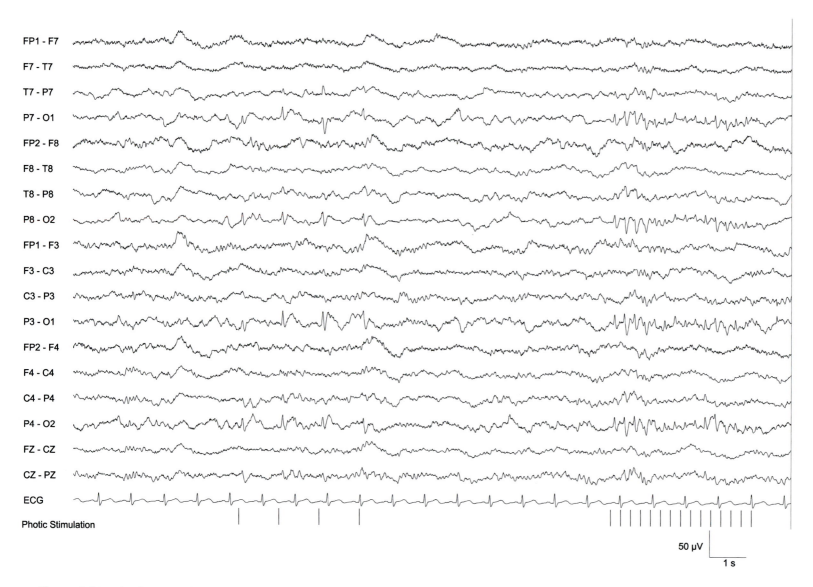

Figure 3.21 **Photic evoked potentials versus spike.** Bipolar longitudinal montage. Photic stimulation at 1 Hz triggers potentials that have the waveform of spike–waves. However, careful analysis reveals that the most prominent component is of positive polarity, strongly suggesting that this is not an epileptiform discharge but, rather, a relatively high-amplitude evoked potential. An analysis of the relationship of the O1/O2 spike with the stimulus artifact showed that, indeed, the occipital spike-waves are time-locked with the stimulus artifact.

Photic evoked potential versus spike

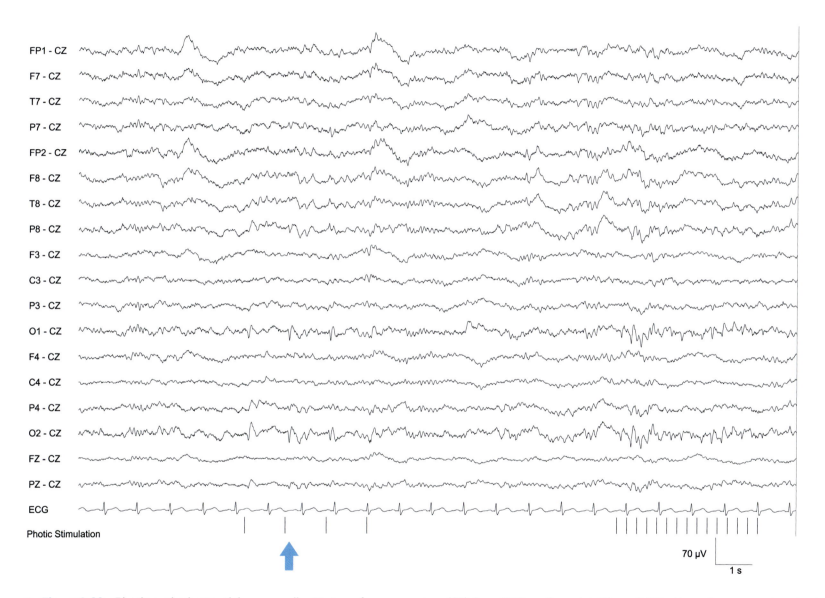

▶ **Figure 3.22** **Photic evoked potential versus spike.** Vertex reference montage (CZ). Same EEG section as in ▶ **Figure 3.21** but in a reference montage to electrode CZ. The deflections in electrodes O1 and O2 point downward (blue arrow), which means that the deflections are positive. See legend to ▶ **Figure 3.21**.

EEG activities can occur continuously or intermittently. In the latter case, this can happen rhythmically (regularly), periodically, or irregularly. It may appear as single intermittent waves or single complexes or in short bursts or paroxysms. This can occur bilaterally and synchronously—that is, almost simultaneously in the right and left hemispheres (alpha rhythm) (▶ Figure 3.23)—or asynchronously (mu rhythm). ▶ Figure 3.24 shows an example of more or less continuous alpha activity that is bilateral synchronous and an asymmetric mu rhythm.

3.3.1.5 Responsiveness/Reactivity

Both physiological and pathological activities can be triggered or blocked by sensory stimuli or maneuvers. Lambda waves occur when the patient looks at images or patterns producing saccadic eye movements (▶ Figure 3.35). K-complexes are triggered by (acoustic) stimuli in light non-REM sleep (▶ Figures 3.58–3.60).

The following responsiveness/reactivity tests can be performed during EEG recordings:

- Blocking the alpha rhythm by eye opening (▶ Figure 3.23).
- Blocking of the mu rhythm by finger movements (▶ Figure 3.24).
- Response to cognitive tasks (mental test; see Sections 3.1 and 3.2) to ensure complete alertness for the assessment of the background activities in normal individuals and also in patients with encephalopathies.
- In comatose patients, changes in the EEG patterns elicited by acoustic, tactile, and pain stimuli should be assessed. EEG responsiveness to these stimuli is a favorable prognostic sign (▶ Figures 3.285 and 3.286).

3.3.2 Reporting of EEG

EEG interpretation is based mainly on a highly subjective visual pattern recognition methodology. The EEG classification defines several EEG patterns that are relatively distinctive, and the EEG reader must determine if the EEG being analyzed shows any of the predetermine categories included in the EEG classification. Unfortunately, classification of any given EEG is, as previously mentioned, a highly subjective endeavor; therefore, EEG reading can be greatly influenced by prior knowledge of the clinical history of the patient being tested.

This is the reason we recommend to initially evaluate the EEG without knowledge of the underlying clinical problem. In addition, the EEG reader should specify, before reviewing the clinical history of the patient being tested, which EEG patterns (classes within the EEG classification) are present in the patient whose EEG is being read. Each EEG class is related with a clearly defined clinical finding. For example, left frontal spikes are closely related to left frontal epilepsy, and left frontal continuous slow is closely related to a left frontal structural lesion. Therefore, the reliability of the reader can be tested by analyzing how often the categories selected by the EEG reader, without prior knowledge of the clinical history, coincide with the actual clinical findings.

It is good practice to read EEGs and decide their classification without knowledge of the clinical history. Too frequent discrepancy between the selected EEG classification and the actual clinical history indicates that the reading is still unreliable. On the other hand, a high percentage of agreement between the selected EEG classification and the corresponding clinical picture indicates that the reader is highly reliable. Reading without knowing the clinical history can also be a powerful learning experience. The reader should review the EEG again in all instances in which the reader's EEG classification is not consistent with the clinical history. This will help the reader determine if they missed an EEG finding or "overinterpreted" a sharp transient as an epileptiform sharp wave. Moreover, the EEG classification can be used as a teaching tool. The teacher can have students classify different EEGs (without revealing the clinical history) and then analyze how often the students classified the EEGs correctly.

An EEG report consists of the following:

A. General information entered by the technologist:
  1. Demographics
  2. Technical characteristics (duration of recording, electrodes used)
  3. Level of consciousness
  4. Brief relevant clinical history
  5. Special events happening during the recording
  The EEG technologist should be instructed to call a senior technologist or an electroencephalographer on call if during the recording there is an unexpected technical problem (e.g., inability to correct an EEG artifact) or the patient experiences signs or symptoms that the technologist would like to have documented by an experienced technician or a physician.
B. General EEG report entered by the EEG reader

Occipital alpha background rhythm

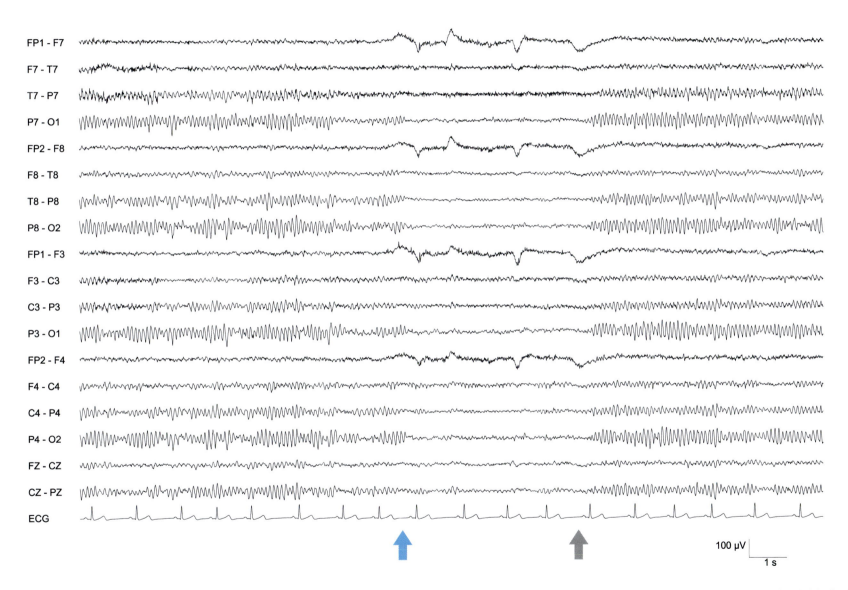

▶ **Figure 3.23** **Occipital alpha background rhythm.** Bipolar longitudinal montage. A well-expressed bilateral occipital background alpha rhythm that is blocked by eye opening (blue arrow) and reappears when the eyes are closed (gray arrow).

Blockage of the mu rhythm

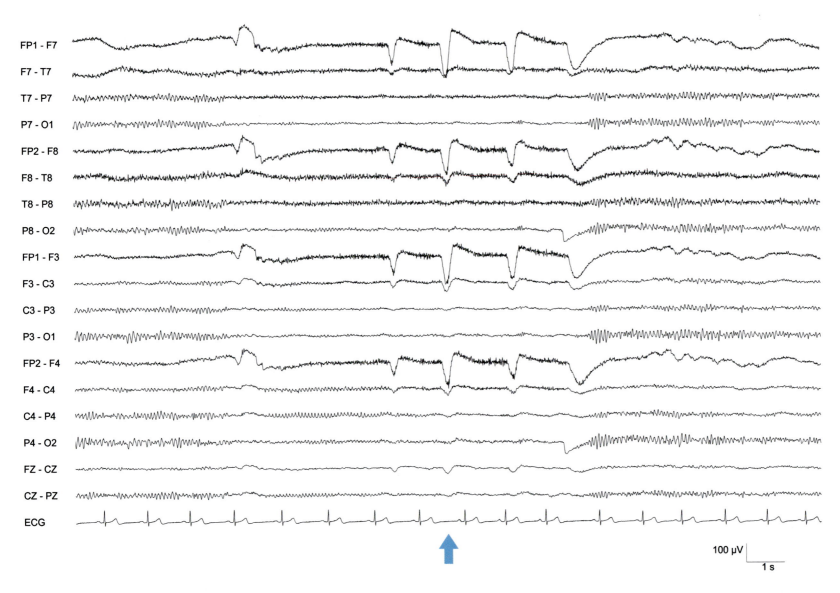

▶ **Figure 3.24** **Blockage of the mu rhythm.** Bipolar longitudinal montage. Eye opening has no influence on the C4 mu rhythm, which is blocked by fist closure (blue arrow).

EEG readers must always specify if the EEG recording shows one or more stages of consciousness (awake, sleep stages 1–4, REM, lethargy, stupor, and coma). Patients in stupor or coma frequently have two and occasionally even more EEG stages of consciousness. These stages of consciousness are labeled as "awake-like" and "sleep-like."

Example: The patient is in deep coma, but two EEG patterns can be distinguished. The sleep-like stage consists of 10–30 μV, diffuse, irregular delta with no blinks or eye movements and minimal EMG or movement artifacts. The awake-like stage consists of 40–120 μV diffuse, irregular delta activity with frequent eye blinks and eye movements and abundant EMG and movement artifacts. Strong stimulation during the sleep-like stage triggers the awake-like stage. An EEG sample that illustrates best the characteristics of each stage of consciousness should be provided.

For normal EEGs, the sample that illustrates best the rhythmical background activity when the patient is awake and has the eyes closed should be attached. In addition, in the description of the stages of consciousness, the frequency of the dominant background activity (if present) should be described.

For patients in stupor or coma, the EEG reader must also specify the approximate percentage of time the patient spends in each stage of consciousness. If there are abnormalities, the EEG reader must define in which stage of consciousness they occur and how frequent they occur in each stage of consciousness.

C. List and describe the abnormal EEG classes (see Section 3.4) entered by EEG reader.

Select EEG samples corresponding to each abnormal EEG class. It is best to describe each of these abnormal findings in a table as discussed above (see ▶ Table 3.4). In the EEG report, it is allowed to use neurophysiological technical terms that are not common to nonspecialists because this part of the report is intended only to be reviewed by neurologists familiar with electroencephalography. Misleading formulations that may result in false clinical conclusions must be avoided (e.g., "high-amplitude phase reversal") (Benbadis, 2013; Kaplan & Benbadis, 2013).

D. EEG classification entered by the EEG reader

The EEG classification provides an assessment of the overall degree of abnormality of the EEG recording. Normal EEG recordings are just classified as normal. Abnormal EEGs are classified as abnormal I, II, or III depending on the degree of abnormality. Each EEG abnormality has a defined degree of abnormality. The overall abnormality of an EEG recoding is determined by the degree of abnormality of the most abnormal EEG category. For example, in ▶ **Figure 3.25**, there are two grade III EEG abnormalities (the epileptiform abnormality and the focal continuous slow). The asymmetry is considered only an abnormality grade II. Therefore, the overall abnormality of the EEG is abnormal III. EEG recordings can also be classified as either "technically difficult" (if the patient is uncooperative) or "technically unsatisfactory" (if the EEG recording cannot be interpreted because of technical deficiencies). A repeat recording without charging the patients should be obtained if the EEG recording is technically unsatisfactory.

In the EEG classification, the overall degree of abnormality is followed by the level of consciousness, which is listed in parentheses.

E. Impression entered by EEG reader

The reader now writes a report that consists of the interpretation of the EEG findings considering the clinical history.

We can expect that clinicians trained in electroencephalography, when receiving an EEG report, will directly integrate the clinical findings with the EEG abnormalities listed in the report. They will also review the EEG samples and decide if they agree with the classification provided by the EEG reader. Clinicians not trained in electroencephalography will need assistance to put the EEG abnormalities listed in the EEG classification in context with the clinical findings. Summarizing, we expect that the detailed EEG report and the EEG samples will be used by clinicians trained in electroencephalography, whereas the impression is addressed to clinicians with no or only limited EEG training and, therefore, with a few exceptions should not contain any EEG terminology.

The report of normal recordings should read as follows: "Normal awake and sleep EEG. No epileptiform or focal abnormality

A 23-year-old patient with post-traumatic left frontal lobe epilepsy

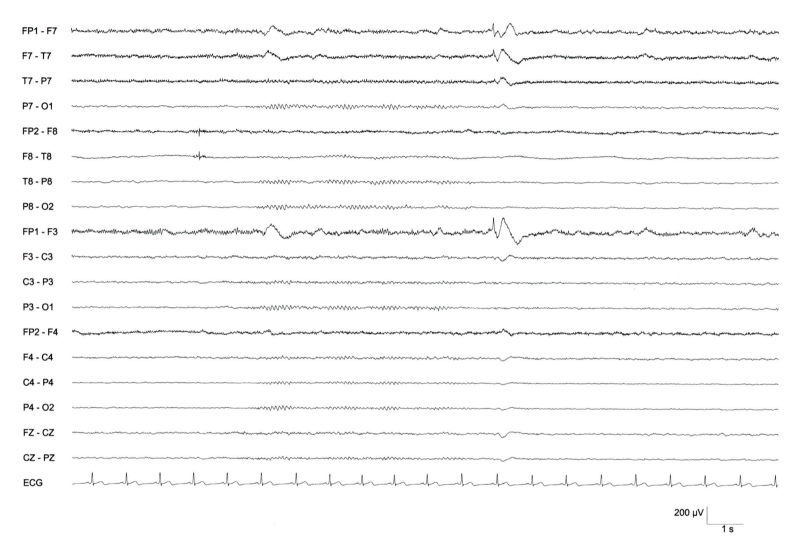

▶ **Figure 3.25** **A 23-year-old patient with post-traumatic left frontal lobe epilepsy.** The seizures consist of nonspecific auras that evolve into either dialeptic seizures or sometimes aphasic seizures. Nocturnal sleep–associated clonic seizures in the right extremities or right versive seizures tend to be followed by generalized convulsive seizures. Invasive epilepsy surgery evaluation localized two epileptogenic zones in the orbitofrontal region and in the post-traumatic gliotic left temporal structures. Resection of the epileptogenic zone sparing language areas led to seizure freedom and a cognitive improvement.

This EEG section shows a spike and a continuous slow with negative potential maximum in the electrode FP1. The amplitude of physiological beta activity is increased in the left frontal region.

EEG classification: Abnormal III (awake)
1. Spikes, FP1 > F7
2. Continuous slow, left frontopolar
3. Asymmetry, increased beta left frontal

EEG report: This EEG supports the diagnosis of post-traumatic left frontal lobe epilepsy and is indicative of a lesion and bone defect in this area.

was recorded." (Assuming that both awake and sleep EEGs were recorded.) Occasionally, the EEG reader may want to make additional recommendations. *Example*: "Patient with possible benign focal epilepsy of childhood. The EEG is normal, but no sleep was recorded." In this case, the EEG reader could add, "Additional sleep recording could be helpful to demonstrate epileptiform abnormalities."

The expression "This EEG supports the diagnosis of . . ." is the most accurate when the patient shows symptoms and/or signs frequently seen with the EEG abnormality the patient showed in this recording. *Example*: "This EEG supports the diagnosis of a left frontal post-traumatic epilepsy" for a patient who showed left frontopolar spikes and slow and left frontal increased beta activity in the EEG (▶ **Figure 3.25**). The expression "is consistent with" is frequently also used in the example mentioned above. However, this is less specific. For example, a normal awake and sleep recording is the most frequent finding when recording a routine EEG in a patient with infrequent generalized tonic–clonic seizures. Notice that in this case, the EEG finding (a normal EEG) is very consistent with the clinical diagnosis. On the other hand, we certainly cannot state that the normal EEG supports the diagnosis of a generalized epilepsy.

▶ **Figure 3.25** illustrates an example of a clinical history, an EEG classification, and the corresponding impression:

EEG classification: Abnormal III (awake/sleep)
1. Spikes, FP1
2. Continuous slow, left frontal
3. Asymmetry, increased beta left frontal

EEG report: This EEG supports the diagnosis of a post-traumatic left frontal lobe epilepsy and a skull defect in that region.

In the following section, the different EEG patterns usually seen in normal individuals are discussed. This is followed by a discussion of the abnormal EEG patterns, including the differential diagnosis with artifacts and other normal EEG patterns.

3.4 EEG Classification

3.4.1 Normal Patterns

Normal EEG patterns are EEG manifestations that have no relationship to pathology and can be seen with some frequency in normal individuals. Many of these patterns, particularly if they occur less frequently, have been considered abnormal. The reason for this mistake is related to the tendency to refer to an EEG lab predominantly patients with paroxysmal disorders. Electroencephalographers then collected EEG recordings with a specific pattern and observed that predominantly patients with clinically suspected paroxysmal disorders presented with that specific EEG pattern. Additional well-designed studies, which considered the bias mentioned above, were then able to demonstrate that these patterns had no pathological significance.

EEG patterns not proven to be diagnostic or predictive through systematic analysis are considered normal. This includes an abundance of physiological EEG patterns that occur during wakefulness or sleep (vertex waves, K-complexes, sleep spindles, etc.). The absence or delayed development of such physiological patterns in pediatric EEG is probably abnormal. However, there are no systematic studies proving the observation. Electroencephalographers must be able to differentiate several sharply contoured normal variants that are easily confused with epileptiform discharges (e.g., wicket spikes, benign epileptiform transients of sleep [BETS], 14 and 6 Hz positive spikes, and 6 Hz "phantom" spike–waves) (Amin & Benbadis, 2019; Benbadis & Lin, 2008; Klass & Westmoreland, 1985; Lüders & Noachtar, 2000a; see Section 3.4.2.4.12).

3.4.1.1 Physiological Wake EEG

The different brain regions are characterized by different background frequencies. In adolescents and adults, beta activity dominates in the frontal lobe, theta activity dominates in the temporal lobe, and alpha activity with a frequency of 8–13 Hz dominates in the parieto-occipital region (▶ Figure 3.26).

3.4.1.1.1 Posterior Alpha Activity

The EEG of premature infants and newborns differs considerably from the EEG of adolescents and adults. A distinction is made between the awake state and active and quiet sleep because the typical sleep signs, which occur in the first months of life, are still missing. The EEG in wakefulness in newborns is characterized by diffusely distributed continuous theta and delta waves with an amplitude of up to approximately 60 µV, whereas in quiet sleep of mature newborns the amplitude increases (200 µV) and alternates with flatter phases. This is called tracé alternant (▶ Figure 3.27). It thus consists of bursts of 3- to 6-s duration (3–6 Hz, 50–200 µV) alternating with low-amplitude activity of approximately the same duration. Tracé alternant is seen at 34 weeks postmenstrual age (PMA) and disappears at 46 weeks PMA. An alpha rhythm of 8–13 Hz and an amplitude of 30–100 µV (measured in a vertex reference) typically dominate in the posterior head regions from school age onwards. From age 10 years, the frequency is usually 10 Hz and remains more or less constant into old age. The amplitude of the alpha rhythm is typically spindle-like modulated, and it has been reported that the alpha rhythm is of higher amplitude on the right occipital region. This observation has not been documented by formal studies. Asymmetries of the alpha rhythm are seen frequently in normal individuals and should only be considered pathological if they are extreme (more than 50%), particularly if they are intermixed with focal slowing. Opening the eyes leads to a blockade of the occipital alpha rhythm. The alpha rhythm is also called the "Berger rhythm" in honor of Hans Berger, who first recorded EEG in humans and also was the first to describe the "alpha rhythm" (Berger, 1930) (▶ Figure 3.26). Starting at age 2 years, delta waves are usually embedded in the occipital background rhythm. Delta waves in the occipital region are referred to as the occipital delta of adolescence (delta de la jeunesse, teenage delta, or posterior slow wave of youth) (▶ Figure 3.28), and as their name suggests occur typically in young patients. As with the alpha rhythm, these delta waves are blocked by eye opening (▶ Figure 3.29). Occipital delta waves of adolescence may persist, even if significantly less prominent, into young adulthood. There is no evidence that the

Berger effect

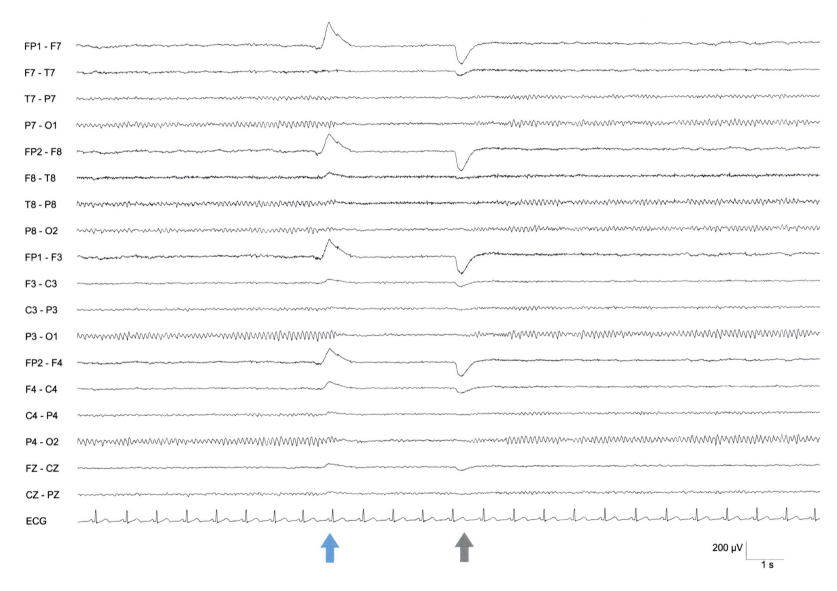

▶ **Figure 3.26** **Berger effect.** Bipolar longitudinal montage. The well-expressed occipital alpha background rhythm is blocked by eye opening (blue arrow) and reappears after eye closure (gray arrow).

Tracé alternant

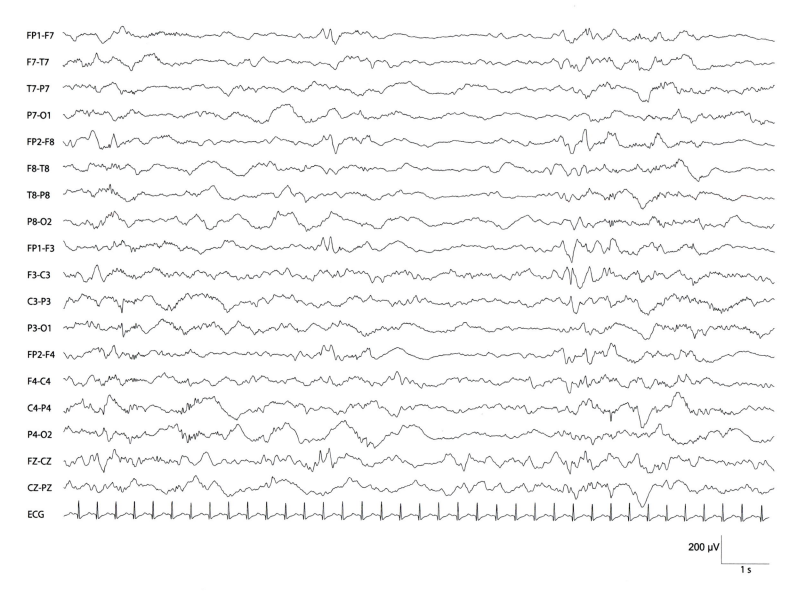

FP1-F7

F7-T7

T7-P7

P7-O1

FP2-F8

F8-T8

T8-P8

P8-O2

FP1-F3

F3-C3

C3-P3

P3-O1

FP2-F4

F4-C4

C4-P4

P4-O2

FZ-CZ

CZ-PZ

ECG

200 µV

1 s

▶ **Figure 3.27** **Tracé alternant.** Bipolar longitudinal montage. Tracé alternant is the typical pattern of quiet sleep in newborns. It consists of 3- to 6-s bursts of high-amplitude slow alternating with 3- to 6-s periods of relatively low-amplitude EEG activity. Frequently, the burst may include multifocal or more generalized sharp transients. Notice the C3 sharp transient in this EEG sample.

Occipital delta waves of youth

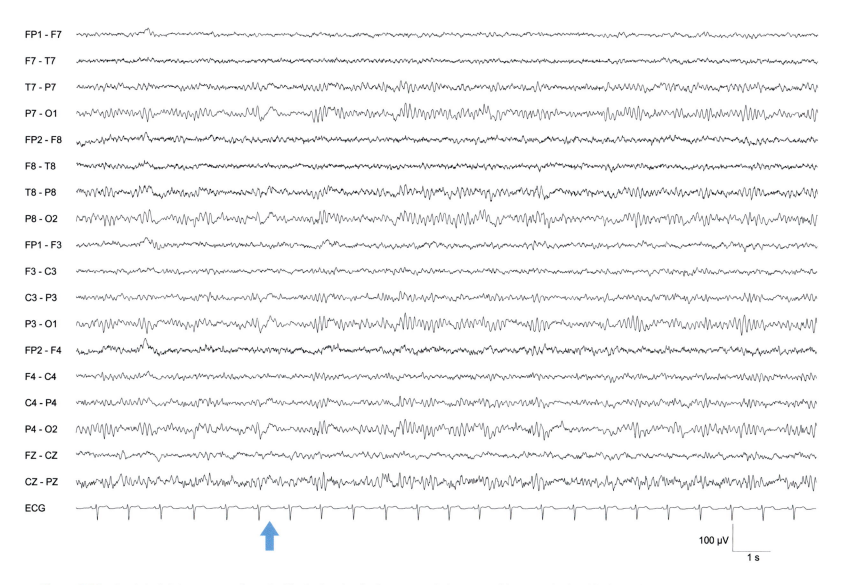

FP1 - F7

F7 - T7

T7 - P7

P7 - O1

FP2 - F8

F8 - T8

T8 - P8

P8 - O2

FP1 - F3

F3 - C3

C3 - P3

P3 - O1

FP2 - F4

F4 - C4

C4 - P4

P4 - O2

FZ - CZ

CZ - PZ

ECG

100 µV

1 s

▶ **Figure 3.28** **Occipital delta waves of youth.** Bipolar longitudinal montage. Delta waves (blue arrow) mix with the well-expressed occipital alpha background rhythm. Occipital slow waves of youth are seen mainly in children and are normal.

Occipital delta waves of youth

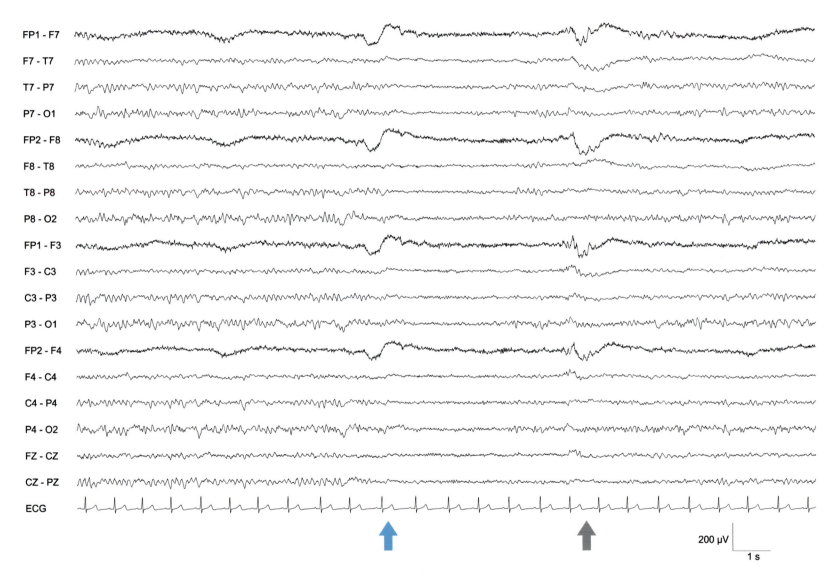

▶ **Figure 3.29** **Occipital delta waves of youth.** Bipolar longitudinal montage. Eye opening (blue arrow) blocks both the occipital alpha background rhythm and the occipital delta waves of youth. Both recur after eye closure (gray arrow).

persistence of occipital delta waves in the second or third decade is related to maturation or developmental delays.

In sleepiness and encephalopathy, however, eye opening may activate the occipital alpha rhythm (paradoxical alpha activation; ▶ **Figure 3.30**). In the first 1 or 2 s after eyelid closure, the frequency of occipital alpha activity can be 1 or 2 Hz faster and then slows down ("squeak phenomenon"; ▶ **Figure 3.31**). Because of the squeak phenomenon, the frequency of the alpha rhythm should not be determined immediately after eye closure.

Physiological variants of the occipital alpha rhythm are a slow (theta) background rhythm variant (▶ **Figures 3.16, 3.32, 3.33,** and **3.36**) and a fast (beta) background rhythm variant (▶ **Figures 3.34** and **3.35**). The theta variant occurs predominantly during relaxation and slight drowsiness, and it is characterized by a subharmonic half frequency of the occipital alpha rhythm of 3–6 Hz. The fast variant corresponds to the beta variant (14–22 Hz) and affects approximately 5% of adults. Both occipital background rhythm variants have the same responsiveness to eye opening and eye closing as the occipital alpha background rhythm (▶ **Figure 3.36**).

The frequency of the predominant physiological occipital background rhythm is age dependent. In the third and fourth months of life, the occipital background rhythm consists of a 3 or 4 Hz activity in approximately 75% of mature born children. This rhythm tends to be inhibited by eye opening. At approximately age 12 months, the occipital background rhythm reaches a frequency of 5 or 6 Hz in approximately two-thirds of healthy children. At approximately age 3 years, more than 80% of healthy children already have an occipital background rhythm of 8 Hz (Noebels & Kellaway, 1989). At age 9 years, the occipital background rhythm of 65% of healthy children reaches 9 Hz (Eeg-Olofsson, 1971b; Eeg-Olofsson, et al., 1971). The occipital background rhythm can be completely blocked in infants and small children with eye opening. Passive eye closure must be performed at least once during the EEG in children who do not close the eyes voluntarily. In general, it is considered that a child has a "background slow" if the background activity is <4 Hz at age 6 months, <5 Hz at age 1 year, <6 Hz at age 3 years, <7 Hz at age 5 years, and <8 Hz at age 8 years (see ▶ **Table 3.9**).

Characteristic EEG patterns allow to assess the gestational age of premature and newborn infants to an accuracy of 1 or 2 weeks (Scher, 2005). Up to the 30th week of gestational age (GA), the EEG is characterized by a discontinuous tracing (tracé discontinu). At a GA of 32–34 weeks, the tracé discontinu is seen during quiet sleep and the discontinuous EEG allows identification of quiet sleep in distinction of the awake state (▶ **Figure 3.37**). At that stage, the duration of the interburst is a function of GA (Pitt & Pressler, 2005). An interburst interval of more than 1 min is considered pathological and is associated with an unfavorable prognosis.

Several EEG patterns are physiological for certain age groups of premature and newborn children. Persistence beyond the physiological age range or occurrence in inadequate vigilance stages, however, are considered abnormal. Temporal sharp transients as well as rhythmic 4–7 Hz theta waves with an amplitude of 100–250 μV are physiological at 29–32 weeks GA. Delta brushes (ripples of prematurity; ▶ **Figure 3.37**) occur predominantly at 31 or 32 weeks GA and only rarely after 42 weeks GA. They have a cockscomb-like appearance, a frequency of 8–22 Hz, and an amplitude of 10–25 μV. These higher frequency rhythms are superimposed on slow subdelta or delta waves located in the occipital or central region. Frontopolar and frontally localized sharp transients (encoches frontales; ▶ **Figure 3.38**) occur from 34 to 36 weeks GA, especially in the transition phase from active to quiet (non-REM) sleep. Encoches frontales typically occur bilaterally but may exhibit somewhat shifting maxima. They normally disappear at age 2 months, and their persistence afterwards, particularly in the awake state, is considered pathological.

The occipital background rhythm varies from 8 to 13 Hz, is approximately 10 Hz in most adolescents and adults, and remains relatively constant throughout their lives. Fluctuations of more than 1 Hz are abnormal. Even with old age, the alpha frequency tends to remain constant. During drowsiness, the alpha frequency tends to gradually decrease. Therefore, the occipital background rhythm must be assessed during mentally active wakefulness. The spindle shape is created by two generators whose frequencies are close to each other (see **Figure 2.4**).

3.4.1.1.2 Central Mu Activity

The characteristic background frequency of the central region (mu rhythm) is often masked by the occipital alpha background activity. The occipital alpha activity and the central mu activity are difficult to differentiate because the frequencies are similar and the localizations are adjacent (▶ **Figure 3.39**). Therefore, the rhythms can be better differentiated if the occipital alpha activity decreases in amplitude after eye opening (▶ **Figure 3.40**). Mu activity occurs uni- or bilaterally (▶ **Figure 3.41**). Typical for mu activity is its blockade by fist closure (▶ **Figure 3.42**). In addition, other activation procedures, such as mental activity and wake-up responses, can also lead to a blockade of mu activity.

Paradoxical alpha activation

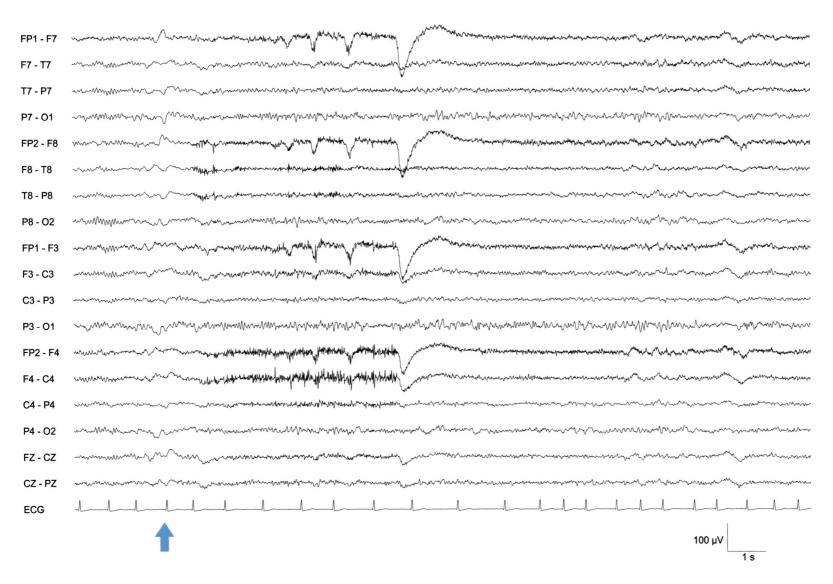

FP1 - F7

F7 - T7

T7 - P7

P7 - O1

FP2 - F8

F8 - T8

T8 - P8

P8 - O2

FP1 - F3

F3 - C3

C3 - P3

P3 - O1

FP2 - F4

F4 - C4

C4 - P4

P4 - O2

FZ - CZ

CZ - PZ

ECG

100 µV

1 s

▶ **Figure 3.30** **Paradoxical alpha activation.** Bipolar longitudinal montage. Calling the patients while he was drowsy leads to an activation of the physiological occipital background activity (blue arrow). This is called "paradoxical" alpha activation because it is the opposite of what happens when the patient opens the eyes when he is awake.

Alpha frequency after eye closure

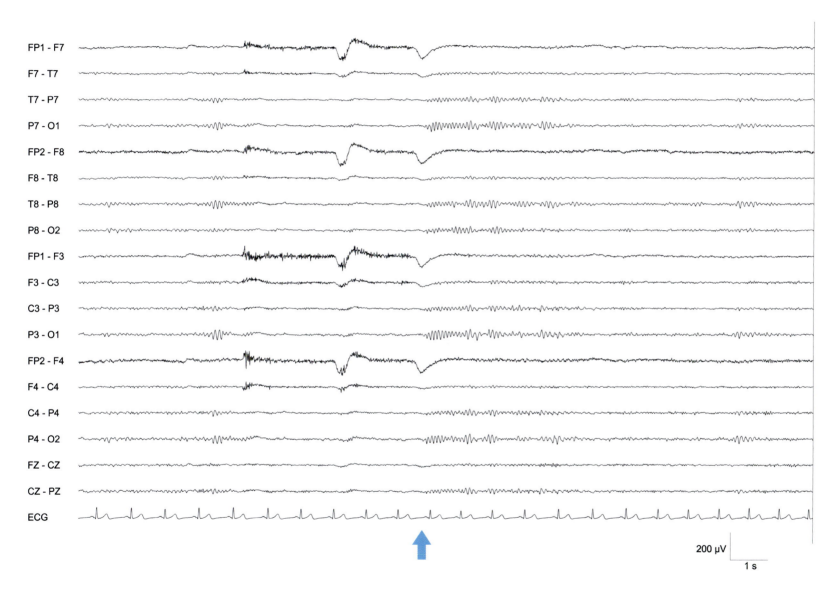

▶ **Figure 3.31** **Alpha frequency after eye closure.** Bipolar longitudinal montage. Immediately after eye closure, for 1 or 2 s, a faster occipital alpha background rhythm occurs (blue arrow). This phenomenon is called the squeak phenomenon.

Occipital slow alpha variant background rhythm

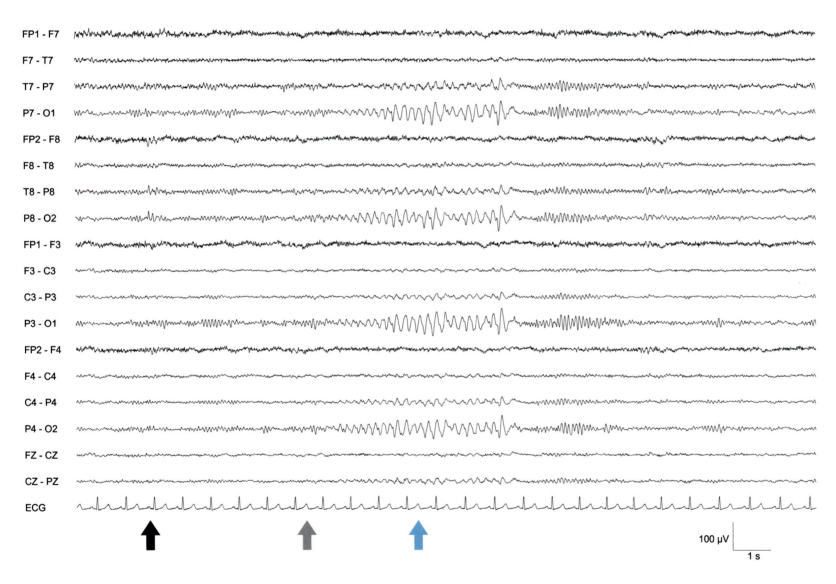

▶ **Figure 3.32** **Occipital slow alpha variant background rhythm.** Bipolar longitudinal montage. This EEG shows the change between occipital 12 Hz alpha (gray arrow) and 6 Hz theta background rhythm (blue arrow). The black arrow marks a small wicket spike.

Occipital slow alpha variant background rhythm

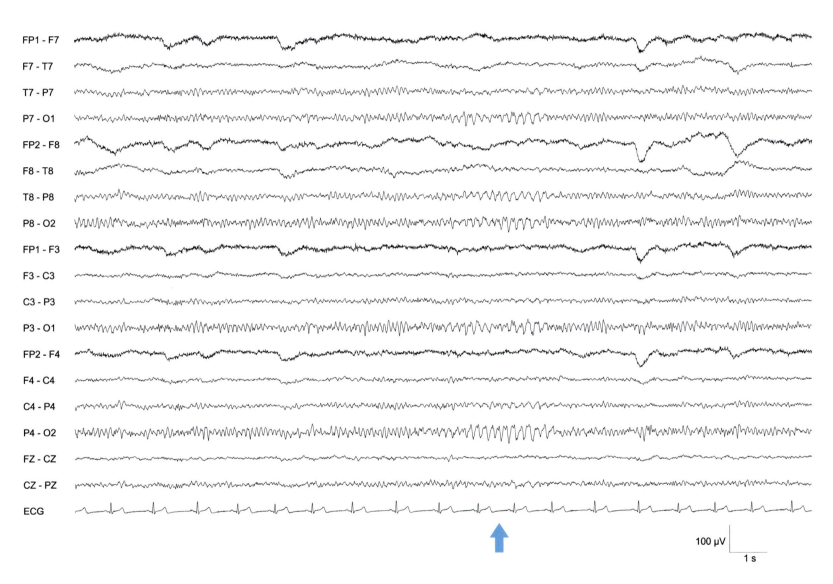

100 µV

1 s

▶ **Figure 3.33** **Occipital slow alpha variant background rhythm.** Bipolar longitudinal montage. The occipital alpha background rhythm (10.5 Hz) is replaced for 2 or 3 s by a theta background rhythm variant (5 Hz) (blue arrow).

"Fast alpha" variant occipital background rhythm

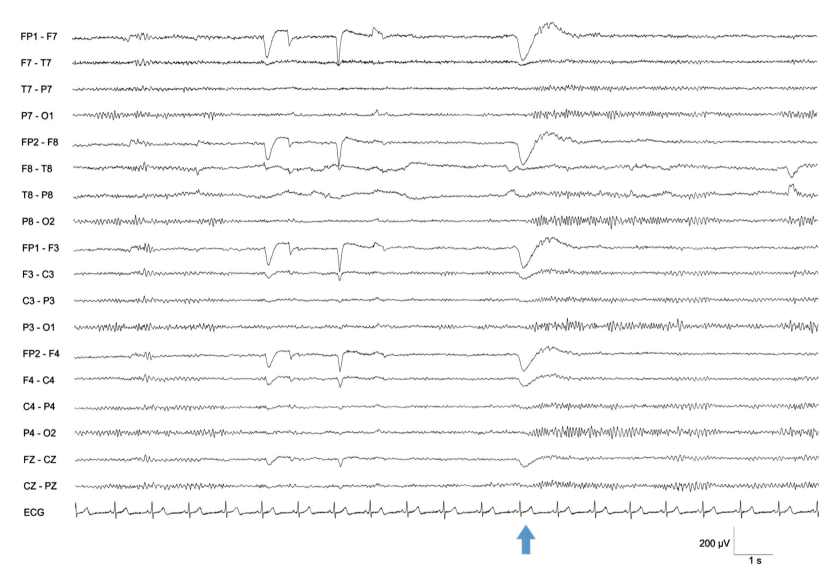

► **Figure 3.34** **"Fast alpha" variant occipital background rhythm.** Bipolar longitudinal montage. After eye closure, a well-pronounced occipital background rhythm of 13 or 14 Hz appears (blue arrow).

"Fast alpha" variant occipital background rhythm

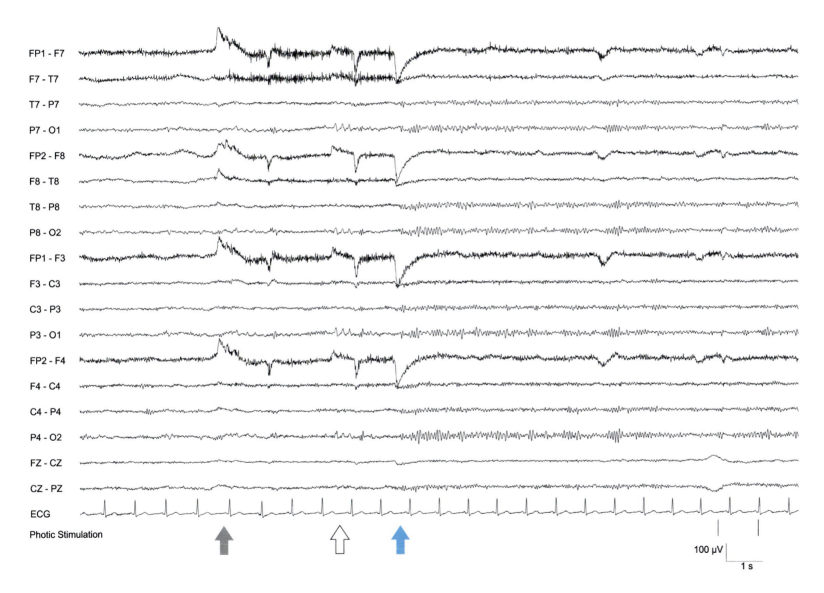

▶ **Figure 3.35** **"Fast alpha" variant occipital background rhythm.** Bipolar longitudinal montage. After eye opening (gray arrow), lambda waves (open arrow) occur in association with fast eye movements. After eye closure, a well-developed occipital beta background rhythm of 13 or 14 Hz occurs (blue arrow).

Blockage of the occipital slow alpha background rhythm

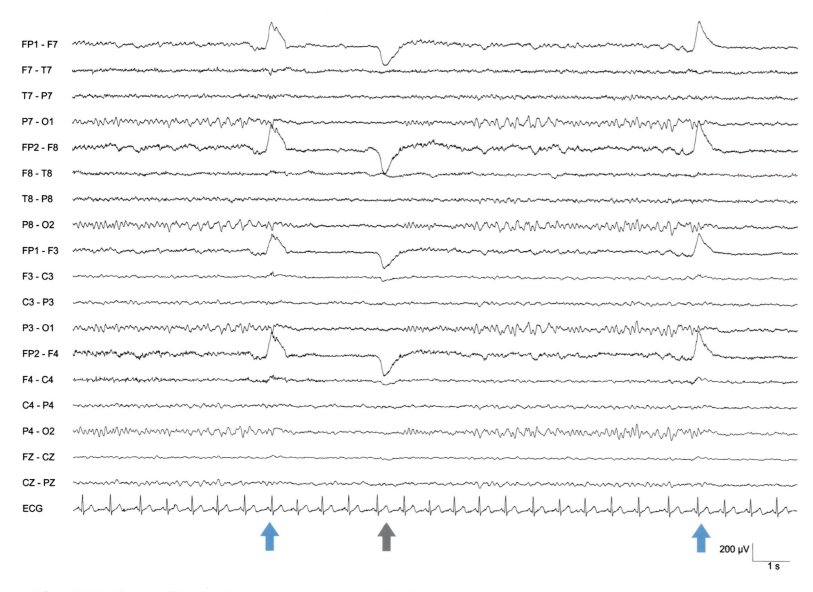

▶ **Figure 3.36** **Blockage of the occipital slow alpha background rhythm.** Bipolar longitudinal montage. After eye opening (blue arrows), the occipital alpha and theta activity disappears and reappears after eye closure (gray arrow).

Tracé discontinu and delta brushes

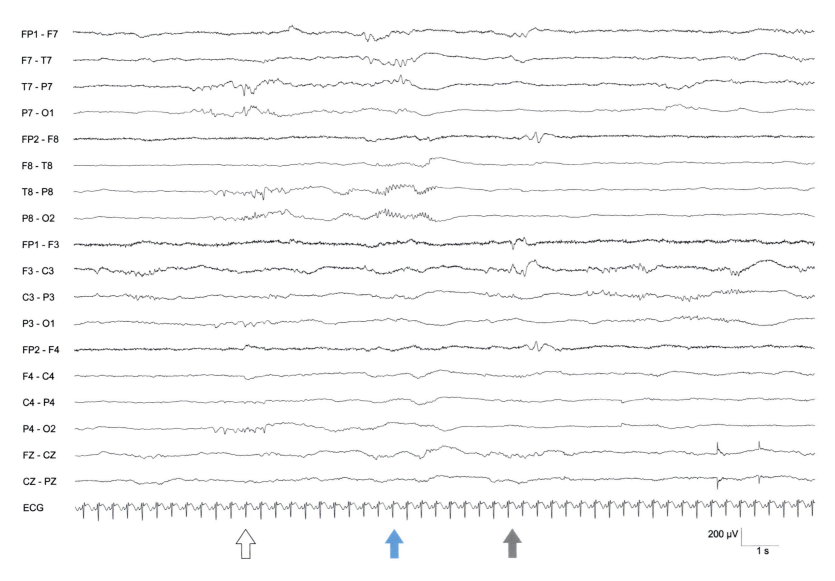

▶ **Figure 3.37** **Tracé discontinu and delta brushes.** Bipolar longitudinal montage. The tracé discontinu is the predominant pattern of the preterm infant in quiet sleep and is characterized by alternation of low-amplitude phases and bursts of slow waves. Delta brushes (blue arrow) and sporadic temporal (open arrow) or frontal sharp transients (gray arrow) are intermixed.

Encoches frontales

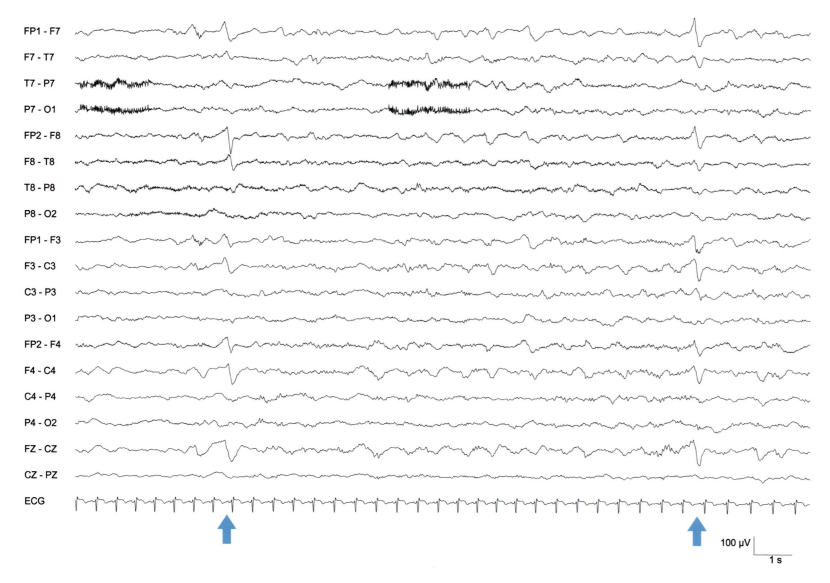

▶ **Figure 3.38** **Encoches frontales.** Bipolar longitudinal montage. High-amplitude frontopolar sharp transients. This pattern occurs in the transition from active to inactive sleep from the 34th to 36th week of gestation (blue arrows).

Central mu and occipital alpha activity

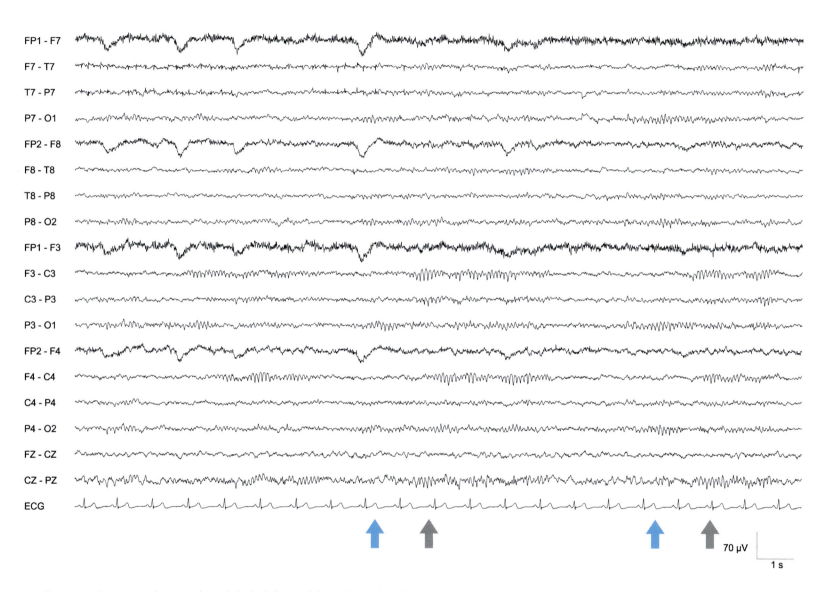

▶ **Figure 3.39** **Central mu and occipital alpha activity.** Bipolar longitudinal montage. This EEG sample illustrates the occipital alpha (blue arrows) and the central mu activity (gray arrows).

Central mu and occipital alpha activity

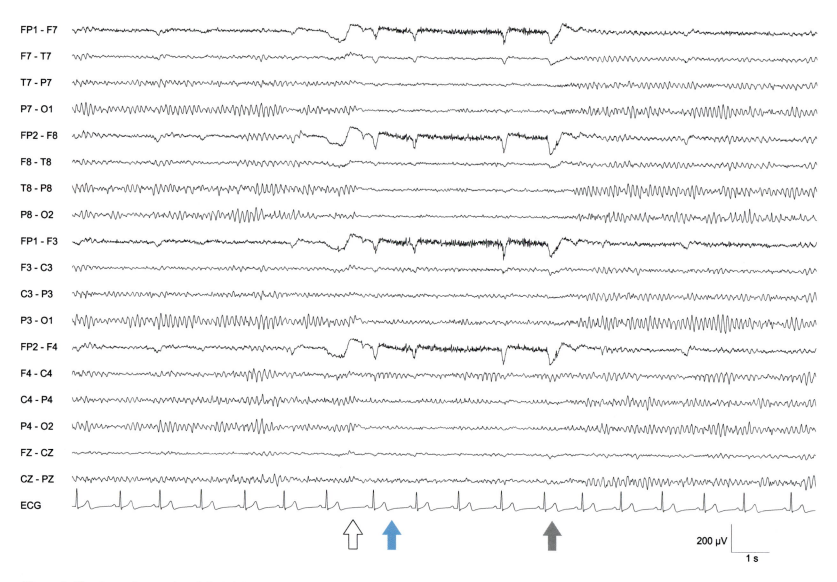

FP1 - F7
F7 - T7
T7 - P7
P7 - O1
FP2 - F8
F8 - T8
T8 - P8
P8 - O2
FP1 - F3
F3 - C3
C3 - P3
P3 - O1
FP2 - F4
F4 - C4
C4 - P4
P4 - O2
FZ - CZ
CZ - PZ
ECG

200 µV

1 s

▶ **Figure 3.40** **Central mu and occipital alpha activity.** Bipolar longitudinal montage. With eye opening (open arrow), the amplitude of the alpha activity is diminished, revealing the central mu activity (blue arrow). After eye closure (gray arrow), it is again difficult to distinguish central mu activity from the occipital alpha rhythm.

Central mu and occipital alpha activity

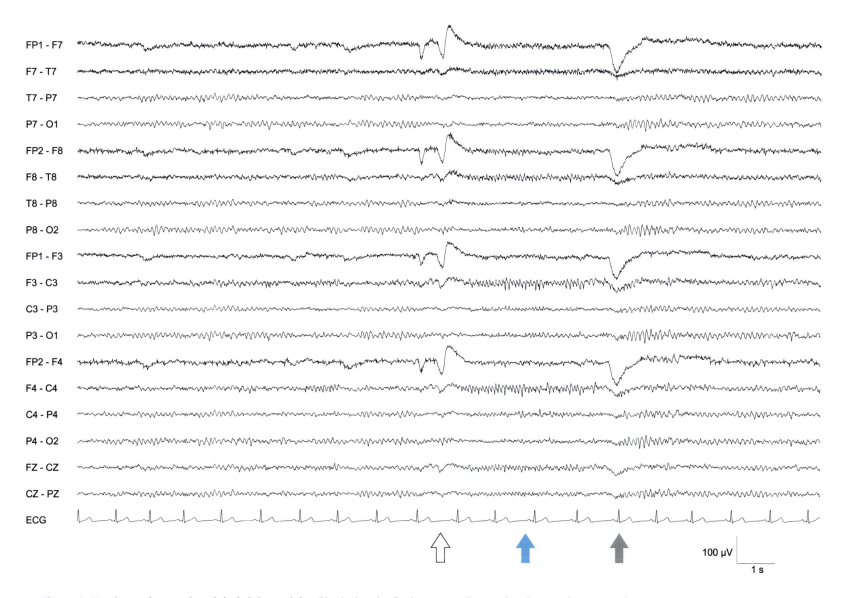

100 µV
1 s

▶ **Figure 3.41** **Central mu and occipital alpha activity.** Bipolar longitudinal montage. By opening the eyes (open arrow), the alpha activity is reduced and thus the central mu activity (blue arrow) is bilaterally pronounced. With eye closure (gray arrow), the occipital alpha activity recurs.

Blockade of the central mu activity by fist closure

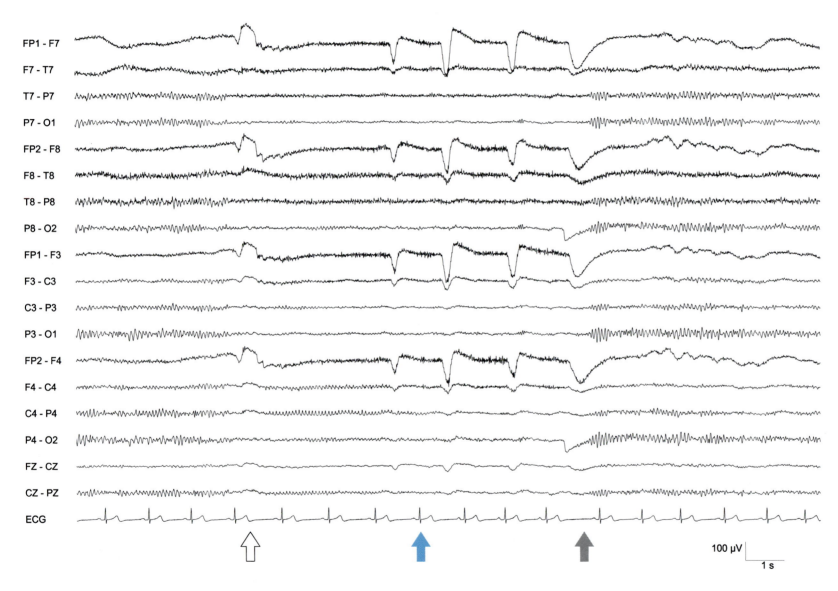

▶ **Figure 3.42** **Blockade of the central mu activity by fist closure.** Bipolar longitudinal montage. The occipital alpha activity is blocked by eye opening (open arrow). The right central mu activity is well-defined after eye opening but blocked by fist closure (blue arrow). The occipital alpha rhythm (gray arrow) resumes after eye closure.

With drowsiness, an "anteriorization" of the alpha rhythm has been described. However, we believe that most likely with drowsiness the alpha activity disappears first and the persistence of the mu activity gives the impression of an anteriorization of the alpha rhythm. The central mu activity typically develops earlier than the occipital alpha rhythm and tends to be more pronounced. Mu activity is not influenced by PS and does not participate in photic driving (▶ **Figure 3.43**).

3.4.1.1.3   Frontal Beta Activity

Relatively low-amplitude (20 μV) beta rhythms with a frequency of 15–25 Hz and spindle-like modulation are often found physiologically in the frontal regions. They become more pronounced with drowsiness (▶ **Figure 3.44**). Sedative drugs such as benzodiazepines, barbiturates, and antipsychotics can increase their expression and distribution so that higher amplitude beta activity may occur diffusely over all brain regions (▶ **Figure 3.45**; see Section 3.4.2.7.1). Bone defects such as those caused by trepanations, skull fractures, or burr holes lead to a higher amplitude of beta activity on the side of the bone defect. This has been referred to as the "breach rhythm." Of course, a bone defect itself cannot generate a rhythm; it only leads to an asymmetric expression of physiological activity with recording of an increased beta rhythm on the side of the bone defect (▶ **Figure 3.46**).

3.4.1.1.4   Temporal Theta Activity

In people older than age 50 years, irregular 2- to 5-s bursts of theta and delta waves are found in the left temporal regions. This is only considered pathological if it exceeds 20% of the recording (▶ **Figure 3.47**) (Kooi et al., 1964; Obrist, 1954). Long bursts (>5 s) of rhythmic theta activity (less frequently delta waves) occur frequently in patients with temporal lobe epilepsy (Reiher et al., 1989). These bursts must be distinguished from the rhythmic temporal bursts of drowsiness ("psychomotor variant" of F. Gibbs et al., 1963). The psychomotor variants are blocked by mental activation (▶ **Figure 3.48**), whereas the rhythmic temporal slow of temporal lobe epilepsy cannot be influenced by mental activation (▶ **Figures 3.49** and **3.50**).

3.4.1.2   Physiological Sleep EEG

The characteristic sleep patterns (sleep spindles, K-complexes, and vertex waves) develop with brain maturation in childhood (▶ **Figure 3.51**, ▶ **Table 3.5**). The classification of sleep stages in the EEG is possible from 33 or 34 weeks of gestation at the earliest. The documentation of body and eye movements and respiration makes it easier to differentiate between the wake state, active sleep, and non-REM quiet sleep in newborns (Watanabe, 1992). The sleep–wake cycles in newborns repeat at intervals of 30–70 min (Stockard-Pope et al., 1992).

The characteristic non-REM sleep pattern of the newborn is the tracé alternant (▶ **Figure 3.27**), which consists of 3- to 6-s bursts of theta waves and steep transients (50–300 μV) alternating with significantly lower amplitude activity of approximately the same duration. Shorter sleep periods are characterized by high-amplitude slow waves, which change into a continuous high-amplitude delta activity from week 44 of gestation. In preterm infants, the tracé discontinu exists, which is characterized by a lower amplitude in the interburst interval (<25 μV) compared with the tracé alternant (▶ **Figure 3.37**). The interburst intervals last longer in the tracé discontinu than in the tracé alternant.

Characteristic for children is the pattern of hypnagogic theta–delta bursts. These rhythms have also been called hypnagogic hypersynchrony, which linguistically is awkward: Because the term synchronous is absolute, there cannot be excessive synchrony ("hyper"). With decreasing vigilance (often still with open eyes), infants aged 3–12 months reveal long runs of high-amplitude, monomorphic 3–5 Hz theta or delta waves (▶ **Figure 3.52**). In young children, similar hypnagogic bursts can be seen but of lower amplitude and shorter duration (▶ **Figure 3.53**). Hypnopompic theta–delta bursts (hypnopompic hypersynchrony) refer to the same pattern in the transition from sleep to awake. Similar patterns also occur in childhood and adulthood in somnambulism from non-REM sleep.

At age 3 or 4 months, vertex waves and sleep spindles appear (▶ **Figure 3.54**). The vertex waves occur usually in groups. The sleep spindles initially are asynchronous between the two hemispheres, and long bursts of up to 10 s can be seen. Between ages 6 and 12 months, the duration of the spindles decreases (to 1-3 seconds) and the asynchrony also decreases (▶ **Figures 3.54** and **3.55**). However, not infrequently some degree of asynchrony between the two hemispheres may persist.

During puberty, POSTS develop in non-REM sleep (▶ **Figure 3.55–3.57**). In adolescents, POSTS and vertex waves usually have higher amplitudes than in adults. POSTS occur in sleep stages 1 and 2. Probably due to their occipital location (sleep polygraphy was traditionally only recorded with a single EEG channel connecting a central electrode to the ear), they were not included in the old sleep classifications (Rechtschaffen & Kales, 1968).

Central mu activity is not influenced by photic stimulation

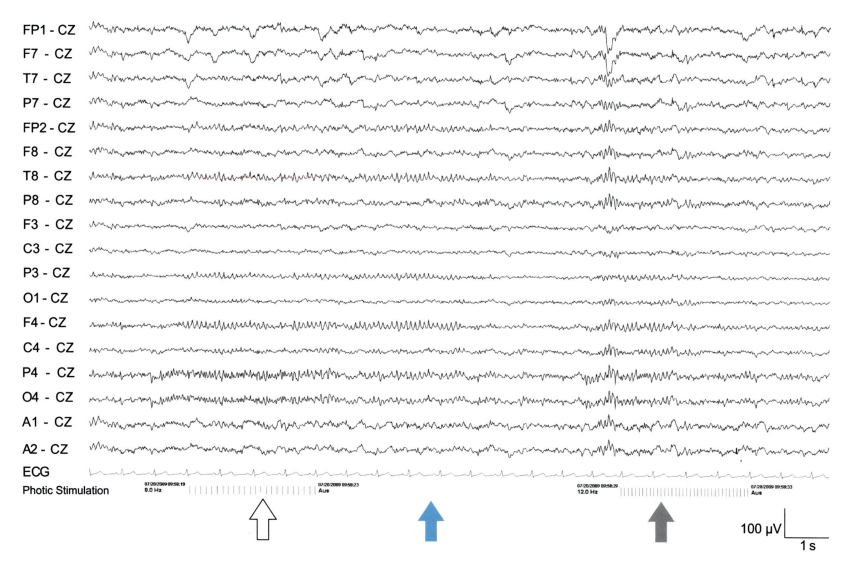

▶ **Figure 3.43** **Central mu activity is not influenced by photic stimulation.** Vertex reference montage. Photic stimulation at 8 Hz (open arrow) and 12 Hz (gray arrow) leads to photic driving. The central mu activity (blue arrow) is unaffected by photic stimulation.

Excessive beta activity

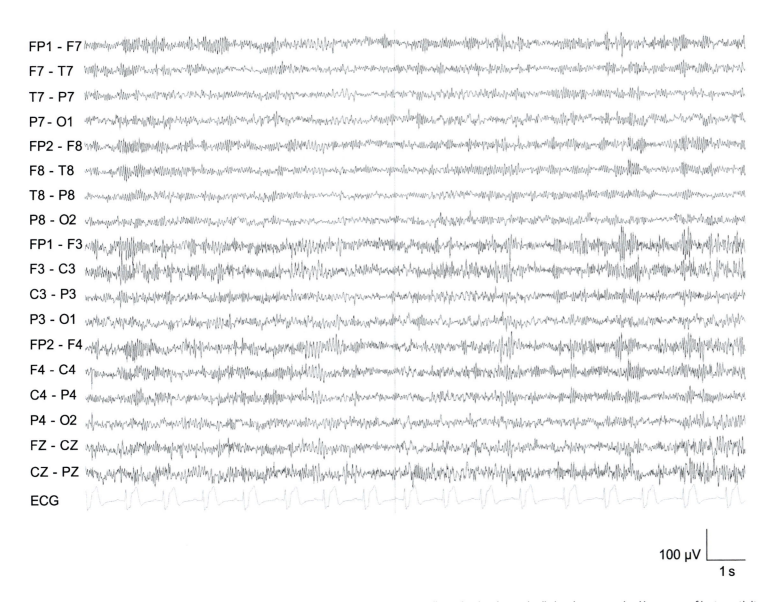

FP1 - F7

F7 - T7

T7 - P7

P7 - O1

FP2 - F8

F8 - T8

T8 - P8

P8 - O2

FP1 - F3

F3 - C3

C3 - P3

P3 - O1

FP2 - F4

F4 - C4

C4 - P4

P4 - O2

FZ - CZ

CZ - PZ

ECG

100 μV

1 s

▶ **Figure 3.44** **Excessive beta activity.** Bipolar longitudinal montage. Benzodiazepine intake typically leads to a marked increase of beta activity.

Excessive beta

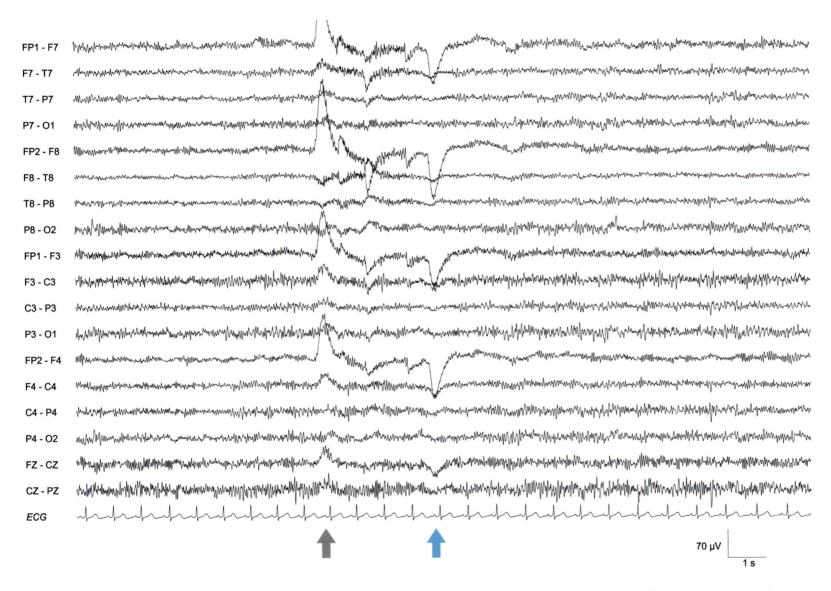

Figure 3.45 **Excessive beta.** Bipolar longitudinal montage. The EEG shows excessive beta activity. Excessive beta activity is defined as generalized beta activity that exceeds 40 μV amplitude. Eye opening (gray arrow) and closure (blue arrow) do not influence the beta activity.

Asymmetry, increased beta right frontal

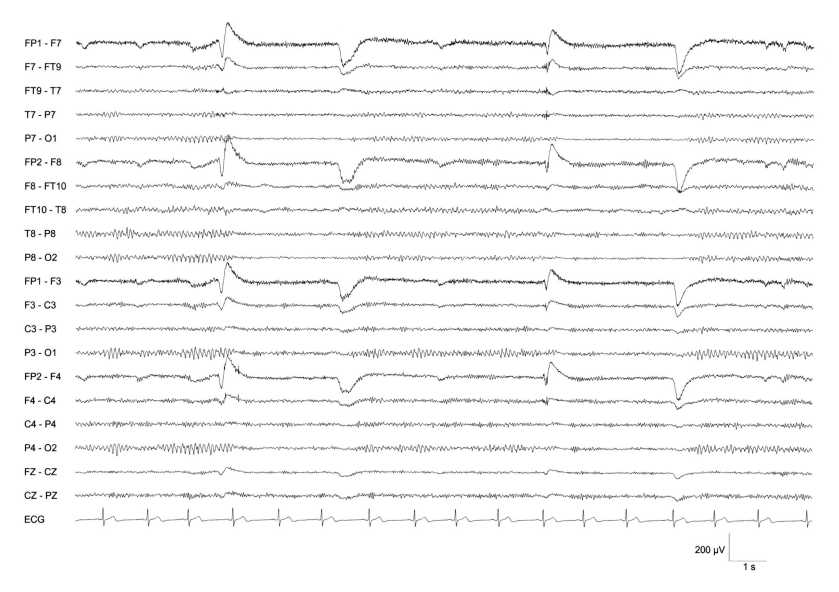

▶ **Figure 3.46** **Asymmetry, increased beta right frontal.** Bipolar longitudinal montage. Due to a right-sided bone defect, the beta activity was increased on the right frontal region. This patient underwent surgery for trigeminal neuralgia on the right side.

EEG classification: Abnormal II (awake)

Asymmetry, increased beta, right frontal

EEG report: This EEG supports the presence of a right-sided trepanation.

Temporal slow of the elderly

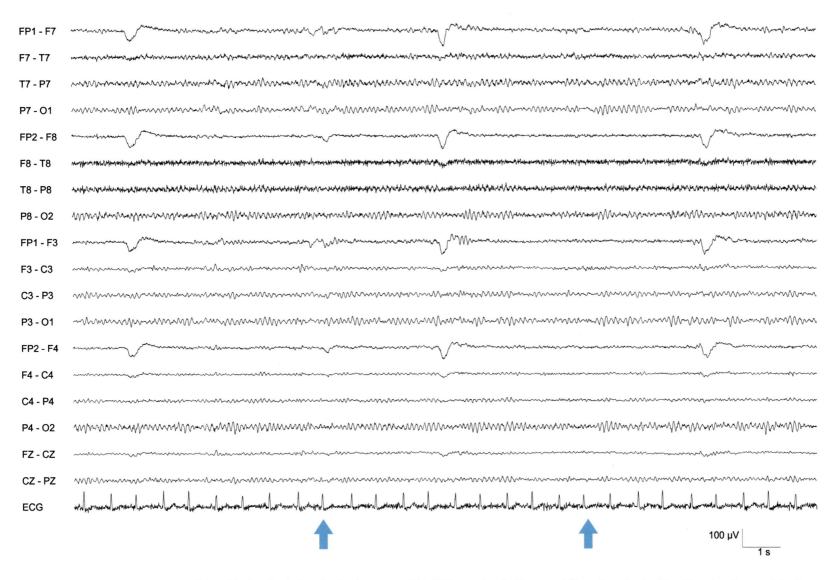

▶ **Figure 3.47** **Temporal slow of the elderly.** Bipolar longitudinal montage. This EEG sample of a 74-year-old female patient with gait unsteadiness, diabetic neuropathy, and heart failure shows short bursts of irregular theta and delta waves (blue arrows) in the left temporal region. The slow was seen in approximately 6% of the recording.

EEG classification: Normal (awake)

EEG report: This EEG is within normal limits.

Rhythmic temporal theta bursts of drowsiness

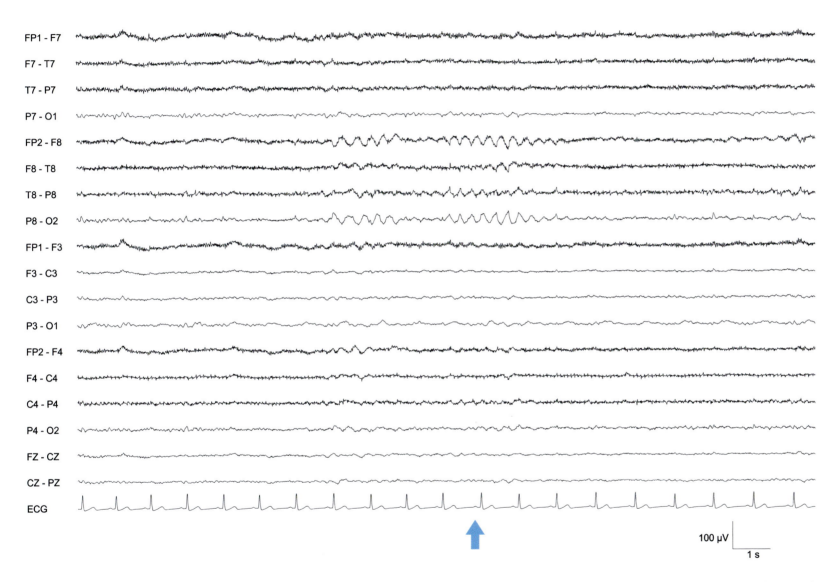

▶ **Figure 3.48** **Rhythmic temporal theta bursts of drowsiness.** Bipolar longitudinal montage. During drowsiness, bursts of approximately 4 Hz, rhythmical waves were seen in the right temporal lobe. These bursts have modulation of amplitude (like spindles) and stop if the patient is spoken to (blue arrow). These bursts can be differentiated from EEG epileptic seizure because there is no progressive evolution of amplitude, distribution, or waveform. This is a normal variant that is also labeled as "psychomotor variant" and not related to temporal lobe epilepsy.

EEG classification: Normal (awake)

EEG report: This EEG is within normal limits.

Sharp wave and rhythmic temporal theta burst

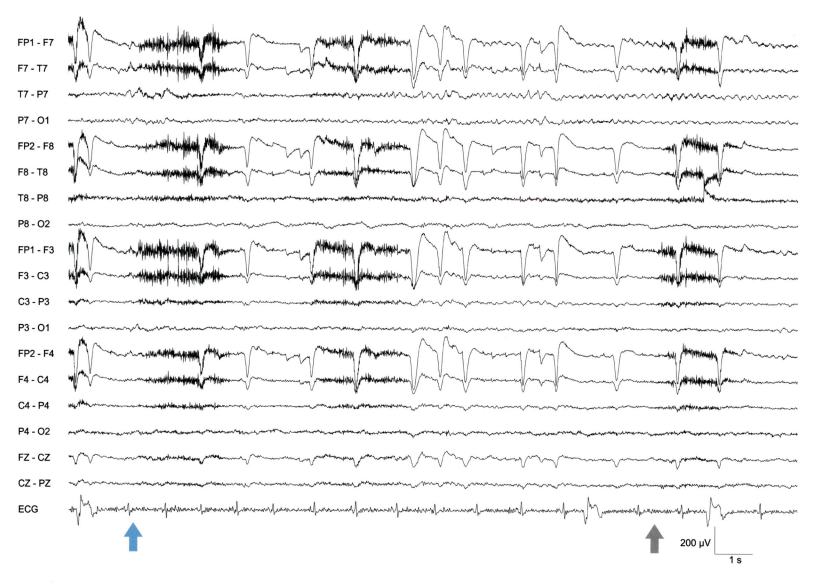

▶ **Figure 3.49** **Sharp wave and rhythmic temporal theta burst.** Bipolar longitudinal montage. A 41-year-old female patient with left temporal lobe epilepsy. This EEG section shows left temporal intermittent rhythmic waves around 5 Hz (gray arrow). The patient is awake and shows frequent eye blinks. The blue arrow marks a left temporal spike.

EEG classification: Abnormal III (awake)
1. Spikes, F 7 > FP1 > T7
2. Intermittent rhythmic slow, left temporal

EEG report: This EEG supports the diagnosis of a left temporal lobe epilepsy.

Spikes and temporal intermittent rhythmic delta activity (TIRDA)

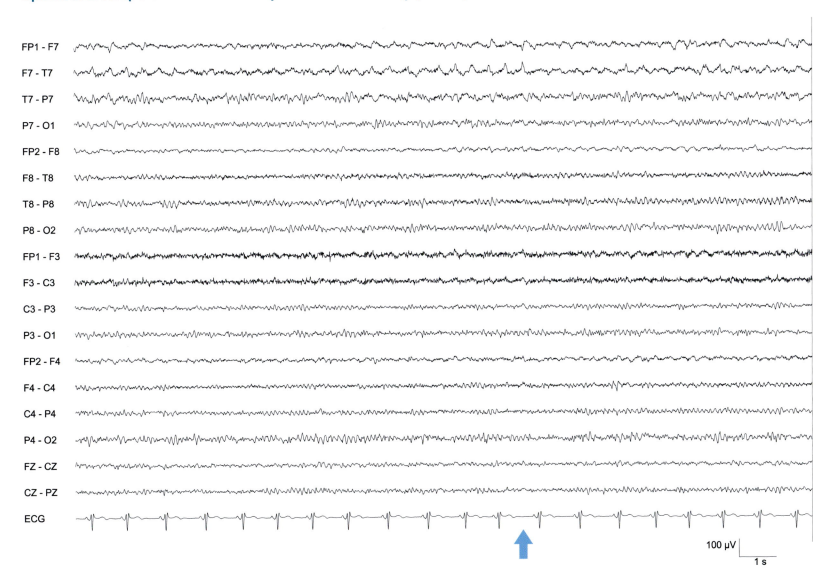

▶ **Figure 3.50** **Spikes and temporal intermittent rhythmic delta activity (TIRDA).** Bipolar longitudinal montage. A 50-year-old female patient who at age 12 years had a left parietal infarct and left mesial temporal sclerosis. The patient now suffers from left temporal epilepsy. This EEG sample shows a spike (blue arrow) and intermittent rhythmic delta activity in the left temporal region.

EEG classification: Abnormal III (awake)
  1. Spikes, F7 > FP1 > T7
  2. Intermittent rhythmic slow, left temporal

EEG report: This EEG supports the diagnosis of a left temporal lobe epilepsy.

Age-dependent development of physiological sleep patterns

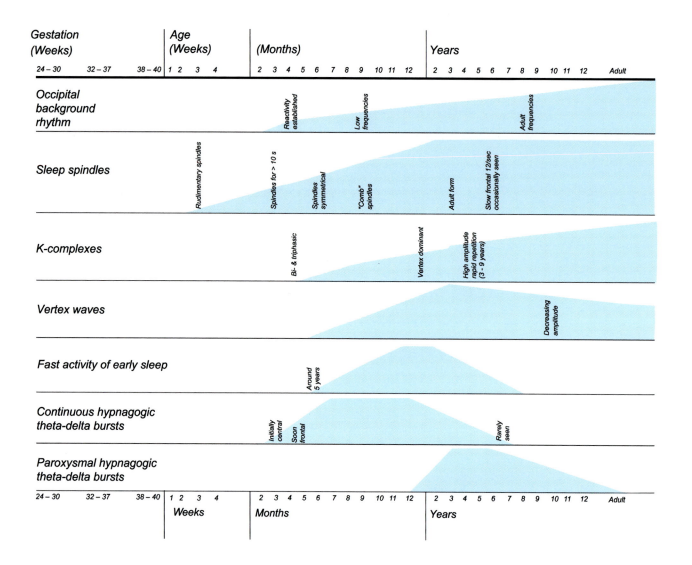

▶ **Figure 3.51 Age-dependent development of physiological sleep patterns.** Temporal sequence of the development of physiological sleep patterns in early childhood.

Source: Modified from Stockard-Pope et al. (1992).

EEG Pattern	Age Limits (Years)	Characteristics	Clinical Significance	References
Slowest normal background activity at	Age ½ 4 Hz Age 1 5 Hz Age 3 6 Hz Age 5 7 Hz Age 8 8 Hz		Background activity of abnormal low frequency is seen in patients with developmental delay and other encephalopathies. Passive eye closure should be performed in toddlers, infants, or disabled patients in order to define the background activity.	Nordli (2012), Petersén & Eeg-Olofsson (1971b)
Central mu	Children >1 year; may precede occurrence of posterior alpha in children <1 year; more frequent in adults	Arcade form (sharp negative); frequency and amplitude similar to posterior alpha rhythm; shifting uni- or bilateral central; best visible when alpha activity is reduced (drowsiness, mental activation); best blocked by contralateral motor activity (fist clenching)	In children with autism spectrum disorder, central mu rhythm is not suppressed during action observation. It has been speculated that this missing suppression reflects dysfunction of the mirror neuron system in autism spectrum disorder.	Dumas et al. (2014), Marshall et al. (2002), Marshall & Meltzoff (2011), Petersén & Eeg-Olofsson (1971b)
Vertex waves (VW)	Usually well developed from the age of 5 months	Sharp transient with maximum over the vertex region indicating sleep stage N1, also occurring in N2; in toddlers and infants—often trains of 100–200 μV VW; usually synchronous and symmetric. At 5–6 months, a few broad (~250 ms) VW are noted, becoming sharper and shorter at 16 months, increasing in frequency until 24 months, and becoming repetitive at 30 months of age. Marked intraindividual variability of VW with respect to symmetry, frequency, amplitude, and duration is common.	Asymmetry of VW: Only pathological if extreme (>50%) and consistent throughout the recording. High-voltage vertex waves in infants might be confused with epileptic spikes, especially when occurring repetitively.	Hrachovy (2000), Hughes (1998), Kellaway & Fox (1952)

3 Clinical Electroencephalography

(continued on next page)

EEG Pattern	Age Limits (Years)	Characteristics	Clinical Significance	References
Sleep spindles	Well developed in children >2–3 months	Frontocentral–central, 12–14 Hz, asynchronous until age 12–24 months; in toddlers, arcade form (sharp negative) occurring for up to 8 s; development to synchronous, non-arcadic appearance and less duration at young school age; spindle-shaped appearance (amplitude increment > amplitude decrement) less pronounced in toddlers	In patients with severe brain damage (i.e., structural or genetic), sleep-related EEG patterns may not be distinguishable at all. In patients with cryptogenic West syndrome, recurrence of sleep spindles under therapy indicates better long-term outcome. Although sleep spindles should appear synchronously from age 24 months, the clinical incidence and clinical significance of persistent asynchrony have not been thoroughly investigated. Only complete absence of spindles in one hemisphere is indicative of a severe cortical lesion.	Hrachovy (2000), Hughes (1985), Spenner et al. (2019), Westmoreland (2009)
K-complexes	May occur as early as 3 months of age, usually well developed from 9 months of age	Frontocentral, biphasic, negative component <1,000 µV, frequently combined with sleep spindle 12–14 Hz	Sharp component intermixed with the slow wave and subsequent sleep spindle may mimic generalized polyspike wave discharges.	Hrachovy (2000), Metcalf et al. (1971)
REM sleep	From birth regardless of gestational age	REM sleep is the predominant sleep state of the premature brain. In premature newborns, tracé discontinue is recorded during REM sleep, and EEG activity gradually develops to more continuous activity at term.	The total amount of REM sleep (in newborns, also called "active sleep") decreases markedly during development from a total amount of sleep time of >70% in premature newborns to 24% at age 8 months.	Stockard-Pope et al. (1992)
Hypnagogic/ hypnopompic theta–delta bursts (discouraged term: hypnagogic/ hypnopompic hypersynchrony)	3 months to 10 years	3- to 10-s bursts of 2–6 Hz slow waves of 200–400 µV; generalized distribution; appear during drowsiness or after awakening; subside with mental activation	Sharp high-frequency components intermixed with the slow waves may mimic generalized spike–waves.	Brandt & Brandt (1955), Eeg-Olofsson et al. (1971b), Mizrahi (1996)

EEG Pattern	Age Limits (Years)	Characteristics	Clinical Significance	References
Lambda waves	Toddlers to adulthood; may occur as early as age 6 months	Associated with saccadic eye movements during visual exploration in bright environment; bi- or triphasic; predominant positive polarity; bilateral occipital; amplitude 10–70 μV; duration 200–300 ms; typically in series	Unilateral or asymmetric localization of lambda waves is not a pathologic finding.	Weber (2005), Westmoreland & Sharbrough (1975)
Positive occipital sharp transients of sleep (POSTS)	From 3 years to adulthood, maximum 15–35 years	Bilateral with variable asymmetries; positive occipital sharp transients of sleep occurring in up to 30% of traces in normal children and adolescence; no subsequent slow wave; often occurs in runs; incidence increases from school age to adolescence	May be confused with posterior epileptic discharges	Hrachovy (2000), Mizrahi (1996), Rey et al. (2009), Dan & Boyd (2006)
14 and 6 Hz positive spikes	May rarely occur in infants, highest peak in adolescence	1- to 3-s bursts of positive spikes at 14 Hz (range, 12–16 Hz) and/or 6–8 Hz; in drowsiness and light sleep with maximum over the posterior temporal leads	May mimic polyspikes	Eeg-Olofsson (1971a), Westmoreland (1996)
Posterior slow waves of youth (POSWY), teenage delta, delta de la jeunesse	Maximal appearance 8–14 years (range, 3–21 years)	1.5–3 Hz posterior slow waves intermixed by occipital background rhythm	Must be differentiated from background slow and intermittent slow; is blocked by eye opening like posterior alpha; intermixed high alpha activity may give the appearance of epileptiform discharges	Hrachovy (2000), Mizrahi (1996)
Frontal beta	School age	Predominant frontal activity changes from theta to beta frequencies at approximately age 8 years.	Usually symmetric, although asymmetry of beta activity of not less than 65% in amplitude is considered as normal	Hrachovy (2000)

(continued on next page)

EEG Pattern	Age Limits (Years)	Characteristics	Clinical Significance	References
Neonates				
Encoches frontales	35–48 weeks of gestational age (maximum 36–41 weeks)	Bilateral synchronous, biphasic (negative > positive) sharp transient followed by a slow wave; maximum over the frontal region; predominantly in active sleep/transition to quiet sleep (syn.: frontal sharp transients)	May predominate in one hemisphere	Ellingson & Peters (1980), Statz et al. (1982), Stockard-Pope et al. (1992)
Anterior slow delta (ASD)	35–48 weeks of gestational age (maximum 36–41 weeks)	Bilateral 2–3 Hz activity, 50–150 µV with maximum over the frontal region (syn.: anterior slow dysrhythmia)	May be confused with encephalopathy; some overlap with encoches frontales	Monod et al. (1972)
Delta brushes	26–38 weeks of gestational age	0.3–1.5 Hz waves of 50–250 µV with superimposed burst of fast activity of 8–22 Hz; seen in active and quiet sleep	Appearance >38 weeks of gestational age is indicative of brain prematurity.	Lombroso (1979), Whitehead et al. (2017)
Temporal sharp transients	29–34 weeks of gestational age	Temporal theta bursts from 100 to 250 µV in amplitude, pattern of prematurity (syn.: temporal sawtooth waves)	Occurrence of temporal sharp transients >36 weeks of gestational age indicates prematurity of the brain	Hughes et al. (1987)
Tracé discontinue	Gradually develops from very premature infants to 34–36 weeks of gestational age	Normal background of quiet sleep interrupted by bursts attenuated or suppressed background activity. Duration of interburst intervals decreases with gestational age. Interburst intervals are usually less than 25 µV. This pattern gradually develops to Tracé alternant.	Persistence of long interburst intervals not appropriate for the gestational age indicates prematurity of the brain	Husain (2005)
Tracé alternant	36–44 weeks of gestational age	Normal background pattern of quiet sleep of mature newborns interrupted by periods of relative background attenuation (25–50 µV)	Persistence of discontinuous pattern in mature newborns >44 weeks of gestational age indicates prematurity of the brain. Discontinuous patterns in term newborns indicate encephalopathy od they persist on awakening.	Husain (2005)
Continuous slow waves sleep	40–44 weeks of gestational age	Pattern of quiet sleep. This pattern emerges once the trace alternant disappears.		Husain (2005)

EEG, electroencephalogram; REM, rapid eye movement.

Source: Courtesy of Ingo Borggräfe.

Hypnagogic delta burst (hypnagogic hypersynchrony)

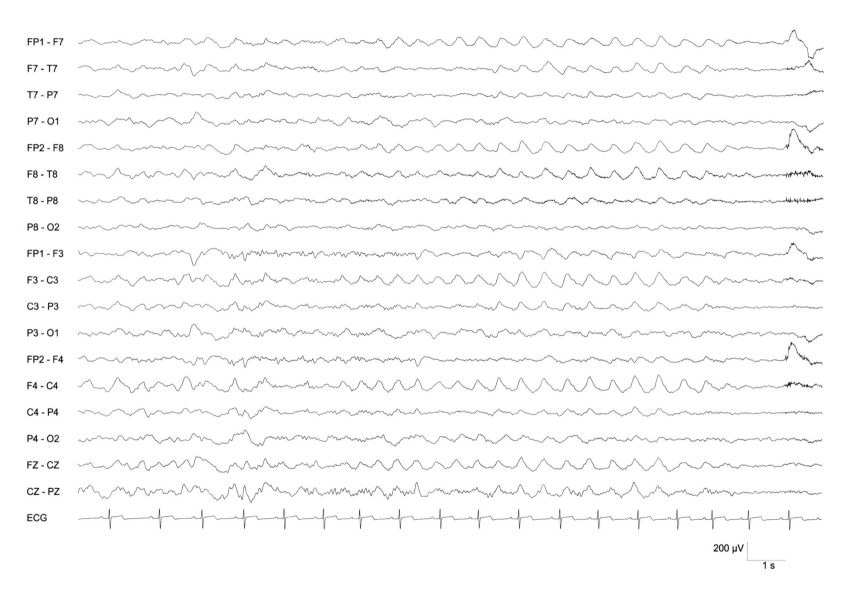

▶ **Figure 3.52** **Hypnagogic delta burst (hypnagogic hypersynchrony).** Bipolar longitudinal montage. This EEG shows high-amplitude rhythmic delta waves in a 4-year-old during drowsiness. This is a typical pattern of drowsiness at this age.

Hypnagogic delta burst (hypnagogic hypersynchrony)

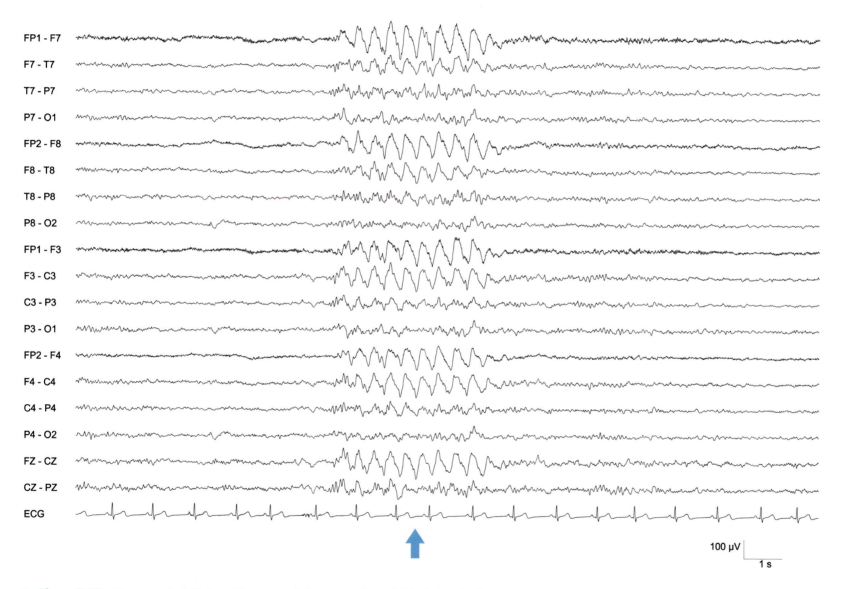

▶ **Figure 3.53** **Hypnagogic delta burst (hypnagogic hypersynchrony).** Bipolar longitudinal montage. High-amplitude, 4-s rhythmic delta burst in a 10-year-old during drowsiness (blue arrow). Notice that intermixed with the delta waves there are faster waves that together with the slow waves may be misdiagnosed as spike–waves. These hypnagogic bursts of delta waves are typical at this age.

Vertex wave and sleep spindle

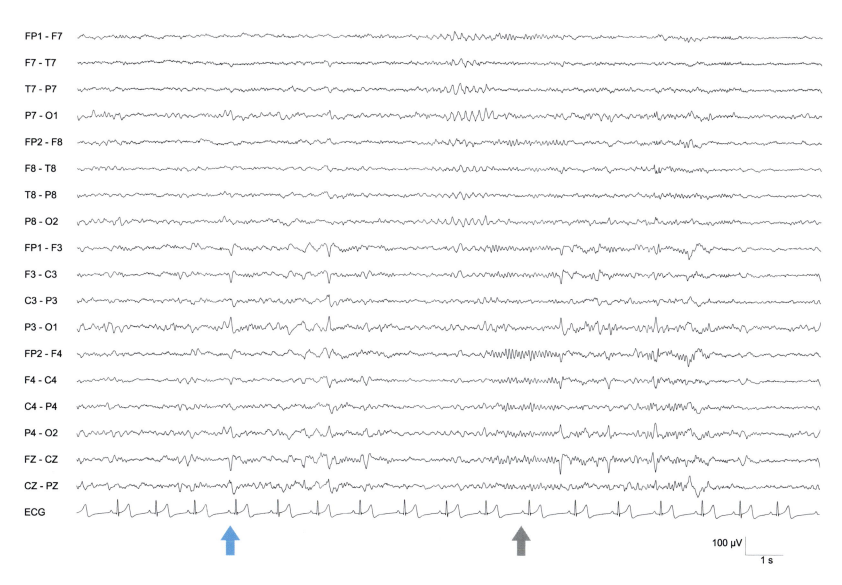

FP1 - F7
F7 - T7
T7 - P7
P7 - O1
FP2 - F8
F8 - T8
T8 - P8
P8 - O2
FP1 - F3
F3 - C3
C3 - P3
P3 - O1
FP2 - F4
F4 - C4
C4 - P4
P4 - O2
FZ - CZ
CZ - PZ
ECG

100 µV

1 s

▶ **Figure 3.54** **Vertex wave and sleep spindle.** Bipolar longitudinal montage. This adult EEG shows vertex waves (blue arrow) and sleep spindles (gray arrow). Sleep spindles occur in non-REM sleep stage N2.

Sleep spindles and positive occipital sharp transients of sleep (POSTS)

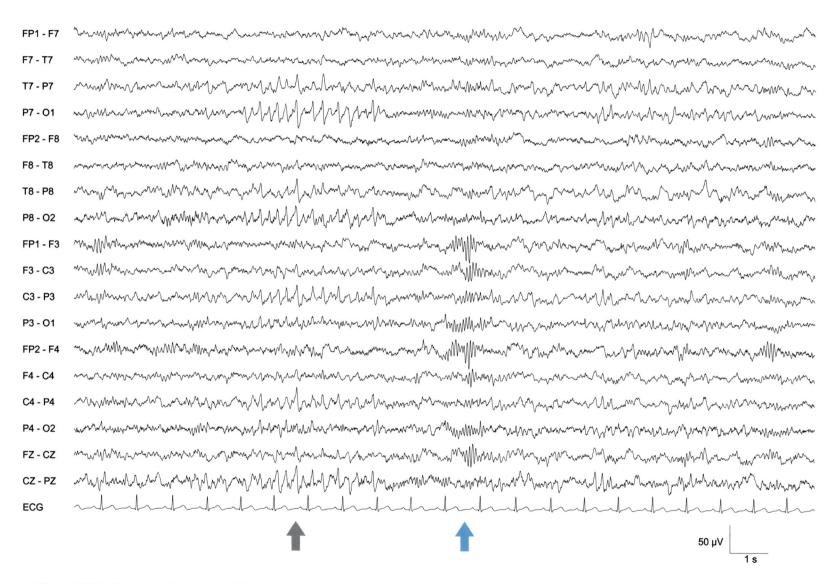

▶ **Figure 3.55** **Sleep spindles and positive occipital sharp transients of sleep (POSTS).** Bipolar longitudinal montage. This EEG of an adolescent shows POSTS (gray arrow) and sleep spindles (blue arrow) during non-REM sleep stage N2.

Positive sharp transients of sleep (POSTS) and sleep spindles

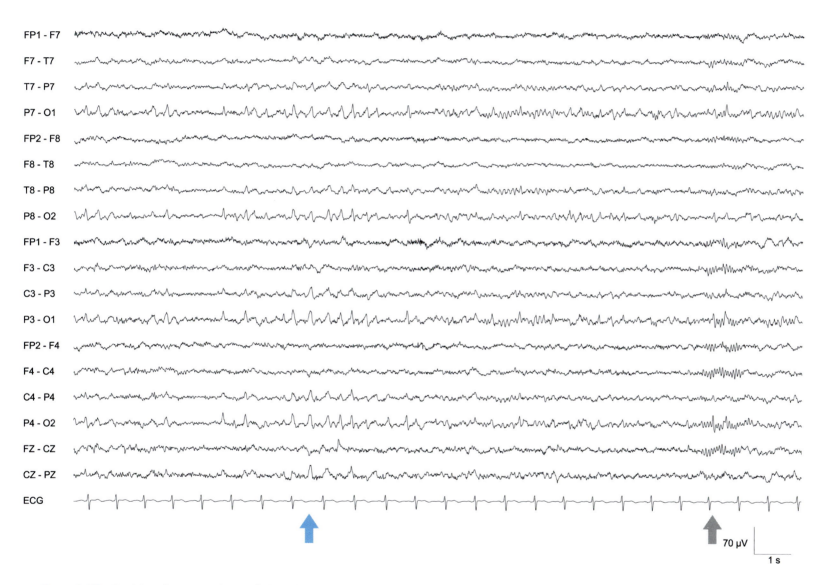

▶ **Figure 3.56** **Positive sharp transients of sleep (POSTS) and sleep spindles.** Bipolar longitudinal montage. This EEG of a young adult shows POSTS (blue arrow) and sleep spindles (gray arrow). These are normal EEG patterns.

Positive sharp transients of sleep (POSTS) and awakening

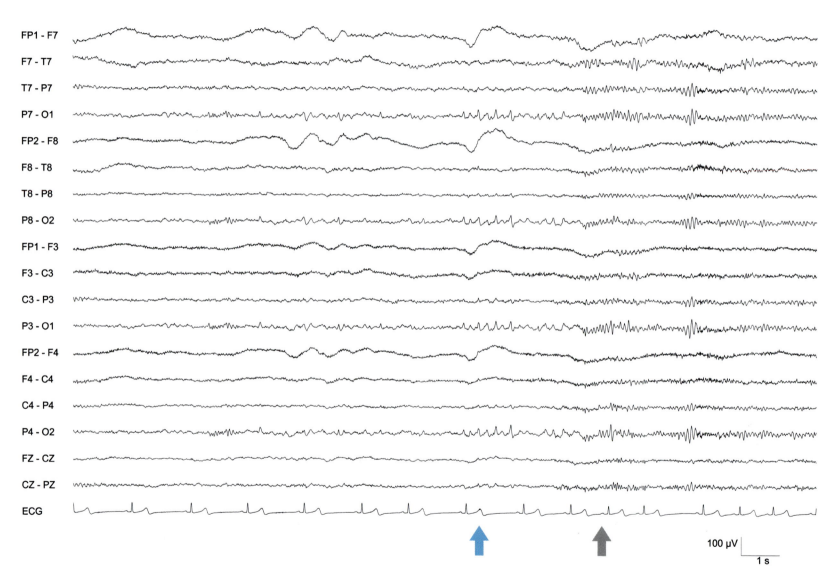

▶ **Figure 3.57** **Positive sharp transients of sleep (POSTS) and awakening.** Bipolar longitudinal montage. POSTS (blue arrow) are replaced by posterior dominant alpha rhythms when the patient wakes up (gray arrow).

At age 5 or 6 months, low-amplitude beta waves of approximately 25 Hz appear during sleep, alternating with vertex waves and high-amplitude K-complexes (▶ Figures 3.58 and 3.59). As the name suggests, the maximum negativity of vertex waves is located at the electrode CZ, whereas the maximum for the first slow component of the K-complex is located frontally. Vertex waves can occur in series, especially in childhood and adolescence (▶ Figure 3.60). Sleep spindles often frame K-complexes—that is, they occur at the beginning or end of a K-complex (Figures 3.58–3.60). The so-called mitten pattern is a variant of the K-complex without pathological significance (▶ Figure 3.61). However, the differential diagnosis between K-complex and epileptic spikes is sometimes difficult. Sleep spindles often trigger K-complexes, and not infrequently the mixture of sleep spindles and K-complexes may give the impression of a spike–wave. K-complexes represent the brain response to external and possibly internal stimuli during sleep. They are easily triggered by acoustic stimuli, which has given them their name. It is said that technical assistants used to knock on a table to wake up patients who were sleeping. This would trigger a K-complex, and the technical assistants documented this by writing a "K" (from knocking) on the EEG recording.

Shut eye waves (slow waves of highest amplitude in occipital derivations) occur 100–500 ms after eye closure at age 6 months to 10 years, with a peak in prevalence in the second or third year of life. Shut eye waves are mono- or biphasic and of relatively high amplitude. They have no pathological significance.

REM sleep is typically not found in routine EEG because it occurs physiologically only approximately 70 min after falling asleep (▶ Figures 3.62 and 3.63). In depressive disorders, REM latency is reduced to approximately 40 min, and in narcolepsy REM sleep occurs within the first 15 min after falling asleep. Strong sleep deprivation, but also a considerably disturbed sleep in severe obstructive sleep apnea, can lead to a similar early occurrence of REM sleep.

3.4.2 Abnormal EEG

This section discusses abnormal EEG categories (▶ Table 3.6). In this classification, each category is consistently related with a distinctive clinical pathology. The assessment of the following categories requires knowledge of the patient's state of consciousness, which must be tested and documented during the EEG. For example, the occipital background rhythm should be assessed when the

patient is fully alert because slowing of the occipital background activity tends to occur even with slight drowsiness.

3.4.2.1 Degree of EEG Abnormality

EEG changes are arranged in the order of their clinical significance and divided into the following categories (Lüders & Noachtar, 2000a):
- Normal EEG
- Abnormal EEG I, II, or III
- Technically difficult
- Technically inadequate

The assignment of the EEG abnormalities to the three degrees of abnormalities (abnormal I, II, or III) is based on (a) the severity of the brain disorder and/or (b) the specificity of the EEG findings. The EEG of a patient with a mild slow of occipital background activity—that is, a mild diffuse brain dysfunction—is classified as "abnormal EEG I" (▶ Figure 3.64), whereas the EEG of a patient in a deep coma and a diffuse delta slow (▶ Figure 3.65) is classified as "abnormal EEG III". On the other hand, the EEG of a neurologically inconspicuous patient showing spikes is also assessed as abnormal EEG III (▶ Figure 3.66) because this EEG finding correlates to a high degree with epilepsy and, therefore, the EEG finding is of highly significant clinical relevance.

3.4.2.2 State of Consciousness

The vigilance of patients during the EEG recording—that is, whether they were awake, asleep, or in different degrees of alteration of consciousness—is shown in brackets followed by the degree of EEG abnormality. The state of consciousness of a patient is essential for the classification of the EEG. EEG findings in patients in coma and stupor are always classified as abnormal III. In ▶ Table 3.7, the abbreviations for the different states of consciousness are listed in brackets.

Technically inadequate and technically difficult EEGs refer to recordings that cannot be adequately assessed because the EEG tech did not correct a technical error (technically inadequate; e.g., uncorrected pulse artifact), the patient was uncooperative (technically difficult; e.g., excessive muscle artifact), or other

Vertex wave and K-complex

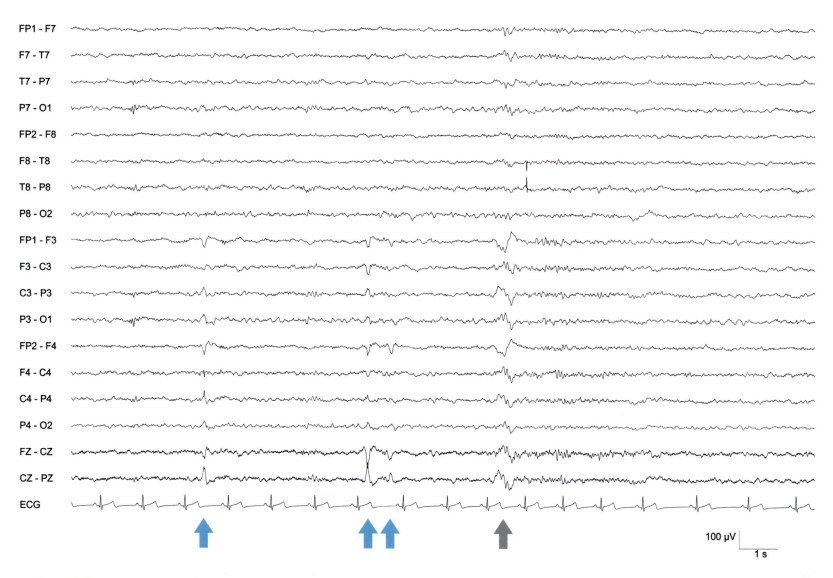

FP1 - F7
F7 - T7
T7 - P7
P7 - O1
FP2 - F8
F8 - T8
T8 - P8
P8 - O2
FP1 - F3
F3 - C3
C3 - P3
P3 - O1
FP2 - F4
F4 - C4
C4 - P4
P4 - O2
FZ - CZ
CZ - PZ
ECG

100 µV
1 s

▶ **Figure 3.58** **Vertex wave and K-complex.** Bipolar longitudinal montage. This EEG of a young adult shows vertex waves (blue arrows) and one K-complex (gray arrow).

K-complex and sleep spindle

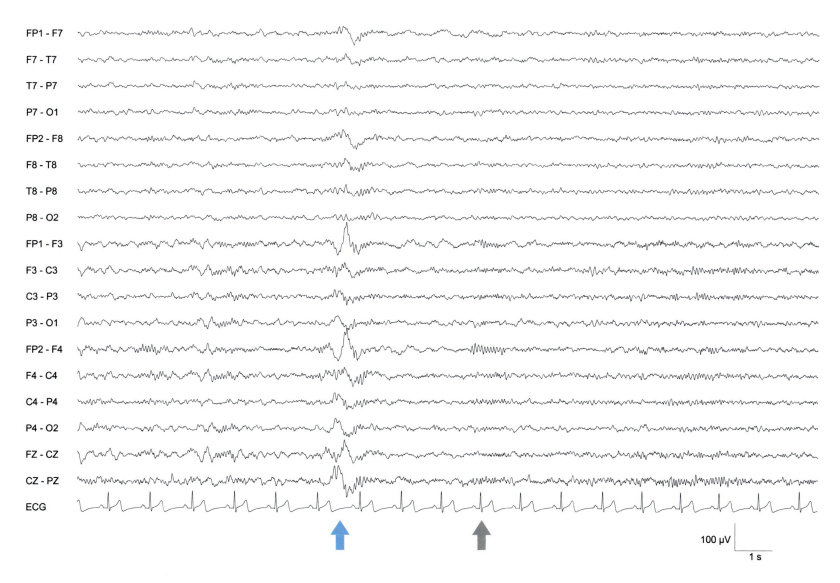

▶ **Figure 3.59** **K-complex and sleep spindle.** Bipolar longitudinal montage. In the sleep of a young adult, K-complexes (blue arrow) and sleep spindles (gray arrow) occur.

Repetitive vertex waves, K-complex, and arousal

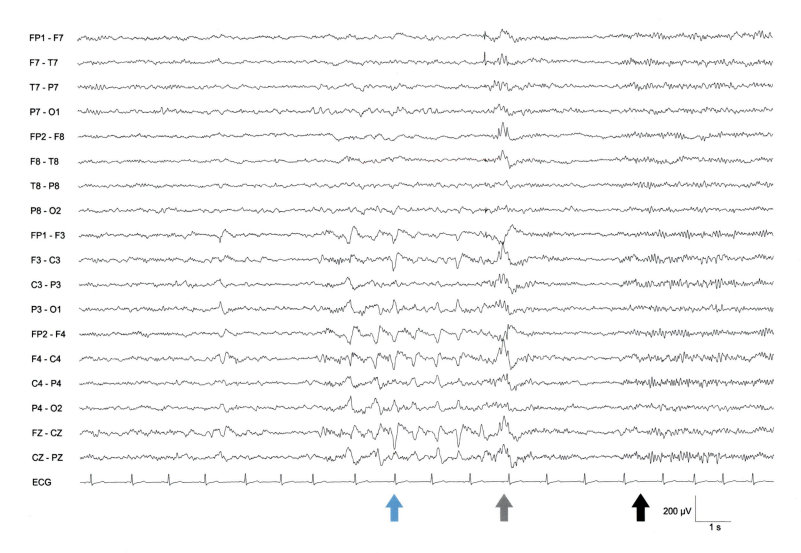

▶ **Figure 3.60** **Repetitive vertex waves, K-complex, and arousal.** Bipolar longitudinal montage. In this 16-year-old patient with vasovagal syncope, repetitive vertex waves (blue arrow) occur during sleep. After a series of vertex waves, a K-complex (gray arrow) appears before an arousal occurs (black arrow).

Mitten pattern and K-complex

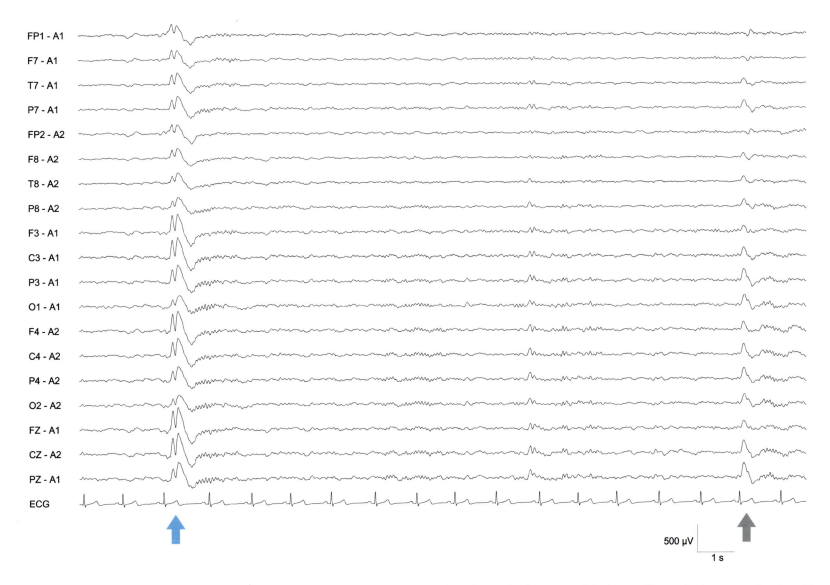

▶ **Figure 3.61** **Mitten pattern and K-complex.** Bipolar longitudinal montage. This EEG sample of a young adult shows a K-complex (gray arrow) and a mitten pattern (blue arrow). Both are normal EEG patterns.

REM sleep

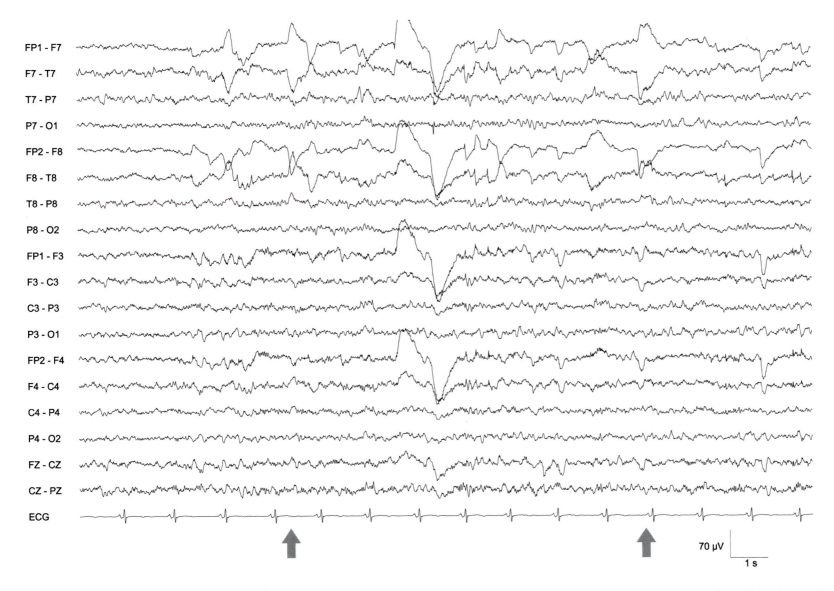

FP1 - F7
F7 - T7
T7 - P7
P7 - O1
FP2 - F8
F8 - T8
T8 - P8
P8 - O2
FP1 - F3
F3 - C3
C3 - P3
P3 - O1
FP2 - F4
F4 - C4
C4 - P4
P4 - O2
FZ - CZ
CZ - PZ
ECG

70 μV
1 s

▶ **Figure 3.62** **REM sleep.** Bipolar longitudinal montage. This EEG sample of a young adult showed REM sleep approximately 70 min after falling asleep. REM sleep is characterized by frequent, predominantly horizontal saccadic eye movements (gray arrows) and relatively little or no EMG artifact. The EEG resembles the EEG of drowsiness, namely low-amplitude theta–delta waves with little or no EMG artifact.

Continuous slow, right temporal and asymmetry, increased beta right temporal

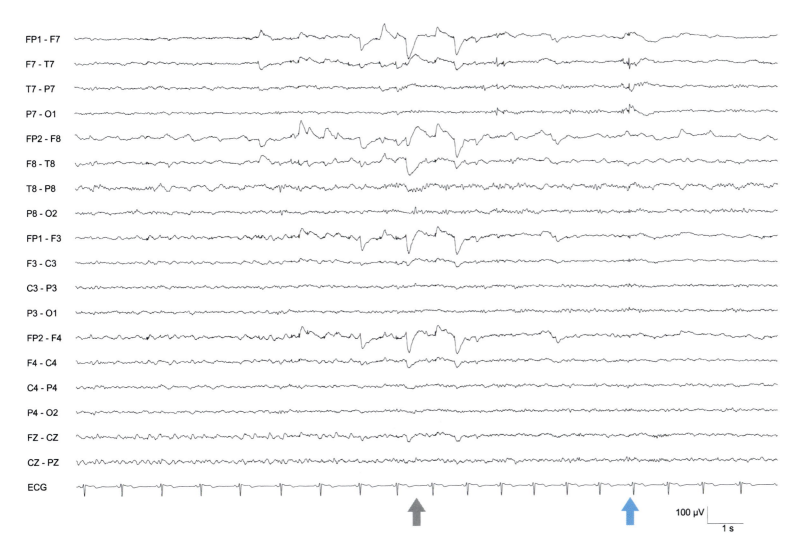

▶ **Figure 3.63** **Continuous slow, right temporal and asymmetry, increased beta right temporal.** REM sleep. Bipolar longitudinal montage. A 36-year-old adult who had a resection of a right temporal low-grade glioma. The EEG shows a right temporal, continuous slow and a slight increase of the amplitude of beta activity in the right temporal region. The frequent saccadic eye movements of REM sleep (gray arrow) make visualization of the EEG abnormality more difficult. The EEG also shows a left temporal muscle spicule (blue arrow). Multifocal muscle spicules also occur frequently during REM sleep. This EEG was performed during continuous EEG video monitoring. REM sleep occurred under physiological conditions during night sleep.

EEG classification: Abnormal III (REM sleep)
1. Continuous slow, right temporal
2. Asymmetry, increased beta right temporal

EEG report: This EEG is the expression of a right anterior temporal lobe resection.

▶ **Table 3.6 Abnormal EEG Categories**

EEG Category	Degree of EEG Abnormality	Figure Numbers
EEG slow and EEG suppression		
1. Background slow (BS)	I–II	3.64, 3.68, 3.69
2. Intermittent slow (IS)	I–II	3.71, 3.72, 3.75
2.1. Intermittent rhythmic slow (IRS)	I–III	3.77–3.82
3. Continuous slow (CS)	I–III	3.101–3.104
4. Background Suppression (BSU)	III	3.113, 3.114
5. Background attenuation (BA)	III	3.111, 3.112
6. Electrocerebral Inactivity (ECI)	III	3.115
Epileptiform discharges		
1. Spikes (SP)	III	3.116–3.123
2. Polyspikes (PSP)		3.132, 3.133, 3.138–3.140
3. Benign epileptiform discharges (BED)	III	2.27, 3.141–3.144
4. Spike–waves		3.145–3.148, 3.150, 3.151, 3.153
5. Polyspike–waves (PSW)	III	3.127
6. 3 Hz spike–waves (3SWC)	III	3.149, 3.152
7. Slow spike–waves (SSW)	III	3.154–3.156
8. Hypsarrhythmia (HYP)	III	3.157–3.159
9. Photoparoxysmal response (PR)	I–III	3.12–3.14

EEG Category	Degree of EEG Abnormality	Figure Numbers
10. Seizure pattern (SEP)	III	3.159, 3.166–3.197
11. Status pattern (STP)	III	3.198–3.205, 3.207–3.231
Periodic pattern		
1. Periodic discharges (PD)	III	3.246–3.252, 3.254
2. Periodic epileptiform discharges (PED)	III	3.253, 3.255–3.259
3. Triphasic waves (TW)	III	3.260–3.266
4. Burst suppression (BUS)	III	3.267–3.270
5. Burst attenuation (BUA)	III	3.271, 3.272
Special patterns		
1. Excessive beta (EB)	I	3.273
2. Asymmetry (ASY)	II	3.274–3.282
3. Sleep-onset REM (SOREM)	III	3.283
Special patterns used only in patients in stupor or coma		
1. Alpha coma (AC)/alpha stupor (AS)	III	3.284, 3.287–3.289
2. Spindle coma (SC)/spindle stupor (SS)	III	3.290, 3.291
3. Beta coma (BC)/beta stupor (BES)	III	3.292
4. Theta coma (TC)/theta stupor (TS)	III	3.293
5. Delta coma (DC) / delta stupor (DS)	III	3.285, 3.286, 3.294, 3.295

EEG, electroencephalogram; REM, rapid eye movement.

Background slow

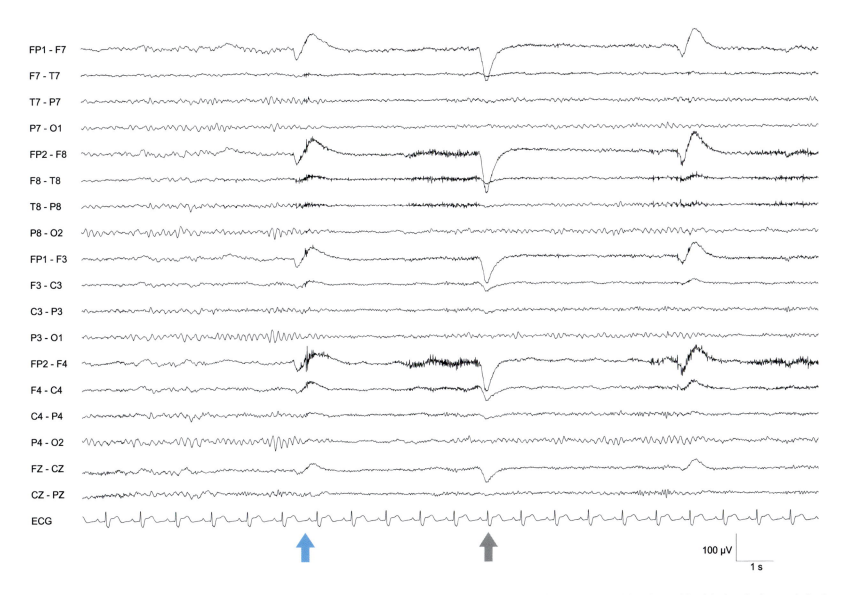

▶ **Figure 3.64**   **Background slow.** Bipolar longitudinal montage. The background occipital rhythm of this 68-year-old patient with Alzheimer's dementia is slowed to 7 Hz. Eye opening (blue arrow) blocks the occipital activity, and after eye closure (gray arrow), the posterior background activity returns.

EEG classification: Abnormal I (awake)

   Background slow

EEG report: This EEG is indicative of a mild diffuse encephalopathy in the context of Alzheimer's dementia.

Delta coma

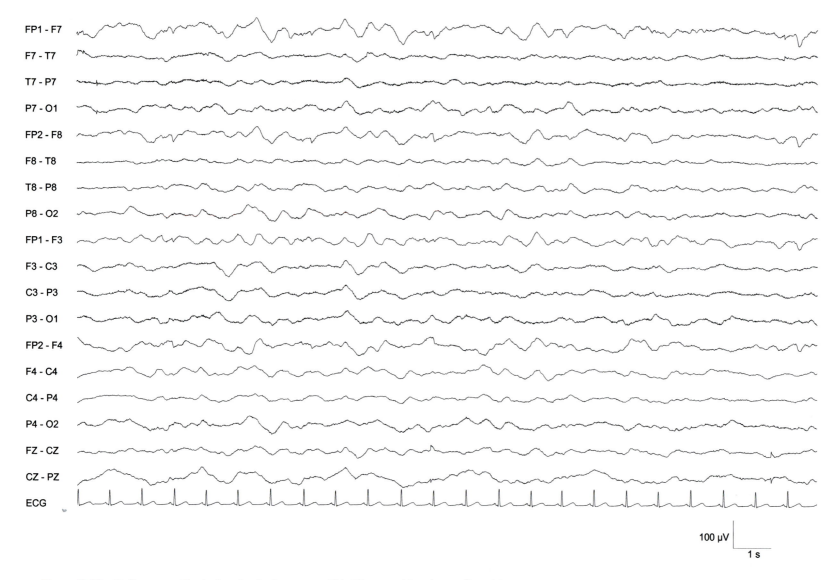

FP1 - F7

F7 - T7

T7 - P7

P7 - O1

FP2 - F8

F8 - T8

T8 - P8

P8 - O2

FP1 - F3

F3 - C3

C3 - P3

P3 - O1

FP2 - F4

F4 - C4

C4 - P4

P4 - O2

FZ - CZ

CZ - PZ

ECG

100 µV

1 s

▶ **Figure 3.65** **Delta coma.** Bipolar longitudinal montage. This 58-year-old patient suffered from severe metabolic encephalopathy due to sepsis and renal failure. The EEG is dominated by diffusely distributed irregular delta waves. There was no EEG or clinical response to external stimuli (passive eye opening, acoustic, tactile, pain).

EEG classification: Abnormal III (coma)

Delta coma

EEG report: This EEG is indicative of a severe metabolic encephalopathy.

Spikes, left frontal, and continuous slow, left frontal

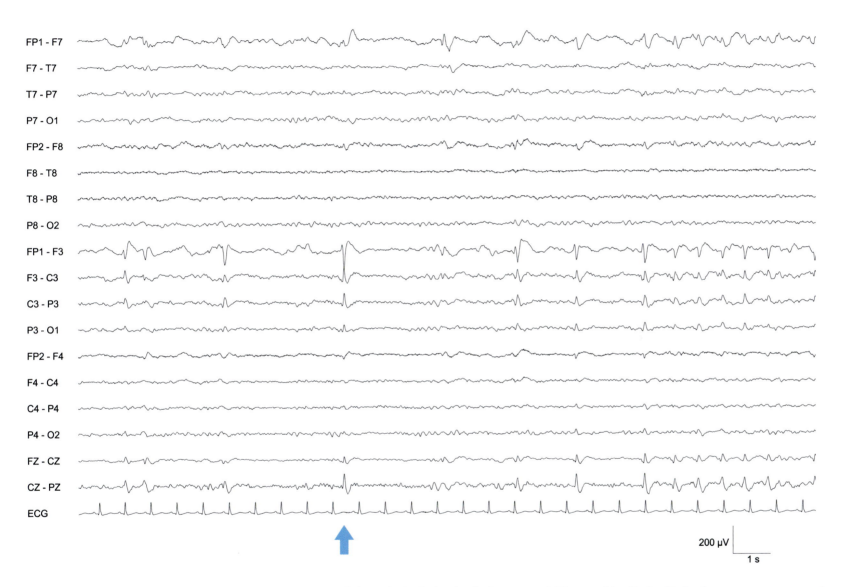

▶ **Figure 3.66** **Spikes, left frontal, and continuous slow, left frontal.** Bipolar longitudinal montage. A 28-year-old patient suffering from a severe open craniocerebral trauma and a left frontal epilepsy. This EEG sample shows frequent left frontal spikes (blue arrow) as well as a continuous left frontal slow. The EEG abnormalities are an expression of the left frontal structural lesion documented in an MRI.

EEG classification: Abnormal III (awake)
1. Spikes, F3 > C3 > FP1
2. Continuous slow, left frontal

EEG report: This EEG supports the diagnosis of highly epileptogenic left frontal lesion.

Wake (W)
Drowsiness (D)
Sleep (S)
Lethargy (L)
Stupor (ST)
Coma (CO)
Anesthesia (AN)
Neuromuscular blockade (NM)

conditions were present that influenced the technical quality of the EEG derivation (e.g., an artifact persists although the EEG tech repeatedly tried to correct the problem). The EEG is classified as technically difficult or technically inadequate, and no other EEG abnormalities are mentioned in the official EEG classification if there is no discernable EEG abnormality. However, technically inadequate or technically difficult EEGs may still contain information that may be mentioned in the clinical evaluation. In the EEG impression, it could then be said, for example, that "the EEG recording does not show epileptiform discharges, as far as it can be assessed in a partially artifact-obscured recording." If despite major portions of technically inadequate EEG, some abnormalities could be identified, they should be classified accordingly.

The EEG is classified as usual if artifacts are present but are not conspicuous enough to not allow adequate evaluation of the EEG.

3.4.2.3   Slow and Suppression

This category includes the following EEG abnormalities:
- Activity abnormally slow for the patient's age
- Regional or lateralized activity slowed down compared to the homotopic contralateral side
- Abnormally attenuated or suppressed background activity

Slow is further subdivided into the following:
1. Background slow (BS)
2. Intermittent slow (IS)
   2.1. Intermittent rhythmic slow (IRS)
3. Continuous slow (CS)

Intermittent rhythmic slow (IRS) is a subgroup of intermittent slow (► **Table 3.8**).

3.4.2.3.1   Background Slow (BS)

Background slow is an EEG whose main awake background frequency is abnormally slow. The normal background rhythm frequency is age dependent. Background slow is diagnosed if the EEG shows background rhythm frequencies that do not reach the values listed in ► **Table 3.9** (Arenas et al., 1986; Eeg-Olofsson, 1971b; Katz & Horowitz, 1982; Torres et al., 1983).

The background activity must be measured when the patient is fully awake. The technologist should have the patient solve some simple cognitive tests to ensure that the patient is fully alert. The task given to the patient should be appropriate for the patient's age. It is important also to be aware that having the patient talk during the test (counting from 1 to 10, answering questions, etc.) frequently leads to tongue movement artifacts (glossokinetic artifacts; ► **Figure 3.67**). In addition to the absolute frequency of the background rhythms, a slowing of the background frequency by more than 1 Hz compared to a previous EEG is considered abnormal. The responsiveness of the patient can also be tested with the "clicker" test (**Fig. 3.150** and **3.194**) (Browne et al., 1974; see Section 3.4.2.4).

The causes of background slow are manifold and usually nonspecific. Background slow is due to disturbances of cortical and/or subcortical mechanisms involved in the generation of background rhythms. Background slow may be caused by any disease that produces a diffuse encephalopathy, such as degenerative, metabolic, or toxic disorders (drug overdose with sedatives, anti-seizure medications, etc.).

The degree of abnormality (encephalopathy) is determined by the degree of slow of the background rhythms. In adults, a background slow at or above 7 Hz is considered abnormal I (mild diffuse encephalopathy). A background slow under 7 Hz is considered abnormal II (moderate diffuse encephalopathy) (► **Figures 3.68** and **3.69**).

▶ **Table 3.8** **Criteria of Slow**

	Background Slow (BS)	Intermittent Slow (IS)	Intermittent Rhythmic Slow (IRS)	Continuous Slow (CS)
Frequency	Theta	Theta and/or delta	Theta and/or delta	Theta and/or delta
Distribution	Similar to the normal occipital background rhythms; may move more frontally	Regional or generalized	Regional or generalized	Regional or generalized
Waveform	Rhythmical	Irregular	Rhythmical	Irregular or rhythmical
Expression	Continuous	Intermittent	Intermittent	Continuous[a]
Responsiveness	Responsive[b]	Responsive[b]	Variable	Variable

[a] Continuous slow for at least 90% of the wake recording.
[b] Responsive = decrease with eye opening and mental activation; increase at the beginning of hyperventilation.

3.4.2.3.2   Intermittent Slow (IS)

This refers to slow that occurs intermittently and irregularly and is not caused by drowsiness. Only EEG recordings in which the degree of slow exceeds the age-related physiological level are classified as abnormal. Intermittent slow can occur generalized or focal. Several relatively specific intermittent slow have been described. Electroencephalographers must recognize these patterns and should be acquainted with their clinical significance.

▶ **Table 3.9** **Lowest Background Frequencies Seen in Normal Children and Adults[a]**

Age (Years)	Background Frequency (Hz)
½	4
1	5
3	6
5	7
8	8

[a] Most children and adults have higher background frequencies. This table shows the lower limit of the background frequencies observed in normal children and adults.

Under certain conditions, intermittent slow may occur physiologically. For example, generalized intermittent slow occurs physiologically under HV and subsides within minutes after the end of HV. It usually has a frontal maximum and is then referred to by the acronym FIRDA (▶ **Figure** 3.70). HV-induced intermittent slow is particularly pronounced in children aged 8–12 years and in adults with a low blood glucose level. Sunder et al. (1980) reported that in children with moyamoya syndrome, HV-induced slow may even increase after the end of HV. This unusual finding has not been confirmed by a systematic study.

Generalized intermittent slow occurs normally during drowsiness. Therefore, it is essential to ask the patient to perform mental tasks to exclude drowsiness as the cause of the intermittent slow. There is discrepancy in the literature regarding the significance of generalized intermittent slow in patients with a normal background activity between bursts of slow activity. Gloor et al. (1968) and Schaul (1990) reported that any intermittent generalized slow, even in patients with a normal background activity, is of abnormal significance. We believe that a short burst of generalized intermittent slow covering less than 10% of the recording is most likely a normal finding, if the background rhythm frequency is within normal limits. These bursts of slow activity most likely reflect slight drowsiness (▶ **Figure** 3.71). Therefore, mental activation at some point during the EEG recording is essential to exclude drowsiness-induced

3 Clinical Electroencephalography

221

Glossokinetic artifact (tongue movement artifact)

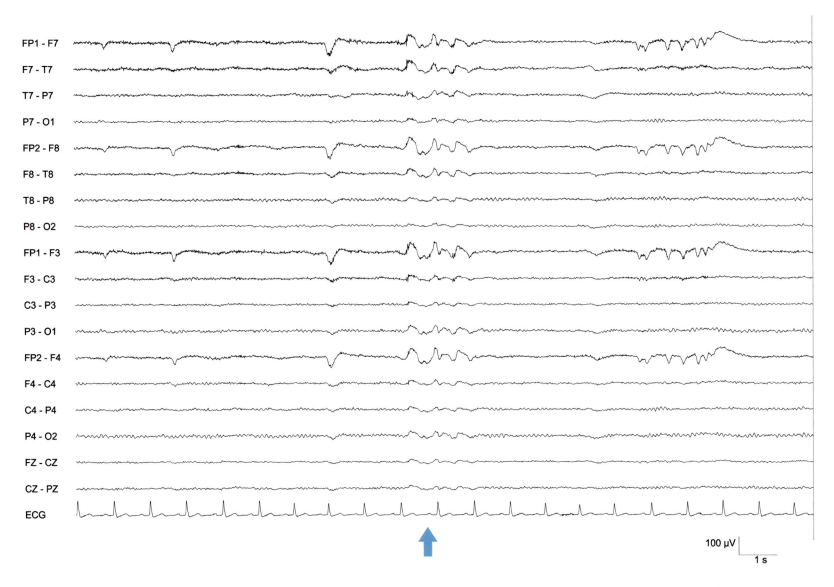

▶ **Figure 3.67** **Glossokinetic artifact (tongue movement artifact).** Bipolar longitudinal montage. This EEG shows a physiological occipital alpha background rhythm and several eye blinks. The blue arrow marks the time when the patient speaks. The artifacts produced by tongue movements are caused by a bipolar generator with the negative pole in the front of the tongue and a positive pole in the back of the tongue. Therefore, if the whole tongue moves up, the frontal electrodes become negative and the occipital electrodes positive. This explains why the frontopolar electrodes show a maximum negativity at FP1/FP2 with an exponential fall off posteriorly and at the same time the occipital electrodes become relatively more positive than more anterior electrodes. This leads to an upward deflection at P4–O2 that is larger than the upward deflection at C4–P4. Eye movements or blinks, however, have a maximum at FP1/FP2 and then fall off exponentially at more posterior electrodes. Therefore, C4–P4 should always be of higher amplitude than P4–O2. In addition, usually the eye artifact is not even detected at channel P4–O2.

Background slow

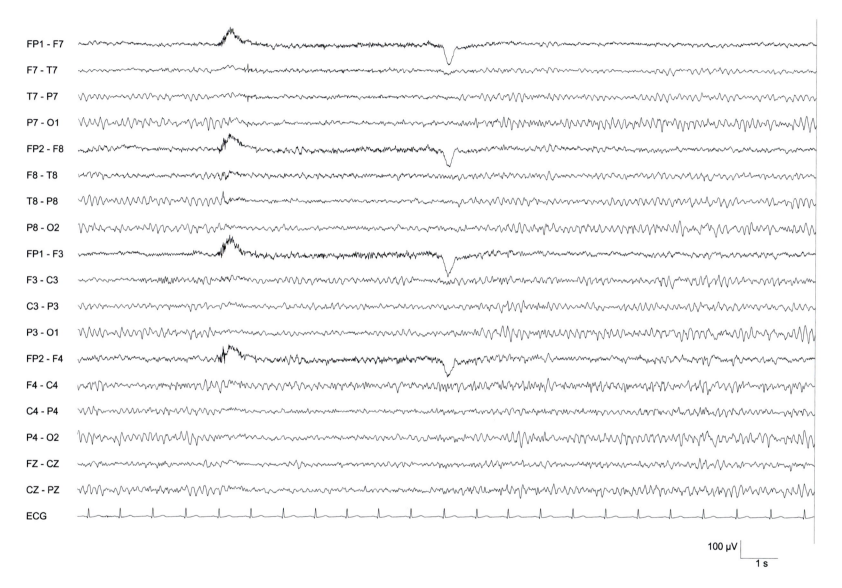

100 µV

1 s

▶ **Figure 3.68** **Background slow.** Bipolar longitudinal montage. A 26-year-old female patient with left focal epilepsy and high-dose medication of topiramate and oxcarbazepine, leading to dizziness, ataxia, and impaired cognition. The occipital background rhythm is at 7 Hz.

EEG classification: Abnormal I (awake)
Background slow

EEG report: This EEG supports the diagnosis of a drug-induced mild diffuse encephalopathy.

Background slow

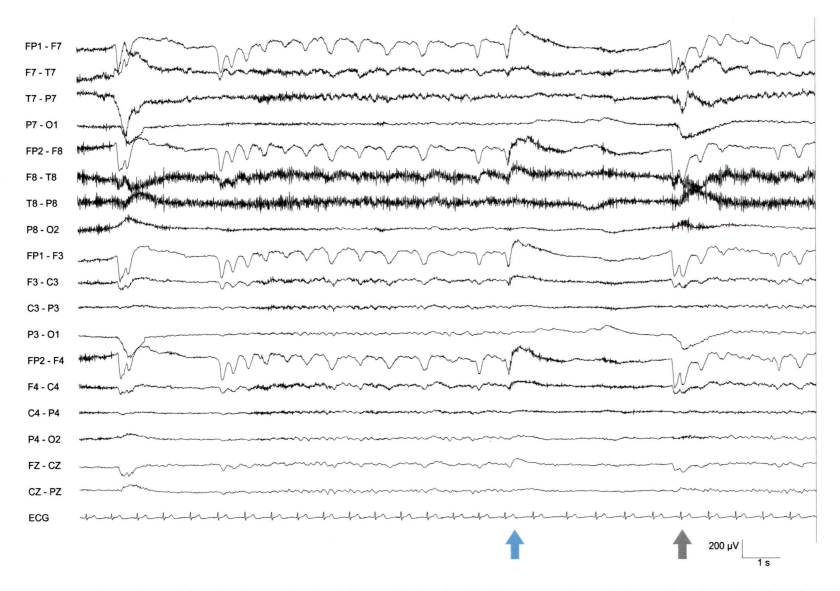

▶ **Figure 3.69**   **Background slow.** Ear reference derivation. A 25-year-old alcoholic patient with new-onset generalized convulsive seizure. During the EEG recording, the patient was still confused. The occipital background rhythm had a frequency of 5 or 6 Hz. Note the inhibition of the occipital background activity by eye opening (blue arrow) and its return after eye closure (gray arrow). Notice also the eyelid flutter, initially at a frequency of 2 Hz and then slowing down progressively to 1 Hz.

EEG classification: Abnormal II (awake)
   Background slow

EEG report: This EEG is indicative of a postictal moderate diffuse encephalopathy.

Generalized maximum frontal intermittent rhythmic slow (FIRDA)

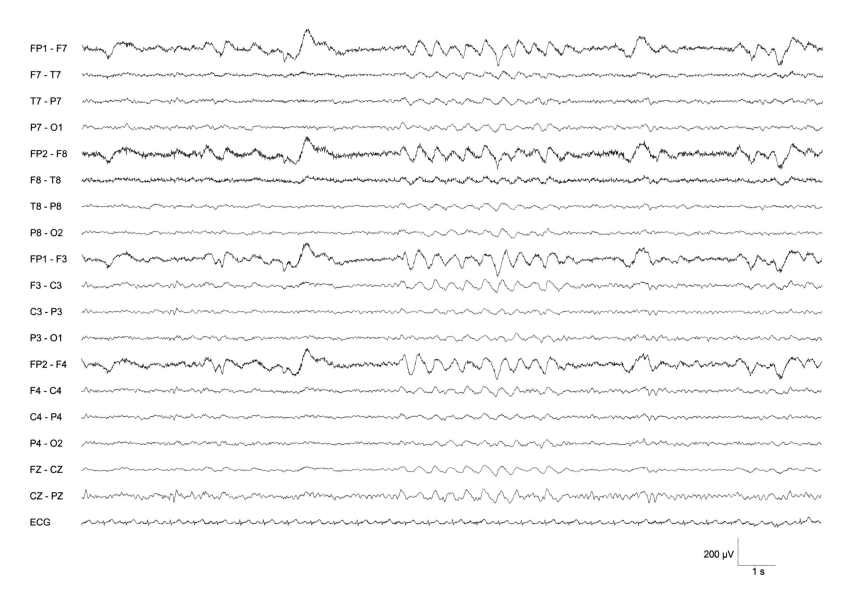

FP1 - F7

F7 - T7

T7 - P7

P7 - O1

FP2 - F8

F8 - T8

T8 - P8

P8 - O2

FP1 - F3

F3 - C3

C3 - P3

P3 - O1

FP2 - F4

F4 - C4

C4 - P4

P4 - O2

FZ - CZ

CZ - PZ

ECG

200 µV

1 s

▶ **Figure 3.70**   **Generalized maximum frontal intermittent rhythmic slow (FIRDA).** Bipolar longitudinal montage. A 37-year-old female patient with dizziness and tension headache. During hyperventilation, a burst of high-amplitude generalized frontal maximum rhythmic delta waves occurred. This pattern, called FIRDA, disappeared within 3 min after hyperventilation.

EEG classification: Normal (awake)

EEG report: This EEG shows a normal finding.

Intermittent slow, generalized. Bipolar longitudinal montage

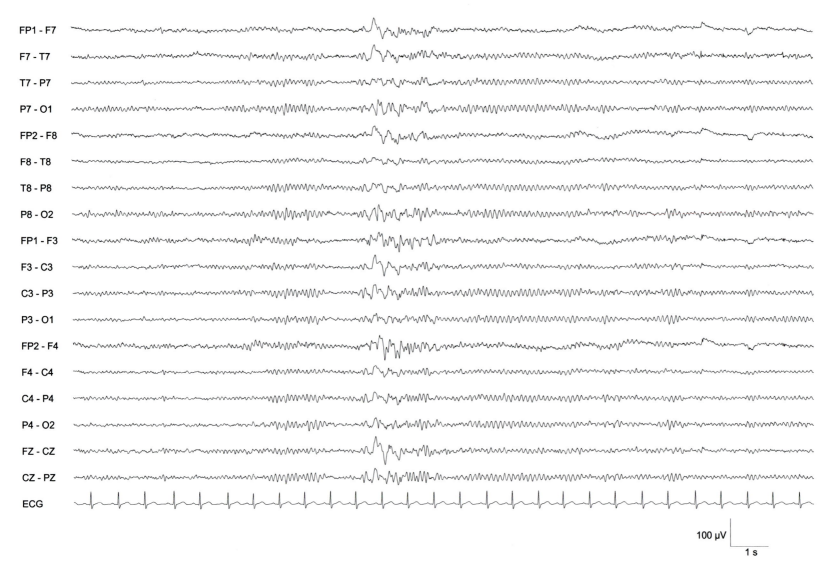

FP1 - F7

F7 - T7

T7 - P7

P7 - O1

FP2 - F8

F8 - T8

T8 - P8

P8 - O2

FP1 - F3

F3 - C3

C3 - P3

P3 - O1

FP2 - F4

F4 - C4

C4 - P4

P4 - O2

FZ - CZ

CZ - PZ

ECG

100 µV

1 s

▶ **Figure 3.71** **Intermittent slow, generalized.** Bipolar longitudinal montage. A 58-year-old obese patient with long-term arterial hypertension, diabetes mellitus II, and severe obstructive sleep apnea syndrome. Repeated groups of high-amplitude frontal rhythmic delta waves occurred. These bursts were unrelated to hyperventilation. They also occurred during cognitive activation. Otherwise, there was a normal alpha EEG.

EEG classification: Abnormal I (awake)
   Intermittent slow, generalized

EEG report: This EEG is indicative of a mild diffuse encephalopathy.

generalized intermittent slow. Generalized intermittent slow of more than 10% is indicative of a mild diffuse encephalopathy if the background rhythms are within normal limits and drowsiness is excluded (▶ Figure 3.72). These EEGs are classified as abnormal EEG I. Usually, generalized intermittent slow occurs together with a mild slowing of the background rhythms (▶ Figure 3.73). In these cases, the degree of abnormality is defined by the degree of slowing of the background rhythms (see above).

In sleep, only regional slow is considered abnormal because sleep itself leads to generalized slow. Regional intermittent slow usually is indicative of regional pathology located approximately in the region of the intermittent slow (▶ Figure 3.74). ▶ Figure 3.75 shows a left temporal intermittent slow that occurs when changing from light sleep to wakefulness.

Occipital intermittent rhythmic delta activity (OIRDA) has been described in children with absence epilepsies, but its epileptiform nature is not well established (▶ Figure 3.76) (Cobb, 1945; Desai et al., 2012; Gullapalli & Fountain, 2003).

3.4.2.3.2.1   Intermittent Rhythmic Slow (IRS)

Temporal intermittent rhythmic delta activity is an example of IRS and has been described in patients with temporal lobe epilepsy (Reiher et al., 1989) (▶ Figures 3.77–3.80). IRS can be also recorded in one frontal lobe in patients with frontal lobe epilepsy (▶ Figure 3.81).

Generalized intermittent rhythmic slow has the same diagnostic implications as generalized intermittent slow (▶ Figure 3.82). As mentioned previously, this nonspecific EEG pattern must be distinguished from the following EEG patterns:

- Hypnagogic theta–delta burst of drowsiness (▶ Figure 3.83) (see below)
- The generalized intermittent rhythmic slow seen in patients with midline frontal lobe epilepsy with secondary bilateral generalization
- OIRDA, which is a normal EEG pattern in children and adolescents (▶ Figure 3.76)

The grade of abnormality depends on the severity of the IRS and is rated abnormal I or II.

3.4.2.3.2.2   Temporal Slow of the Elderly

Normal individuals older than age 50 years frequently show 2- to 4-s burst of irregular theta–delta waves localized to the temporal region., especially on the left hemisphere (Katz & Horowitz, 1982; Torres et al., 1983) (▶ Figures 3.84 and 3.85). These bursts of slow activity have no relationship to any temporal lobe pathology and, therefore, are considered a normal EEG pattern.

3.4.2.3.2.3   Hypnagogic/Hypnopompic Theta–Delta Bursts

In children, generalized bursts of theta–delta activity tend to occur in the transition from awake to sleep state and also in the transition from sleep to awake. These theta–delta bursts usually are maximum in the frontal region. The maximum amplitude tends to alternate between the two hemispheres. The bursts are rhythmic and can last for minutes in toddlers. In older children and adolescents, they usually occur in shorter bursts (▶ Figures 3.86 and 3.87). They are also called hypnagogic or hypnopompic hypersynchrony, depending on whether the phenomenon occurs when falling asleep (hypnagogic) or waking up (hypnopompic). Hypersynchrony, however, is an awkward term because an increase of the absolute term synchronous is conceptually impossible.

3.4.2.3.2.4   Occipital Slow of Youth

In normal adolescents, individual or short bursts of delta waves occur in the occipital region (occipital delta waves of adolescence, delta de la jeunesse, teenage delta, and posterior slow waves of youth). Bursts of delta waves occur mainly in younger adolescents, whereas individual delta waves are typical of older adolescents (▶ Figures 3.88–3.90). They behave like the occipital alpha background rhythm—that is, the amplitude tends to be slightly higher on the right hemisphere and the slow waves are blocked by eye opening. Irregular occipital slow that does not follow these characteristics has to be differentiated.

Sometimes a higher amplitude alpha wave precedes the occipital slow wave, possibly giving the impression of a sharp wave (▶ Figure 3.91).

3.4.2.3.2.5   Eye Closure Activity

In normal individuals, occasionally rhythmic delta waves occur after eye closure (▶ Figure 3.92). Eyelid closure activity must be distinguished from "fixation-off" sensitivity, in which occipital and occasionally also generalized spikes occur if the eyes are kept closed. The spikes, however, disappear when the patient opens the eyes and fixes the gaze (▶ Figure 3.93). Prevention of gaze fixation by Frenzel goggles leads to the appearance of the spikes even with open eyes. Conversely, the spikes do not reappear if the patient is placed in a dark room and is asked to fixate the gaze on a small red target. Fixation-off sensitivity

Intermittent slow, generalized

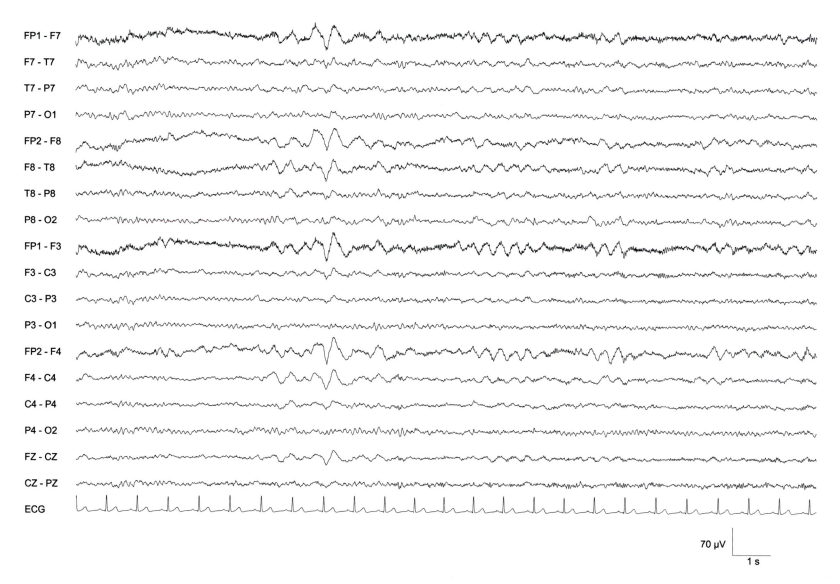

FP1 - F7

F7 - T7

T7 - P7

P7 - O1

FP2 - F8

F8 - T8

T8 - P8

P8 - O2

FP1 - F3

F3 - C3

C3 - P3

P3 - O1

FP2 - F4

F4 - C4

C4 - P4

P4 - O2

FZ - CZ

CZ - PZ

ECG

70 μV

1 s

▶ **Figure 3.72** **Intermittent slow, generalized.** Bipolar longitudinal montage. A 43-year-old patient with multiple sclerosis and anxiety disorder. Frequent bursts of generalized, irregular slow waves occur.

EEG classification: Abnormal I (awake)
    Intermittent slow, generalized

EEG report: This EEG supports the diagnosis of a mild diffuse encephalopathy due to multiple sclerosis.

Background slow and intermittent slow, generalized

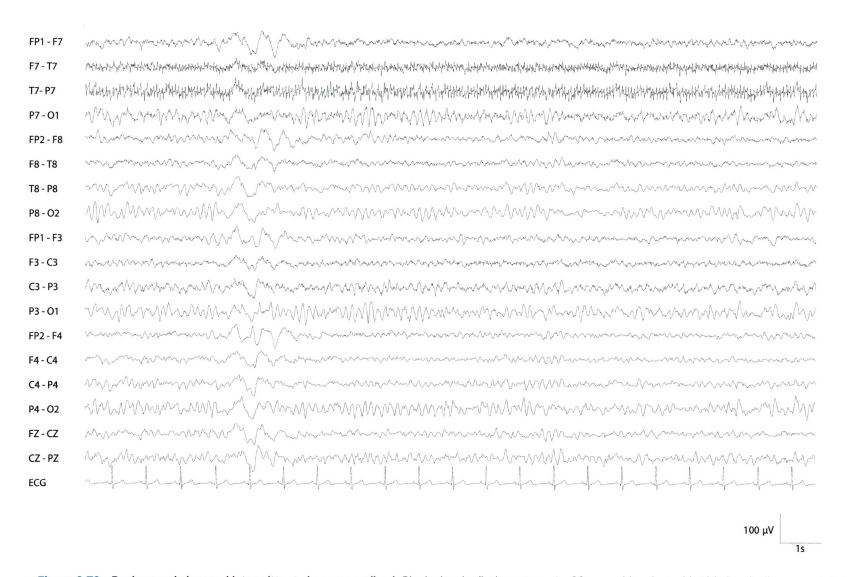

100 µV

1s

▶ **Figure 3.73** **Background slow and intermittent slow, generalized.** Bipolar longitudinal montage. An 80-year-old patient with Alzheimer's disease and status post fall with mild traumatic subarachnoid hemorrhage and bifrontal mild hemorrhagic encephalomalacia. During mental activation, a burst of generalized high amplitude delta waves occurs. The occipital background rhythm is slow at 6 Hz.

EEG classification: Abnormal II (awake)
1. Background slow
2. Intermittent slow, generalized

EEG report: This EEG is indicative of a moderate diffuse encephalopathy.

Intermittent slow, left temporal

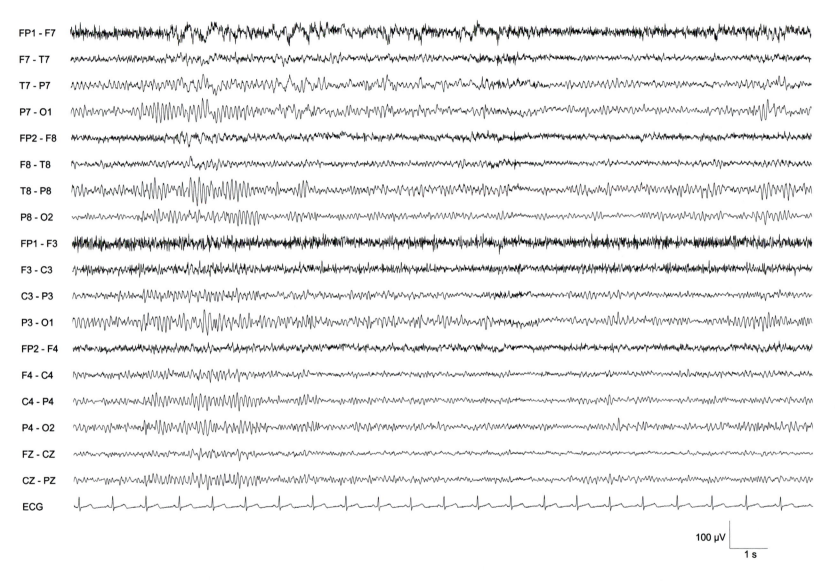

FP1 - F7

F7 - T7

T7 - P7

P7 - O1

FP2 - F8

F8 - T8

T8 - P8

P8 - O2

FP1 - F3

F3 - C3

C3 - P3

P3 - O1

FP2 - F4

F4 - C4

C4 - P4

P4 - O2

FZ - CZ

CZ - PZ

ECG

100 μV

1 s

▶ **Figure 3.74** **Intermittent slow, left temporal.** Bipolar longitudinal montage. In this 59-year-old female patient with transitory ischemic attacks, irregular theta and delta waves occur intermittently in the left temporal region. Otherwise, the EEG shows a normal occipital alpha background rhythm.

EEG classification: Abnormal I (awake)

EEG report: This EEG shows a left temporal dysfunction associated with left hemisphere transient ischemic attack.

Intermittent slow, left temporal

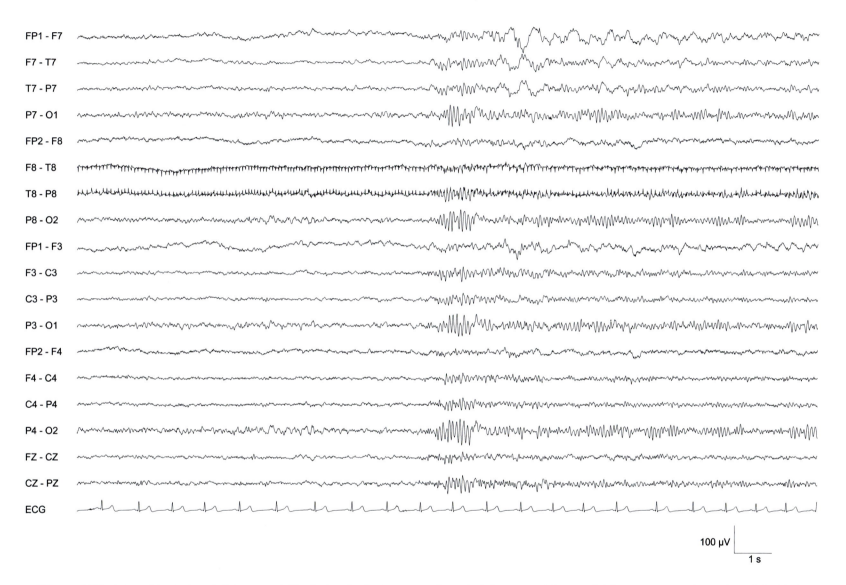

FP1 - F7
F7 - T7
T7 - P7
P7 - O1
FP2 - F8
F8 - T8
T8 - P8
P8 - O2
FP1 - F3
F3 - C3
C3 - P3
P3 - O1
FP2 - F4
F4 - C4
C4 - P4
P4 - O2
FZ - CZ
CZ - PZ
ECG

100 µV

1 s

▶ **Figure 3.75 Intermittent slow, left temporal.** Bipolar longitudinal montage. Irregular left temporal theta and delta waves occur intermittently in this 34-year-old female patient with left temporal lobe epilepsy of unknown etiology when she wakes up from a mild non-REM sleep (with slow eye movements). During wakefulness, there is an occipital 11 Hz background rhythm. Note the EMG artifact in T8.

EEG classification: Abnormal II (awake and sleep)
    Intermittent slow, left temporal

EEG report: This EEG supports the diagnosis of left temporal lobe epilepsy.

Occipital intermittent rhythmic delta activity (OIRDA)

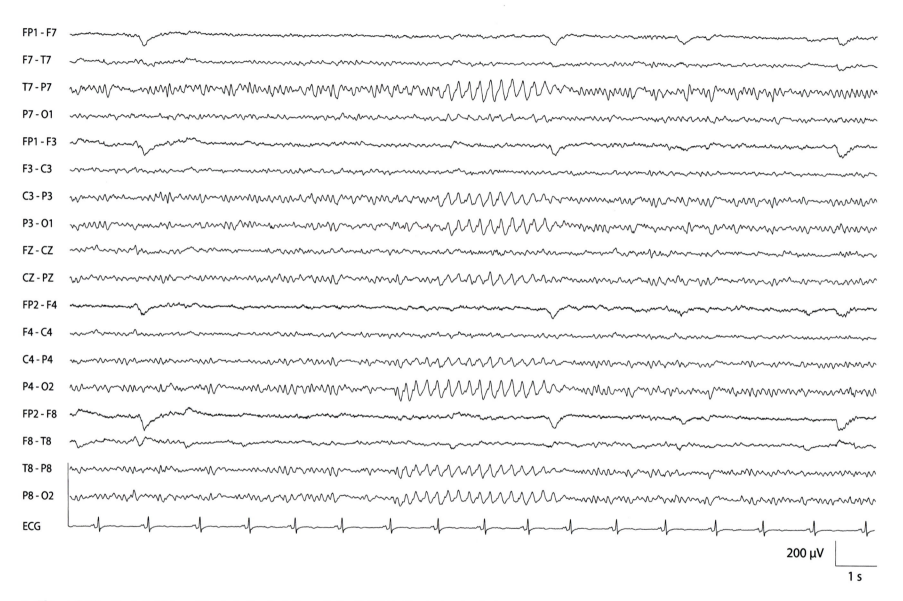

FP1 - F7
F7 - T7
T7 - P7
P7 - O1
FP1 - F3
F3 - C3
C3 - P3
P3 - O1
FZ - CZ
CZ - PZ
FP2 - F4
F4 - C4
C4 - P4
P4 - O2
FP2 - F8
F8 - T8
T8 - P8
P8 - O2
ECG

200 µV

1 s

▶ **Figure 3.76** **Occipital intermittent rhythmic delta activity (OIRDA).** Bipolar longitudinal montage. A 12-year-old patient with childhood absence epilepsy. A 4-s burst of occipital 4 Hz delta waves replaces the background alpha activity. Rhythmical delta occipital bursts are seen relatively frequently in patients with absence epilepsy. However, in isolation, they have no diagnostic value. You cannot diagnose absence epilepsy, and certainly they are not an index of encephalopathy.

EEG classification: Normal (awake)

EEG report: Normal EEG.

Intermittent rhythmic slow, right temporal

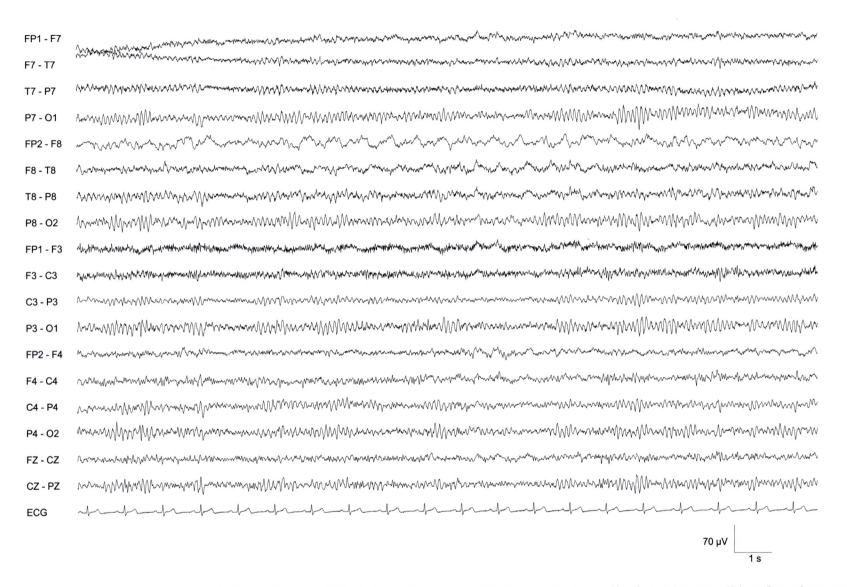

70 µV

1 s

▶ **Figure 3.77** **Intermittent rhythmic slow, right temporal.** Bipolar longitudinal montage. This 68-year-old patient suffers from right temporal lobe epilepsy due to mesial temporal sclerosis. Temporal intermittent rhythmic delta activity is typical for patients with temporal lobe epilepsies (Reiher et al., 1989). Otherwise, the EEG shows a normal occipital alpha background rhythm.

EEG classification: Abnormal II (awake)
Intermittent rhythmic slow, right temporal

EEG report: This EEG supports the diagnosis of right temporal lobe epilepsy.

Intermittent rhythmic slow, left temporal

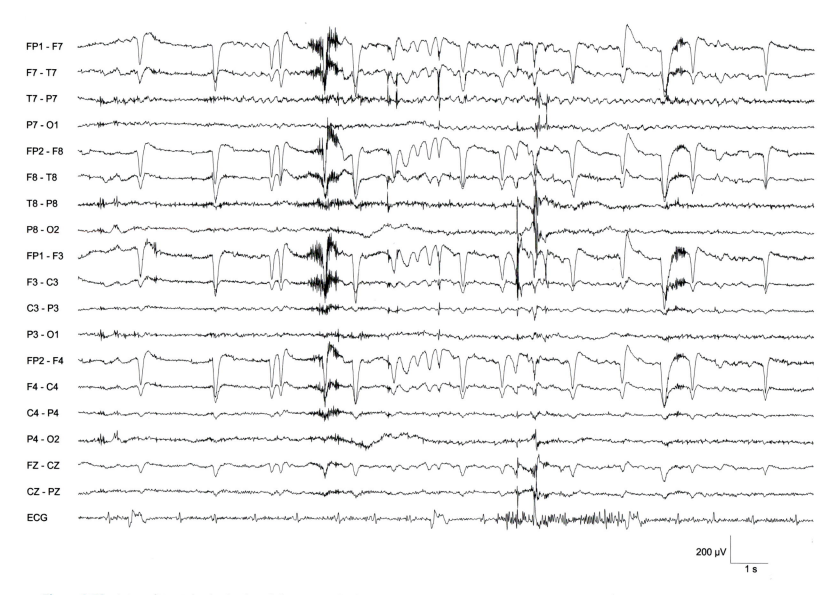

200 μV

1 s

▶ **Figure 3.78** **Intermittent rhythmic slow, left temporal.** Bipolar longitudinal montage. A 41-year-old patient with left mesial temporal lobe epilepsy. This EEG shows rhythmical, 4 or 5 Hz, 10- to 15-s bursts of theta activity in the left temporal region.

EEG classification: Abnormal III (awake)

Intermittent rhythmic slow, left temporal

EEG report: This EEG shows a left temporal dysfunction typical for temporal lobe epilepsies.

Intermittent rhythmic slow, left temporal

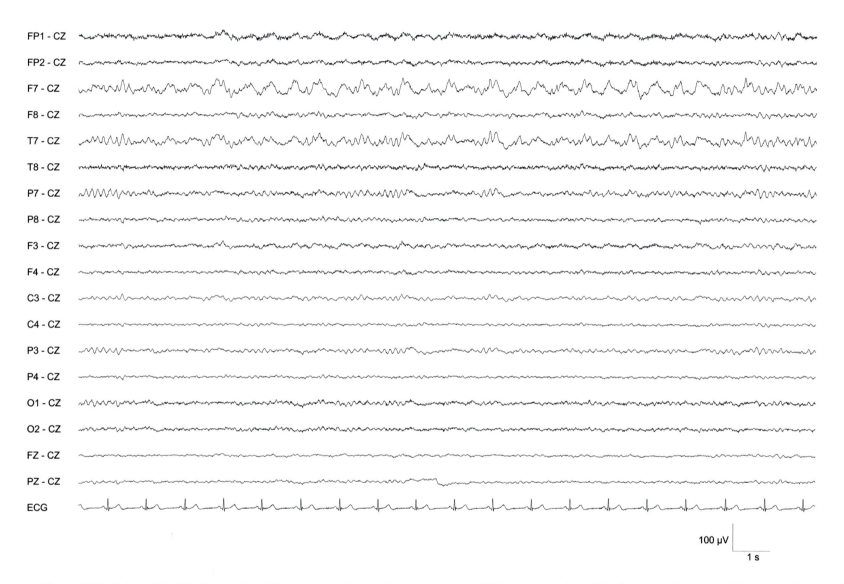

100 µV

1 s

▶ **Figure 3.79** **Intermittent rhythmic slow, left temporal.** Vertex reference montage. A 70-year-old patient with a first generalized convulsive seizure 19 years after resection and radiotherapy of a left temporoparietal xantho-astrocytoma (World Health Organization grade III).

EEG classification: Abnormal III (awake)
1. Intermittent rhythmic slow, left temporal
2. Asymmetry, increased background left temporal

EEG report: This EEG reflects a left temporal epileptogenic lesion after trepanation and resection of the left temporoparietal xantho-astrocytoma.

Intermittent rhythmic slow, left temporal. Bipolar longitudinal montage

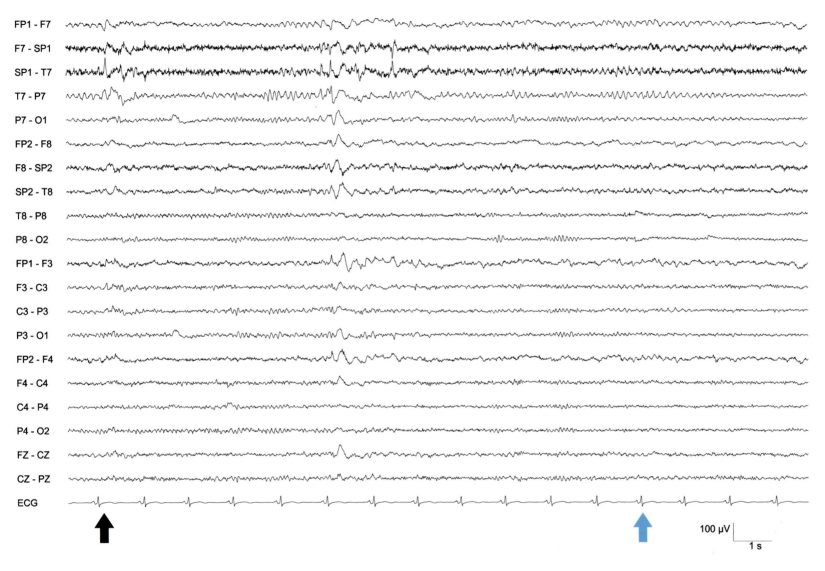

▶ **Figure 3.80** **Intermittent rhythmic slow, left temporal.** Bipolar longitudinal montage. A 41-year-old patient with left mesial temporal lobe epilepsy. This EEG section shows an intermittent rhythmic slow in the left temporal region (blue arrow) and left temporal spikes with maximum amplitude at electrode SP1 (black arrow).

EEG classification: Abnormal III (awake)
1. Spikes, SP1 > F7 > T7
2. Intermittent rhythmic slow, left temporal

EEG report: This EEG supports the diagnosis of left temporal lobe epilepsy.

Intermittent rhythmic slow, left frontal

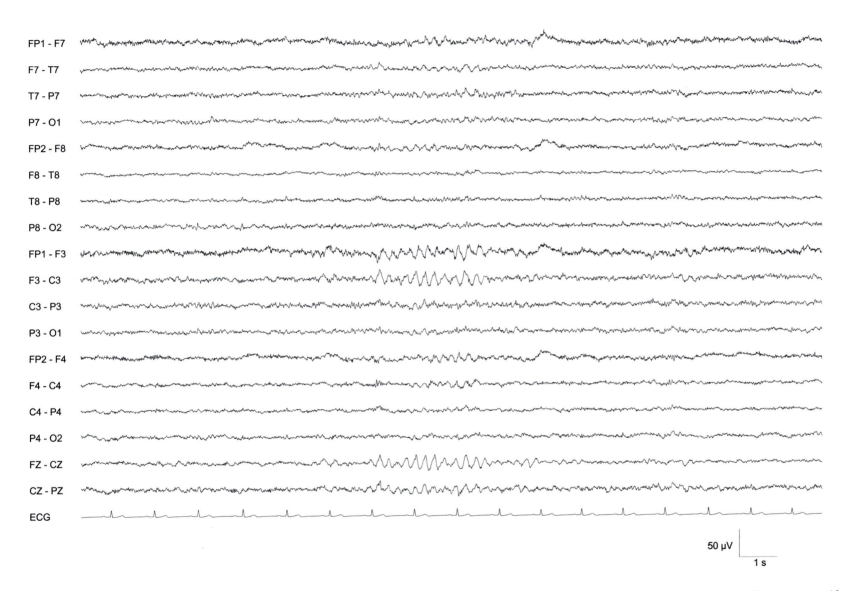

FP1 - F7

F7 - T7

T7 - P7

P7 - O1

FP2 - F8

F8 - T8

T8 - P8

P8 - O2

FP1 - F3

F3 - C3

C3 - P3

P3 - O1

FP2 - F4

F4 - C4

C4 - P4

P4 - O2

FZ - CZ

CZ - PZ

ECG

50 µV

1 s

▶ **Figure 3.81** **Intermittent rhythmic slow, left frontal.** Bipolar longitudinal montage. A 59-year-old patient with a left frontal chronic subdural hematoma and focal epilepsy. There was a continuous diffuse slow intermixed with bursts of high-amplitude rhythmic slow in the left frontal region.

EEG classification: Abnormal II (awake)
1. Intermittent rhythmic slow, left frontal
2. Continuous slow, left frontal

EEG report: This EEG reflects the focal epilepsy due to left frontal subdural hematoma.

Intermittent rhythmic slow, generalized

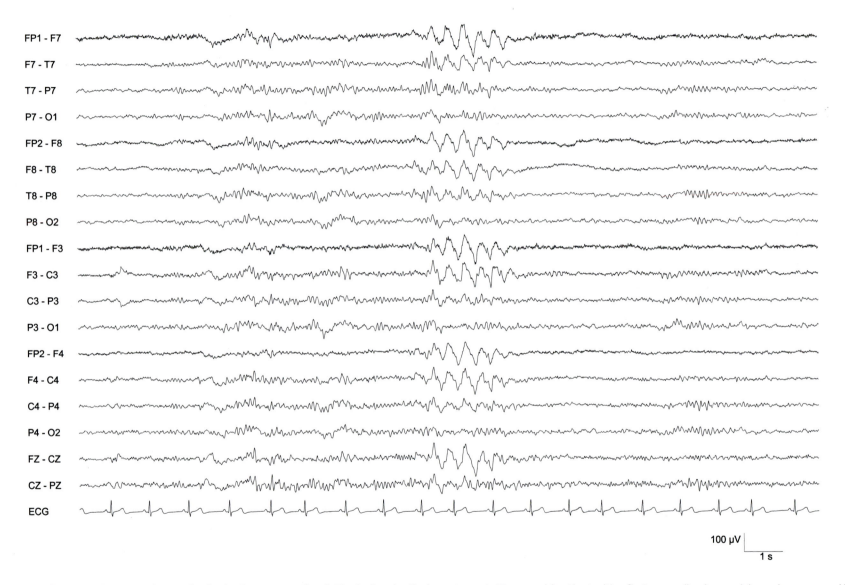

100 µV

1 s

▶ **Figure 3.82** **Intermittent rhythmic slow, generalized.** Bipolar longitudinal montage. A 43-year-old patient with a first generalized convulsive seizure caused by relapsing–remitting multiple sclerosis. The EEG shows a generalized, intermittent rhythmic delta slow (with a bifrontal maximum).

EEG classification: Abnormal I (awake)
Intermittent rhythmic slow, generalized

EEG report: This EEG reflects a mild diffuse encephalopathy in a patient with multiple sclerosis.

Hypnagogic theta bursts

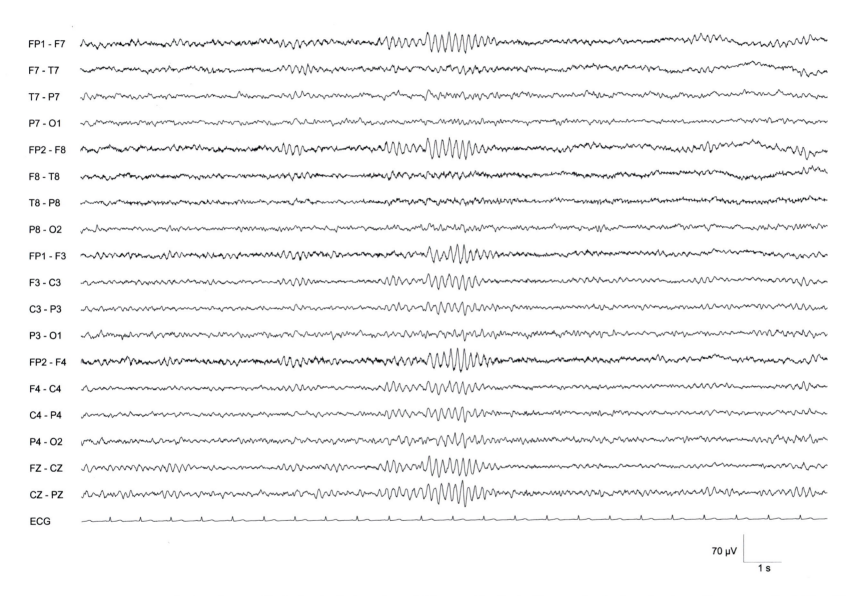

70 μV

1 s

▶ **Figure 3.83** **Hypnagogic theta bursts.** Bipolar longitudinal montage. A 36-year-old patient with excessive daytime sleepiness. These generalized, intermittent rhythmic bursts of theta waves occurred only during drowsiness.

EEG classification: Normal (awake/drowsy)

EEG report: This EEG is normal.

Intermittent temporal slow of the elderly

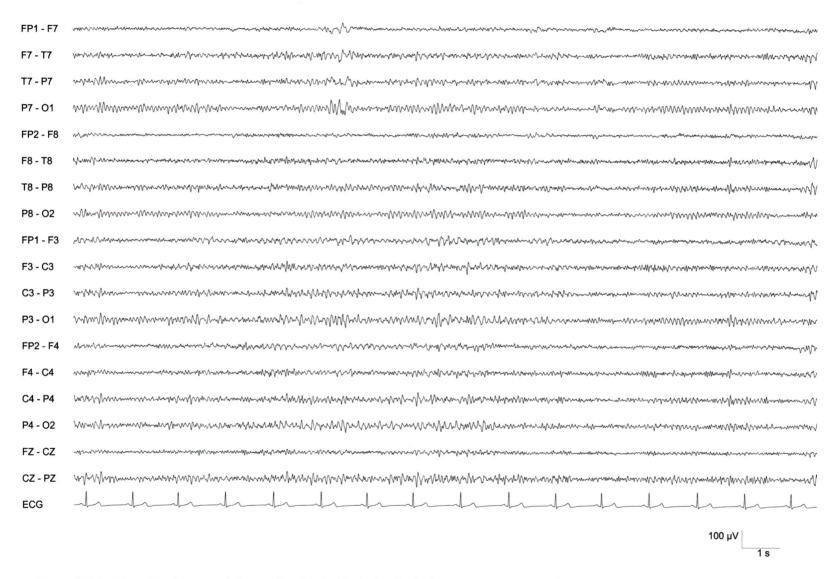

FP1 - F7

F7 - T7

T7 - P7

P7 - O1

FP2 - F8

F8 - T8

T8 - P8

P8 - O2

FP1 - F3

F3 - C3

C3 - P3

P3 - O1

FP2 - F4

F4 - C4

C4 - P4

P4 - O2

FZ - CZ

CZ - PZ

ECG

100 µV

1 s

▶ **Figure 3.84** **Intermittent temporal slow of the elderly.** Bipolar longitudinal montage. A 64-year-old patient with dizziness and impairment of concentration of unknown etiology. A 1- or 2-s burst of irregular theta–delta waves is seen in the left temporal region. The slow accounts for approximately 5% of the EEG recording. Otherwise, there is an occipital 10 Hz background rhythm.

EEG classification: Normal (awake)

EEG report: This EEG shows an age-related normal finding.

Intermittent temporal slow of the elderly

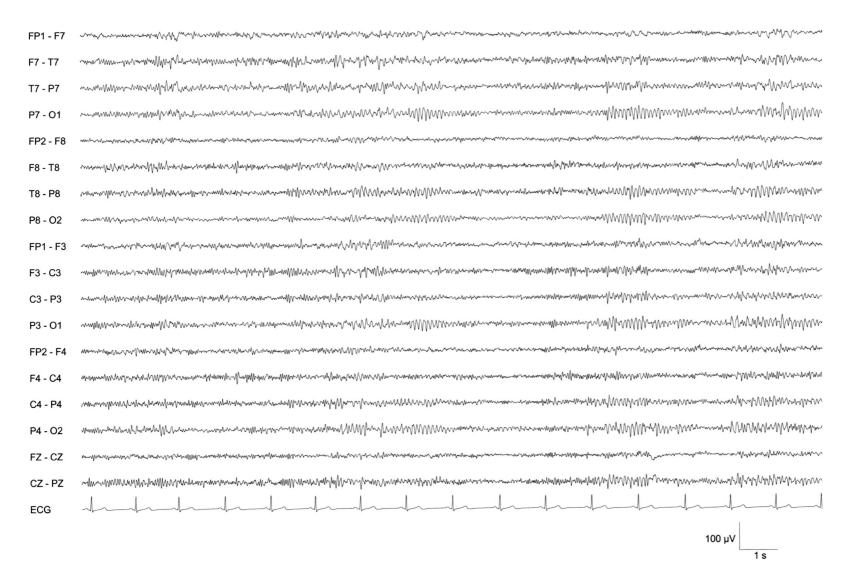

▶ **Figure 3.85** **Intermittent temporal slow of the elderly.** Bipolar longitudinal montage. An 86-year-old patient with gait difficulty and dizziness. Irregular theta bursts and delta activity is seen intermittently in the left temporal region for 3 or 4 s. The slow accounts for approximately 10% of the recording. Otherwise, there is an occipital 10 Hz background rhythm.

EEG classification: Normal (awake)

EEG report: This EEG is normal.

Hypnopompic theta–delta burst (hypnapompic hypersynchrony)

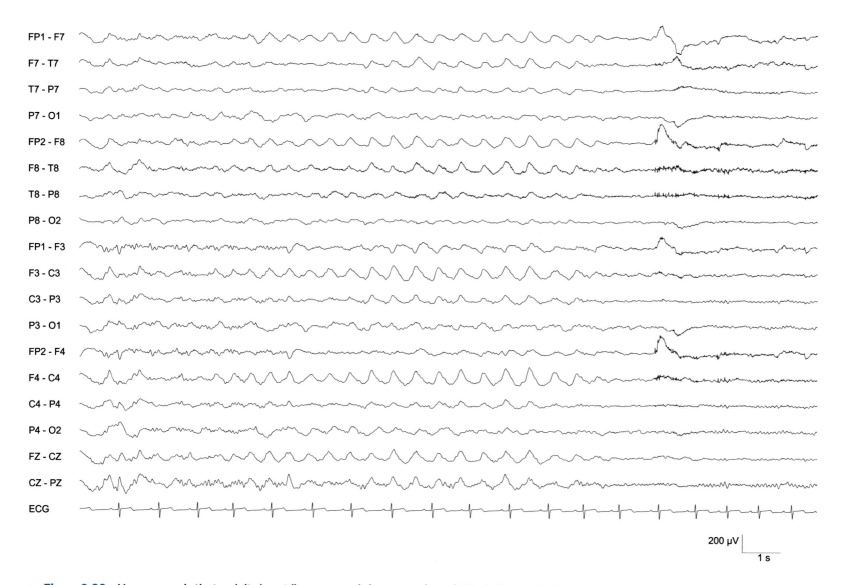

FP1 - F7

F7 - T7

T7 - P7

P7 - O1

FP2 - F8

F8 - T8

T8 - P8

P8 - O2

FP1 - F3

F3 - C3

C3 - P3

P3 - O1

FP2 - F4

F4 - C4

C4 - P4

P4 - O2

FZ - CZ

CZ - PZ

ECG

200 µV

1 s

▶ **Figure 3.86**   **Hypnopompic theta–delta burst (hypnapompic hypersynchrony).** Bipolar longitudinal montage. An 11-year-old boy with grand mal epilepsy. During light sleep, approximately 10-s bursts of high-amplitude rhythmic delta waves with a frontal maximum occur. The EEG then flattens out, and an approximately 11 Hz occipital alpha background rhythm develops as an expression of the waking state.

EEG classification: Normal (awake and sleep)

EEG report: This EEG is normal.

Hypnagogic theta–delta bursts (hypnagogic hypersynchrony)

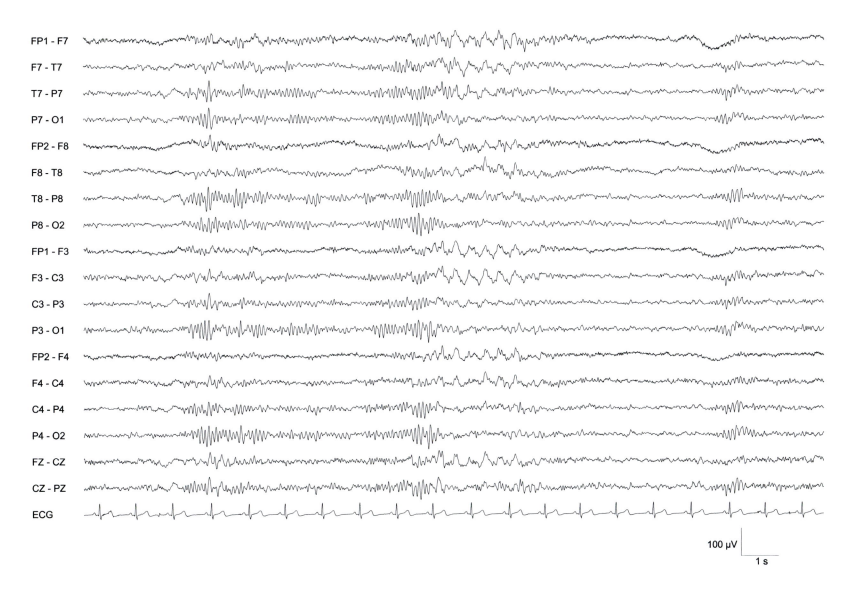

▶ **Figure 3.87**   **Hypnagogic theta–delta bursts (hypnagogic hypersynchrony).** Bipolar longitudinal montage. This teenager shows poorly developed alpha background rhythm as an indication of drowsiness. A 2-s burst of high-amplitude frontal rhythmic delta waves occurs. These waves did not occur during wakefulness and mental activation. There is an F8 sweat artifact.

EEG classification: Normal (awake)

EEG report: This EEG is normal.

Occipital delta waves of youth

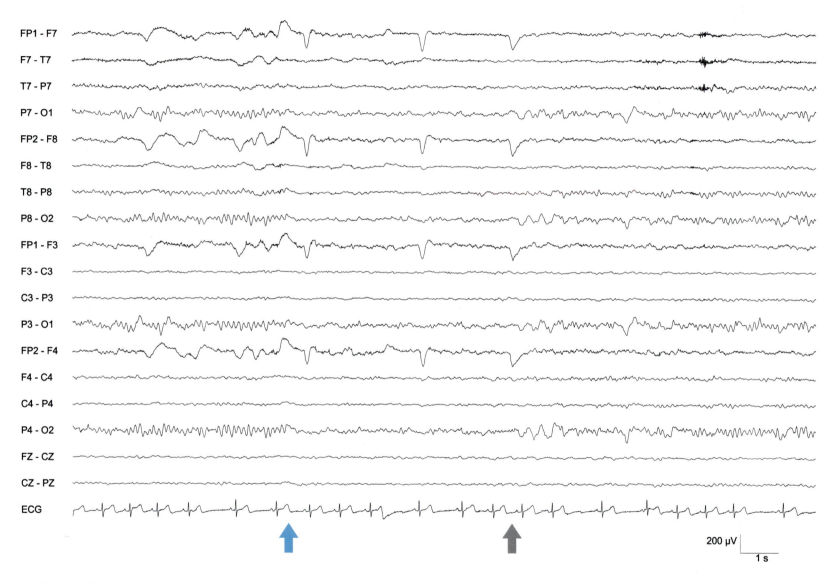

▶ **Figure 3.88** **Occipital delta waves of youth.** Bipolar longitudinal montage. After eye closure (gray arrow), 3- or 4-s bursts of occipital rhythmic delta waves intermix with alpha background activity. The occipital alpha rhythm and delta waves are blocked by eye opening (blue arrow).

EEG classification: Normal (awake)

EEG report: This EEG is normal.

Occipital delta waves of youth

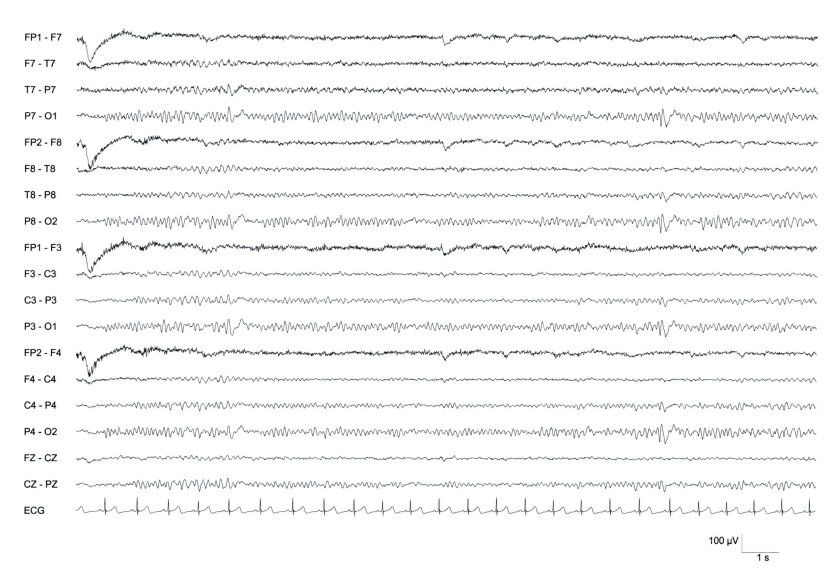

FP1 - F7

F7 - T7

T7 - P7

P7 - O1

FP2 - F8

F8 - T8

T8 - P8

P8 - O2

FP1 - F3

F3 - C3

C3 - P3

P3 - O1

FP2 - F4

F4 - C4

C4 - P4

P4 - O2

FZ - CZ

CZ - PZ

ECG

100 µV

1 s

▶ **Figure 3.89** **Occipital delta waves of youth.** Bipolar longitudinal montage. The occipital delta waves of youth become less frequent with age. In addition, the characteristic intermixed, irregular delta activity seen in children tends to disappear in adolescence. Notice that the sharp transient occurring at the end of the sample has negative polarity, making it more difficult to recognize its benign nature.

EEG classification: Normal (awake)

EEG report: This EEG is normal.

Occipital delta waves of youth

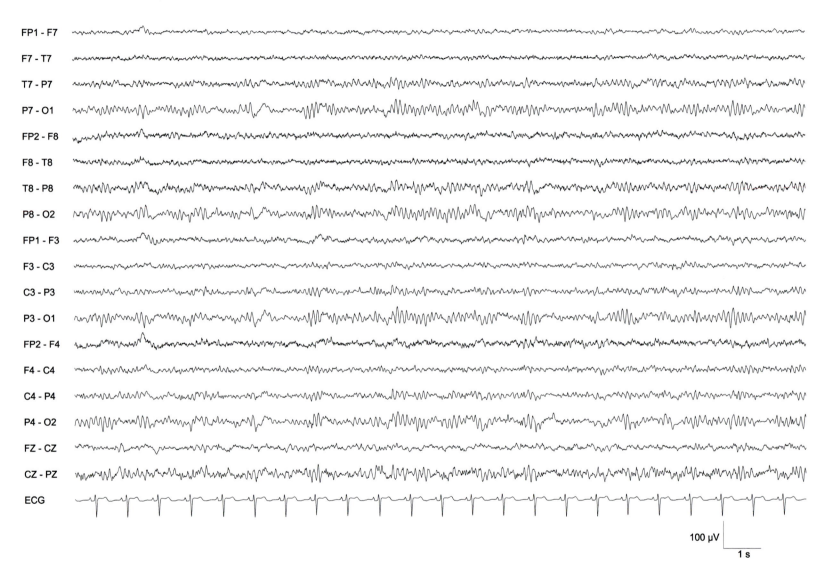

FP1 - F7	
F7 - T7	
T7 - P7	
P7 - O1	
FP2 - F8	
F8 - T8	
T8 - P8	
P8 - O2	
FP1 - F3	
F3 - C3	
C3 - P3	
P3 - O1	
FP2 - F4	
F4 - C4	
C4 - P4	
P4 - O2	
FZ - CZ	
CZ - PZ	
ECG	

100 μV

1 s

▶ **Figure 3.90** **Occipital delta waves of youth.** Bipolar longitudinal montage. This EEG shows occipital delta waves intermixed with the occipital alpha background rhythm. The patient is a normal adolescent.

EEG classification: Normal (awake)

EEG report: This EEG is normal.

Occipital delta waves of youth

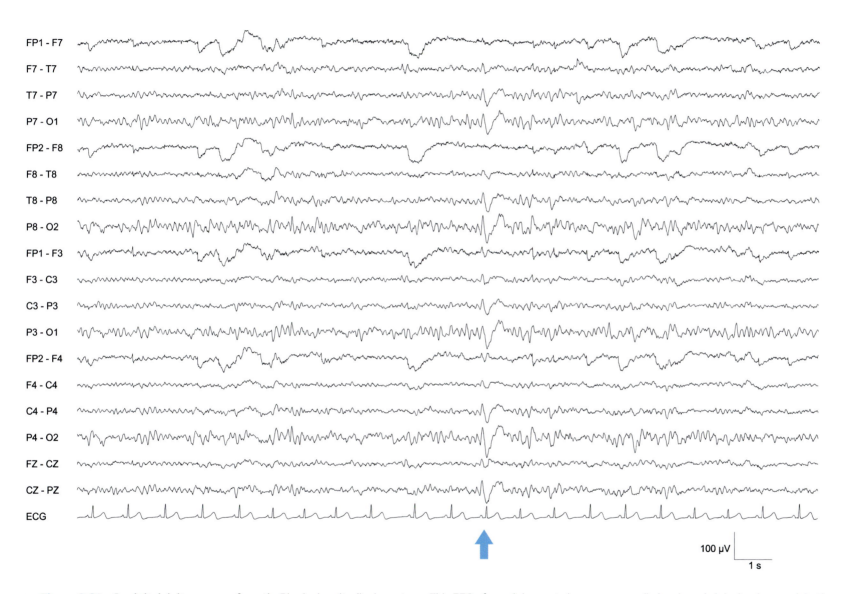

100 µV

1 s

▶ **Figure 3.91** **Occipital delta waves of youth.** Bipolar longitudinal montage. This EEG of an adolescent shows a very well-developed alpha background rhythm with intermingled delta waves. These occipital delta waves may give the impression of sharp waves if they occur directly after slightly higher amplitude alpha waves (blue arrow). Notice also that the sharp transient pointing upward (blue arrow) is of positive polarity. Epileptiform discharges recorded with scalp electrodes almost always are of negative polarity.

EEG classification: Normal (awake)

EEG report: This EEG is normal.

Eye closure activity

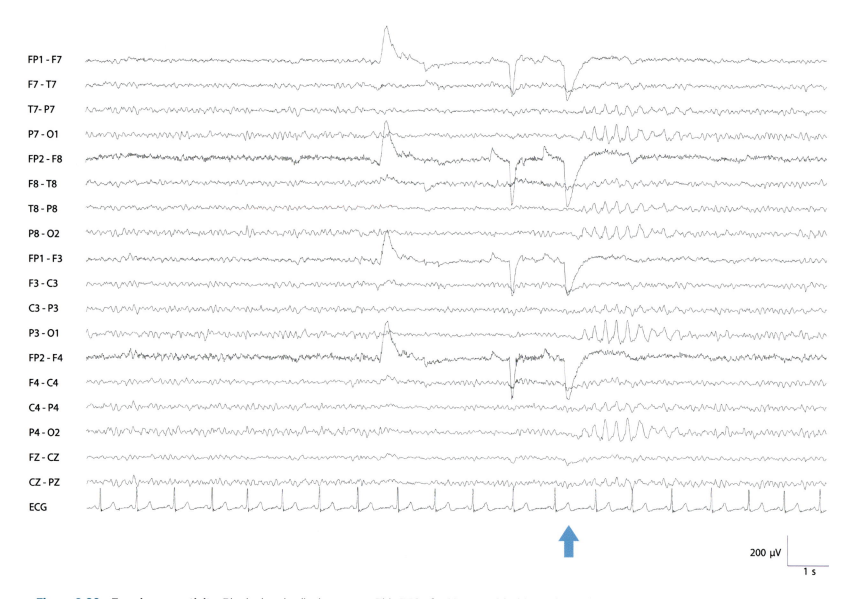

▶ **Figure 3.92** **Eye closure activity.** Bipolar longitudinal montage. This EEG of a 22-year-old with tension headaches and concentration deficit disorders shows a 2- or 3-s burst of spindle-modulated, occipital, rhythmic delta waves after eye closure (blue arrow). This is a normal finding at this age.

EEG classification: Normal (awake)

EEG report: This EEG is normal.

Fixation-off sensitivity

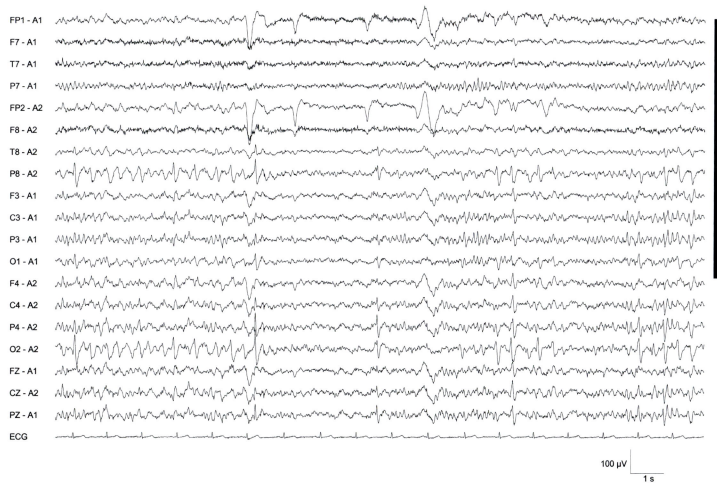

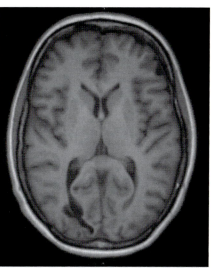

▶ **Figure 3.93** **Fixation-off sensitivity.** Ear reference montage. A 55-year-old female patient with right occipital lobe epilepsy due to an intracerebral hemorrhage caused by a skiing accident. Opening of the eyes ends the repetitive spikes. After eye closure, the spikes resume. Prevention of fixation by Frenzel glasses has the same effect as eye closure. This rare phenomenon indicates an increased epileptogenicity of the occipital lobe but also occurs in patients with generalized epilepsies. The MRI shows the right occipital post-hemorrhagic lesion.

EEG classification: Abnormal III (awake)
1. Spikes, right occipital (fixation-off)
2. Continuous slow, right occipital

EEG report: This EEG reflects a right occipital epileptogenic zone secondary to the traumatic right occipital hemorrhage.

is very rare and found in children with benign occipital lobe epilepsy and adults with focal (sometimes occipital) and generalized epilepsies (▶ Figures 3.93 and 3.94) (Das Pektezel et al., 2023; Fattouch et al., 2013). It rarely disappears with successful epilepsy treatment (▶ Figure 3.94) (Das Pektezel et al., 2023).

3.4.2.3.2.6 Rhythmical Temporal Theta Bursts of Drowsiness

Rhythmic temporal theta bursts of drowsiness, formerly also known as the psychomotor variant (Gibbs & Gibbs, 1952), occur in approximately 0.5% of healthy adults and are characterized by rhythmic theta waves of a frequency of 5–7 Hz. The bursts are localized to the temporal region, and they tend to alternate between the left and right hemisphere (▶ Figures 3.95–3.98). The waves are monomorphic, spindle-like modulated, and the negative waves tend to be sharply contoured. These bursts occur during drowsiness, decrease with increasing sleep depth, and can be interrupted by mental activation (▶ Figure 3.96) This pattern has to be distinguished from intermittent temporal slow, which may occur in the same temporal lobe (▶ Figure 3.97). The bursts are not influenced by PS as long as the vigilance does not change (▶ Figure 3.98).

For a long time, there was controversy about the clinical significance of this pattern, classifying it as pattern of uncertain clinical significance. In 1963, the famous neurophysiologist and epileptologist Frederik Gibbs, acting as an expert in the murder trial against Jack Ruby (Jack Ruby killed Lee Harvey Oswald, who was accused of killing John F. Kennedy), declared that the EEG of Jack Ruby showed bursts of "psychomotor variant." He concluded that this EEG pattern was an indication of an abnormal dysfunction of the temporal lobes (Weinmann, 2007). The neurological expert of the public prosecutor's office, Frank Foster, did not agree with this opinion and held the position that the "psychomotor variant" is a normal variant without any correlation to abnormal temporal lobe function. This interpretation is still valid (Weinmann, 2007; Westmoreland & Klass, 1990).

3.4.2.3.2.7 Rhythmical Midline Theta

This pattern consists of 4- to 20-s bursts of rhythmic theta activity at 4–7 Hz located in the frontocentral region (▶ Figures 3.99 and 3.100). It must be distinguished from similar activities in healthy individuals during cognitive tasks, from drowsiness patterns in children (hypnagogic theta–delta bursts or hypnagogic hypersynchrony; ▶ Figures 3.86 and 3.87) (Westmoreland & Klass, 1986), and from subclinical rhythmic electrographic discharges in adults (SREDA; Westmoreland & Klass, 1981, 1997) (▶ Figure 3.176 and Table 3.11).

The association of this pattern with epilepsies was recognized early, but originally the pattern was correlated to temporal lobe epilepsies (Cigánek, 1961). However, at that time, today's concepts of frontal lobe epilepsy were not yet established.

More recent studies have shown that only 4% of patients with rhythmical midline theta suffer from temporal lobe epilepsy. On the other hand, 48% of patients showing this EEG pattern suffer from frontal lobe epilepsy (Beleza et al., 2009).

3.4.2.3.3 Continuous Slow (CS)

Continuous slow means slow activity that occurs continuously, is not responsive to external stimuli, and clearly exceeds the proportion of continuous, irregular slow that is normal (▶ Figure 3.101). It is usually irregular (polymorphic), and its frequency is in the delta–theta frequency range. With the severity of encephalopathy, the generalized polymorphic slow becomes more pronounced, and at the same time, the rhythmical background activity diminishes and eventually disappears completely. In severe encephalopathy, there is typically no rhythmical background activity.

Regional, unilateral, continuous slow is always abnormal (▶ Figure 3.102 and 3.103), pointing to a structural lesion in the affected region. In general, if there is continuous slow with preserved rhythmical background activity (even when the rhythmical background activity is slow), the underlying cortical damage is usually relatively mild (▶ Figure 3.104). Abnormal slow cannot be influenced by activation, such as eye opening and closing (▶ Figure 3.104). On the other hand, normal slow waves such as slow alpha variant background rhythm can be influenced by activation procedures (▶ Figure 3.105). Continuous focal slow may also occur together with intermittent focal slow (▶ Figure 3.106). The intermittent slow reflects a functional abnormality typically distant to the lesion. Continuous slow may also combine with a periodic pattern in the same region (▶ Figure 3.107).

A one-sided or circumscribed amplitude decrease of a physiological activity in the case of a slowing is classified as asymmetry, reduced background (▶ Figures 3.106 and 3.108–3.110; see Section 2.2.3.4, and Section 3.4.2.7.2). A continuous regional slow in combination with a reduced amplitude of the background activity in the same region or hemisphere usually indicates a severe regional structural lesion (▶ Figures 3.108–3.110). A unilateral reduced background may also involve a physiological pattern such as an arousal pattern on the affected hemisphere (▶ Figure 3.110). The combination of continuous regional slow with

Continuous slow, right occipital

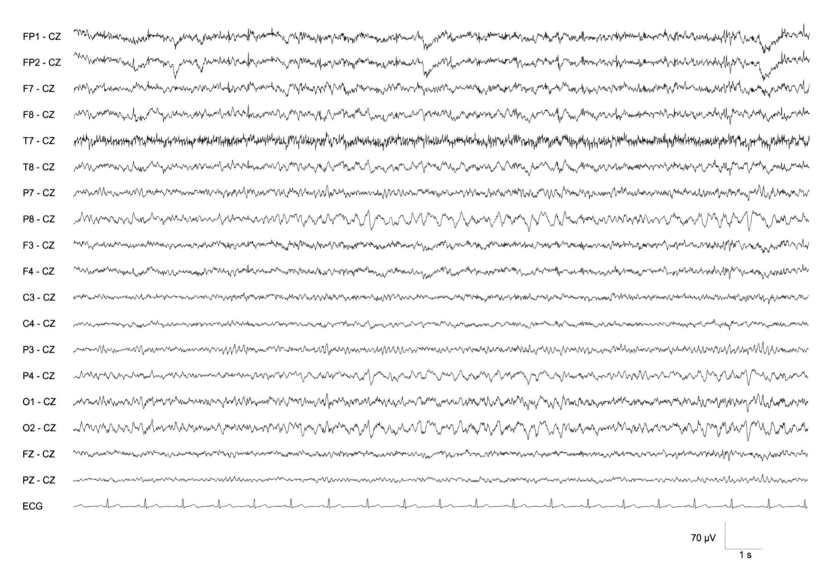

70 μV

1 s

▶ **Figure 3.94** **Continuous slow, right occipital.** Vertex reference montage. Same patient as ▶ **Figure 3.93**. Right occipital lobe epilepsy after intracerebral hemorrhage. The fixation-off sensitivity subsided with anti-seizure medication, leading to seizure freedom. Right occipital slow prevails.

EEG classification: Abnormal III (awake)
　　　Continuous slow, right occipital

EEG report: This EEG reflects the right occipital lesion.

Rhythmic temporal theta burst of drowsiness

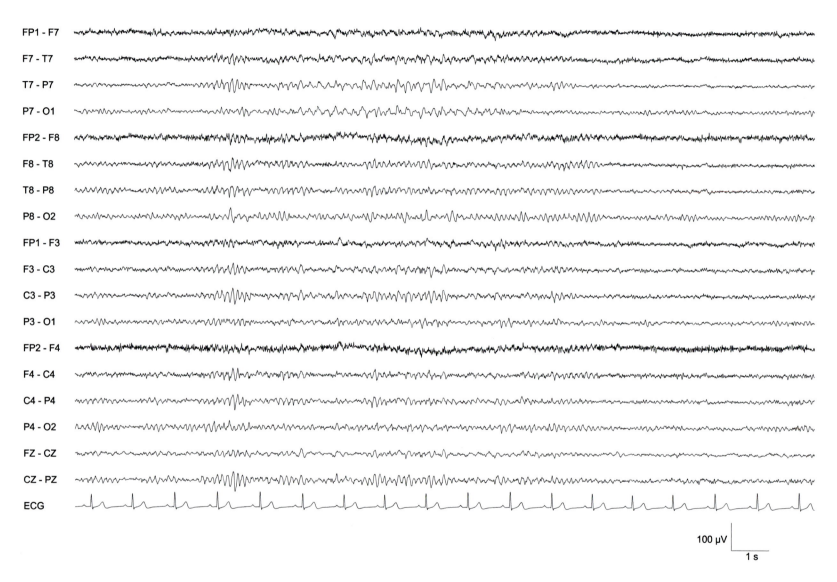

FP1 - F7

F7 - T7

T7 - P7

P7 - O1

FP2 - F8

F8 - T8

T8 - P8

P8 - O2

FP1 - F3

F3 - C3

C3 - P3

P3 - O1

FP2 - F4

F4 - C4

C4 - P4

P4 - O2

FZ - CZ

CZ - PZ

ECG

100 µV

1 s

▶ **Figure 3.95**   **Rhythmic temporal theta burst of drowsiness.** Bipolar longitudinal montage. EEG of a 24-year-old woman with daytime sleepiness and depression. A 7- or 8-s burst of rhythmic theta waves occurs in the left temporal region ("psychomotor variant"). Toward the end of the figure, the background alpha rhythm wanes as a sign of drowsiness.

EEG classification: Normal (awake)

EEG report: This EEG is normal.

Rhythmic temporal theta burst of drowsiness

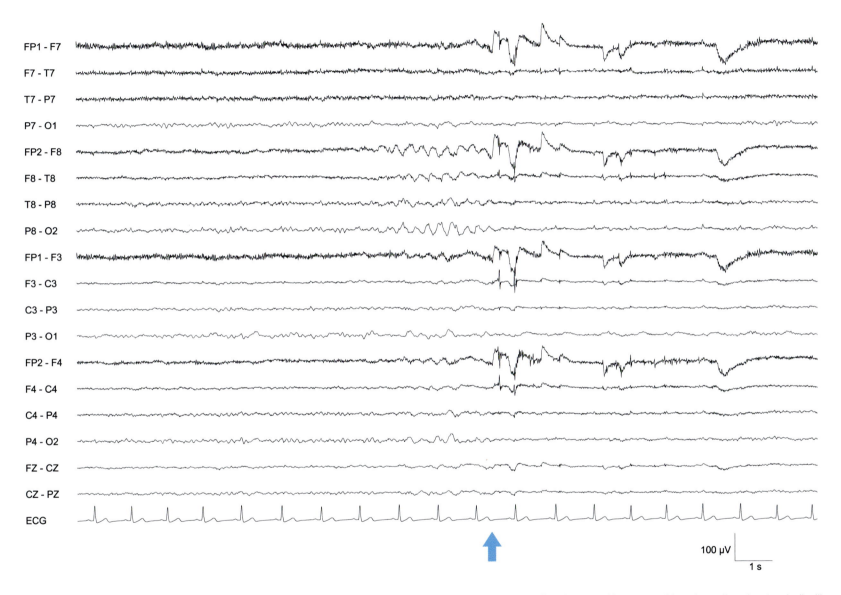

▶ **Figure 3.96** **Rhythmic temporal theta burst of drowsiness.** Bipolar longitudinal montage. EEG of a 30-year-old woman with a sleep disorder. A spindle-like modulated burst of right temporal rhythmic, approximately 3 Hz waves appears that immediately stops when calling the patient (blue arrow). With eye opening, the bursts disappear. Although the pattern, also called psychomotor variant, was later named after the predominant theta waves, at times the rhythmical waves are slower, as in this case.

EEG classification: Normal (awake)

EEG report: This EEG is normal.

Rhythmic temporal theta burst of drowsiness

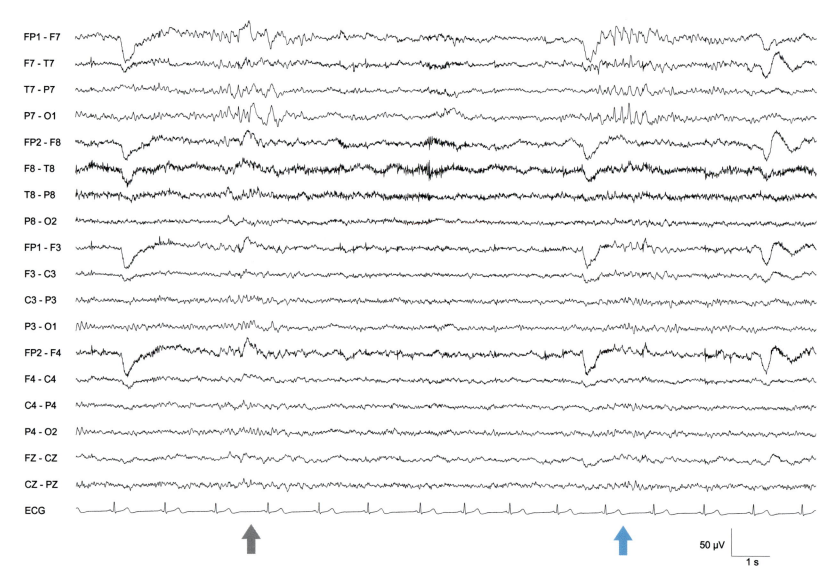

▶ **Figure 3.97** **Rhythmic temporal theta burst of drowsiness.** Bipolar longitudinal row. The EEG of this 42-year-old patient showed 2- or 3-s bursts of left temporal rhythmic theta waves during drowsiness (blue arrow). When alerted by being spoken to, these theta bursts stopped immediately. This pattern is also called psychomotor variant and represents a physiological variant. In addition, there is a left temporal intermittent irregular slow (gray arrow), which reflects his pseudo-migraine with temporary neurological symptoms and lymphocytic pleocytosis (pseudomyxoma peritonei syndrome: global aphasia and right sensory and motor hemisyndrome).

EEG classification: Abnormal I (awake)
Intermittent slow, left temporal

EEG report: This EEG shows a left temporal dysfunction in a drowsy patient.

Rhythmic temporal theta burst of drowsiness and photic driving

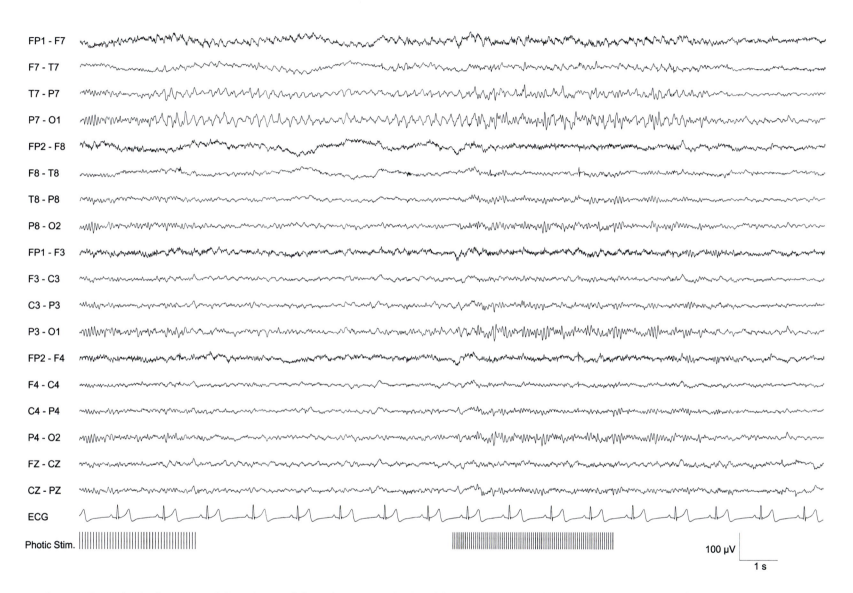

▶ **Figure 3.98** **Rhythmic temporal theta burst of drowsiness and photic driving.** Bipolar longitudinal montage. A 17-year-old female patient with absence epilepsy. Slow horizontal eye movements indicate drowsiness. A left temporal spindle-like modulated burst of rhythmic theta waves occurs for approximately 12 s. Photic stimulation at 15 and 20 Hz leads to photic driving but does not affect the psychomotor variant.

EEG classification: Normal (awake)

EEG report: This EEG is normal.

Rhythmic midline theta activity

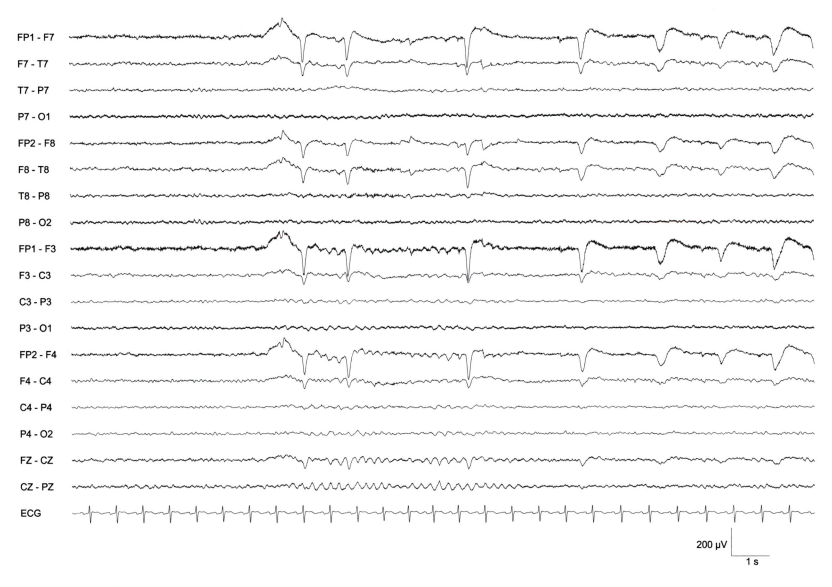

▶ Figure 3.99 **Rhythmic midline theta activity.** Bipolar longitudinal montage. A 22-year-old patient with left mesial frontal lobe epilepsy and symmetrical bilateral tonic, myoclonic, and generalized convulsive seizures secondary to a left frontal, probably post-encephalitic gliosis. A 7- or 8-s burst of CZ maximum rhythmic theta waves (approximately 5 Hz).

EEG classification: Abnormal II (awake)

Intermittent rhythmic slow, CZ

EEG report: This EEG shows midline maximum theta burst. This EEG pattern has been described as a normal variant (see Ciganek's midline rhythm) as also in patients suffering from frontal epilepsy (Beleza et al., 2009).

Rhythmic midline theta activity

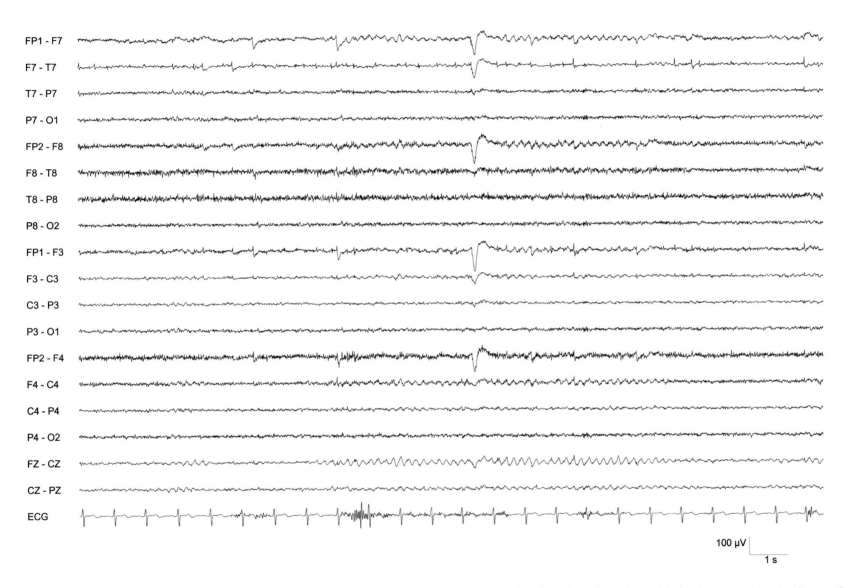

FP1 - F7
F7 - T7
T7 - P7
P7 - O1
FP2 - F8
F8 - T8
T8 - P8
P8 - O2
FP1 - F3
F3 - C3
C3 - P3
P3 - O1
FP2 - F4
F4 - C4
C4 - P4
P4 - O2
FZ - CZ
CZ - PZ
ECG

100 µV

1 s

▶ **Figure 3.100** **Rhythmic midline theta activity.** Bipolar longitudinal montage. A 33-year-old female patient with right occipital epilepsy who had visual auras, right versive, and gener-alized convulsive seizures. The EEG shows FZ maximum, 8- or 9-s rhythmic theta waves with a frequency of 5.5 Hz. During this EEG sample, the patient was awake and responsive. Note the frequent left-sided rectus lateralis and the superior rectus muscle spicules.

EEG classification: Abnormal II (awake)
Intermittent rhythmic slow, FZ

EEG report: This EEG shows midline maximum theta burst. This EEG pattern has been described as a normal variant (see Ciganek's midline rhythm) as also in patients suffering of frontal epilepsy (Beleza et al., 2009).

Background slow and continuous slow, generalized

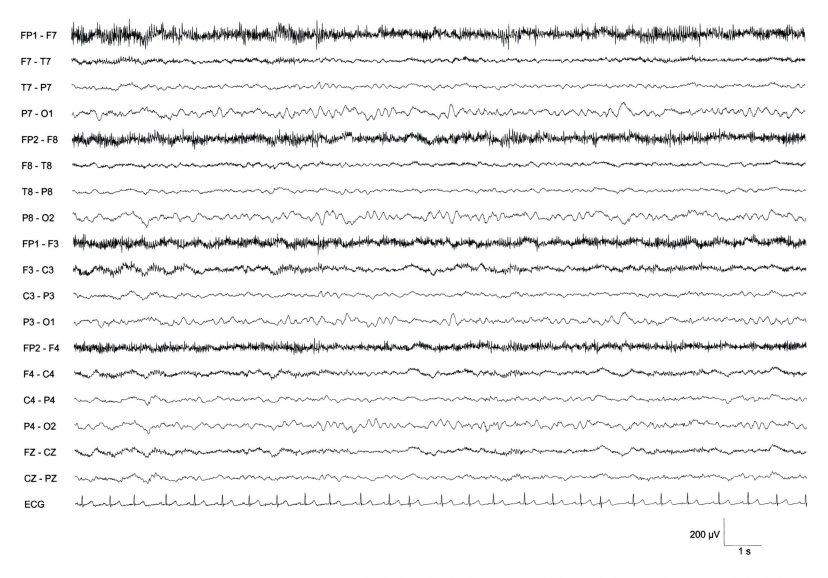

200 μV

1 s

▶ **Figure 3.101 Background slow and continuous slow, generalized.** Bipolar longitudinal montage. A 72-year-old female patient with confusion in the context of febrile infection. The occipital background rhythm is slowed to 5 Hz. In addition, there is diffusely distributed, irregular delta activity.

EEG classification: Abnormal II (awake)
1. Background slow
2. Continuous slow, generalized

EEG report: This EEG shows evidence of a moderate diffuse encephalopathy.

Continuous slow, left temporofrontal

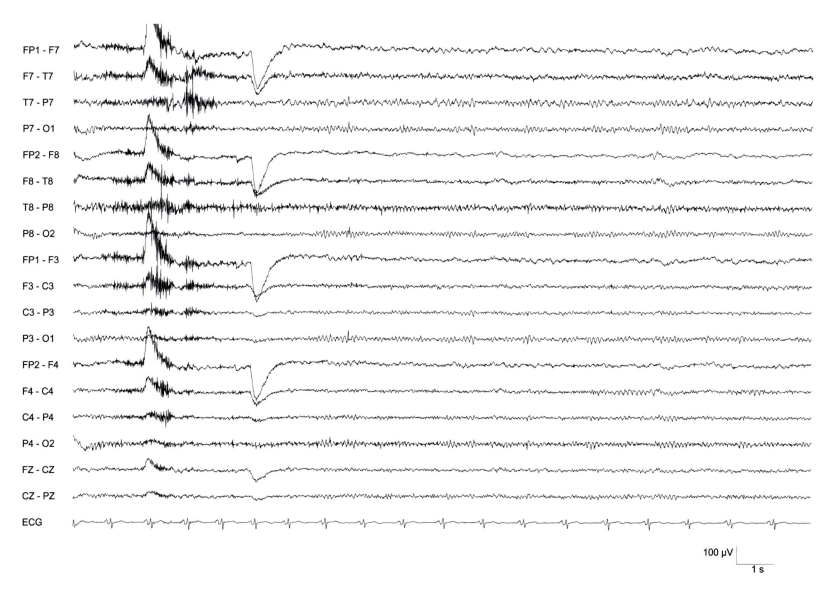

100 µV

1 s

▶ **Figure 3.102** **Continuous slow, left temporofrontal.** Bipolar longitudinal montage. A 41-year-old female patient with left temporal lobe epilepsy. In the left temporofrontal region, there is a rhythmical, continuous, 5 or 6 Hz theta activity and also some irregular, continuous slow activity.

EEG classification: Abnormal III (awake)
Continuous slow, left temporofrontal

EEG report: This EEG shows evidence of a left temporal lesion.

Continuous slow, left temporal

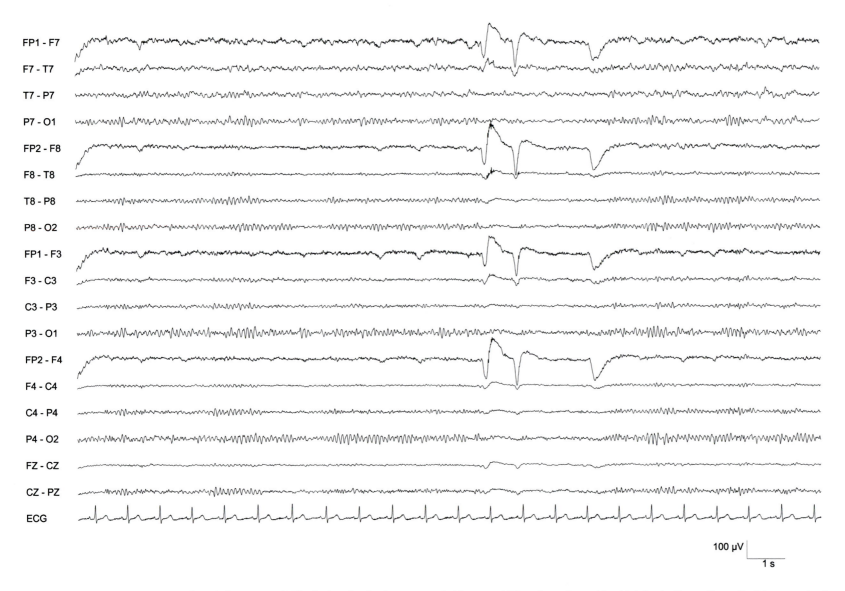

FP1 - F7

F7 - T7

T7 - P7

P7 - O1

FP2 - F8

F8 - T8

T8 - P8

P8 - O2

FP1 - F3

F3 - C3

C3 - P3

P3 - O1

FP2 - F4

F4 - C4

C4 - P4

P4 - O2

FZ - CZ

CZ - PZ

ECG

100 µV

1 s

▶ **Figure 3.103** **Continuous slow, left temporal.** Bipolar longitudinal montage. A 49-year-old female patient with a histologically confirmed left temporal astrocytoma (WHO grade II). There is a slow activity at F7–T7. A well-developed, relatively symmetrical, spindle-like modulated 11 Hz alpha background rhythm prevails over the occipital region.

EEG classification: Abnormal III (awake)
Continuous slow, left temporal

EEG report: This EEG reflects the left temporal astrocytoma.

Continuous slow, left occipital

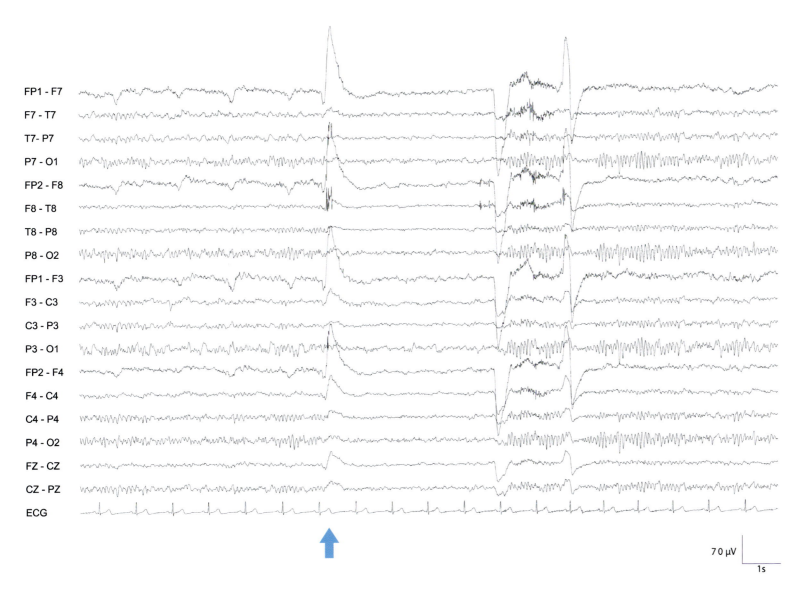

FP1 - F7

F7 - T7

T7- P7

P7 - O1

FP2 - F8

F8 - T8

T8 - P8

P8 - O2

FP1 - F3

F3 - C3

C3 - P3

P3 - O1

FP2 - F4

F4 - C4

C4 - P4

P4 - O2

FZ - CZ

CZ - PZ

ECG

70 µV

1s

▶ **Figure 3.104** **Continuous slow, left occipital.** Bipolar longitudinal montage. A 68-year-old patient with posterior infarct on the left side. Above the occipital region, a very well-developed, spindle-like modulated 11 Hz alpha background rhythm is visible. In the left occipital region, there is a continuous irregular theta–delta slow, which persists after opening the eyes (blue arrow). There is no blocking of slow activity due to the left occipital lesion. Notice that with eye closure, the alpha background activity is as well developed at O1 as at O2.

EEG classification: Abnormal III (awake)

Continuous slow, left occipital

EEG report: This EEG reflects the left posterior cerebral artery infarct.

Slow alpha variant background rhythm

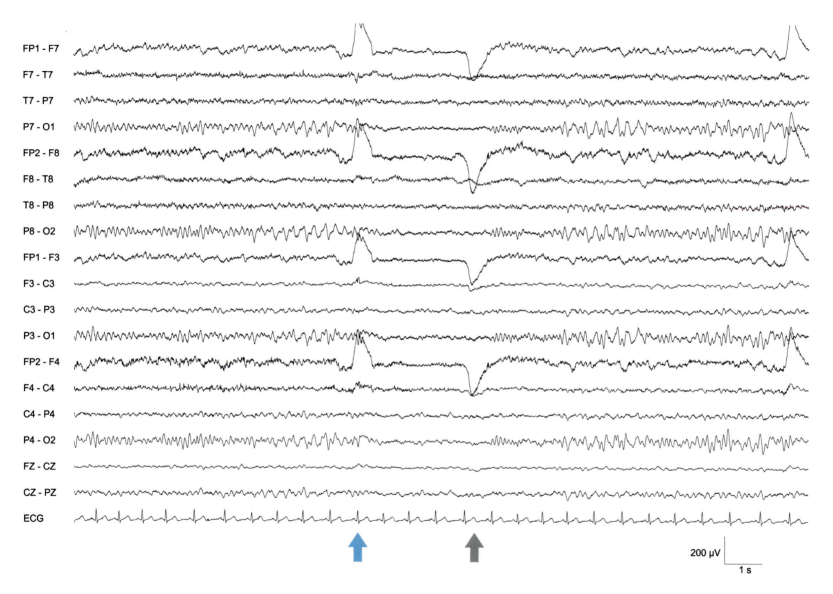

▶ **Figure 3.105** **Slow alpha variant background rhythm.** Bipolar longitudinal montage. A 36-year-old patient with attacks of dizziness. The occipital alpha background rhythm alternates with rhythmic waves of approximately 4 Hz. This EEG pattern has been labeled "slow alpha background variant rhythm." Both the alpha background activity and its slow variant are blocked by eye opening (blue arrow) and reappear after eye closure (gray arrow).

EEG classification: Normal EEG (awake)

EEG report: Normal EEG.

Continuous slow, left temporal and intermittent slow, left frontal

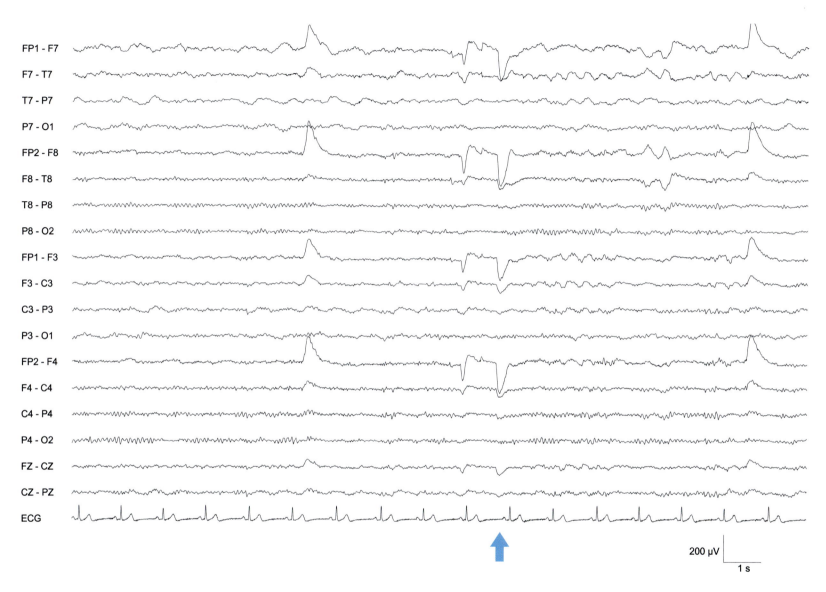

200 µV

1 s

▶ **Figure 3.106** **Continuous slow, left temporal and intermittent slow, left frontal.** Bipolar longitudinal montage. This 57-year-old patient with aphasia due to a low-grade glioma in the left temporal lobe has continuous irregular delta waves in the left temporal region. After eye closure (blue arrow), there is a 3- or 4-s burst of intermittent, left frontal rhythmic delta waves. There is also an almost complete absence of background alpha activity on the left side.

EEG classification: Abnormal III (awake)
1. Continuous slow, left temporal
2. Intermittent rhythmic slow, left frontal
3. Asymmetry, decreased background rhythms left

EEG report: This EEG reflects the left temporal glioma.

Continuous slow, right occipital and periodic discharge, right occipital

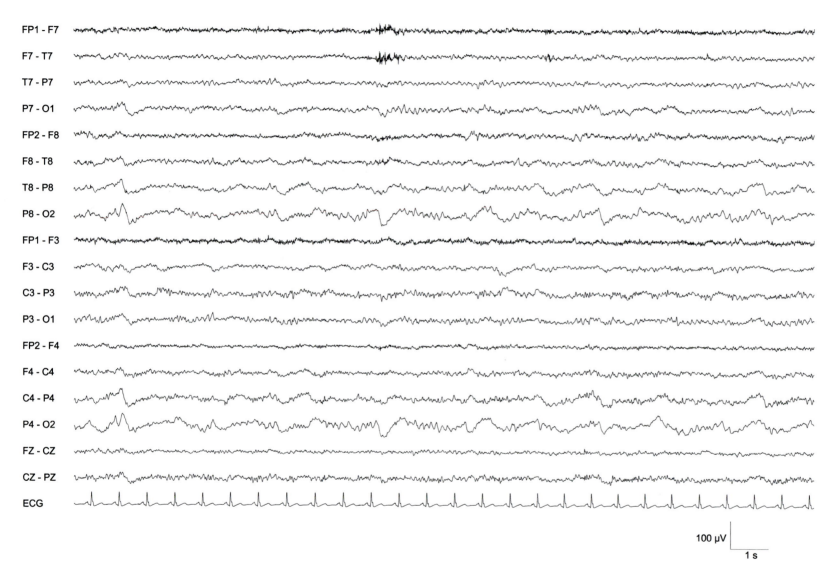

100 μV

1 s

▶ **Figure 3.107** **Continuous slow, right occipital and periodic discharge, right occipital.** Bipolar longitudinal montage. A 76-year-old patient with right posterior cerebral artery infarction. The occipital region shows a background alpha rhythm of approximately 9 Hz. On the right occipital side, there is a continuous slow of delta and subdelta waves. In addition, there is a periodic discharge with intervals of 2-3 seconds.

EEG classification: Abnormal III (awake)
1. Continuous slow, right occipital
2. Periodic discharges, right occipital

EEG report: This EEG reflects the right occipital infarct.

Continuous slow left frontotemporal and asymmetry, decreased background left

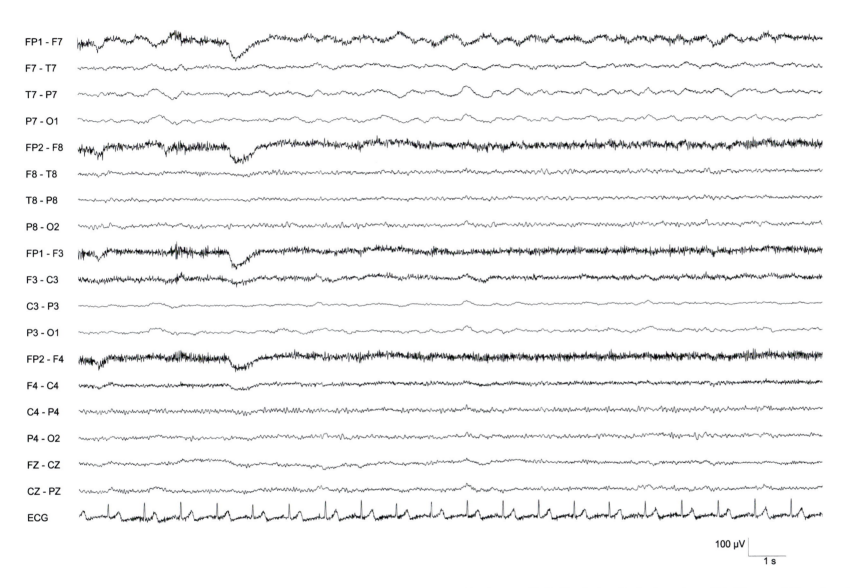

100 µV

1 s

▶ **Figure 3.108** **Continuous slow left frontotemporal and asymmetry, decreased background left.** Bipolar longitudinal montage. This 78-year-old female patient had a fluctuating aphasia due a hemorrhage and infarct in the left middle cerebral artery territory. The EEG shows continuous delta activity and almost complete absence of background alpha activity on the left hemisphere.

EEG classification: Abnormal III (awake)
1. Continuous slow, left
2. Asymmetry, reduced background left

EEG report: This EEG reflects the extensive left infarct and hemorrhage.

Continuous slow, left hemisphere; asymmetry, decreased background rhythm left and background slow

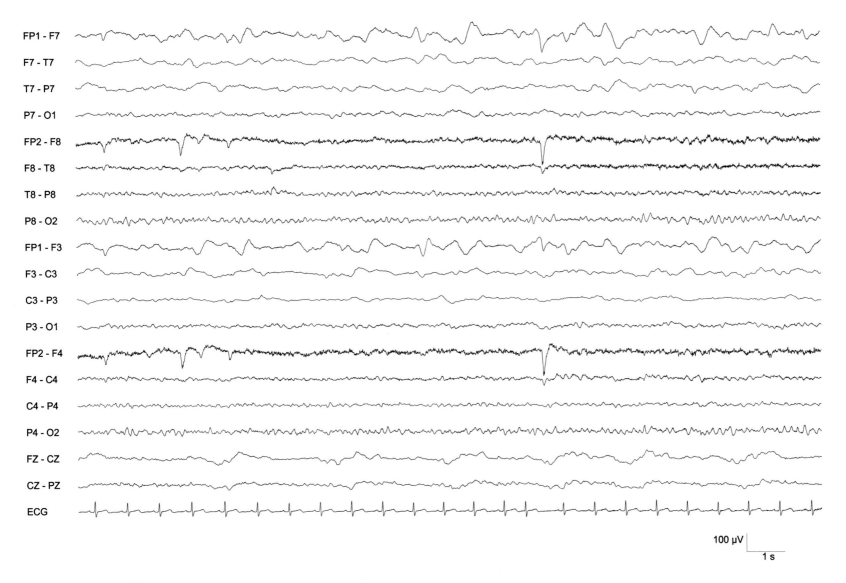

▶ **Figure 3.109** **Continuous slow, left hemisphere; asymmetry, decreased background rhythm left and background slow.** Bipolar longitudinal montage. This 58-year-old patient suffered from a hypertensive left basal ganglia and intraventricular hemorrhage. The right occipital background rhythm is slowed to 7 Hz. The left hemisphere shows irregular delta slow. The occipital background rhythm and frontal beta waves are reduced in amplitude on the left side.

EEG classification: Abnormal III (awake)
1. Continuous slow, left maximum frontal
2. Asymmetry, reduced background left
3. Background slow

EEG report: This EEG reflects the extensive left-brain bleeding and shows evidence of a mild diffuse encephalopathy.

Continuous slow, right temporoparietal and asymmetry, decreased right arousal pattern

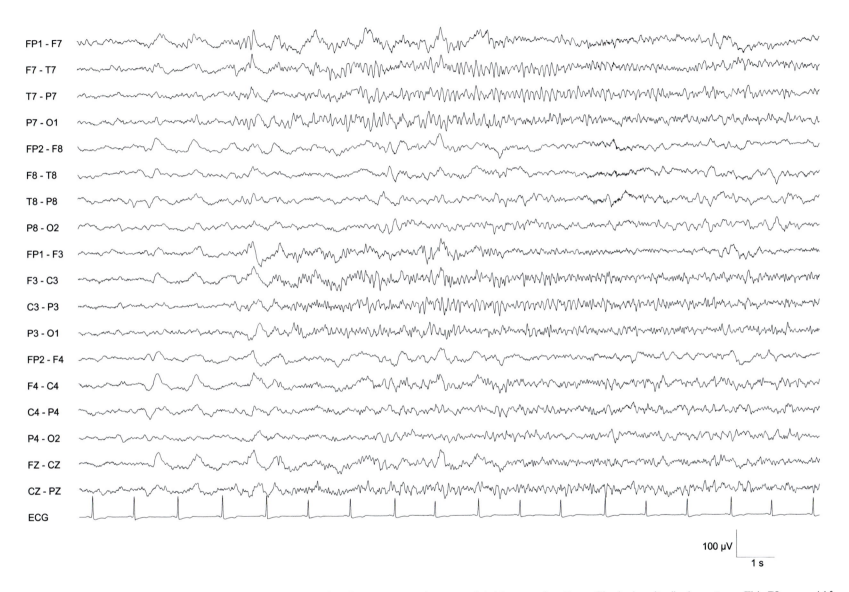

100 µV

1 s

▶ **Figure 3.110** **Continuous slow, right temporoparietal and asymmetry, decreased right arousal pattern.** Bipolar longitudinal montage. This 72-year-old female patient had a right parietal meningeoma. The EEG shows an arousal from sleep stage 2, with beta and alpha background activity of significantly higher amplitude on the left side, whereas the right temporoparietal region shows continuous slow.

EEG classification: Abnormal II (awake and sleep)
1. Continuous slow, right temporoparietal
2. Asymmetry, decreased right arousal pattern

EEG report: This EEG reflects the right parietal meningioma.

an asymmetry with increased background rhythm on the same hemisphere suggests a lesion with a skull defect (trepanation; e.g., a cleared bleeding or a tumor biopsy) (see Section 2.2.3.4, and Section 3.4.2.7.2).

After lesions in the upper brainstem and diencephalon of cats, high-amplitude delta waves could be recorded (Lindsley et al., 1949). The EEG, however, remained unchanged after lesions of the lower brainstem. After pontine lesions, isolated bursts of spindles occurred in these animals.

In order to clarify the mechanisms leading to slow in the EEG, the spatial relationship between the location of thermocoagulation lesions and the location of the continuous slow was investigated in cats (Gloor et al., 1977). The results can be summarized as follows:

- Cortex: Isolated lesions of the cortex did not slow down the EEG. There was only a regional amplitude reduction (asymmetry).
- Subcortical white matter: Delta slow occurs above the lesion immediately after placing the lesion.
- Thalamus: Focal or unilateral delta activity.
- Hypothalamus: Bilateral lesion led to bilateral slow activity.

From these investigations, it was concluded that the slow activity is not caused by damage to the generators (cortical neurons) but, rather, by their deafferentiation from deeper structures. These experimental studies in animals are supported by clinical observations. In patients with tumors in the cortex, white matter, diencephalon, brainstem, or cerebellum, it was observed that polymorphic delta activity only occurred in those patients in whom the white matter or deeper structures were also affected by the tumor (Jasper & Van Buren, 1955). It was assumed that the interruption of cortical afferences is necessary for the development of regional slow. Studies on diffuse encephalopathies have also shown that continuous slow was more common in patients with processes involving the medullary bedding than in patients with diffuse processes involving only the gray matter (Gloor et al., 1968).

The localization of regional slow does not necessarily have to match the localization of the lesion (Goldensohn, 1979). Typically, the EEG tends to show temporal changes even if the lesion is extratemporal (Rémi et al., 2011a). However, the lateralization of the slowing is usually correlated with the lateralization of the lesion.

Regional continuous slows are classified as abnormal III because of the high association with regional structural lesions. Generalized continuous slows are classified as abnormal I–III. Generalized continuous slow is classified as abnormal I when it occurs together with mild slowing (>7 Hz) of background rhythms. It is classified as abnormal II if there still is rhythmical background activity, but it is of <7 Hz. It is classified as abnormal III if there is no rhythmical background activity. Patients showing a continuous slow grade III are usually in stupor or coma.

3.4.2.3.4 Background Attenuation (BA)

The EEG shows no activity of more than 20 µV during the whole recording or, if the patient has more than one EEG pattern, during one of the EEG coma/stupor patterns. As previously mentioned, it is not so infrequent that a normal individual may show background attenuation. However, the two conditions can easily be differentiated. Background attenuation is only classified for EEGs that show no rhythmical background activity and mostly in patients who are in stupor or coma. EEGs with rhythmical background of less than 20 µV seen in normal individuals, who are awake and alert and usually show a normal rhythmical background activity suppressed by eye opening, are reported as normal. Pathological diffuse background attenuation only occurs in patients who clinically are suffering from a severe diffuse encephalopathy (▶ **Figures 3.111** and **3.112**). If the reduction of the background amplitude affects only one hemisphere, it is classified as asymmetry, decreased background (see Section 3.4.2.7.2). However, it is classified as background attenuation or background suppression (BSU) if the amplitude on the affected side is less than 10 µV (BSU) or less than 20 µV (BA).

We classify an EEG as "background attenuation" when the EEG shows only very low-amplitude brain activity (between 10 and 20 µV). This EEG is seen mainly in patients with a severe encephalopathy but is still a reversible EEG pattern.

Background attenuation is classified as abnormal EEG III because it is associated with severe encephalopathies or hemispheric lesions.

3.4.2.3.5 Background Suppression (BSU)

EEG recordings that do not show any brain activity of more than 10 µV are classified as background suppression (▶ **Figures 3.113** and **3.114**). Patients with background suppression almost always are in coma or stupor. However, we have seen normal individuals who have an extremely low-amplitude EEG of less than 10 µV. These EEGs should be classified as normal. It is not rare that normal individuals have EEGs of less than 20 µV; EEG of less than 10 µV, however, is extremely infrequent in normal individuals.

Background attenuation

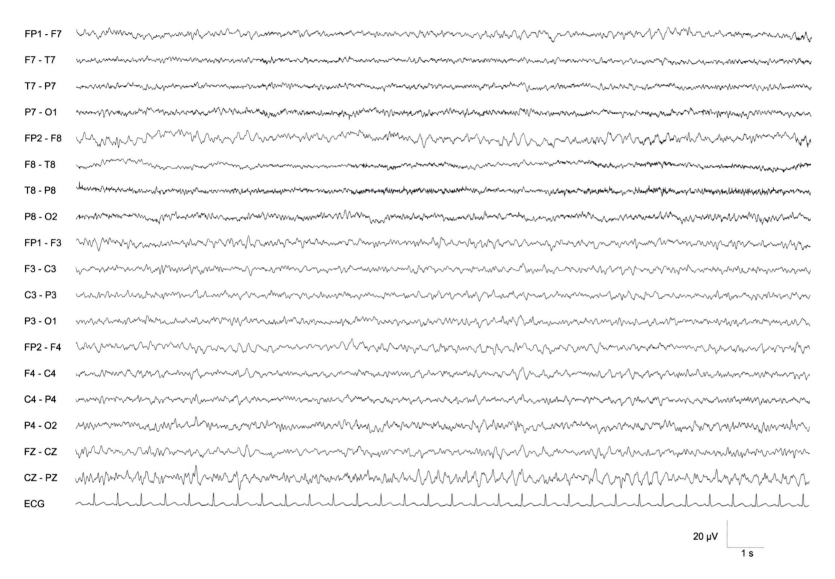

20 µV

1 s

▶ **Figure 3.111** **Background attenuation.** Bipolar longitudinal montage. A 76-year-old stuporous patient post cardiopulmonary resuscitation due to a central pulmonary embolism. The EEG shows a diffuse low-amplitude theta activity below 20 µV.

EEG classification: Abnormal III (stupor)
Background attenuation, generalized

EEG report: This EEG reflects a severe encephalopathy due to cardiopulmonary arrest with resuscitation.

Background attenuation, left; theta stupor

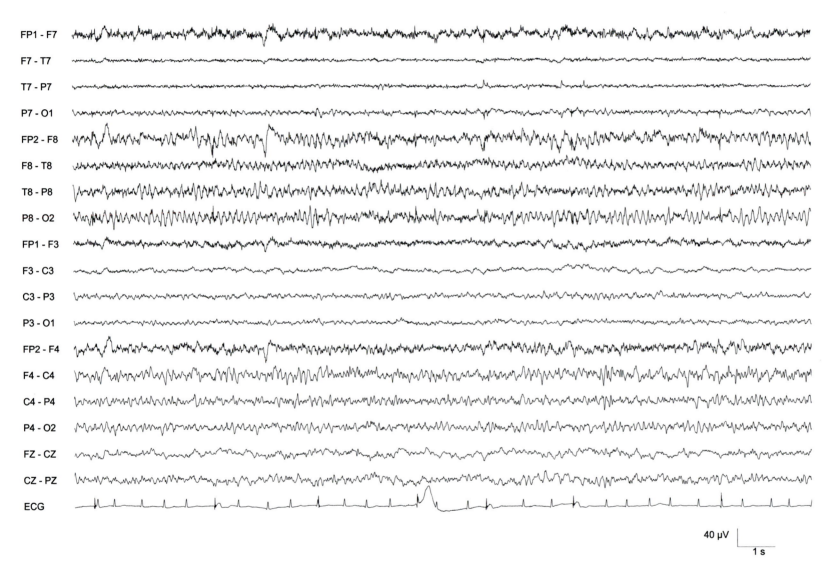

FP1 - F7

F7 - T7

T7 - P7

P7 - O1

FP2 - F8

F8 - T8

T8 - P8

P8 - O2

FP1 - F3

F3 - C3

C3 - P3

P3 - O1

FP2 - F4

F4 - C4

C4 - P4

P4 - O2

FZ - CZ

CZ - PZ

ECG

40 µV

1 s

▶ **Figure 3.112** **Background attenuation, left; theta stupor.** Bipolar longitudinal montage. An 84-year-old stuporous patient with complete left internal carotid embolic stroke was in an ICU. The EEG was filtered at 50 Hz due to extensive mains artifacts. He has had atrial fibrillation. The right hemisphere shows predominant diffuse theta activity. The left hemisphere has no activity above 20 µV. Note the artifact in the ECG and less prominent in the EEG, mainly channel P7–O1, likely due to one of the electrical devices in the ICU.

EEG classification: Abnormal III (stupor)
1. Theta stupor
2. Background attenuation, left

EEG report: This EEG reflects a severe diffuse encephalopathy and an extensive left hemisphere infarction.

Background suppression, generalized

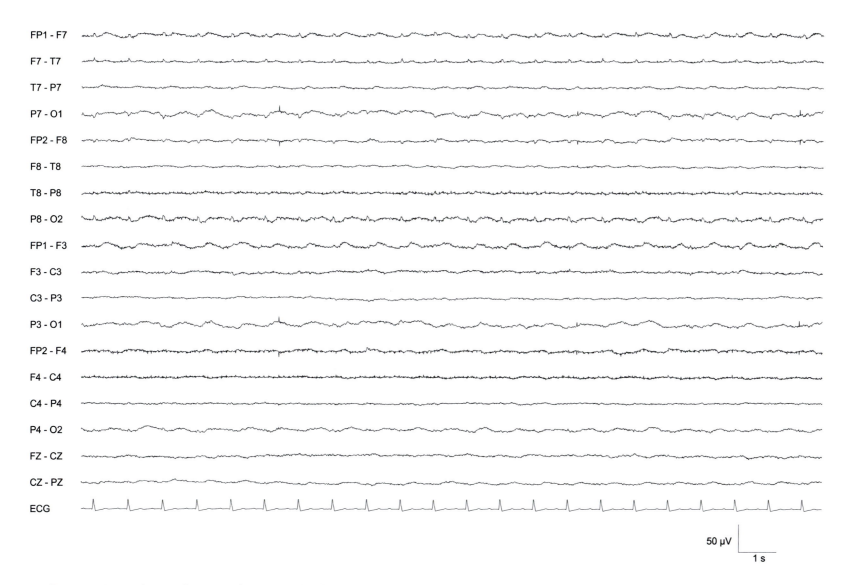

FP1 - F7
F7 - T7
T7 - P7
P7 - O1
FP2 - F8
F8 - T8
T8 - P8
P8 - O2
FP1 - F3
F3 - C3
C3 - P3
P3 - O1
FP2 - F4
F4 - C4
C4 - P4
P4 - O2
FZ - CZ
CZ - PZ
ECG

50 µV

1 s

▶ **Figure 3.113** **Background suppression, generalized.** Bipolar longitudinal montage. A 73-year-old patient with anoxic encephalopathy after resuscitation due to cardiorespiratory arrest. The EEG is flat, and an occipital background rhythm cannot be identified. Only diffuse low-amplitude beta and alpha activity can be identified. Pulse and ECG artifacts dominate.

EEG classification: Abnormal III (coma)
Background suppression, generalized

EEG report: This EEG contains no evidence of brain activity. Absence of brain activity after an anoxic encephalopathy and in the absence of sedative medication or hypothermia is of guarded prognosis and usually is an irreversible EEG pattern. To diagnose "electrocerebral silence," an EEG following the guidelines of the American Neurophysiological Society should be obtained.

Background suppression, right; continuous slow, left frontal and generalized, and background slow

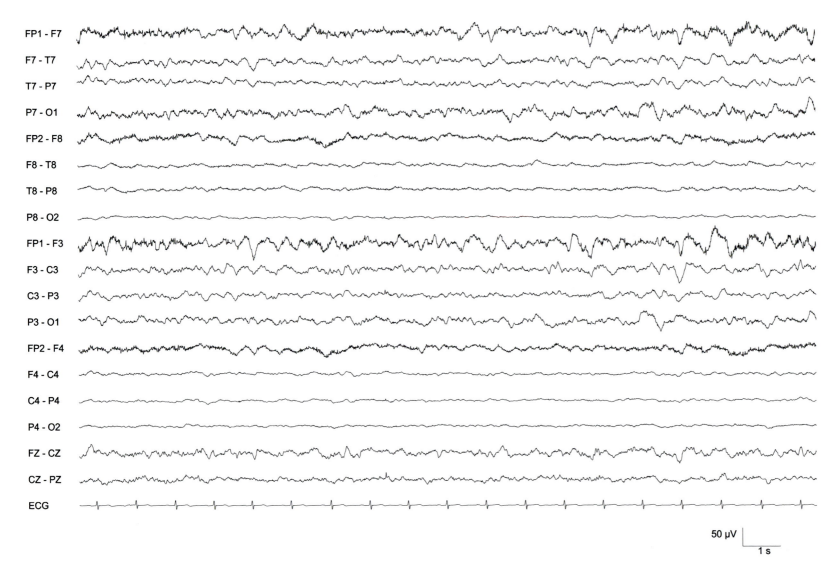

FP1 - F7
F7 - T7
T7 - P7
P7 - O1
FP2 - F8
F8 - T8
T8 - P8
P8 - O2
FP1 - F3
F3 - C3
C3 - P3
P3 - O1
FP2 - F4
F4 - C4
C4 - P4
P4 - O2
FZ - CZ
CZ - PZ
ECG

50 μV

1 s

▶ **Figure 3.114** **Background suppression, right; continuous slow, left frontal and generalized, and background slow.** Bipolar longitudinal montage. An 80-year-old male patient with severe Alzheimer's dementia and a recent right media infarction who now presented with an acute right subdural hematoma. The EEG shows no activity above 10 μV over the right hemisphere. The posterior background is hardly visible at 4 or 5 Hz. In addition, there is a diffuse and left frontal continuous slow.

EEG classification: Abnormal III (awake)
1. Background suppression, right
2. Continuous slow, left frontal and generalized
3. Background slow

EEG report: This EEG reflects the acute right subdural hematoma, the old right media infarction, and the moderate to severe encephalopathy due to Alzheimer's dementia.

Temporary postictal flattening of the background activity, as it can occur temporarily after an epileptic seizure, is not classified as background suppression.

Background suppression can also occur regionally and then indicates a severe regional cortical brain lesion or absence of brain tissue (▶ Figure 3.114), such as a porencephalic cyst with no brain tissue under the recording electrodes.

The typical ballistic pulse artifacts, frequently seen in patients with background suppression, are caused by an increased blood flow via the external carotid artery, when the flow via the internal carotid artery is reduced. In addition, the EEG of patients with background suppression is always reviewed with higher sensitivity, making ballistic artifacts more obvious.

Background suppression is classified as abnormal III.

3.4.2.3.6 Electrocerebral Silence (ECS)

EEG recordings in which the amplitude of brain activity does not exceed 2 μV (▶ Figure 3.115) are classified as electrocerebral silence. Usually, such EEGs are displayed with very high sensitivity and, therefore, they show a high-amplitude ECG and ballistic artifact (see above). Brain death is defined as the state of irreversible extinction of all the functions of the cerebrum, cerebellum, and brainstem (irreversible loss of brain function) while cardiovascular function is still maintained by controlled ventilation.

The diagnosis of brain death is based on the guidelines for determining brain death agreed on by several national and international medical associations (Wijdicks, 2002; Wijdicks et al., 2010). There are, however, some discrepancies in the definitions of cerebral death. These discrepancies involve particularly the need to include or not the death of the brainstem in the determination of brain death (Wijdicks, 2002).

The following EEG recording technique is recommended by the ACNS to detect electrocerebral silence (Stecker et al., 2016):

1. A complete set of scalp electrodes should be utilized.
2. Inter-electrode impedances should be less than 10,000 Ω but more than 100 Ω.
3. The integrity of the entire recording system should be tested.
4. Montages for electrocerebral inactivity interpretation should include electrode pairs at least 10 cm apart.
5. Sensitivity must be increased to a maximum of 2 μV/mm for at least 30 min of the recording.

6. Filter settings should be appropriate (1–70 Hz).
7. Additional monitoring techniques should be employed when the electroencephalographer cannot decide if certain waves are brain activity or artifacts.
8. There should be no EEG reactivity to intense somatosensory, auditory, or visual stimuli.
9. Recordings should be performed only by a qualified technologist.
10. A repeat EEG should be performed when electrocerebral inactivity is in doubt.
11. Vital parameters and medications should be noted.

Note that each country may have its own slightly varying recommendations in place.

3.4.2.4   Epileptiform Discharges (ED)

EEG in epilepsy patients is usually performed during seizure intervals (i.e., interictally). However, the presence of interictal epileptiform discharges is closely related to epilepsy; additionally, focal interictal discharges point to the location of the epileptogenic zone. The term epileptiform discharges is used as an umbrella term lumping together all the EEG patterns that are an expression of epileptogenicity—that is, sharp waves, spikes, polyspikes, spike–waves, slow spike–waves, typical EEG seizure patterns, and so on.

It is important to recognize that essentially all "interictal" epileptiform discharges represent epileptic activity such as "little" seizures. However, most spikes are of short duration and most likely produce so subtle clinical signs that neither the observers nor the patients realize that a "small seizure" occurred. However, if the same spike of the same intensity occurs over the primary motor area, it may trigger a clinical seizure (myoclonic jerk). Moreover, in many instances, an epileptiform discharge may be labeled as "interictal" because the deficit produced by the epileptiform discharge may only become obvious if appropriate testing is done during the epileptiform discharge (Beniczky et al., 2016).

The expression "subclinical seizure" refers to epilepsy patients who, in the "interictal period," show no clinical symptomatology but the EEG reveals EEG patterns that usually occur with clear epileptic symptomatology (Weil et al., 2005). The transition from a seizure to a status epilepticus is fluid.

Electrocerebral silence, generalized

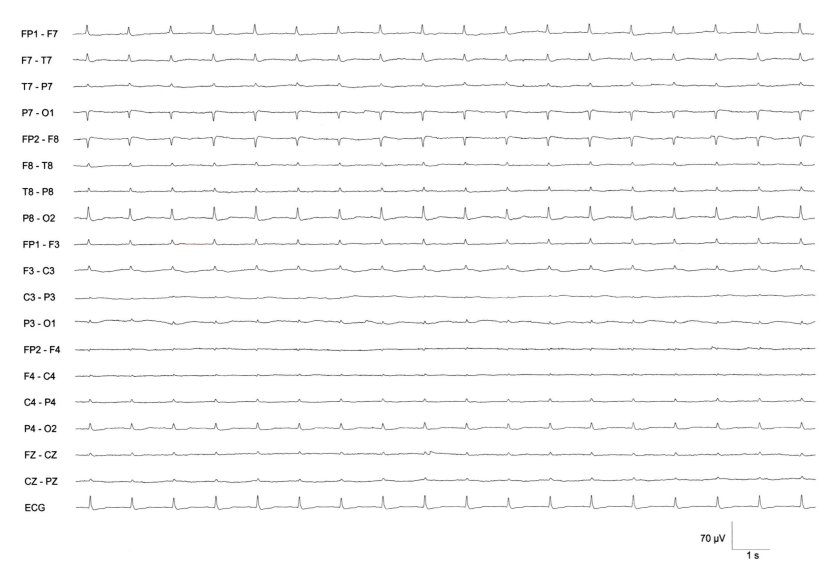

70 µV

1 s

▶ **Figure 3.115** **Electrocerebral silence, generalized.** Bipolar longitudinal row. A 56-year-old polytraumatized patient with massive brain edema after severe bilateral brain concussion with subarachnoid hemorrhage and left subdural hematoma. The EEG shows no brain activity above 2 µV and is dominated by ECG artifacts. Notice the bipolar distribution of the ECG artifact with a positive pole at P7 > T7 and a negative pole at F8 > T8 > P8. Usually, in routine EEGs, the cardiac vector is maximum negativity at A2 > FP2 = F8 and the positive pole is at A1 > P7 = O1. The difference of ECG distribution is determined by head rotations: The cardiac vector is fixed in space. However, with head rotations, the vector will project on different scalp electrodes. In this particular case, the patient had the head rotated to the left.

EEG classification: Abnormal III (coma)
    Electrocerebral silence, generalized

EEG report: This EEG shows electrocerebral silence. The EEG was obtained following the recommendations of the American Neurophysiology Society for the recording of cerebral inactivity. The absence of brain activity, in the absence of any sedative medication and/or hypothermia, is an irreversible condition.

In summary, we believe that any epileptiform discharge represents clinical seizure activity with a fluid transition between "apparently asymptomatic" interictal spikes, "subclinical" epileptic seizures, epileptic seizures, and status epilepticus.

Interictal epileptiform abnormalities occur almost exclusively in patients who also have well-documented epileptic seizures (Gregory et al., 1993). Note that the identification of epileptiform discharges is not objectively but, rather, subjectively determined by the electroencephalographer (Grant et al., 2014). Some children have epileptiform discharges without suffering from epileptic seizures. There is relative consensus that approximately 2–3.5% of healthy children have benign epileptiform discharges and that only a very small proportion of these children (approximately 8%) suffer from clinical epileptic seizures (Eeg-Olofsson et al., 1971; Gregory et al., 1993; Lüders et al., 1987). Interictal epileptiform discharges are found even less frequently among healthy adults or individuals with brain disorder but no epileptic seizures (0.5–2.2%) (Gregory et al., 1993; Zivin & Marsan, 1968).

The EEG provides answers to the following questions (Noachtar & Rémi, 2009):

- Is it epilepsy?
- What epilepsy syndrome?
- What is the localization of the epileptogenic zone?
- Is epilepsy surgery an option?

The sensitivity and specificity of interictal epileptiform discharges for epilepsy depend on various factors. The epilepsy syndrome, the etiology of epilepsy, and the duration of epilepsy influence the sensitivity of interictal epileptiform discharges for epilepsy (Desai et al., 1988; Selvitelli et al., 2010). The first EEG after an epileptic seizure shows interictal epileptiform discharges in 12–55% of patients (Baldin et al., 2014; Goodin et al., 1990; Hopkins et al., 1988; M. King et al., 1998; Shinnar et al., 1990; Van Donselaar et al., 1992). The EEG after a first epileptic seizure is most sensitive in the first 12 hr after the seizure (Sofat et al., 2016).

When an EEG shows epileptiform discharges, the following formulation is often found in the EEG impression: ". . . this EEG is compatible with epilepsy." This formulation is not very meaningful and rather clumsy because (a) an interictal EEG is most frequently normal in patients with epilepsy and (b) essentially any EEG is compatible with epilepsy except electrocerebral inactivity. A more meaningful impression is to report that the "EEG is supportive" of epilepsy when the EEG indeed shows epileptiform discharges.

Epilepsy patients with temporal lesions very often show interictal epileptiform discharges in the EEG (▶ **Figure 3.116**) (Rémi et al., 2011a). Often, there is a more or less pronounced slow in the same region (▶ **Figure 3.116**). In contrast, extratemporal epilepsies of adults, especially when they have epileptogenic zones in the central and frontal region, often do not show epileptiform discharges despite continuous EEG recordings over several days (Rémi et al., 2011a). Children and adolescents with absence epilepsy (▶ **Figure 3.117**) or benign focal epilepsy of childhood (▶ **Figure 3.141**), on the other hand, if untreated usually show epileptiform EEG patterns. This indicates that the sensitivity of the EEG strongly depends on the epilepsy syndrome (Baldin et al., 2014). A short latency from the last seizure to the EEG recording significantly increases the chances to detect interictal epileptiform discharges (Ajmone-Marsan & Zivin, 1970; Baldin et al., 2014; Gotman & Koffler, 1989; Gotman & Marciani, 1985; King et al., 1998; Sofat et al., 2016; Sundaram et al., 1990). Repeated recordings also significantly improve the chance to record interictal epileptiform discharges (80–90%; Ajmone-Marsan & Zivin, 1970; Betting et al., 2006; Goodin & Aminoff, 1984; Salinsky et al., 1987; Sundaram et al., 1990).

Prolonged EEG recordings capturing waking and sleep greatly increase the chance of detecting epileptiform discharges and epileptic seizures (Ives, 1975). The introduction of digital EEG machines allowing electronic storage of the EEG recordings has greatly simplified long-term EEG recordings.

There are reports that recordings during sleep after partial sleep deprivation increase the probability to detect abnormal EEG findings. Sleep deprivation has been reported to be most effective in triggering interictal epileptiform discharges in patients with idiopathic generalized epilepsies (Ferrillo et al., 2000; Foldvary-Schaefer & Grigg-Damberger, 2009; Fountain et al., 1998). Some patients have difficulty falling asleep in the EEG laboratory without previous sleep deprivation. The external conditions regarding comfort and rest should therefore be designed to make it as easy as possible for patients to fall asleep. For this reason, we conduct all EEGs in comfortable beds. The EEG room for sleep recordings must be quiet and darkened. One can also take advantage of postprandial fatigue to facilitate sleep.

Spikes and continuous slow, left anterior temporal

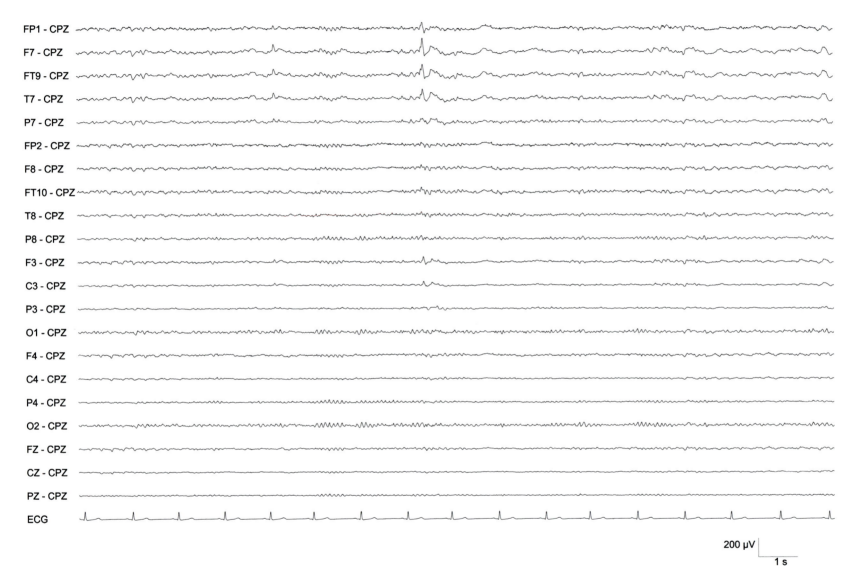

FP1 - CPZ
F7 - CPZ
FT9 - CPZ
T7 - CPZ
P7 - CPZ
FP2 - CPZ
F8 - CPZ
FT10 - CPZ
T8 - CPZ
P8 - CPZ
F3 - CPZ
C3 - CPZ
P3 - CPZ
O1 - CPZ
F4 - CPZ
C4 - CPZ
P4 - CPZ
O2 - CPZ
FZ - CPZ
CZ - CPZ
PZ - CPZ
ECG

200 μV

1 s

▶ **Figure 3.116** **Spikes and continuous slow, left anterior temporal.** Reference derivation to CPZ. This 27-year-old female patient with left mesial temporal lobe sclerosis and left temporal lobe epilepsy shows left anterior temporal spikes during drowsiness. The spikes show maximum negativity at electrode F7 > FT9. In the same region, there is also a continuous slow with irregular theta and delta waves.

EEG classification: Abnormal III (awake)
1. Spikes, F7 > FT9 > T7
2. Continuous slow, left anterior temporal

EEG report: This EEG supports the diagnosis of a left temporal lobe epilepsy.

Spike–waves, generalized

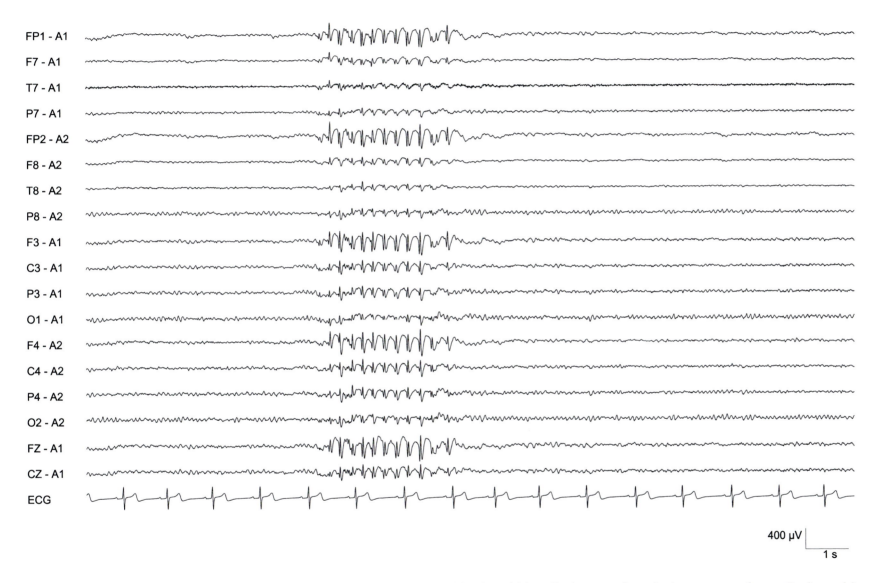

FP1 - A1
F7 - A1
T7 - A1
P7 - A1
FP2 - A2
F8 - A2
T8 - A2
P8 - A2
F3 - A1
C3 - A1
P3 - A1
O1 - A1
F4 - A2
C4 - A2
P4 - A2
O2 - A2
FZ - A1
CZ - A1
ECG

400 µV

1 s

▶ **Figure 3.117** **Spike–waves, generalized.** Ear reference montage. This 17-year-old patient with juvenile absence epilepsy had a recurrence of generalized convulsive seizures after discontinuing medication. He had been seizure-free for 2 years on medication. The EEG shows a burst of generalized spike–waves with a repetition rate of approximately 4 Hz for 3 s.

EEG classification: Abnormal III (awake)
Spike–waves, generalized

EEG report: This EEG supports the diagnosis of juvenile absence epilepsy.

It is also important to remember that the percentage of epilepsy in the studied cohort will greatly influence the chances of recording interictal epileptiform discharges (Pedley et al., 2003). The positive predictive value (PPV) for interictal epileptic discharges in collectives is derived from the ratio of the number of patients with epilepsy who have interictal epileptiform discharges to all people (with and without epilepsy) who show epileptiform discharges in the EEG. The following example illustrates how strongly the PPV for epileptiform discharges depends on the probability of encountering patients with epilepsy in an investigated collective. Let us assume that the probability of recording interictal epileptiform discharges in the first EEG of a patient with epilepsy is 55% and that the probability of recording epileptiform discharges in the first EEG of a person without epilepsy is 2% (Zivin & Marsan, 1968). If a random collective of 1,000 unselected patients from a defined geographical region were studied, the prevalence rate for epilepsy would be approximately 0.5%. In such a collective, 5 people would be expected to have epilepsy, 3 of whom would also have epileptiform discharges in the EEG, but there would be another 20 people without epilepsy whose EEG would show epileptiform discharges. In this setting, the PPV for epileptiform discharges for the diagnosis of epilepsy would be only 3/23 (i.e., 13%). Let us now consider a collective as is typically referred for EEG examination. In this constellation, the probability of finding epilepsy patients in the group will be much higher. Let's assume that half of the patients assigned to the EEG laboratory suffer from epilepsy. Out of 1,000 patients, 500 would then have epilepsy and 275 (55%) of these would also show epileptiform discharges in the EEG. Of the 500 patients without epilepsy, 10 (i.e., 2%) would show interictal epileptiform discharges. In this setting, the PPV for epileptiform discharges would be 275/285 (i.e., 96%) (Pedley et al., 2003). When assessing the sensitivity and specificity of the EEG, we must consider which patient sample is involved—that is, how many epilepsy patients are examined in a given collective.

The different interictal epileptic EEG patterns and seizure and status patterns are listed below. Use the terms "spikes" and "polyspikes" when the negative spike is not followed by a negative slow wave that clearly exceeds the amplitude of the presiding negative spike. Use the terms "spike–wave" or "polyspike–wave" if the negative slow wave following the negative spike clearly exceeds the amplitude of the preceding spike or polyspike. Use the expressions "polyspike" or "polyspike–wave" if the epileptiform discharge preceding a prominent slow wave consists of two or more spikes.

All following epileptiform EEG categories are classified as abnormal III because of their high association with epilepsy. The only exception to this rule is the photoparoxysmal response (see below):

- Spikes (SP)
- Polyspikes (PSP)
- Benign epileptiform discharges (BED)
- Spike–waves (SW)
- Polyspike–waves (PSW)
- 3 Hz spike–waves (3SW)
- Slow spike–waves (SSW)
- Hypsarrhythmia (HYP)
- Photoparoxysmal response (PR)
- Seizure pattern (SEP)
- Status pattern (STP)

3.4.2.4.1   Spikes (SP)

This refers to "steep waves" and "spikes" or "sharp waves" that clearly stand out in amplitude and wave duration from the background activity, are almost only recorded in patients with epilepsy, and can be differentiated from "sharp transients" that can often be observed in patients without epilepsy. Historically, spikes and sharp waves were differentiated by their duration—that is, spikes were sharp transients of a duration of less than 70 ms. However, it was never specified exactly how to measure the duration of a sharp wave or spike. We recognized also that the clinical significance of sharp waves and spikes was essentially the same (i.e., both spikes and sharp waves support the diagnosis of epilepsy), and their distribution was an index of the localization of the epileptogenic zone. Therefore, we now use the term spikes for all sharp transients that we believe are epileptogenic; thus, the term sharp waves will not be used anymore when dealing with epileptiform discharges. The term sharp transients should be used to identify "sharply contoured waves" when the EEG reader is not sure if the wave is epileptiform or not.

It is also important to realize that diagnosis of spikes is subjective and, therefore, strongly investigator-dependent (Williams et al., 1985). The problem is illustrated with the following definition of spikes: "Like a familiar face, a spike is easy to recognize but difficult to describe to someone else" (Daly, 1990). Unfortunately, quantitative criteria describing spikes are not available. The following subjective criteria are applied to determine whether or not sharply contoured waves are epileptiform discharges, and the contribution of each parameter has been investigated (Kural et al., 2020):

- Sharp transients that stand out from the background activity. Because there is no generally valid limit for this, we use the rule that the spike exceeds the background activity in an uncontaminated referential montage by at least twice.
- The duration of spikes (sharp waves) is by definition 20–200 ms (Noachtar et al., 1999). As mentioned previously, this distinction is certainly also subjective because there is no definition of how to measure the duration of spikes.
- Subsequent slow waves disrupt the background rhythms. The following slow wave is caused by inhibitory mechanisms, which is why some have called it the "brake wave."
- The polarity of the main component of epileptiform discharges recorded with scalp electrodes is usually negative, and only in very rare exceptional cases can a positive spike or dipole be recorded with scalp electrodes (Franco et al., 2018; Matsuo & Knott, 1977). Positive spikes in adults are mainly found in patients who have had a craniotomy and a cortical resection (Franco et al., 2018).
- Determination of the polarity and field distribution of sharp transients helps identify epileptiform discharges and differentiate spikes from artifacts or physiological potentials, such as POSTS.
- Regional epileptiform discharges are frequently associated with intermittent or continuous (rhythmic) slow (IS/IRS or CS/CRS) in the same region. Generalized epileptiform discharges are often associated with generalized intermittent (rhythmic) slow.

Spikes and sharp waves can occur regionally over any brain region or may have a generalized distribution. EEGs not infrequently show clearly defined spikes in a specific brain location and nonspecific slow waves of a similar distribution. Some of these waves (nonspecific sharp transients) probably also are epileptogenic but, due to the filtering of the skull, appear as nonspecific sharp transients (▶ Figure 3.118). It is important to note that the different montages can considerably influence the representation of spikes and their differentiation from non-epileptiform transients (▶ Figures 3.119 and 3.120). In ▶ Figure 3.119, there is a clearly distinguishable right temporal spike. However, in a bipolar montage, only the slow wave of the spike–wave is visible because the potential differences for the spike between adjacent electrodes do not exceed sufficiently the amplitude of the background activity (▶ Figures 3.119 and 3.120).

Most electroencephalographers, however, only diagnose spikes in the standard montage with bipolar longitudinal chains of electrodes. Electroencephalographers get used to recognizing spikes in this montage and, by this approach, avoid the additional variable given by the use of different montages. Spikes particularly change greatly on waveform when using referential montages. On the other hand, the electroencephalographer will use all the other montages to define characteristics of the spike, such as a detailed distribution.

Patients with mesial temporal lobe epilepsies usually have mesial temporal epileptiform discharges, which—like slow in these regions—can occur uni- or bilaterally (▶ Figure 3.121). Bilateral temporal epileptiform discharges do not exclude epilepsy surgical treatment if the seizures start from one temporal lobe. However, the chance of postoperative seizure freedom in these patients is somewhat less favorable than in patients with exclusively unitemporal interictal discharges (Rémi 2011a; Schulz et al., 2000). If all interictal epileptiform discharges are unitemporal and magnetic resonance imaging shows a lesion in the same temporal lobe, ictal recordings will usually not add any additional information for epilepsy surgery (Vollmar et al., 2018). In extratemporal epilepsies, interictal epileptiform discharges can also provide valuable information regarding the localization of the epileptogenic zone (▶ Figures 3.122 and 3.123) (Rémi et al., 2011a). In addition to the spikes and slow activity recorded from the region of the epileptogenic zone, the background activity frequently is decreased or absent in the same region if the patient has a structural lesion in that area (▶ Figure 3.124). Extratemporal epileptogenic lesions are often associated with interictal epileptiform discharges in the temporal region (Hartl et al., 2016). In addition, in half of the cases with lesions in the central region, no interictal spikes are recorded (Rémi et al., 2011a). This may be related to the fact that a significant percentage of extratemporal lobe epilepsies have epileptogenic zones in the mesial frontal region, and in many cases these epileptic foci do not generate interictal epileptiform discharges that can be recorded with scalp electrodes.

Generalized spikes often have a frontal maximum that may shift between the two sides (▶ Figure 3.125). However, patients with generalized idiopathic epilepsies may also have regional epileptiform discharges (▶ Figure 3.126) (Lombroso, 1997). During sleep, generalized epileptiform discharges tend to occur with K-complexes (▶ Figure 3.127). A muscle artifact of the forehead

Spikes, right temporo-occipital and intermittent slow, right temporo-occipital

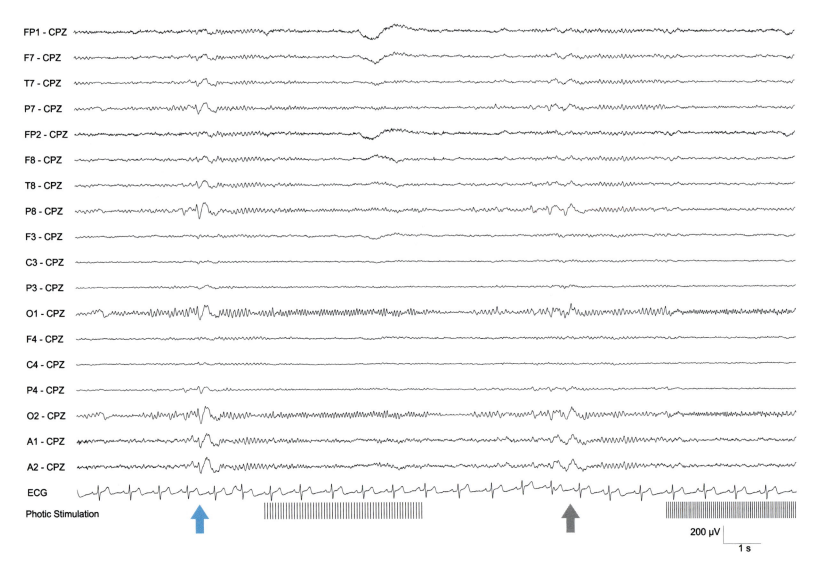

▶ **Figure 3.118** **Spikes, right temporo-occipital and intermittent slow, right temporo-occipital.** Reference derivation to CPZ. A 36-year-old patient with right occipital lobe epilepsy due to a focal cortical dysplasia. The electrodes P8 and O2 show spikes (blue arrow) and slow waves (gray arrow). Note that the slow waves have the same distribution as the temporo-occipital spikes. Most likely, the intermittent slow waves also represent epileptiform discharges that would be evident with depth recording but cannot be visualized with scalp electrodes. Photic stimulation leads to photic driving.

EEG classification: Abnormal III (awake)
1. Spikes, P8 = O2
2. Intermittent slow, right temporo-occipital

EEG report: This EEG supports the diagnosis of a right occipital lobe epilepsy.

Spikes, right temporal. Reference derivation to CZ

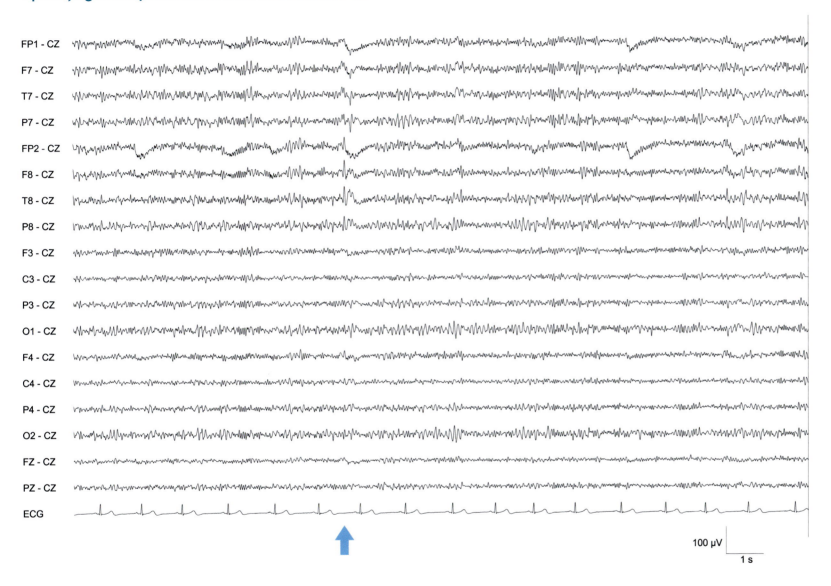

FP1 - CZ

F7 - CZ

T7 - CZ

P7 - CZ

FP2 - CZ

F8 - CZ

T8 - CZ

P8 - CZ

F3 - CZ

C3 - CZ

P3 - CZ

O1 - CZ

F4 - CZ

C4 - CZ

P4 - CZ

O2 - CZ

FZ - CZ

PZ - CZ

ECG

100 µV

1 s

▶ **Figure 3.119** **Spikes, right temporal.** Reference derivation to CZ. A 47-year-old female patient with juvenile absence epilepsy. The spike with a maximum at the electrodes F8 and T8 was followed by a slow wave and is not accompanied by further slow waves in the same region. In other sections of this EEG, the patient had generalized spikes. The EEG classification refers to the entire EEG.

EEG classification: Abnormal III (awake)
1. Spikes, generalized
2. Spikes, F8 = T8

EEG report: This EEG supports the diagnosis of juvenile absence epilepsy.

Visualization of spikes in different montages

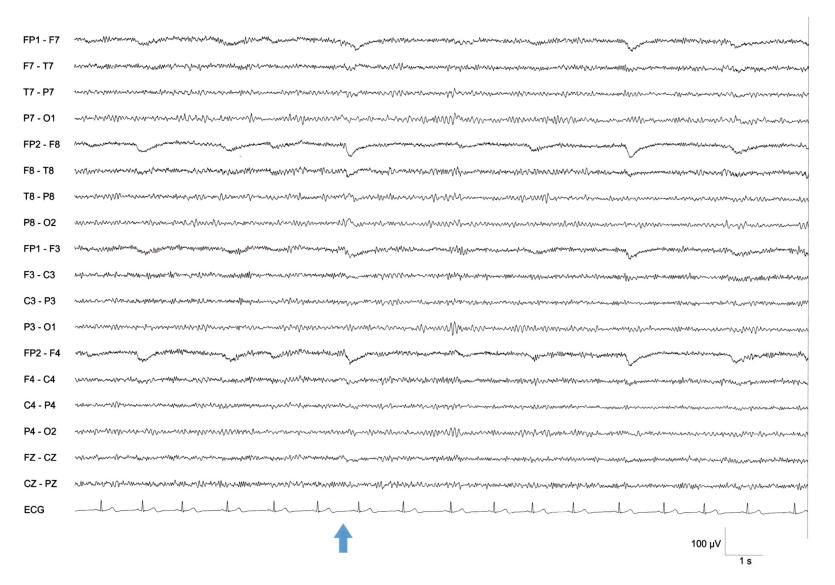

FP1 - F7

F7 - T7

T7 - P7

P7 - O1

FP2 - F8

F8 - T8

T8 - P8

P8 - O2

FP1 - F3

F3 - C3

C3 - P3

P3 - O1

FP2 - F4

F4 - C4

C4 - P4

P4 - O2

FZ - CZ

CZ - PZ

ECG

100 µV

1 s

▶ **Figure 3.120   Visualization of spikes in different montages.** Same EEG section as in ▶ **Figure 3.119** reformatted in a bipolar longitudinal montage. The spike, well represented in ▶ **Figure 3.119**, with a maximum at the electrodes F8, and T8, is no longer definable. Only a short right temporal slow remains. The distinction between spikes and slow requires the use of the optimal montage for appropriate representation of the EEG potential. This EEG would be classified as normal if no additional abnormalities would be detected. We know, however that this patient had generalized epileptiform discharges in other portions of the recording. Therefore, the complete recording would be classified as follows:

EEG classification: Abnormal III (awake)

Spikes, generalized

EEG report: This EEG supports the diagnosis of juvenile absence epilepsy.

Spikes, left and right temporal, and intermittent slow, left temporal

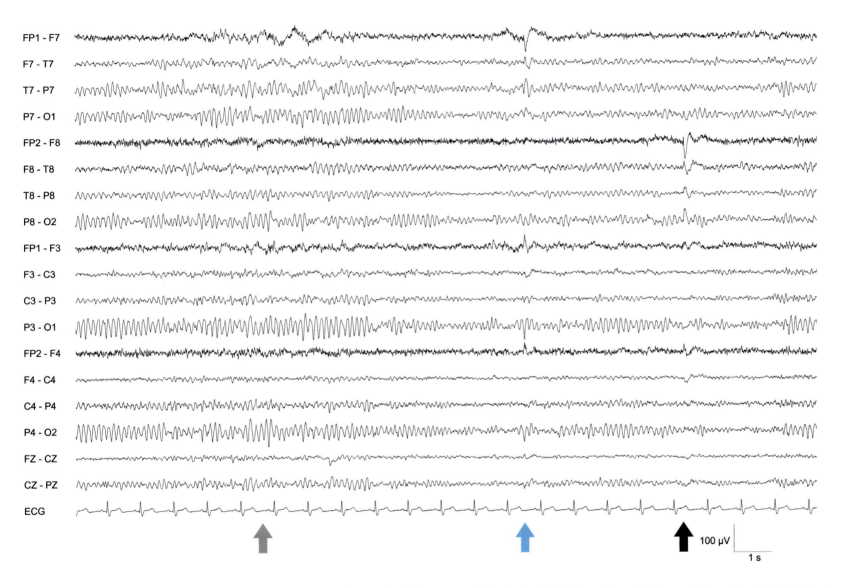

▶ **Figure 3.121** **Spikes, left and right temporal, and intermittent slow, left temporal.** Bipolar longitudinal montage. A 76-year-old female patient with focal epilepsy due to bilateral partial middle cerebral artery infarctions. There is one left (blue arrow) and one right (black arrow) temporal spike. In the left temporal and frontal region, an intermittent delta slow occurs (gray arrow). The occipital alpha background rhythm is well developed bilaterally.

EEG classification: Abnormal III (awake)
1. Spikes, F7 > T7
2. Spikes, F8 > T8
3. Intermittent slow, left temporofrontal

EEG report: This EEG supports the diagnosis of a bitemporal lobe epilepsy.

Spikes, left frontal

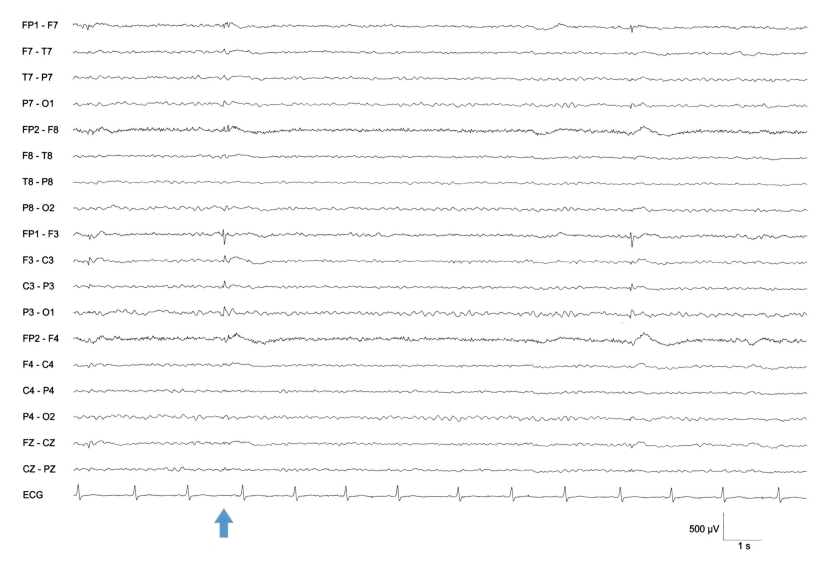

FP1 - F7
F7 - T7
T7 - P7
P7 - O1
FP2 - F8
F8 - T8
T8 - P8
P8 - O2
FP1 - F3
F3 - C3
C3 - P3
P3 - O1
FP2 - F4
F4 - C4
C4 - P4
P4 - O2
FZ - CZ
CZ - PZ
ECG

500 µV

1 s

▶ **Figure 3.122 Spikes, left frontal.** Bipolar longitudinal montage. This 34-year-old female patient suffered from left frontal lobe epilepsy. Spikes (blue arrow) appear in the left frontal region.

EEG classification: Abnormal III (awake)

Spikes, F3 > C3

EEG report: This EEG supports the diagnosis of a left frontal lobe epilepsy.

Spikes, left occipital; left occipital continuous slow; asymmetry, decreased alpha rhythm left occipital and background slow

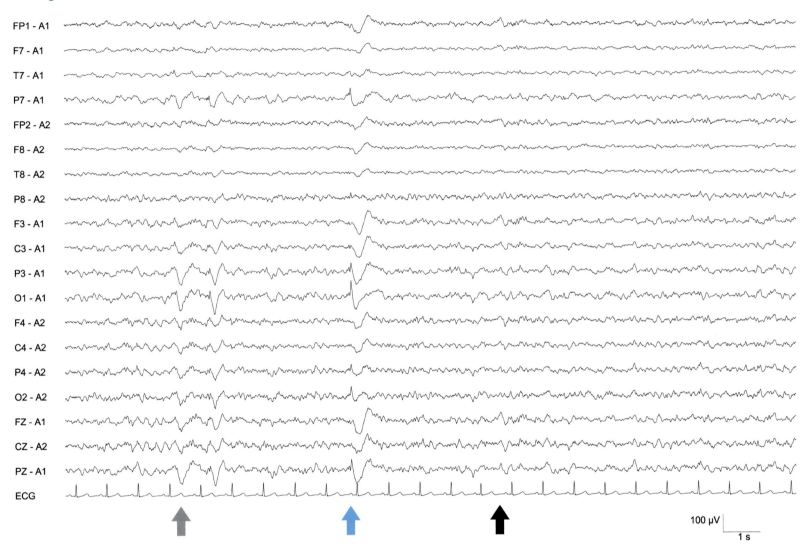

▶ **Figure 3.123** **Spikes, left occipital; left occipital continuous slow; asymmetry, decreased alpha rhythm left occipital and background slow.** Ear reference derivation. This 26-year-old female patient with late-onset Rasmussen's encephalitis at the age of 22 years suffered from aphasic and right-sided motor seizures. The MRI showed a slowly progressing left hemisphere atrophy. The medication, including several anti-seizure drugs, had been significantly increased after an aphasic status that led to sedation.

Spikes (blue arrow) and a continuous slow (gray arrow) are visible in the left occipital region. In addition, there is a posterior-dominant background activity of approximately 7 Hz that is absent on the left side (black arrow). In earlier EEGs, there were also left temporal and left frontal spikes.

EEG classification: Abnormal III (awake)
1. Spikes, O1 > PZ
2. Continuous slow, left occipital
3. Asymmetry, decreased alpha rhythm left occipital
4. Background slow

EEG report: This EEG supports the diagnosis of Rasmussen's encephalitis with a currently active left occipital epileptogenic lesion.

Right central periodic epileptiform discharges; continuous slow, right central and asymmetry, decreased background rhythm on the right

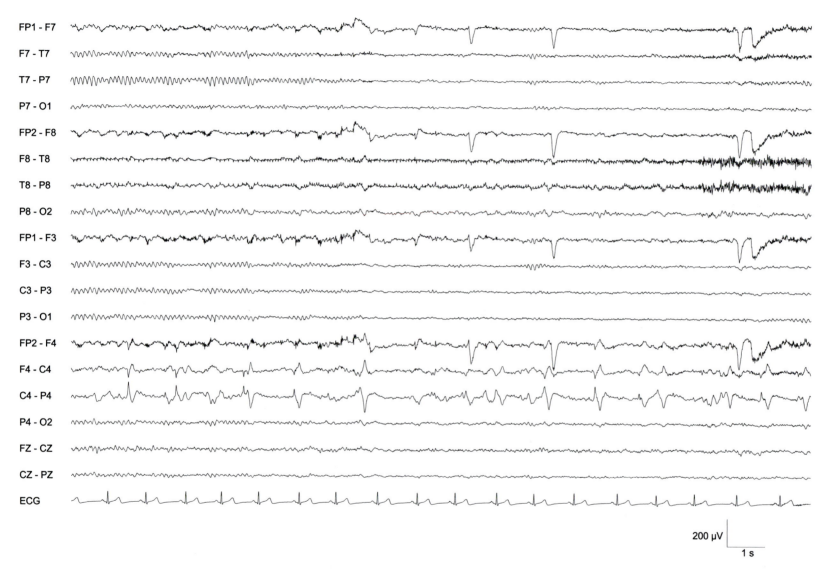

200 µV

1 s

▶ **Figure 3.124** **Right central periodic epileptiform discharges; continuous slow, right central and asymmetry, decreased background rhythm on the right.** Bipolar longitudinal montage. This 23-year-old female patient with an extensive right central glioma and a left spastic hemiparesis suffered from frequent motor seizures of the left side of her body.

In the right central region, periodic epileptiform discharges are seen. In addition, there is a continuous slow in this region. The amplitude of the background alpha rhythm is reduced on the right.

EEG classification: Abnormal III (awake)
1. Periodic epileptiform discharges, C4 > F4
2. Continuous slow, right central
3. Asymmetry, reduced background rhythm on the right

EEG report: This EEG supports the diagnosis of an extensive, highly epileptogenic right central lesion.

Spikes, generalized

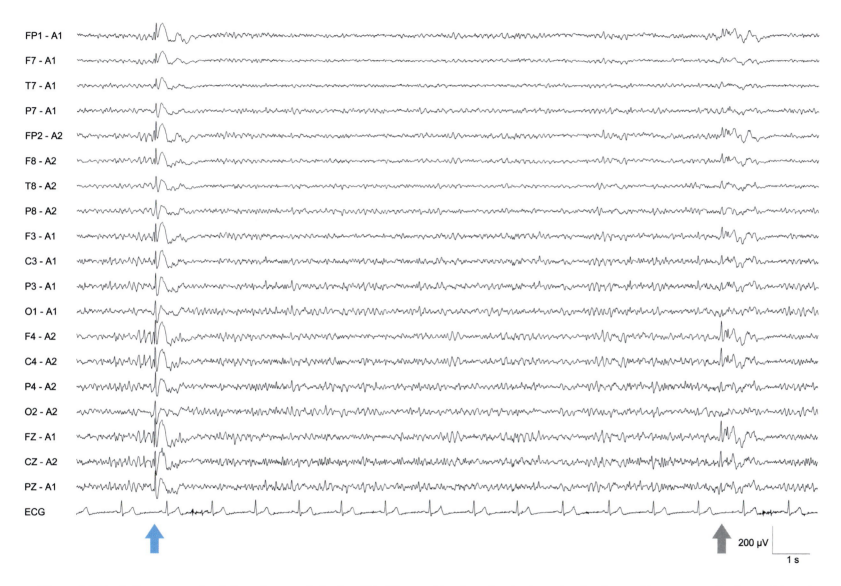

FP1 - A1
F7 - A1
T7 - A1
P7 - A1
FP2 - A2
F8 - A2
T8 - A2
P8 - A2
F3 - A1
C3 - A1
P3 - A1
O1 - A1
F4 - A2
C4 - A2
P4 - A2
O2 - A2
FZ - A1
CZ - A2
PZ - A1
ECG

200 µV

1 s

▶ **Figure 3.125** **Spikes, generalized.** Ear reference derivation. This 57-year-old male patient had grand mal epilepsy with rare generalized convulsive seizures. The generalized spike shows a right frontal maximum (blue arrow) in this EEG section. The maxima of the spikes shift between electrodes F4 and F3, with FZ almost always lying within the 90% field of the maximum amplitude. The gray arrow points to a spike of smaller amplitude. The spike does not stand out from the background and by itself would not have been labeled as an epileptiform discharge. This illustrates the difficulty of EEG interpretation.

EEG classification: Abnormal III (awake)
Spikes, generalized

EEG report: This EEG supports the diagnosis of a generalized epilepsy.

Spikes, left occipital

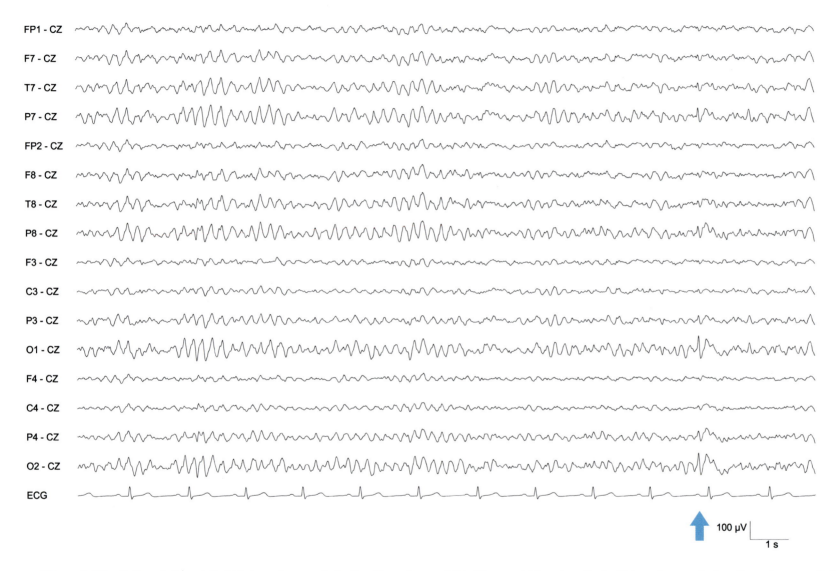

FP1 - CZ
F7 - CZ
T7 - CZ
P7 - CZ
FP2 - CZ
F8 - CZ
T8 - CZ
P8 - CZ
F3 - CZ
C3 - CZ
P3 - CZ
O1 - CZ
F4 - CZ
C4 - CZ
P4 - CZ
O2 - CZ
ECG

100 µV

1 s

▶ **Figure 3.126** **Spikes, left occipital.** Vertex reference derivation. The seizures of this 22-year-old female patient with juvenile myoclonic epilepsy increased after sleep deprivation and alcohol consumption. The spike in this EEG section shows a more or less symmetrical distribution at O1 and O2. The EEGs of patients with generalized epilepsies not infrequently show, in addition to generalized spikes, spike "fragments" with variable degrees of focality. In this example, biooccipital spikes have been recorded (blue arrow). Elsewhere in this EEG, she had generalized spikes. The EEG report refers to the entire EEG.

EEG classification: Abnormal III (awake)

Spikes, generalized and multifocal left and right hemisphere

EEG report: This EEG supports the diagnosis of a juvenile myoclonic epilepsy.

Polyspike–waves, generalized

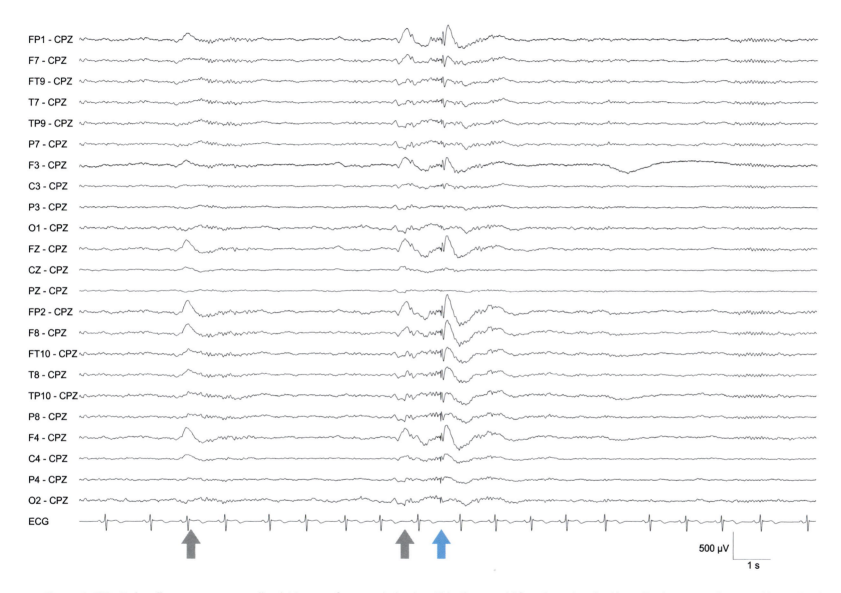

▶ **Figure 3.127   Polyspike–waves, generalized.** Vertex reference derivation. This 19-year-old female patient had juvenile absence epilepsy. With medication, generalized spikes only occurred during sleep. The distribution of the generalized polyspikes–waves (blue arrow) shifted between right and left frontal or frontopolar region. The K-complexes (gray arrows) have a similar potential field.

EEG classification: Abnormal III (Sleep)
    Polyspike–waves, generalized

EEG report: This EEG supports the diagnosis of juvenile absence epilepsy.

or eye muscles in combination with eye movement occasionally can be misjudged as an epileptiform discharge (▶ Figure 3.128). The muscle artifact in ▶ Figure 3.128 is at electrode FP2 and also much smaller at electrode F4. In the reformatting to the ear reference, the amplitude with regard to the background is reduced and, thus, it seems now limited to the right frontopolar electrode (▶ Figure 3.129). In ▶ Figure 3.129, the gain is much lower and, thus, relatively low-amplitude high frequencies are less well appreciated. The muscle spicule should be almost identical in size at FP2 and F4 if one increases the gain in the ear reference recording. This is an extreme example of a muscle spicule preceding eye opening.

3.4.2.4.2 Polyspikes (PSP) and Paroxysmal Fast (PF)

Groups of two or more consecutive spikes with a frequency of more than 10 Hz are called polyspikes (▶ Figure 3.130). They can be generalized or regional. The transition to paroxysmal fast is fluid. If polyspikes are followed by a slow wave that clearly exceeds the amplitude of the preceding spike, they are called polyspike–waves (▶ Figure 3.131; see Section 3.4.2.4.5). Patients with idiopathic generalized epilepsies who have generalized spikes in the wake state often show generalized polyspikes or polyspike–waves during sleep (▶ Figure 3.132).

Generalized polyspikes are typically found in juvenile myoclonic epilepsy (Janz & Christian, 1957) and in Lennox–Gastaut syndrome (Brenner & Atkinson, 1982; Gastaut et al., 1966). Patients with generalized epilepsies may also show some regional spikes in addition to generalized polyspikes (▶ Figure 3.133).

The transition to generalized low-amplitude paroxysmal activity and the so-called electrodecremental pattern is fluid, especially in patients with Lennox–Gastaut syndrome, in which the boundary between ictal and interictal EEG pattern is blurred (▶ Figure 3.134). At night during sleep, paroxysmal fast or electrodecremental EEG seizure patterns may occur as a subclinical manifestation or may be associated with generalized tonic seizures. Sometimes the clinical ictal character can only be recognized with the help of additional methods (e.g. the recording of respiration) because otherwise the apnea or irregular breathing during the generalized polyspikes may go unnoticed (▶ Figure 3.135) (Tezer et al., 2009).

Regional polyspikes are typical for patients with focal cortical dysplasia (▶ Figures 3.136 and 3.137) (Noachtar et al., 2008). It has been demonstrated that the frequencies of such epileptic discharges in invasive discharges can be very high (100–500 Hz; Urrestarazu et al., 2007). The use of filters can make the distinction between polyspikes and EMG artifacts more difficult or impossible (▶ Figures 3.138–3.140). A "ringing artifact" due to a notch filter may mimic high-frequency discharges in invasive recordings (▶ Figure 2.20 and Section 2.2.2.1) (Kirac et al., 2016). One must be very careful with the use of filters in these settings.

Polyspikes are classified as abnormal III because of their strong association with epilepsy. It is very likely that due to the phenomenon of "temporal summation," polyspikes are more epileptogenic than just spikes.

3.4.2.4.3 Benign Focal Epileptiform Discharges (BFED)

Benign focal epileptiform discharges occur most frequently in patients with benign focal epilepsy of childhood (▶ Figure 3.141) (Lüders et al., 1987). They typically occur in children aged 3–15 years in different brain regions, with the potentials in the central region being most common and leading some to use the term Rolando spikes for all these discharges regardless of their localization (Drury & Beydoun, 1991). However, more than one-third of the BFED have a localization outside the centrotemporal region (Drury & Beydoun, 1991). Younger children often have these spikes in the occipital region (▶ Figures 3.142 and 3.143), whereas older children have them in the central, temporal, and frontal region on one or both sides (▶ Figures 3.141 and 3.144) (Lüders et al., 1987). In addition, BFED also occur in midline derivations (PZ > CZ). The waveform of these potentials is very characteristic with a low-amplitude positive wave followed by a relatively high-amplitude negative spike. The main negative spike is then followed by a relatively large positive wave and finally a negative slow wave that almost never exceeds the amplitude of the preceding negative spike (▶ Figure 3.141). BFED often are generated in the anterior bank of the central sulcus, with scalp electrodes recording a dipole. BFED increase significantly in frequency during drowsiness or light sleep and then often occur in series. These discharges usually disappear spontaneously in adolescence. It is important to note also that approximately 2–4% of healthy children also have these discharges (Cavazzuti, 1980; Eeg-Olofsson et al., 1971). Only a very small proportion (8%) of children presenting BFED will have epileptic seizures (Blom et al., 1972; Lüders et al., 1987).

BFED are classified as abnormal III because of their association with benign focal epilepsy of childhood.

Muscle artifact

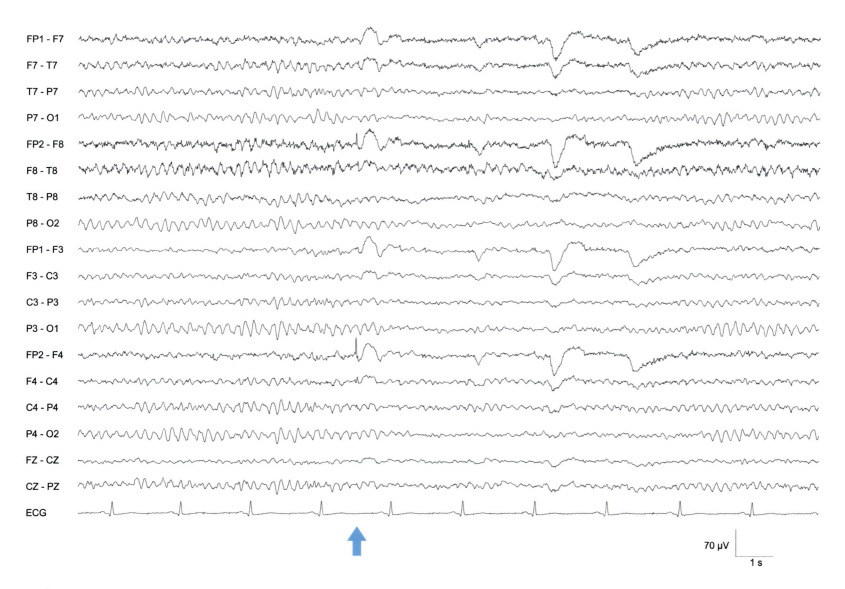

FP1 - F7
F7 - T7
T7 - P7
P7 - O1
FP2 - F8
F8 - T8
T8 - P8
P8 - O2
FP1 - F3
F3 - C3
C3 - P3
P3 - O1
FP2 - F4
F4 - C4
C4 - P4
P4 - O2
FZ - CZ
CZ - PZ
ECG

70 µV

1 s

▶ **Figure 3.128**   **Muscle artifact.** Bipolar longitudinal montage. The EEG of this 42-year-old patient with concentration deficits due to depression shows a muscle artifact in the FP2 electrode and with lower amplitude in the channels F8–T8 and F4–C4 immediately before eye opening (blue arrow). The shape of the spike and the following slow wave could be misjudged as an epileptiform discharge by "pattern recognition." Note the pulse artifact at electrode P8.

Muscle artifact

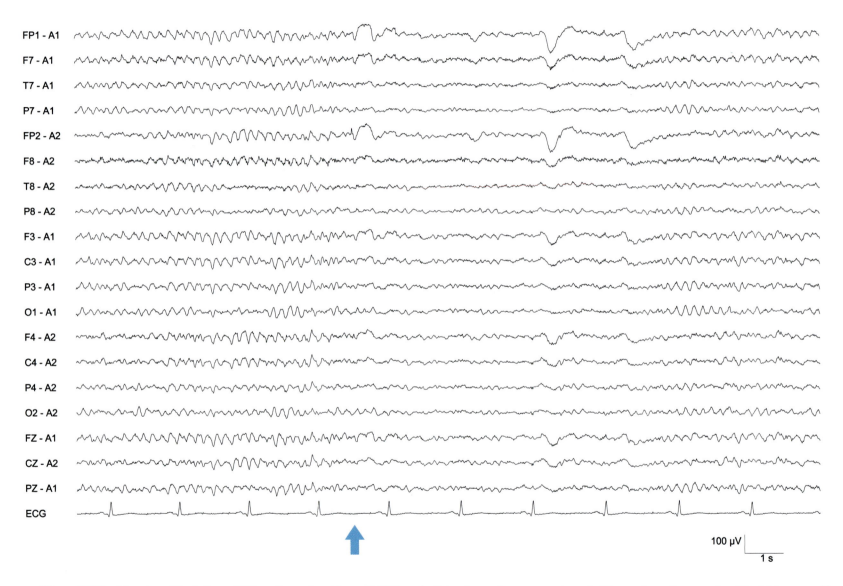

▶ **Figure 3.129** **Muscle artifact.** Same EEG section as in ▶ **Figure 3.128** in an ipsilateral ear reference montage. In this montage, the muscle artifact (blue arrow) is exclusively represented in the electrode FP2 because the sensitivity is reduced and the small deflections in the other channels, which are visualized in ▶ **Figure 3.128**, cannot be differentiated from the baseline activity. Such muscle artifacts are typically caused by forehead or eye muscles and must be differentiated from epileptiform discharges.

Paroxysmal fast, generalized. Ear reference derivation

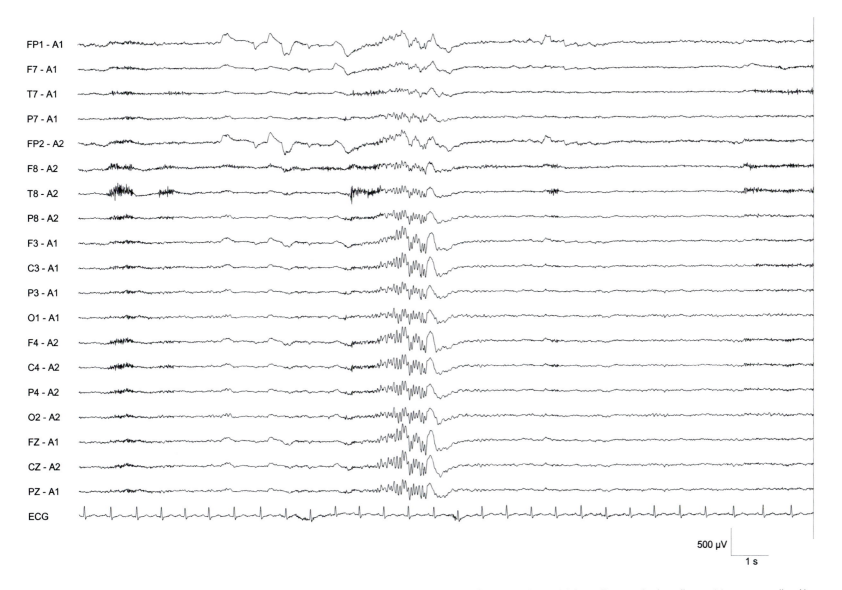

500 μV

1 s

▶ **Figure 3.130** **Paroxysmal fast, generalized.** Ear reference derivation. A 21-year-old female patient with juvenile myoclonic epilepsy. Many generalized bursts of paroxysmal fast were recorded when she was not taking medication. The occipital background rhythm is normal.

EEG classification: Abnormal III (awake)

Seizure: EEG seizure pattern, generalized (paroxysmal fast)
No clinical signs

EEG report: This EEG supports the diagnosis of juvenile myoclonic epilepsy.

Paroxysmal fast, generalized

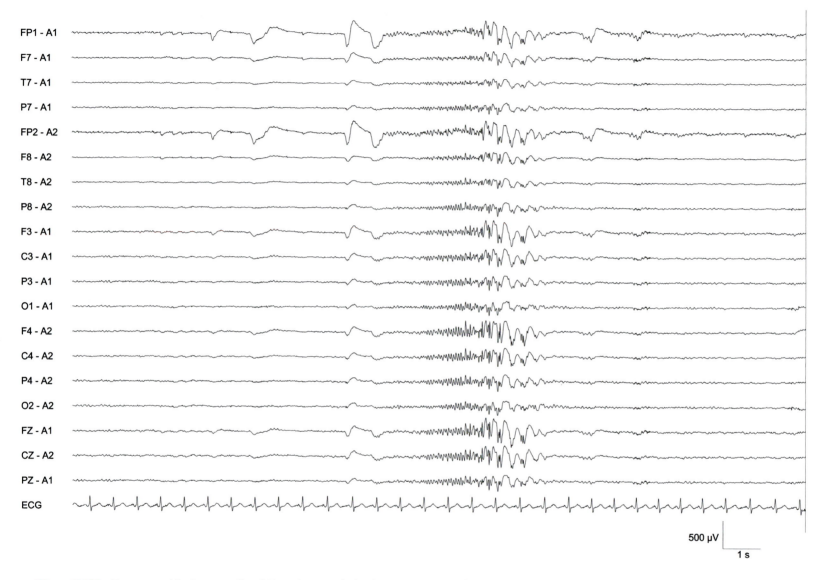

500 µV

1 s

▶ **Figure 3.131 Paroxysmal fast, generalized.** Ear reference derivation. A 29-year-old female patient with juvenile myoclonic epilepsy. During wakefulness, paroxysmal fast of increasing amplitude evolves into irregular polyspike–waves. The background occipital rhythm is normal.

EEG classification: Abnormal III (awake)

Seizure: EEG seizure pattern, generalized (paroxysmal fast)
No clinical signs

EEG report: This EEG supports the clinical diagnosis of juvenile myoclonic epilepsy. The patient's responsiveness was not tested during the generalized discharge.

Spikes during wakefulness, polyspikes during sleep

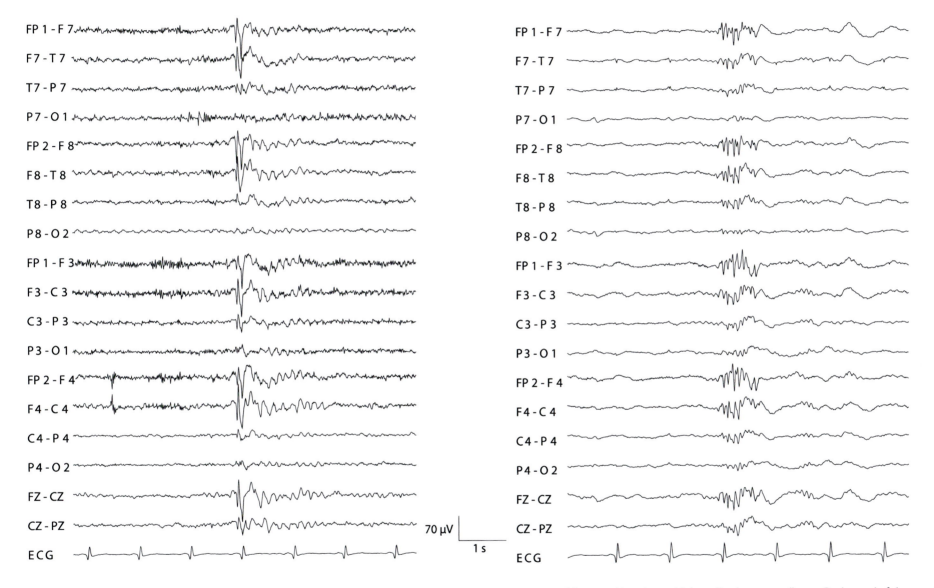

► **Figure 3.132** **Spikes during wakefulness, polyspikes during sleep.** Bipolar longitudinal montage. A 58-year-old patient with juvenile absence epilepsy. During wakefulness, single generalized spikes followed by a 1.5-s burst of generalized theta waves appeared. During sleep, generalized polyspikes prevailed. Notice that only the polyspikes are included in the EEG classification. This follows the EEG classification rule that only the most epileptogenic epileptiform discharge is included in the EEG classification when different types of epileptiform discharges of equal distribution are recorded.

EEG classification: Abnormal III (awake and sleep)
    Polyspikes, generalized

EEG report: This EEG supports the diagnosis of juvenile absence epilepsy.

Polyspikes, generalized; spikes right and left right temporal

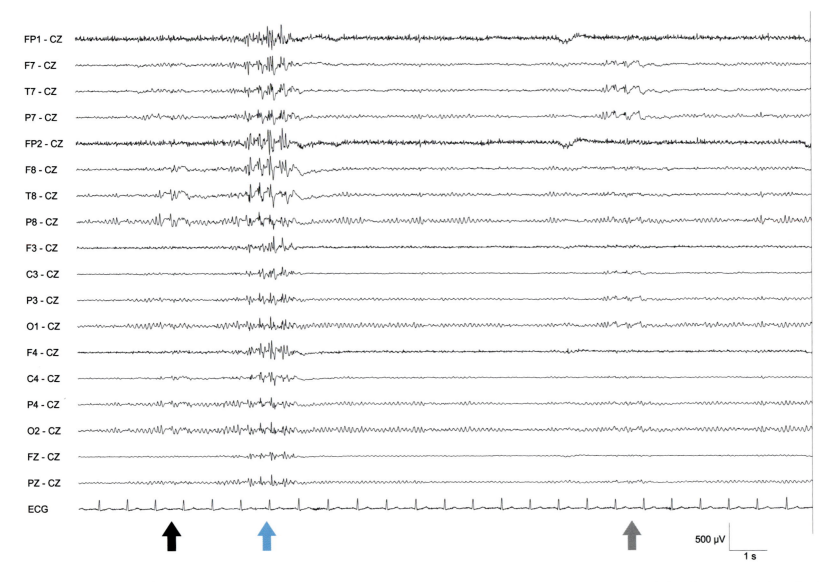

▶ **Figure 3.133** **Polyspikes, generalized; spikes right and left right temporal.** Vertex reference derivation. A 62-year-old female patient with juvenile absence epilepsy. In addition to frequent generalized polyspikes (blue arrow), there were also spikes in the right (black arrow) and left (grey arrow) temporal regions. The vertex reference CZ allows good display of the temporal spikes, but the generalized polyspikes show phase reversal. The generalized polyspikes would be better displayed without phase reversal in an ear reference. An ear reference, however, would be contaminated by temporal spikes.

EEG classification: Abnormal III (awake)
1. Polyspikes, generalized
2. Spikes, P8 > T8
3. Spikes T7 = P7

EEG report: This EEG supports the diagnosis of juvenile absence epilepsy.

Paroxysmal fast, generalized

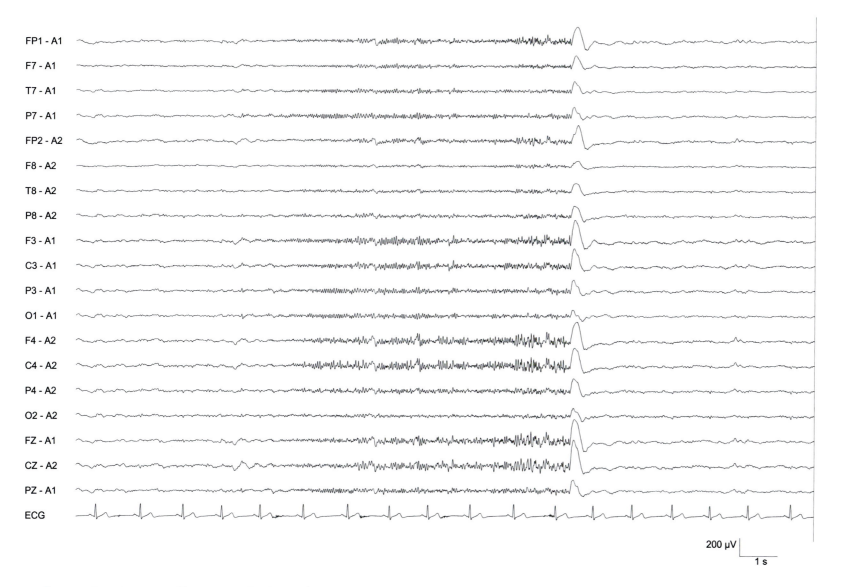

200 µV

1 s

▶ **Figure 3.134 Paroxysmal fast, generalized.** Ear reference derivation. This 19-year-old mentally challenged patient with Lennox–Gastaut syndrome had up to 8-s bursts of generalized paroxysmal fast activity, especially during sleep but also during wakefulness. In this case, the bursts of paroxysmal fast ended with a high-amplitude frontocentral slow wave. These bursts were not associated with any clinical signs. Long bursts of paroxysmal fast or electrodecremental episodes are frequently associated with tonic or atonic seizures.

EEG classification: Abnormal III (awake)

Seizure: EEG seizure pattern, generalized (paroxysmal fast)
No clinical signs

EEG report: This EEG supports the diagnosis of Lennox–Gastaut syndrome.

EEG seizure pattern, generalized; irregular breathing

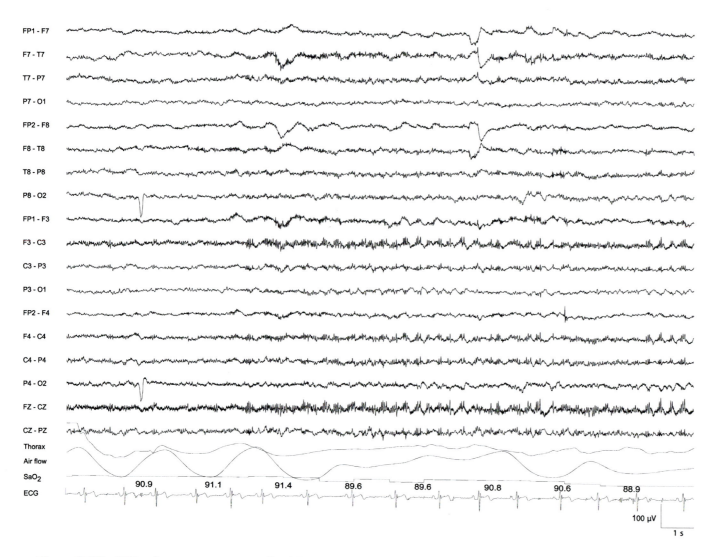

▶ **Figure 3.135** **EEG seizure pattern, generalized; irregular breathing.** Bipolar longitudinal montage. A 17-year-old mentally challenged patient with Lennox–Gastaut syndrome had a burst of paroxysmal fast activity lasting several seconds. These episodes of paroxysmal fast appeared to be asymptomatic. However, recording of nasal airflow, chest excursions, and percutaneous measurement of oxygen saturation showed that the episodes or paroxysmal fast activity were associated with hypopnea and mild oxygen desaturation. The hypopnea was probably triggered by a mild tonic seizure not visible because the patient was covered with a blanket.

EEG classification: Abnormal III (awake)
1. Seizure: EEG seizure pattern, generalized (paroxysmal fast)
   Tonic seizure
2. Background slow
3. Continuous slow, generalized

EEG report: This EEG documents a mild tonic seizure associated with irregular breathing during night sleep in a patient with Lennox–Gastaut syndrome.

Paroxysmal fast, left hemisphere

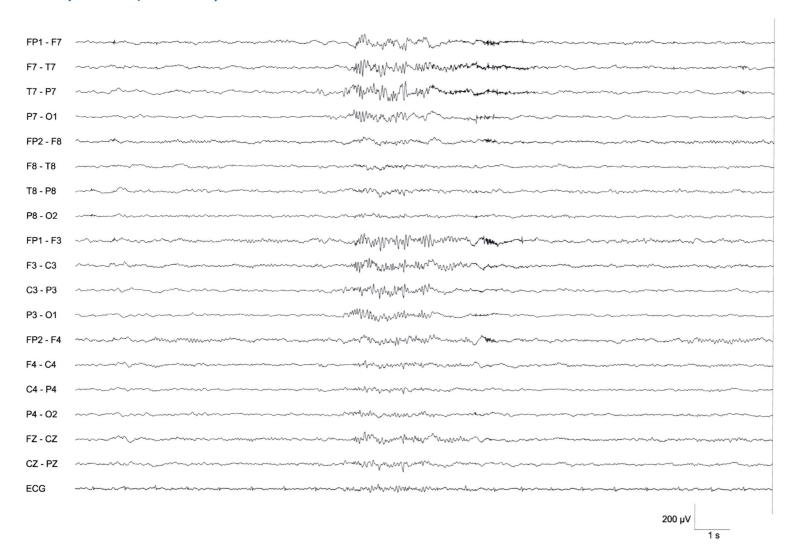

200 µV

1 s

▶ **Figure 3.136** **Paroxysmal fast, left hemisphere.** Bipolar longitudinal montage. A 28-year-old mentally challenged patient with bilateral multifocal epilepsy of unknown etiology. This EEG sample shows a 2-s burst of left hemisphere paroxysmal fast. In other parts of the EEG, there was an occipital background activity of 6 Hz, intermittent generalized slow, and multiregional spikes over both hemispheres. The EEG classification below and report refer to the entire EEG and not only the sample shown here.

EEG classification: Abnormal III (awake, sleep)
1. Seizure: EEG seizure pattern, left hemisphere (paroxysmal fast)
   No clinical signs
2. Spikes, bilateral multiregional
3. Background slow
4. Intermittent slow, generalized

EEG report: This EEG supports the diagnosis of a highly epileptogenic generalized epilepsy and moderate encephalopathy.

Paroxysmal fast, right frontal

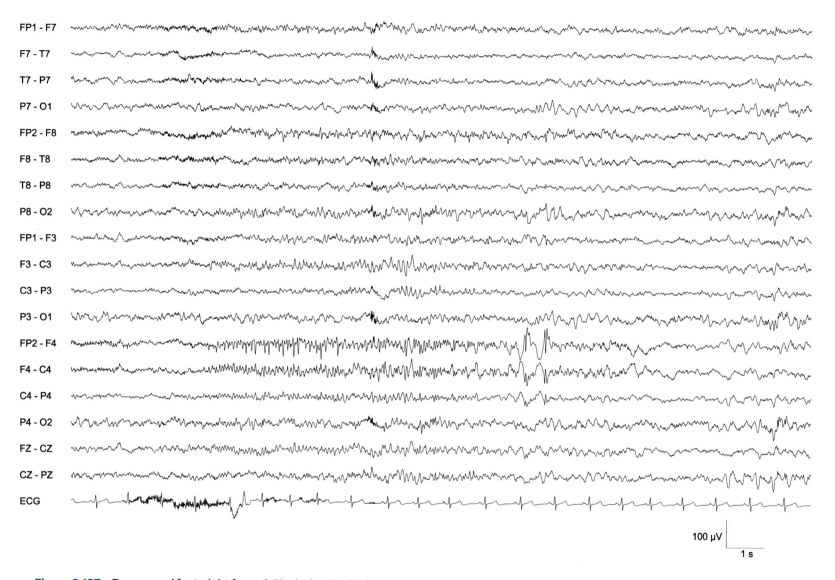

FP1 - F7

F7 - T7

T7 - P7

P7 - O1

FP2 - F8

F8 - T8

T8 - P8

P8 - O2

FP1 - F3

F3 - C3

C3 - P3

P3 - O1

FP2 - F4

F4 - C4

C4 - P4

P4 - O2

FZ - CZ

CZ - PZ

ECG

100 μV

1 s

▶ **Figure 3.137   Paroxysmal fast, right frontal.** Bipolar longitudinal montage. A 24-year-old female patient with right frontal lobe epilepsy due to focal cortical dysplasia. Frequent right frontal burst of paroxysmal fast occurred during wakefulness.

EEG classification: Abnormal III (awake)

Seizure: EEG seizure pattern, F4>C4>FP2
No clinical manifestation

EEG report: This EEG supports the diagnosis of a right frontal lobe epilepsy.

Polyspikes, left temporoparietal and EMG artifact

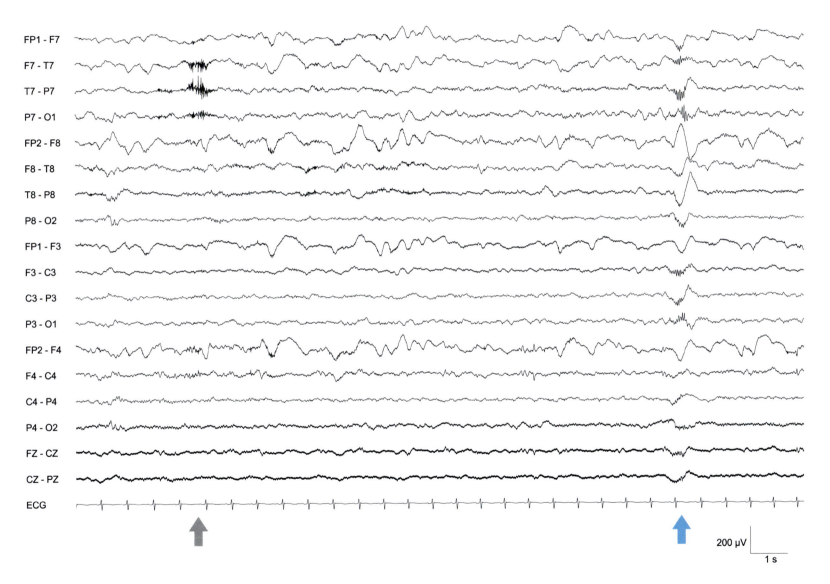

▶ **Figure 3.138** **Polyspikes, left temporoparietal and EMG artifact.** Bipolar longitudinal montage. An 11-year-old mentally challenged patient with bilateral cortical dysplasia. With 1–70 Hz filtering, the polyspikes (blue arrow) can be distinguished from the EMG artifact (gray arrow).

Polyspikes, left temporoparietal and EMG artifact; 30 Hz filter

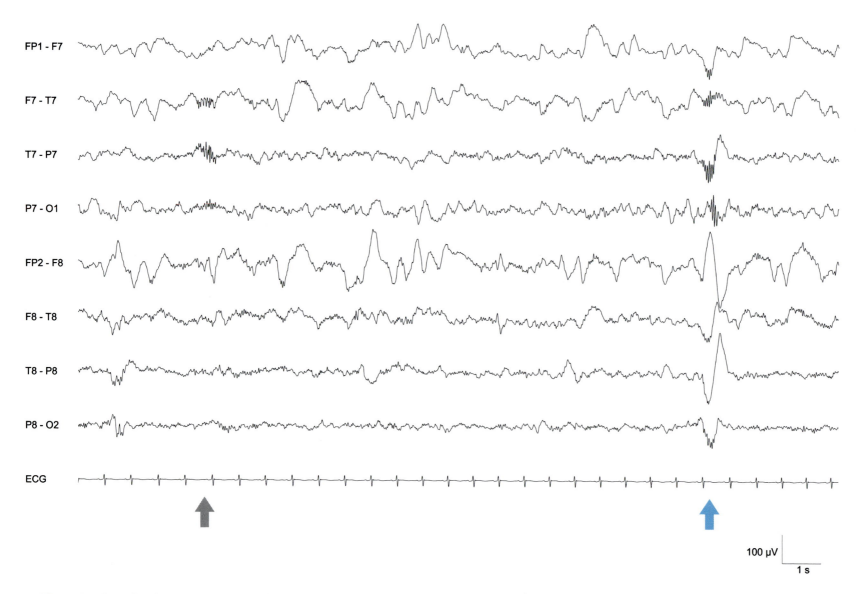

▶ **Figure 3.139** **Polyspikes, left temporoparietal and EMG artifact; 30 Hz filter.** Eight-channel EEG cutout (for better illustration) of the same EEG section as in ▶ **Figure 3.138** with 1–30 Hz filtering. The polyspikes (blue arrow) can hardly be distinguished from the high-frequency EMG artifact (gray arrow).

Polyspikes, left temporoparietal and EMG artifact; 15 Hz filter

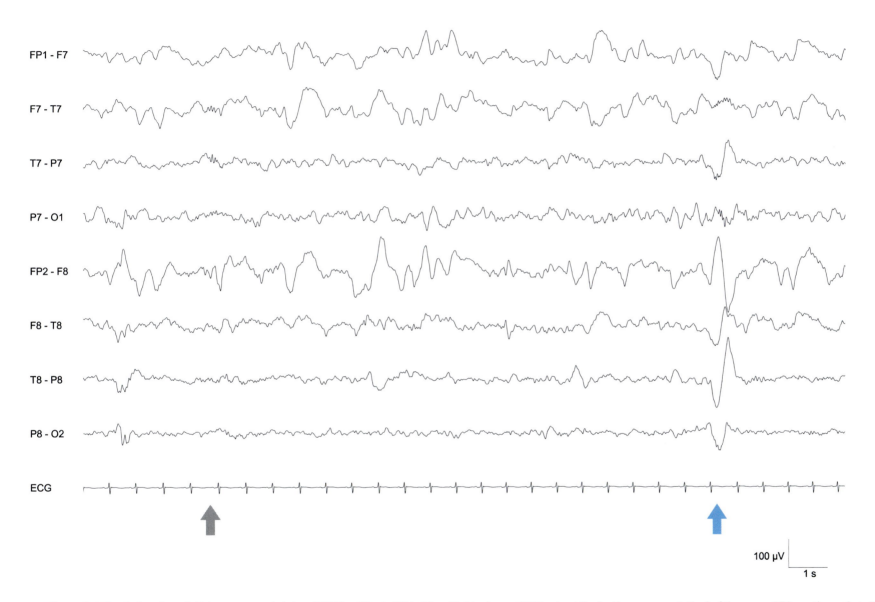

▶ **Figure 3.140**   **Polyspikes, left temporoparietal and EMG artifact; 15 Hz filter.** Eight-channel EEG cutout (for better representation) of the same EEG section as in ▶ **Figures 3.138** and 3.139 with 1–15 Hz filtering. The polyspikes (blue arrow) and the EMG artifact (gray arrow) are barely visible.

Benign focal epileptiform discharges, left temporocentral

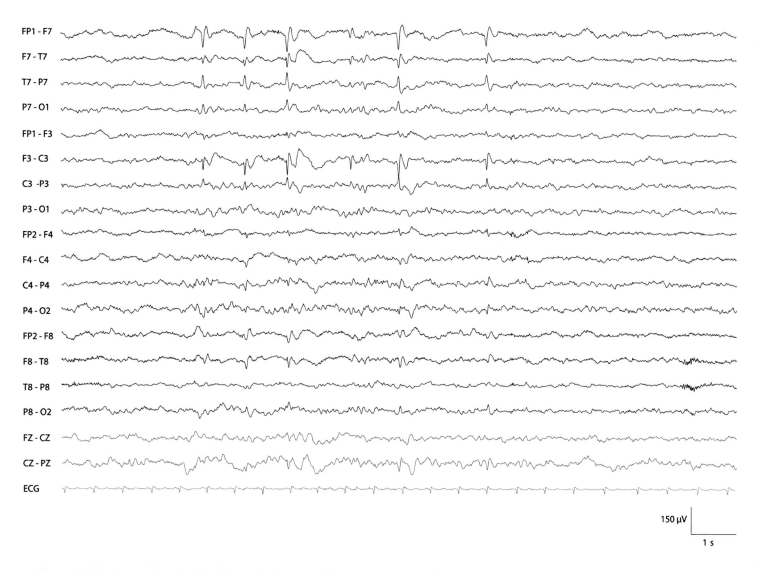

FP1 - F7
F7 - T7
T7 - P7
P7 - O1
FP1 - F3
F3 - C3
C3 - P3
P3 - O1
FP2 - F4
F4 - C4
C4 - P4
P4 - O2
FP2 - F8
F8 - T8
T8 - P8
P8 - O2
FZ - CZ
CZ - PZ
ECG

150 μV

1 s

▶ **Figure 3.141** **Benign focal epileptiform discharges, left temporocentral.** Bipolar longitudinal montage. A 12-year-old girl with rare nocturnal clonic seizures of the right face that evolved to generalized convulsive seizures.

The sharp waves seen in benign focal epilepsy of childhood have a typical waveform with a relatively large negative spike followed by a prominent positive slow wave and a small negative slow wave that usually does not exceed the initial spike.

In the parasagittal row, the spike is of relatively high amplitude in channel F3–C3 compared with all the other channels in that row. This is because the spike shows a large deflection when the row of electrodes crosses the dipole and F3 is close to the positive pole and C3 is close to the negative pole. This is different in the longitudinal temporal row of electrodes. Notice that here, the deflections at F7–T7 are similar to the deflections at T7–P7. This is the typical distribution of spikes generated at the crown of the sulcus, and there is a more or less symmetrical, exponential fall-off in all directions.

EEG classification: Abnormal III (sleep)
 Benign focal epileptiform discharges, T7 > F7

EEG report: This EEG supports the diagnosis of a benign focal epilepsy of childhood.

Benign focal epileptiform discharges, right occipital

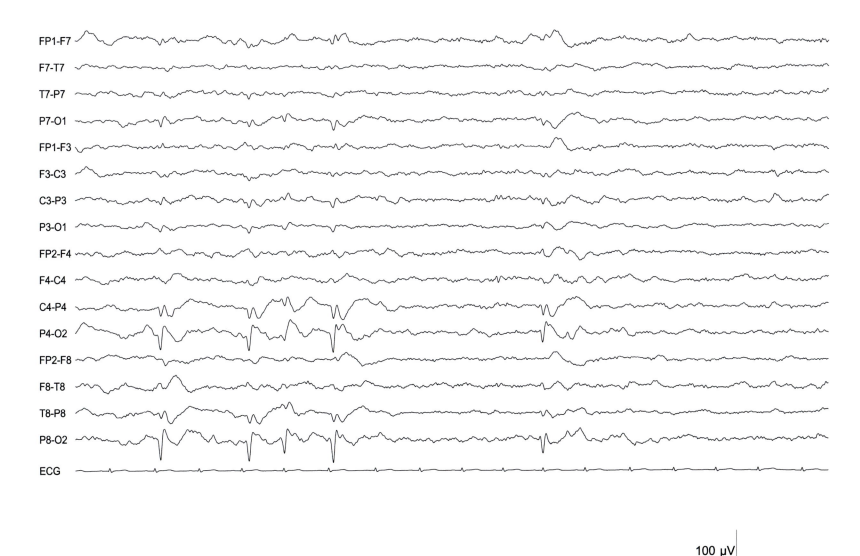

100 μV

1 s

▶ **Figure 3.142** **Benign focal epileptiform discharges, right occipital.** Bipolar longitudinal montage. A 6-year-old boy, so far with one nocturnal, generalized convulsive seizure. The EEG shows right occipital spikes during light sleep. This tracing also reveals a bipolar distribution with a maximum negativity at O2 and a maximum positivity at F4–C4. The relatively low amplitude of the positive pole and the higher amplitude of the negative pole probably indicate that the dipole vector is such that the negative pole points more to the cortical surface, whereas the positive pole points more to the brain middle.

EEG classification: Abnormal III (sleep)
   Benign focal epileptiform discharges, O2

EEG report: This EEG supports the diagnosis of a benign focal epilepsy of childhood.

Benign focal epileptiform discharges, right occipital

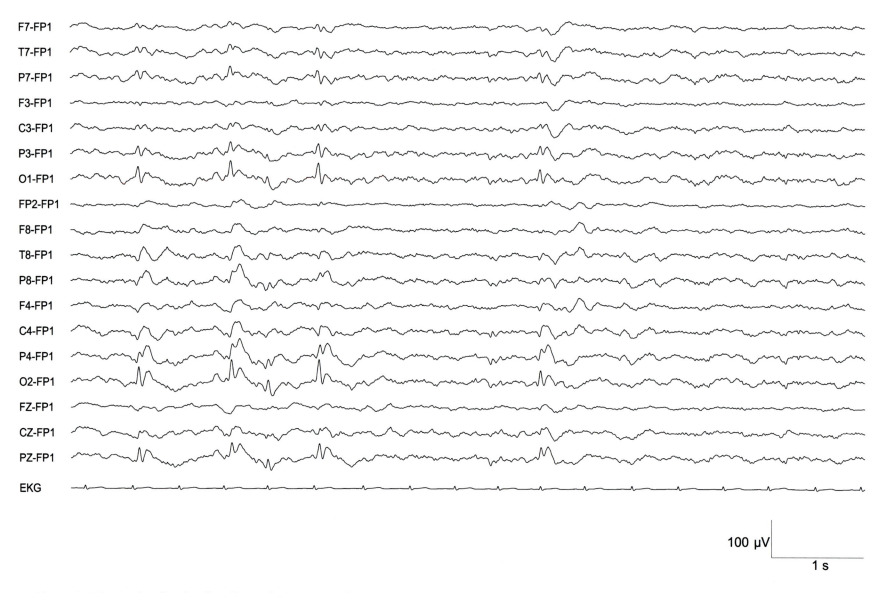

F7-FP1

T7-FP1

P7-FP1

F3-FP1

C3-FP1

P3-FP1

O1-FP1

FP2-FP1

F8-FP1

T8-FP1

P8-FP1

F4-FP1

C4-FP1

P4-FP1

O2-FP1

FZ-FP1

CZ-FP1

PZ-FP1

EKG

100 µV

1 s

▶ **Figure 3.143** **Benign focal epileptiform discharges, right occipital.** Same EEG section as in ▶ **Figure 3.142** in an FP1 reference. For EEG classification and report, see ▶ Figure 3.142.

Benign focal epileptiform discharges, right and left temporal

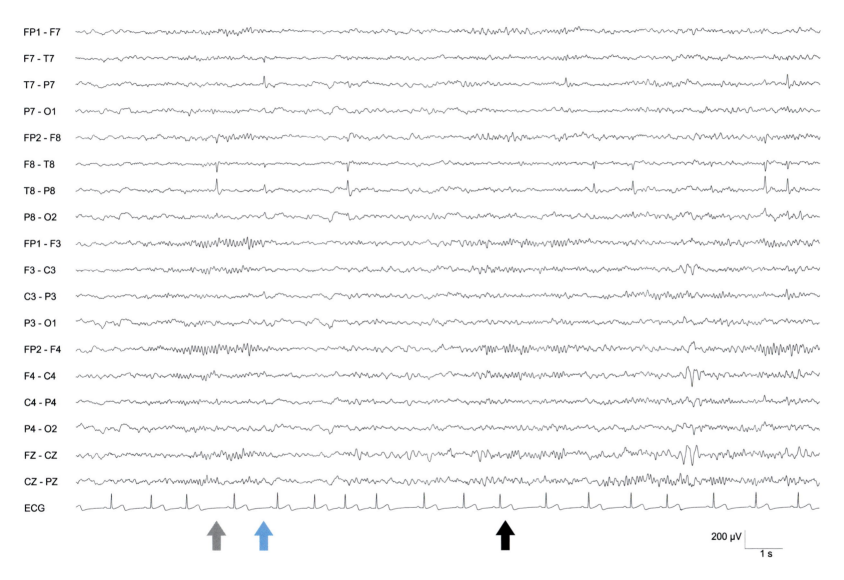

▶ **Figure 3.144** **Benign focal epileptiform discharges, right and left temporal.** Bipolar longitudinal montage. A 10-year-old boy with learning difficulties. No evidence of epilepsy. In sleep stage 2, characterized by sleep spindles (black arrow), spikes appear more in the right (gray arrow) than in the left (blue arrow) temporal region.

EEG classification: Abnormal III (sleep)
    Benign focal epileptiform discharges, T8 > F8 and T7 > F7

EEG report: This EEG shows benign focal epileptiform discharges (BFED), which are found in approximately 2% of healthy children. Only approximately 8% of patients with BFED have clinical seizures.

3.4.2.4.4 Spike–Waves (SW)

Spike–waves are repetitive, consecutive spikes followed by a relatively prominent slow wave (▶ **Figures 3.117** and **3.145**). They can be further subdivided into 3 Hz spike–waves or slow spike–waves (see below). By tradition, single-occurring spikes are not called spike–waves, even when the spike is followed by a prominent slow wave. Spike–waves often occur together with K-complexes (▶ **Figure 3.146**). The transition between interictal and ictal spike–wave patterns is fluid and depends on the duration of the discharge. Most patients are no longer able to respond promptly to external stimuli when bursts of 3 Hz spike–waves have a duration of more than 3 s (▶ **Figure 3.147**; see also ▶ **Figure 3.167**). However, some patients are already unable to respond adequately to external stimuli with spike–wave bursts of only 1- or 2-s duration (▶ **Figures 3.145** and **3.147**) (Rémi et al., 2011a). Some patients, for example, may only show a delayed response to the clicker (▶ **Figure 3.148**) (Rémi et al., 2011b). This implies that the neuronal networks involved in perception of the sound produced by the clicker are functioning normally but that the patient, for a short period of time, was unable to respond to the sound of the clicker. The ictal inability to initiate a movement is certainly not a "loss of consciousness" ("absence") but, rather, more appropriately an "akinetic seizure" (Rémi et al., 2011b). The duration of spike–waves is not the only factor that determines responsiveness. Some patients can react adequately despite discharges of 5 s or more (▶ **Figure 3.149**). Targeted reaction time measurements are required to make reliable statements on the ability to respond (Browne et al., 1974). This is particularly important when assessing driving ability.

Spike–waves are often generalized, with maximum amplitude shifting between the right and left frontal regions. However, there are also regional spike–waves—that is, spike–wave bursts consistently of higher amplitude in a specific brain localization rather than shifting (▶ **Figures 3.150** and 3.151).

3.4.2.4.5 Polyspike–Waves (PSW)

This EEG pattern is very similar to spike–waves, but the spike is replaced by two or more spikes followed by a prominent negative slow wave (▶ **Figure 3.131**). Generalized polyspike–waves, similar to generalized polyspikes (not followed by a slow wave), are typically found in juvenile myoclonic epilepsy (Janz & Christian, 1957) and in Lennox–Gastaut syndrome (Brenner & Atkinson, 1982; Gastaut et al., 1966).

Polyspikes are classified as abnormal III because of their strong association with epilepsy. In general, it is reasonable to assume that polyspikes or polyspike–waves are an expression of relatively stronger epileptogenicity than spikes or spike–waves.

3.4.2.4.6 3 Hz Spike–Waves (3SW)

This EEG pattern consists of bursts of 3 Hz spike–waves that have a duration of 3 s or more (▶ **Figures 3.117** and **3.147**). To increase the specificity of this EEG pattern, only bursts of 3 s or more are required to classify the EEG pattern as 3 Hz spike–waves. At the initial part of the burst of 3 Hz spike–waves, the repetition rate of the spike is slightly faster than 3 s. During the burst, the repetition rate of the spike–waves and also the amplitude of the spikes tend to decrease. Occasionally, the spike component of the burst of 3 Hz spike–waves disappears completely toward the end of the discharge (▶ **Figure 3.152**). The duration and the morphology of the spike–wave discharge do not permit prediction of the degree of cognitive impairment the patient is going to have during the burst of 3 Hz spike–waves. The example in ▶ **Figure 3.152** shows that during the first 4 s of the generalized spike–wave, the patient is able to push a button, but not afterwards, whereas in Figure 3.147 no response is available in the first second of the discharge.

The 3 Hz spike–wave is the classic EEG pattern seen in patients with childhood absence epilepsy (Gibbs et al., 1935). With increasing age, generalized spike–wave complexes typically become more irregular in patients with idiopathic generalized epilepsy (▶ **Figure 3.153**). The EEG of these patients during sleep frequently shows bursts of generalized polyspikes (▶ **Figure 3.132**).

The 3 Hz spike–waves are classified as abnormal III because of their strong association with generalized epilepsy, particularly childhood absence epilepsy.

3.4.2.4.7 Slow Spike–Waves (SSW)

Bursts of generalized spike–waves with a repetition frequency below 2.5 Hz are typical for patients with Lennox–Gastaut syndrome (▶ **Figure 3.154**). Bursts of more than 3-s duration of slow spike–waves are required to diagnose slow spike–wave. The duration and the morphology of the bursts of slow spike–wave do not permit prediction of the degree of cognitive impairment these patients suffer during the occurrence of the burst of slow spike–waves (▶ **Figures 3.155** and **3.156**) (Holmes et al., 1987). Lennox–Gastaut patients almost always, in addition to the slow spike–waves, show background slow. This is related to

Spike–waves, generalized; akinetic seizure

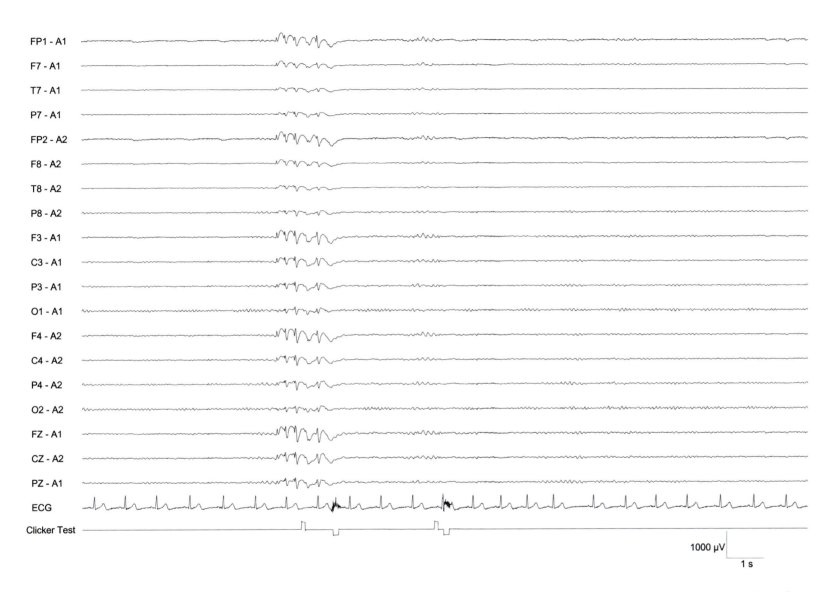

▶ **Figure 3.145** **Spike–waves, generalized; akinetic seizure.** Ear reference derivation. A 34-year-old female patient with juvenile absence epilepsy. One-second burst of spike–waves of 2 or 3 Hz. The burst interrupts the alpha background activity, which, however, returns as soon as the burst is finished. Note that the reaction time to an acoustic stimulus during the spike–waves is delayed compared to the response a few seconds later (short akinetic seizure). Such delays in reaction time are of clinical significance regarding driving restrictions. Notice that the patient responds as soon as the burst of spike–waves is completed. This suggests that the delayed response is not only a slowing of response time but also possibly a complete akinesia that lasts as the epileptiform discharge continues. Note the artifact in the ECG due to the movement to push a button in the clicker test.

EEG classification: Abnormal III (awake)

Seizure: EEG seizure pattern, generalized
Akinetic seizure

EEG report: This EEG supports the diagnosis of a juvenile absence epilepsy. It also documents the occurrence of akinetic seizures triggered by bursts of spike–waves.

Spike–waves, generalized

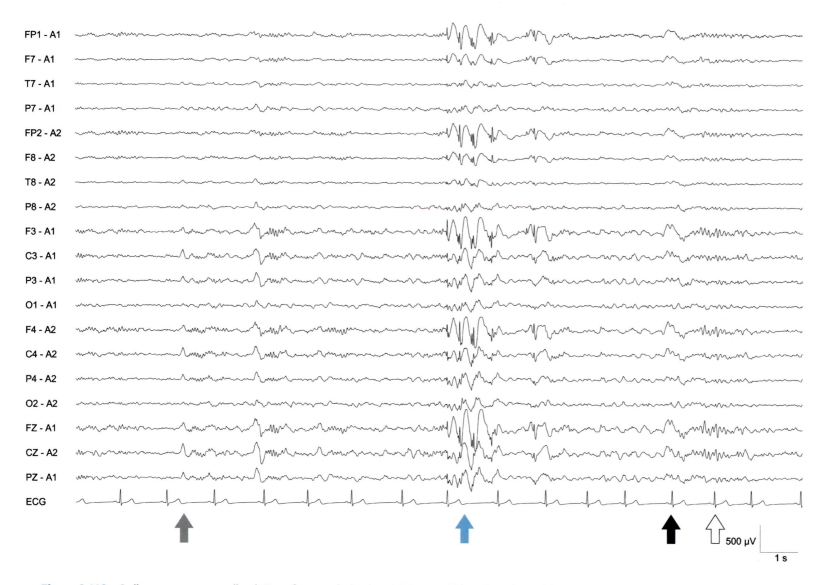

▶ **Figure 3.146** **Spike–waves, generalized.** Ear reference derivation. A 27-year-old female patient with grand mal epilepsy in whom generalized spike–waves (blue arrow) could only be recorded during sleep. The EEG sample shows vertex waves (gray arrow), K-complexes (black arrow), and sleep spindles (open arrow) typical of sleep stage 2.

EEG classification: Abnormal III (sleep)

    Spike–waves, generalized

EEG report: This EEG supports the diagnosis of generalized epilepsy.

Spike–waves, generalized; dialeptic seizure

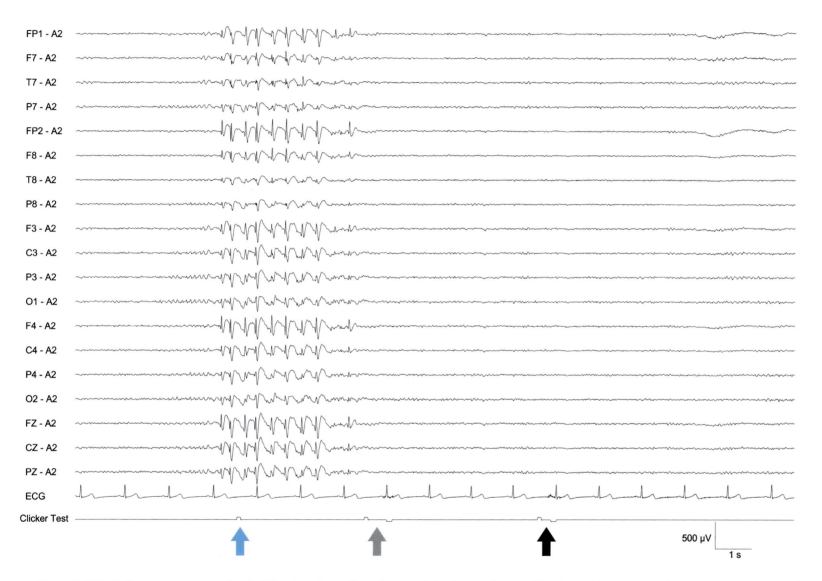

▶ **Figure 3.147** **Spike–waves, generalized; dialeptic seizure.** Ear reference derivation. A 42-year-old patient with absence epilepsy. During a 3-s burst of generalized spike–waves, the patient is not able to press a button (clicker test) in response to an acoustic stimulus (blue arrow). After the spike–waves, the reaction time is still somewhat delayed (gray arrow) compared to the reaction a few seconds later (black arrow). No test word was given during the discharge.

EEG classification: Abnormal III (awake)

Seizure: EEG seizure pattern, generalized (3 Hz spike-wave)
Dialeptic seizure

EEG report: This EEG documents a dialeptic seizure in a patient with absence epilepsy.

Spike–waves, generalized; akinetic seizure

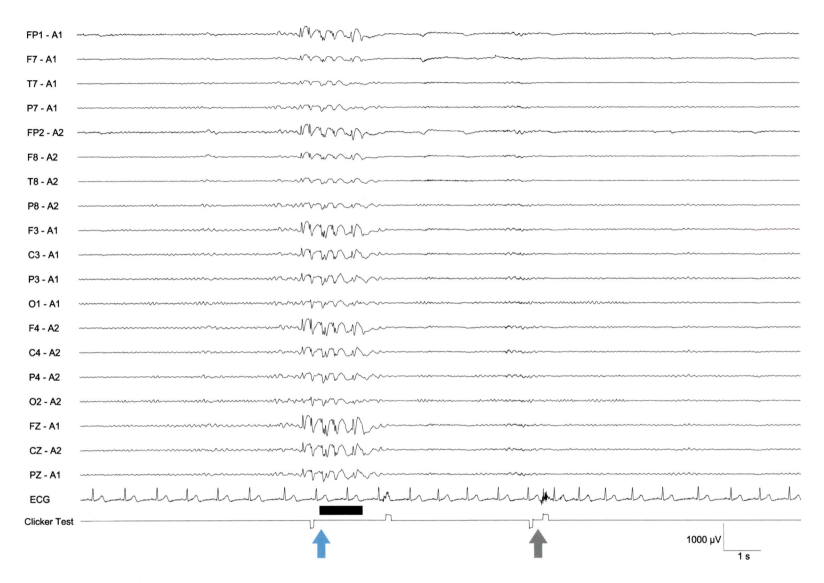

▶ **Figure 3.148** **Spike–waves, generalized; akinetic seizure.** Ear reference derivation. A 22-year-old female patient with absence epilepsy. During a 1.5-s burst of generalized spike–waves, the patient is unable to press a button (clicker test) in response to an acoustic stimulus (blue arrow). A few seconds after the spike–waves, she can react in time (gray arrow). She could, however, remember the test word given to her during the spike–waves (horizontal black bar). A review of the video obtained during the testing revealed that indeed the word was given to the patient immediately after the beginning of the epileptiform discharge and before the discharge had finished (horizontal black bar). The fact that the patient remembered a word (indicating that she was not dialeptic) but was unable to push the clicker documents that she was suffering from a pure akinetic seizure (Rémi et al., 2011b).

EEG classification: Abnormal III (awake)

Seizure: EEG seizure pattern, generalized (3 Hz spike–wave)
Akinetic Seizure

EEG report: This EEG documents an akinetic seizure in a patient with absence epilepsy.

3 Hz spike–waves, generalized

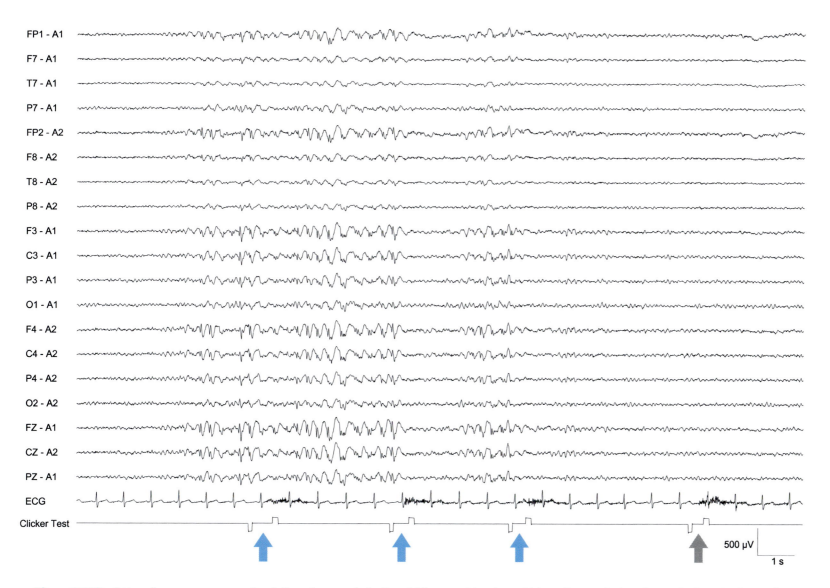

▶ **Figure 3.149**   **3 Hz spike–waves, generalized.** Ear reference derivation. A 68-year-old patient with juvenile myoclonic epilepsy. During a 5-s burst of generalized 3 Hz spike–waves, the patient can press a button in response to an acoustic stimulus (blue arrows) with only a slightly delayed reaction time (clicker test). The gray arrow marks the response when no spike–waves are recorded.

EEG classification: Abnormal III (awake)

    3 Hz spike–waves, generalized

EEG report: This EEG supports the clinical diagnosis of juvenile myoclonic epilepsy.

Spike–waves, right frontal

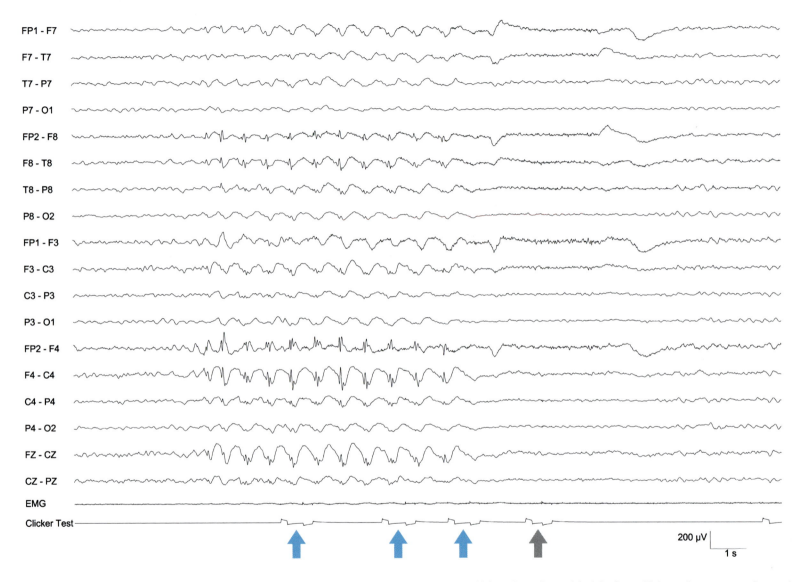

FP1 - F7

F7 - T7

T7 - P7

P7 - O1

FP2 - F8

F8 - T8

T8 - P8

P8 - O2

FP1 - F3

F3 - C3

C3 - P3

P3 - O1

FP2 - F4

F4 - C4

C4 - P4

P4 - O2

FZ - CZ

CZ - PZ

EMG

Clicker Test

200 µV

1 s

▶ **Figure 3.150** **Spike–waves, right frontal.** Bipolar longitudinal montage. A 19-year-old female patient with right frontal lobe epilepsy secondary to bacterial meningitis. During a 7-s burst of right frontal spike–waves, the patient can press a button (blue arrows) in response to acoustic stimuli with only a slightly delayed reaction time (clicker test). The gray arrow marks the response without spike–waves.

EEG classification: Abnormal III (awake)

Spike–waves, F4 > FP2

EEG report: This EEG supports the diagnosis of a right frontal lobe epilepsy.

Spike–waves, left occipital and continuous slow left temporal

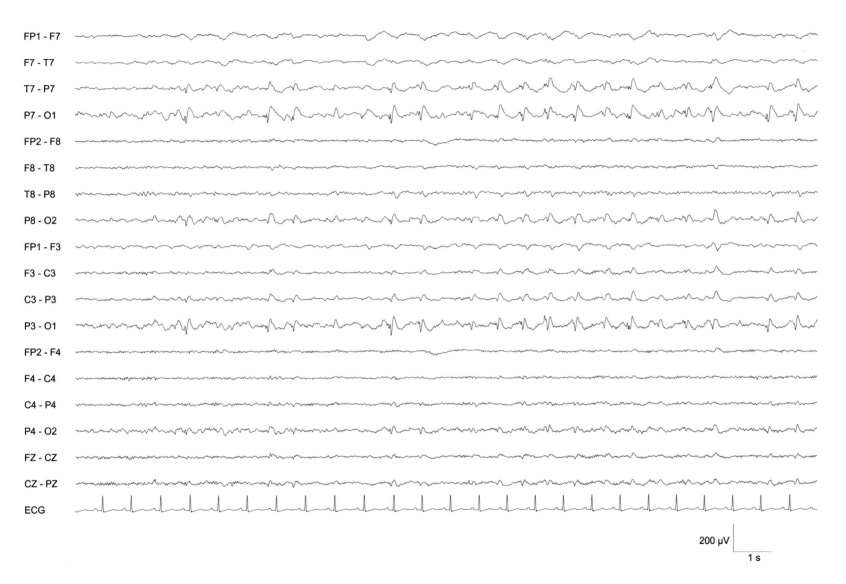

FP1 - F7
F7 - T7
T7 - P7
P7 - O1
FP2 - F8
F8 - T8
T8 - P8
P8 - O2
FP1 - F3
F3 - C3
C3 - P3
P3 - O1
FP2 - F4
F4 - C4
C4 - P4
P4 - O2
FZ - CZ
CZ - PZ
ECG

200 µV

1 s

▶ **Figure 3.151** **Spike–waves, left occipital and continuous slow left temporal.** Bipolar longitudinal montage. A 26-year-old female patient with left Rasmussen's encephalitis. Notice that the main slowing is in the left temporal leads, whereas the epileptiform discharges are very localized to O1.

EEG classification: Abnormal III (awake)
1. Spike–waves, O1 > O2
2. Continuous slow, left temporal

EEG report: This EEG supports the diagnosis of a left hemisphere Rasmussen's encephalitis with a highly epileptogenic left occipital lesion.

3 Hz spike–waves, generalized; dialeptic seizure

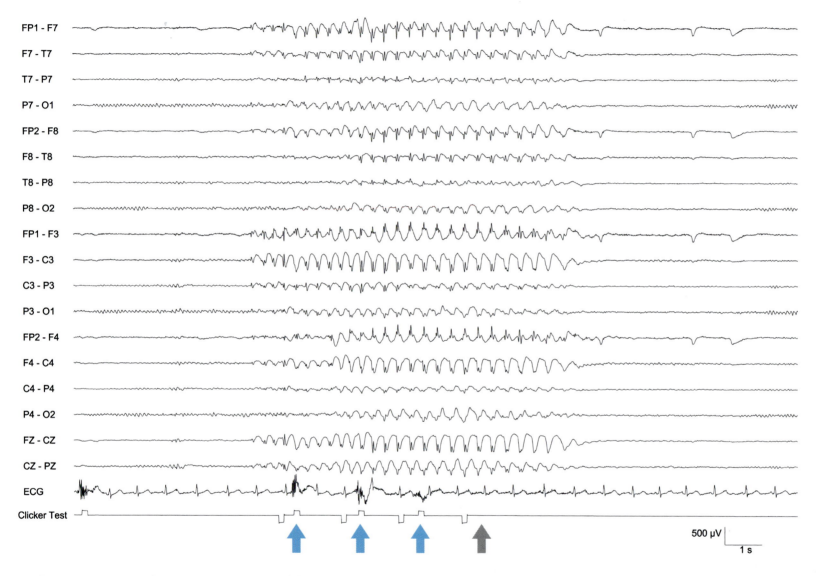

▶ **Figure 3.152** **3 Hz spike–waves, generalized; dialeptic seizure.** Bipolar longitudinal montage. A 31-year-old female patient with juvenile absence epilepsy. In the initial part of the burst of 3 Hz spike–waves, the patient is able to press a button (blue arrows) in response to acoustic stimuli (clicker test). However, during the latter part of the discharge, she becomes unresponsive (gray arrow). Toward the end of the burst of spike–waves, the amplitudes of the spikes, but not of the slow waves, become lower.

EEG classification: Abnormal III (awake)

Seizure: EEG seizure pattern, generalized (3 Hz spike–waves)
Dialeptic seizure

EEG report: This EEG supports the diagnosis of a juvenile absence epilepsy.

Spike–waves, generalized

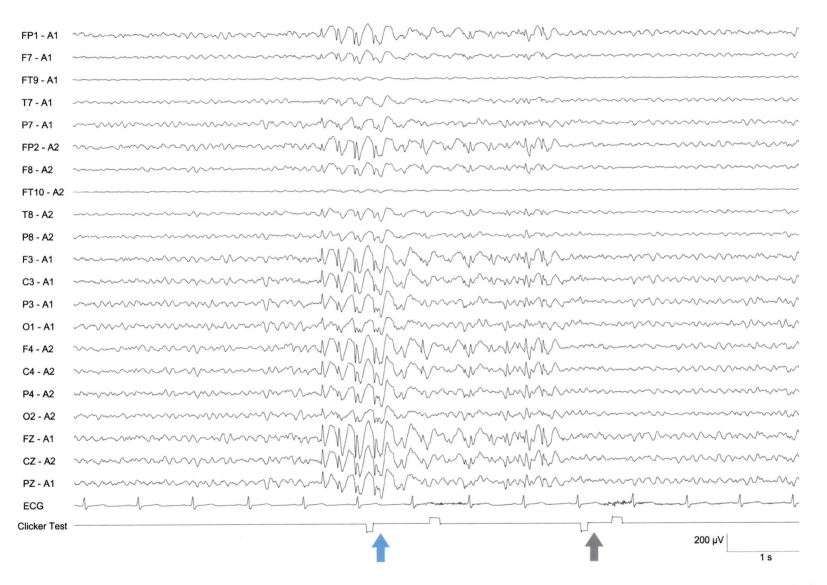

▶ **Figure 3.153** **Spike–waves, generalized.** Ear reference derivation. A 68-year-old patient with juvenile absence epilepsy. The patient's reaction to the first acoustic stimulus (blue arrow) occurring during the burst of generalized spike–waves (clicker test) is markedly delayed. After the burst of spike–waves is over, he responds promptly to the clicker (gray arrow). No test word was given during the discharge. The spike–waves are more regular at the beginning of the burst compared with the spike–waves in the later part of the burst.

EEG classification: Abnormal III (awake)

Seizure: EEG seizure pattern, generalized (3 Hz spike–wave)
Akinetic seizure

EEG report: This EEG documents an akinetic seizure in a patient with juvenile absence epilepsy.

Slow spike–waves, generalized

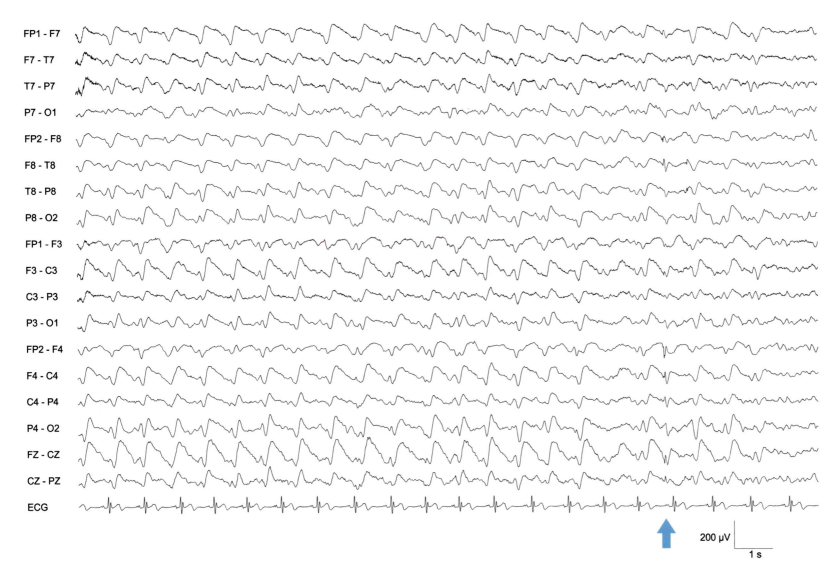

▶ **Figure 3.154** **Slow spike–waves, generalized.** Bipolar longitudinal montage. This mentally severely challenged 27-year-old patient with Lennox–Gastaut syndrome had frequent dialeptic, automotor, and bilateral tonic seizures despite high doses of several anti-seizure drugs. This EEG shows monomorphic slow spike–waves with a repetition rate of 1.3 Hz. Note a right frontal spike (blue arrow) in the later part of this EEG sample. In other EEG samples, not shown here, multiregional spikes in both hemispheres were also observed. In addition, the background occipital rhythm was slowed to 6 Hz (not shown in this EEG sample). The EEG classification below refers to the entire EEG.

EEG classification: Abnormal III (awake)
1. Slow spike–waves, generalized
2. Spikes, bilateral multiregional
3. Background slow

EEG report: This EEG supports the diagnosis of a Lennox–Gastaut syndrome.

the fact that patients with Lennox–Gastaut syndrome by definition also have intellectual disability. In addition, during sleep, patients with Lennox–Gastaut syndrome also have bursts of generalized polyspikes or polyspike–waves or 3- to 10-s runs of almost complete absence of brain activity ("electrodecremental" episodes). These electrodecremental episodes are frequently associated with generalized tonic seizure. Occasionally, bursts of slow spike–waves occur despite a normal background activity (▶ Figure 3.156). Such a combination suggests that the patient does not have Lennox–Gastaut syndrome. It is also important to remember that sometimes, complete abolishment of slow spike–waves may not be associated with a simultaneous improvement of cognitive function. This may be because the slow spike–waves are not producing any clinically significant change of mental functioning. Sometimes, however, days after abolishing the slow spike–wave status, there may be a major improvement of cognitive function. This delayed improvement is likely due to the fact that the cortex was exhausted and, therefore, a Todd's equivalent phenomenon persisted immediately after stopping the EEG status.

3.4.2.4.8 Hypsarrhythmia (HYP)

The typical EEG of West syndrome is called hypsarrhythmia (Gibbs & Gibbs, 1952). It occurs in the first year of life and consists of generalized, high-amplitude, irregular delta and theta activity (>300 μV) with multiregional bilateral and rarely generalized spikes (▶ Figure 3.157). During sleep, a pattern of burst attenuation may occur (▶ Figure 3.158). During infantile spasms, the EEG usually flattens, giving rise to the "electrodecremental" EEG seizure pattern (▶ Figure 3.159). (The common spelling used here is linguistically not correct: hypsarhythmia would be correct.)

▶ Table 3.10 summarizes several epileptic EEG patterns and their association with certain epilepsy syndromes.

3.4.2.4.9 Photoparoxysmal Response (PR)

Photoparoxysmal response refers to the triggering of epileptiform discharges by PS. This was discovered very early in the development of the EEG (Walter et al., 1946). Photoparoxysmal responses can occur regionally—mostly in the posterior brain regions (▶ Figure 3.12)—or have a generalized distribution (▶ Figures 3.13, 3.14, 3.160 and 3.161). Photic driving—that is, synchronization of the occipital background rhythm with the stimulation frequency—must be distinguished from the photoparoxysmal response as a normal response to PS (▶ Figures 3.162 and 3.163). It may have a different localization in connatal amaurosis (▶ Figure 3.164).

PS-induced occipital spikes are not considered abnormal if they are stimulus bound—that is, synchronous to the stimulus (▶ Figure 3.165). The only exceptions are "giant photic evoked responses," which are an index of slightly elevated epileptogenesis (abnormal I). These "giant" spike–wave complexes are actually spikes triggered by the photic stimulus.

Generalized photoparoxysmal responses are considered a typical EEG findings of generalized epilepsies (Jayakar & Chiappa, 1990; Newmark & Penry, 1979). The stimulation frequency at which epileptiform discharges are usually triggered by PS is approximately 15 Hz in adolescents and adults and somewhat lower at 10 Hz in children. However, such discharges can rarely (0.3%) also be found in patients who do not suffer from epileptic seizures (Gregory et al., 1993). Photoparoxysmal responses, surprisingly, are rarely found in patients with occipital epilepsy. Photoparoxysmal responses that outlast the end of PS have been described as particularly typical for epilepsy (▶ Figure 3.166) (Reilly & Peters, 1973), but this has not gone unchallenged (Jayakar & Chiappa, 1990). Patients with neonatal amaurosis show photoparoxysmal responses maximum in superior frontal electrodes (▶ Figure 3.164). The duration of PS probably also plays a role in the duration of the photoparoxysmal response.

The degree of EEG abnormality of EEGs with photoparoxysmal responses is classified as follows: Posterior dominant, non-time-locked photoparoxysmal responses (▶ Figure 3.12) and also time-locked giant occipital evoked responses are assessed as abnormal I (▶ Figure 3.165). Generalized, photoparoxysmal discharges (whether time-correlated or not) are assessed as abnormal II (▶ Figures 3.160 and 3.161). Self-sustaining photoparoxysmal discharges (i.e., those that persist after the end of stimulation) are classified as abnormal III (▶ Figure 3.166).

3.4.2.4.10 Seizure Patterns (SEP)

The recording of seizures with EEG—usually simultaneously with video—typically only succeeds in long-term recordings; due to the short recording time in routine EEG, it is an exception to record seizures. In outpatients, a postictal recording is more often performed. Postictally, patients are frequently obtunded and confused (Rémi & Noachtar, 2010), and the EEG shows regional or generalized slow. The localization of the focal slow is closely related to

Slow spike–waves generalized

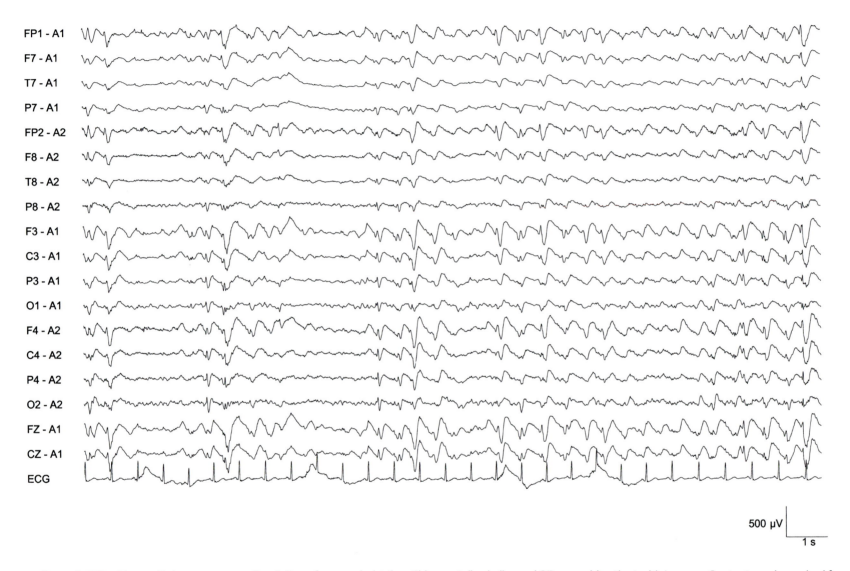

500 µV

1 s

▶ **Figure 3.155** **Slow spike–waves generalized.** Ear reference derivation. This mentally challenged 25-year-old patient with Lennox–Gastaut syndrome had frequent dialeptic, myo-clonic, and bilateral tonic seizures. This EEG shows monomorphic slow spike–waves with a repetition rate of 2 Hz. The background occipital rhythm was 7 Hz.

EEG classification: Abnormal III (awake)
1. Slow spike–waves, generalized
2. Background slow

EEG report: This EEG supports the diagnosis of a Lennox–Gastaut syndrome.

Slow spike–waves, generalized and continuous slow, bilateral frontal

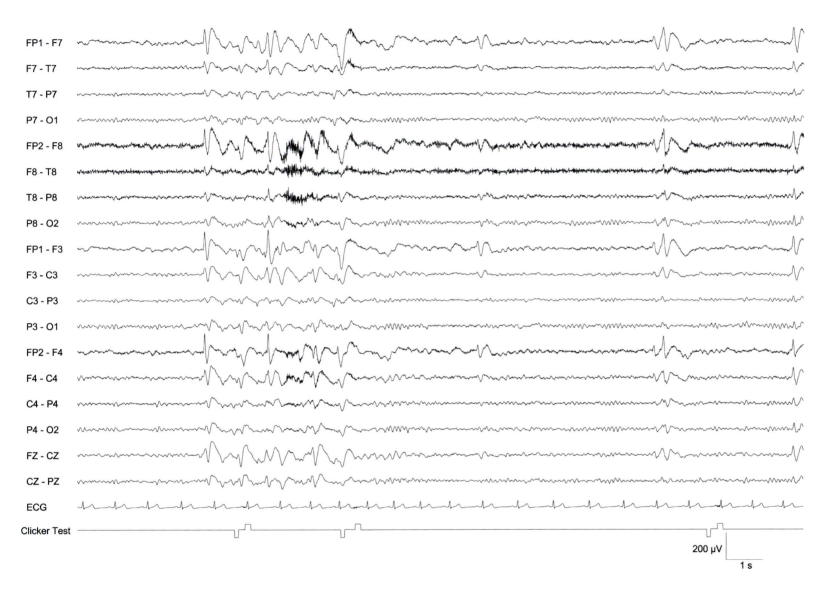

▶ **Figure 3.156** **Slow spike–waves, generalized and continuous slow, bilateral frontal.** Bipolar longitudinal montage. This 24-year-old patient with frontal lobe epilepsy due to bifrontal cortical dysplasias shows generalized slow spike–waves with a repetition rate of 2 Hz. Note the normal occipital rhythm, bifrontal slow, and normal responsiveness during generalized slow spike–waves.

EEG classification: Abnormal III (awake)
1. Slow spike–waves, generalized
2. Continuous slow, bilateral frontal

EEG report: This EEG supports the diagnosis of bilateral frontal lobe epilepsy.

Hypsarrhythmia

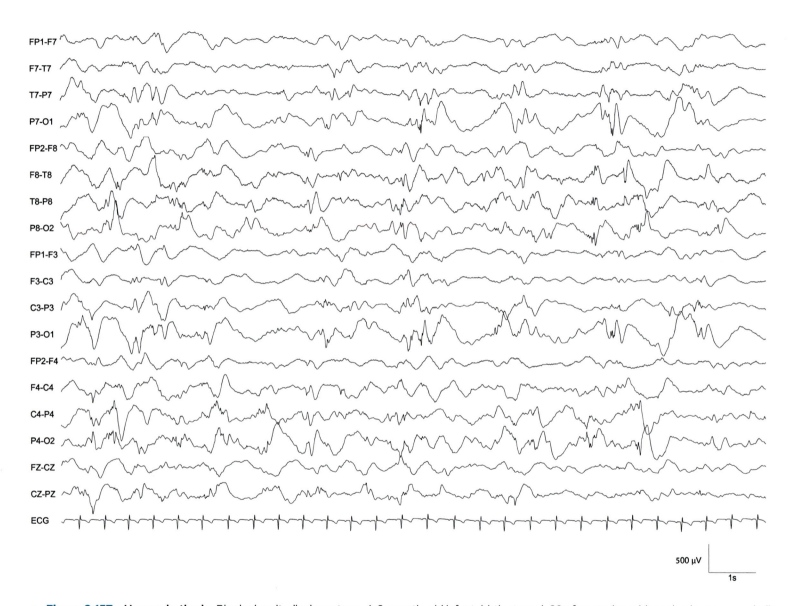

FP1-F7
F7-T7
T7-P7
P7-O1
FP2-F8
F8-T8
T8-P8
P8-O2
FP1-F3
F3-C3
C3-P3
P3-O1
FP2-F4
F4-C4
C4-P4
P4-O2
FZ-CZ
CZ-PZ
ECG

500 μV

1s

▶ **Figure 3.157** **Hypsarrhythmia.** Bipolar longitudinal montage. A 9-month-old infant; birth at week 29 of gestation with asphyxia, porencephalic cysts, and cerebral palsy. There is a generalized, high–amplitude slow delta activity of more than 300 μV with frequent bilateral multiregional spikes (maxima at electrodes P4, O1, T8, P8, and PZ).

EEG classification: Abnormal III (awake)

   Hypsarrhythmia, generalized

EEG report: This EEG supports the diagnosis of West syndrome.

Hypsarrhythmia during sleep

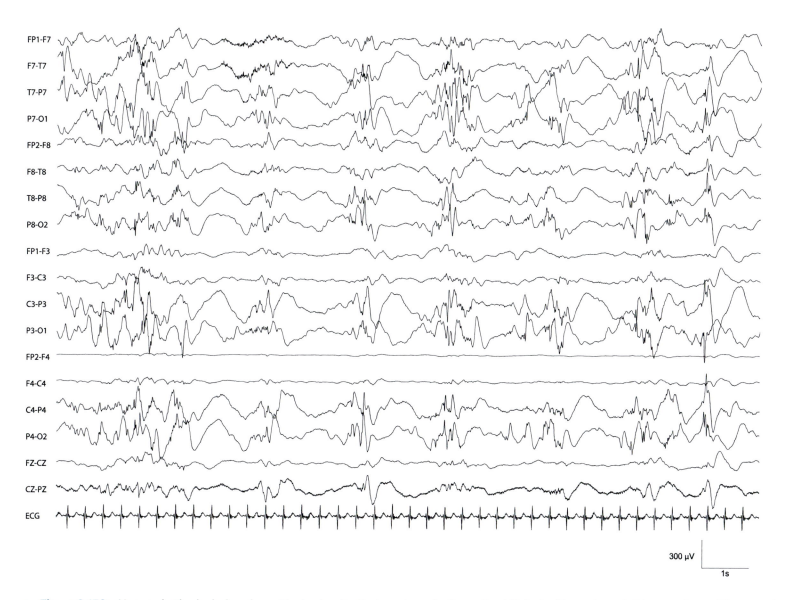

300 µV

1s

▶ **Figure 3.158 Hypsarrhythmia during sleep.** Bipolar, longitudinal montage. An 8-month-old infant with cryptogenic West syndrome. There was hypsarrhythmia during wakefulness. This recording was obtained when the patient was asleep. It shows periodic epileptiform discharges of a generalized distribution, maximum in posterior derivations. The recording shows a high-amplitude (>300 µV), generalized, irregular delta activity. These slow waves are interrupted every 2 or 3 s by a 1- to 3-s burst of bilateral, multifocal spikes. This burst-attenuation pattern of generalized periodic epileptiform discharges during sleep is characteristic for patient with West syndrome.

EEG classification: Abnormal III (sleep)
    Periodic epileptiform discharges, generalized maximum posterior head regions

EEG report: This EEG supports the diagnosis of West syndrome.

Flattening during seizure in hypsarrhythmia

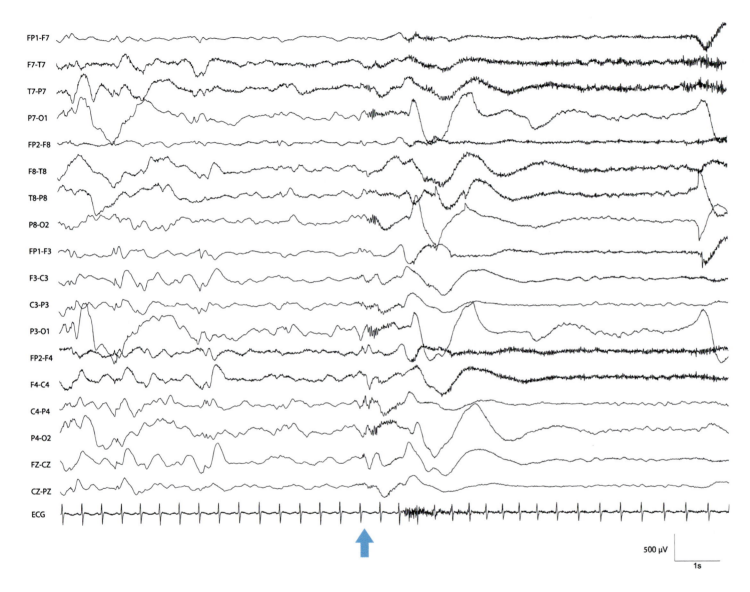

▶ **Figure 3.159**   **Flattening during seizure in hypsarrhythmia.** Bipolar longitudinal montage. A 21-month-old, severely mentally challenged girl with idiopathic West syndrome. After a short high-amplitude burst of slow waves (blue arrow), the EEG flattens, which is the typical EEG pattern of epileptic spasms. Electrodes T7 and F4 are artifactuous. The spasms reflect in the ECG with a short high-amplitude EMG artifact that later subsides.

EEG classification: Abnormal III (awake)
1. Hypsarrhythmia
2. Seizure: EEG seizure pattern, (electrodecrement), generalized
      Epileptic spasm

EEG report: This EEG documents an epileptic spasm in West syndrome.

▶ **Table 3.10   Typical EEG Patterns in Several Epilepsy Syndromes**

EEG Pattern	Figures	Epilepsy Syndrome
3 Hz spike–waves, generalized	3.149, 3.152	Absence epilepsy
4 Hz (irregular) generalized spike–waves and polyspikes	3.127, 3.132	Juvenile myoclonic epilepsy
Photoparoxysmal response	3.12–3.14, 3.160, 3.161, 3.166	Idiopathic generalized epilepsy (juvenile myoclonic epilepsy; absence epilepsy)
Slow spike–waves, generalized	3.154–3.156	Lennox–Gastaut syndrome
Generalized paroxysmal fast	3.130, 3.131	Lennox–Gastaut syndrome
Hypsarrhythmia	3.157–3.159	West syndrome
Anterior temporal spikes	3.116, 3.121	Mesial temporal lobe epilepsy
Benign epileptiform discharges	2.27, 3.141–3.144	Benign focal epilepsy of childhood
Regional polyspikes	3.138–3.140	Cortical dysplasia

EEG, electroencephalogram.

the location of the epileptogenic zone. However, these changes can disappear within minutes to hours so that the EEG can be normal again depending on how long after the seizure the recording is obtained. Continuous recordings of EEG simultaneously with video has been possible since the 1960s. Our electroclinical knowledge of epileptic seizures has since decisively expanded. The simultaneous recording of clinical seizures with EEG and video allows detailed classification of epilepsies and epileptic seizures (Noachtar et al., 2004). Ictal recordings primarily serve the following purposes:

- The differential diagnostic of epileptic seizures from non-epileptic syndromes, such as syncope and functional (psychogenic non-epileptic) seizures
- Precise classification of epileptic seizures

The chances of recording a habitual seizure depend on the frequency of the seizures. Typically, at least one seizure per week should occur to have a realistic chance to record a seizure during a 1-week EEG video monitoring. In most cases, however, the chances of recording a seizure are greatly increased by reducing or discontinuing anti-seizure medication (Noachtar et al., 2004). Digital processing of the EEG signal using multichannel recordings has been introduced (Scherg et al., 2002, 2012).

The first seizure patterns in EEG were detected in absence epilepsies (Gibbs et al., 1935). The typical pattern of these patients is the generalized 3 Hz spike–waves (▶ **Figure 3.167**). If these bursts of spike–waves last longer than 3 s, most patients are not able to respond appropriately during the discharge (▶ **Figures 3.147** and **3.167**). For clinical classification, it is important to know whether a patient remembers a word called during spike–wave discharge. Some patients remember a test word but cannot press a button during the discharge to document their response (▶ **Figures 3.148** and **3.168**) (Rémi et al. 2011b). These patients describe the inability to press the button. In such cases, there is no disturbance of consciousness, but there is an inability to initiate a movement. In this setting, we speak of an akinetic seizure (Noachtar & Lüders, 2000; Rémi et al., 2011b).

Photoparoxysmal response II

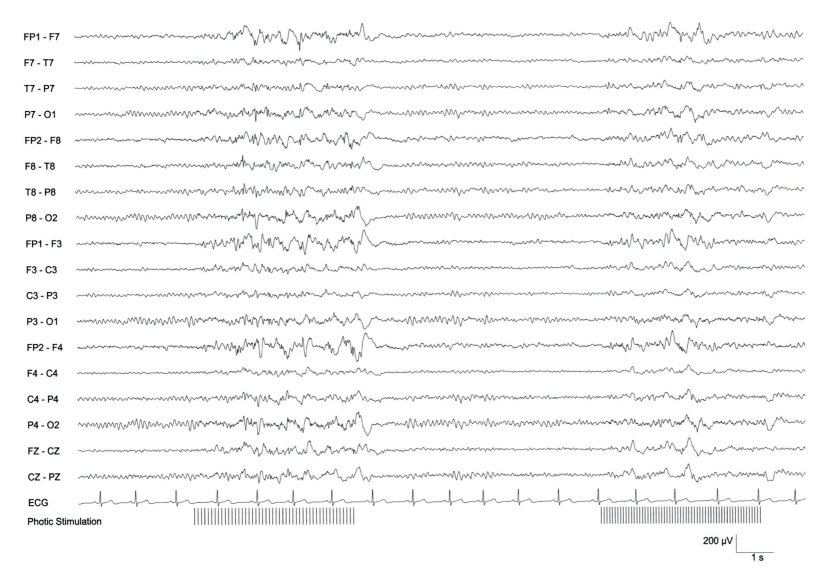

▶ **Figure 3.160** **Photoparoxysmal response II.** Bipolar longitudinal montage. Untreated 14-year-old female patient with juvenile myoclonic epilepsy. During photic stimulation at 12 Hz, generalized spikes with maximum at FP2 more than FP1 and at 15 Hz stimulation bifrontal slow waves occur. The spikes do not outlast the stimulation.

EEG classification: Abnormal II (awake)
    Photoparoxysmal response, generalized

EEG report: This EEG demonstrates photosensitivity in juvenile myoclonic epilepsy.

Photoparoxysmal response II

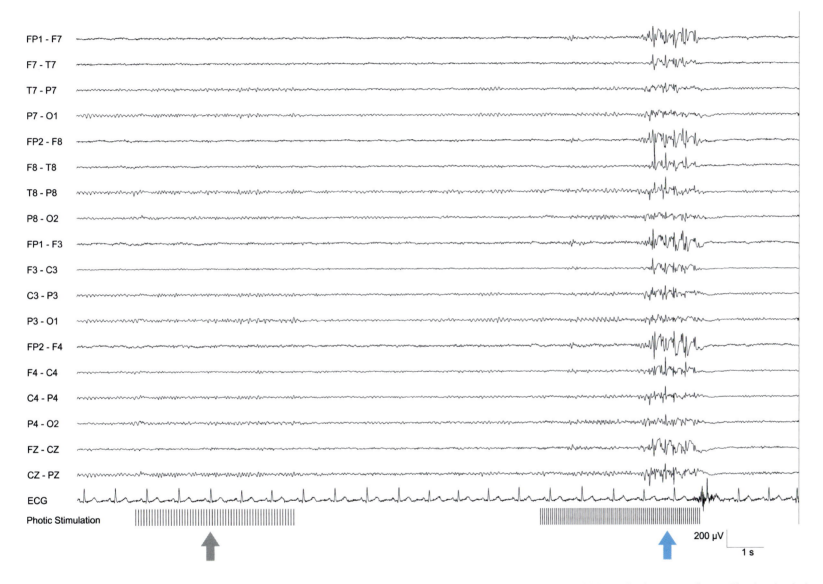

▶ **Figure 3.161** **Photoparoxysmal response II.** Bipolar longitudinal montage. A 30-year-old female patient with juvenile absence epilepsy. Photic stimulation at 20 Hz triggered generalized polyspikes (blue arrow), whereas stimulation at 15 Hz led to photic driving (gray arrow).

EEG classification: Abnormal II (awake)
Photoparoxysmal response, generalized

EEG report: This EEG supports the diagnosis of juvenile absence epilepsy.

Photic driving

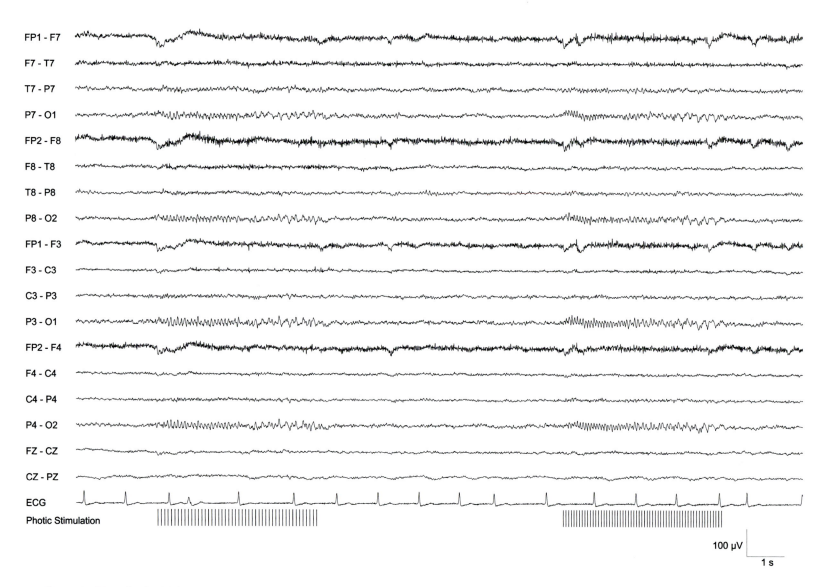

FP1 - F7

F7 - T7

T7 - P7

P7 - O1

FP2 - F8

F8 - T8

T8 - P8

P8 - O2

FP1 - F3

F3 - C3

C3 - P3

P3 - O1

FP2 - F4

F4 - C4

C4 - P4

P4 - O2

FZ - CZ

CZ - PZ

ECG

Photic Stimulation

100 µV

1 s

▶ **Figure 3.162** **Photic driving.** Bipolar longitudinal montage. A 42-year-old female patient with migraine. Photic stimulation with 12 and 15 Hz leads to occipital photic driving, which initially has a 1:1 ratio and then slows down to a 1:4.5 ratio.

EEG classification: Normal (awake)

EEG report: This EEG is normal.

Photic driving

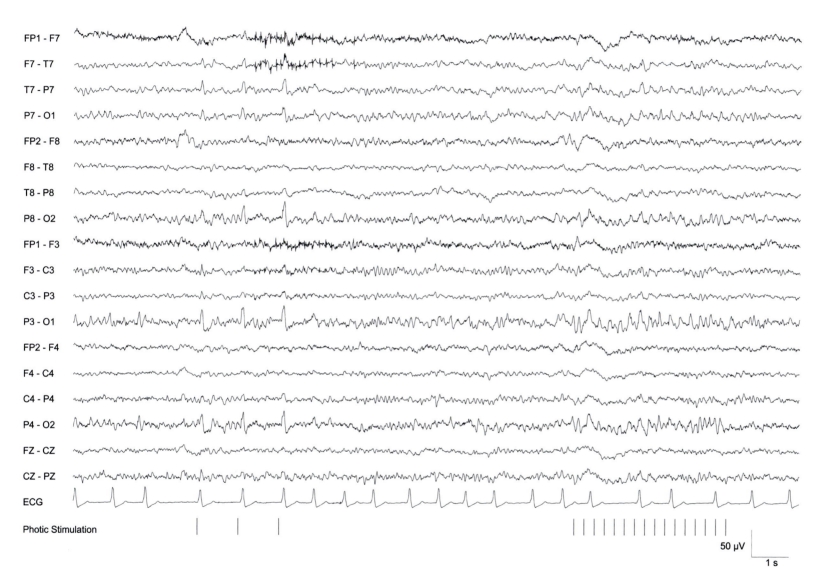

FP1 - F7

F7 - T7

T7 - P7

P7 - O1

FP2 - F8

F8 - T8

T8 - P8

P8 - O2

FP1 - F3

F3 - C3

C3 - P3

P3 - O1

FP2 - F4

F4 - C4

C4 - P4

P4 - O2

FZ - CZ

CZ - PZ

ECG

Photic Stimulation

50 μV

1 s

▶ **Figure 3.163** **Photic driving.** Bipolar longitudinal montage. An 87-year-old female patient with mild Alzheimer's dementia. Photic stimulation with 1 and 4 Hz leads to photic driving, which occurs in a 1:1 ratio. The background occipital rhythm is 9 Hz and is superimposed on a generalized, low-amplitude continuous slow.

EEG classification: Abnormal I (awake)

Continuous slow, generalized

EEG report: This EEG shows mild diffuse encephalopathy and supports the diagnosis of Alzheimer's disease.

Photic driving in congenital amaurosis

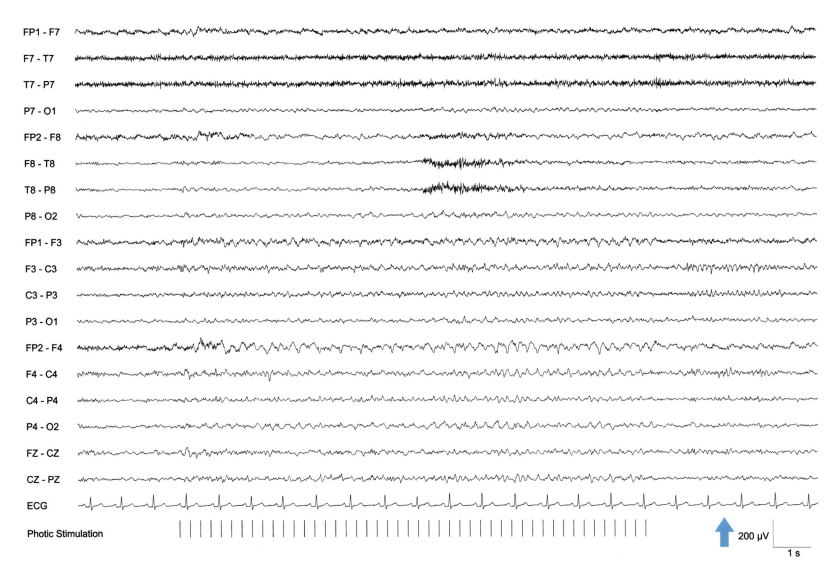

FP1 - F7

F7 - T7

T7 - P7

P7 - O1

FP2 - F8

F8 - T8

T8 - P8

P8 - O2

FP1 - F3

F3 - C3

C3 - P3

P3 - O1

FP2 - F4

F4 - C4

C4 - P4

P4 - O2

FZ - CZ

CZ - PZ

ECG

Photic Stimulation

200 µV

1 s

▶ **Figure 3.164** **Photic driving in congenital amaurosis.** Bipolar longitudinal montage. A 33-year-old female patient with congenital amaurosis and a concentration disorder. Photic stimulation with 4 Hz leads to photic driving in a 1:1 ratio with a F3 and F4 maximum. Note mu activity in the left central region (blue arrow).

EEG classification: Normal (awake)

EEG report: This EEG shows a photic driving of an atypical distribution (maximum in the superior frontal electrodes) in connatal amaurosis.

Giant photic evoked responses in coma

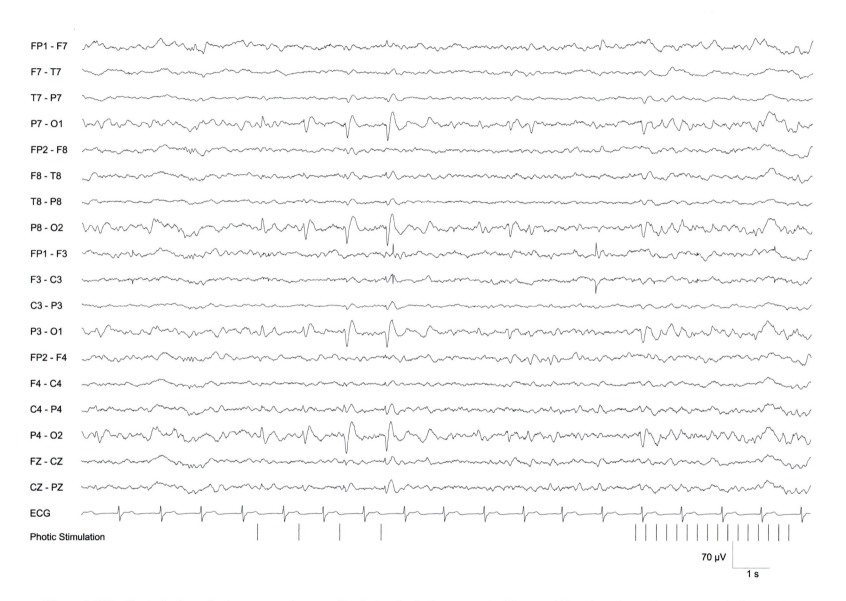

FP1 - F7

F7 - T7

T7 - P7

P7 - O1

FP2 - F8

F8 - T8

T8 - P8

P8 - O2

FP1 - F3

F3 - C3

C3 - P3

P3 - O1

FP2 - F4

F4 - C4

C4 - P4

P4 - O2

FZ - CZ

CZ - PZ

ECG

Photic Stimulation

70 µV

1 s

▶ **Figure 3.165** **Giant photic evoked responses in coma.** Bipolar longitudinal montage. An 89-year-old female patient with severe metabolic encephalopathy. Photic stimulation with 1 Hz triggered biphasic negative occipital spikes corresponding to visual evoked potentials. Stimulation with 4 Hz results in relatively low-amplitude photic driving. The waveform of the spikes generated by 1 Hz stimulation is identical to occipital benign focal epileptiform discharges usually seen in young children with benign focal epilepsy of childhood.

EEG classification: Abnormal III (coma)
Delta coma

EEG report: This EEG is indicative of a severe diffuse encephalopathy.

Photoparoxysmal response III

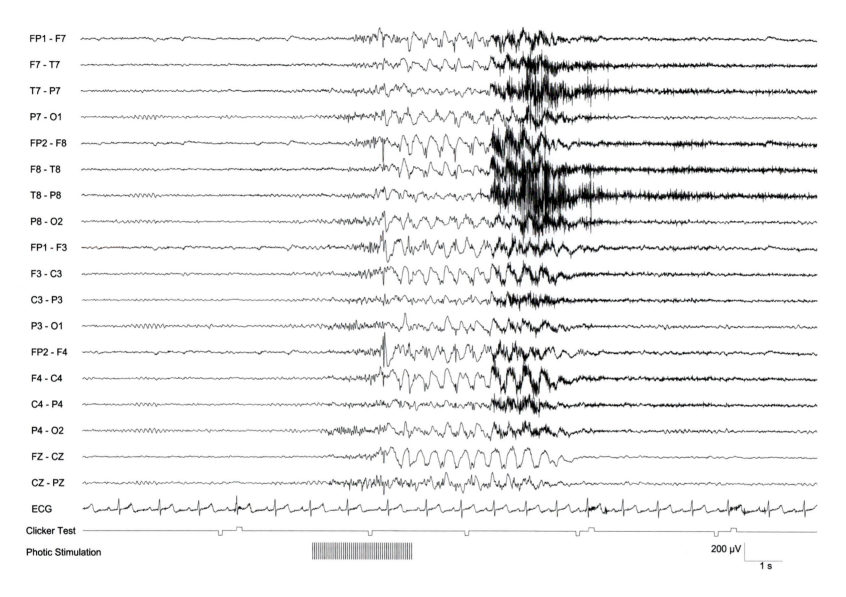

▶ **Figure 3.166** **Photoparoxysmal response III.** Bipolar longitudinal montage. A 34-year-old female patient with juvenile myoclonic epilepsy. Photic stimulation with 20 Hz leads initially to a progressively higher amplitude photic driving. Thereafter, still during photic stimulation, generalized spike–waves appear that outlast the end of photic stimulation. The patient is not able to respond to an acoustic stimulus (clicker test) given at the beginning and in the middle of the burst of spike–waves.

EEG classification: Abnormal III (awake)
1. Photoparoxysmal response, generalized
2. Seizure: EEG seizure pattern, generalized (spike-waves)
   Dialeptic seizure

EEG report: This EEG documents a dialeptic seizure elicited by photic stimulation in a patient with juvenile myoclonic epilepsy.

EEG seizure pattern, generalized; dialeptic seizure

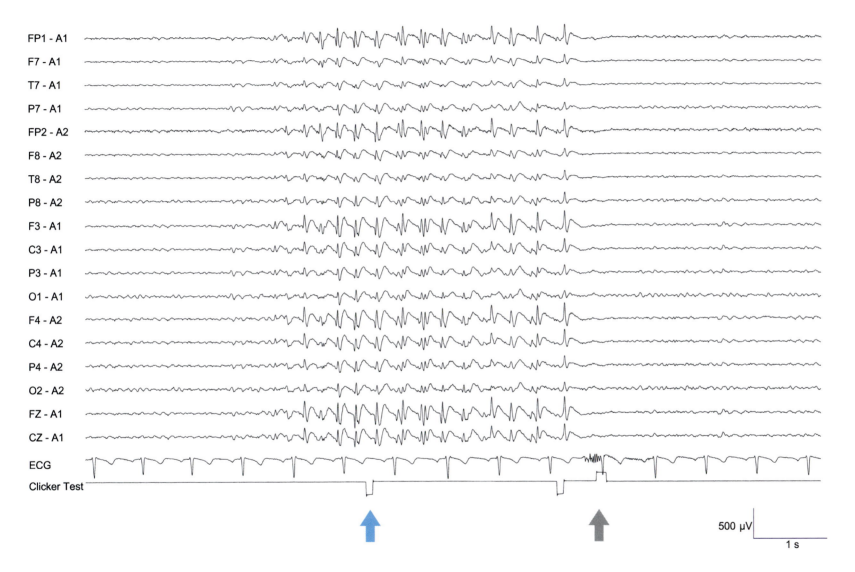

FP1 - A1
F7 - A1
T7 - A1
P7 - A1
FP2 - A2
F8 - A2
T8 - A2
P8 - A2
F3 - A1
C3 - A1
P3 - A1
O1 - A1
F4 - A2
C4 - A2
P4 - A2
O2 - A2
FZ - A1
CZ - A1
ECG
Clicker Test

500 µV

1 s

▶ **Figure 3.167** **EEG seizure pattern, generalized; dialeptic seizure.** Ear reference derivation. A 27-year-old female patient with juvenile absence epilepsy. The patient did not respond (press a button) to the presentation of an acoustic stimulus (beep tone; blue arrow) during the generalized spike–waves. Toward the end of the discharge, the patient responds (gray arrow).

EEG classification: Abnormal III (awake)

Seizure: EEG seizure pattern, generalized (3 Hz spike–wave)
Dialeptic seizure

EEG report: This EEG documents a dialeptic seizure and supports the diagnosis of juvenile absence epilepsy.

EEG seizure pattern, generalized; dialeptic seizure

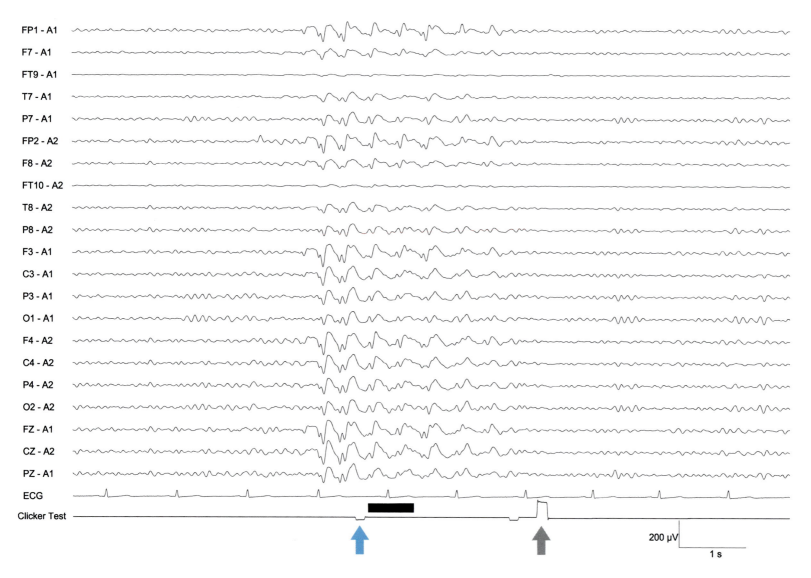

▶ **Figure 3.168** **EEG seizure pattern, generalized; dialeptic seizure.** Bipolar longitudinal montage. A 21-year-old female patient with absence epilepsy. The patient failed to respond (push a button) to an acoustic stimulus (beep tone; blue arrow) presented by an EEG tech during the spike–waves but could remember the word ("auto") that was presented to her during this phase. Review of the video in slow motion confirmed that the word "auto" was given during the burst of spike–waves. The marks in the figure show the exact time the tech started and completed the word "auto" to the patient. Soon afterward (gray arrow), the patient responded adequately (i.e., pressed a button in response to the acoustic stimulus). Thus, there is no disturbance of consciousness (dialeptic seizure; "absence seizure") but, rather, the ictal inability to initiate a motor response (akinetic seizure) (Rémi et al., 2011).

EEG classification: Abnormal III (awake)

Seizure: EEG-seizure pattern, generalized (spike–waves)
        Akinetic seizure

EEG report: This EEG documents an akinetic seizure and supports the diagnosis of juvenile absence epilepsy.

Bilateral tonic seizures in generalized epilepsies are usually accompanied by a generalized, low- to medium-amplitude, high-frequency EEG seizure pattern called paroxysmal fast (pattern) (▶ **Figure 3.169**). This paroxysmal fast pattern may not be associated with clinical signs if it lasts only 1 or 2 s (▶ **Figure 3.130** and **3.131**). Sometimes the ictal high-frequency activity can be of so low amplitude that it appears almost as a flattening compared to the preictal background activity (▶ **Figure 3.170**). Polygraphic recordings including, for example, EMG or respiration are sometimes necessary to recognize the ictal character of epileptiform discharges (Lüders & Noachtar, 2000a, 2001). EMG recordings are usually required to distinguish a negative myoclonic seizure from a ("positive") myoclonic seizure; the negative myoclonic seizure occurs during an unusually prolonged silent period (Noachtar et al., 1997). Atonic or akinetic seizures can also be documented by simultaneous EMG recordings (Noachtar & Lüders, 1999). Recording respiration by means of thoracic/abdominal belts, nasal thermistors and pulse oximeters is particularly helpful if an ictal apnea occurs during sleep (▶ **Figure 3.171**) (Lacuey et al., 2017; Tezer et al., 2009). However, it is usually unclear whether the ictal apnea is an expression of reduced respiratory drive or results from tonic contraction of the diaphragm or other respiratory muscles (Tezer et al., 2009). A relatively high percentage of patients with mesial temporal epilepsy show initially a central apnea that consistently precedes other clinic manifestations and occurs before the initiation of the ictal pattern recorded with scalp electrodes, including sphenoidal electrodes. Generalized myoclonic seizures are usually accompanied by generalized polyspikes (▶ **Figure 3.172**). Generalized tonic–clonic seizures are associated with typical EEG changes and artifacts (▶ **Figures 3.173–3.175**). At the beginning, the patient remains motionless until a tonic muscular tension occurs, which gradually turns into clonic movements of increasing amplitude. The intervals between the clonic movements gradually becomes longer. After the seizure, the EEG is flat.

There is a generalized EEG pattern that resembles seizure patterns but has no clinical significance. It is called the subclinical rhythmic electrographic discharge of adults (SREDA) (▶ **Figure 3.176**) (Westmoreland & Klass, 1981).

The localization of the first recognizable ictal EEG discharge is of particular importance in the evaluation of focal epilepsies because it indicates the localization of the seizure-onset zone that is closely related to the epileptogenic zone. In the EEG seizure classification used in this book, the different ictal patterns are not further subdivided because only the initial localization of the EEG pattern is of clinical relevance.

Regional EEG seizure patterns are identified because they are characterized by a continuously evolving change in localization, amplitude, morphology, and frequency of the ictal discharge (▶ **Figures 3.177–3.182**) (Noachtar & Rémi, 2009). It is essential to also remember that many regional seizures start with a low-amplitude, well-localized paroxysmal fast activity (▶ **Figures 3.177** and **3.178**). This pattern is particularly frequent in extratemporal neocortical epilepsies. Therefore, it is important not to filter out high-frequency components even if the EEG is highly contaminated by high-frequency EMG artifacts. In temporal lobe epilepsies and especially mesial temporal lobe epilepsies, theta–delta frequencies typically dominate the initial EEG ictal manifestations (▶ **Figure 3.182**). The scalp ictal EEG in these patients is often diffusely slowed bilaterally in the first 30 s and only then shows a unilateral temporal seizure pattern with rhythmic theta and delta waves (Risinger et al., 1989). It can also begin with somewhat faster frequencies and change into repetitive spikes (▶ **Figures 3.182** and **3.183**). Recording from additional electrodes, such as the anterior temporal electrodes FT10 and FT9 or the sphenoidal electrodes SP2 and SP1, is essential because mesial temporal interictal spikes and mesial temporal EEG seizure patterns usually are of highest amplitude at these electrodes (▶ **Figures 3.184** and **3.185**). Repetitive spikes/sharp waves at the beginning of an EEG seizure pattern are rare and tend to be observed more frequently in extratemporal seizures onset. Occasionally, frontal EEG seizure patterns, which were nonlateralized at the beginning, may spread to one temporal lobe (▶ **Figure 3.186**).

When localizing EEG seizure patterns, it must be considered that the initial EEG seizure pattern recorded with scalp electrodes usually is an expression of seizure propagation. Therefore, we may miss the actual seizure onset, which can be detected with invasive electrodes (▶ **Figures 3.187** and **3.188**). Regional flattening at the beginning of the seizure is rare and usually evolves into slow rhythmic waves of decreasing frequency and increasing amplitude (▶ **Figures 3.189–3.193**).

The EEG derived from the scalp sometimes shows no seizure pattern despite clinical seizure symptoms. This happens because the epileptically excited cortex region is either too small or lies too deep to be noticed with scalp electrodes. Approximately half of all auras show no seizure patterns in scalp EEG recordings (Lieb et al., 1976). In such situations, electrodes placed at the appropriate depth will record an EEG seizure pattern that cannot be detected with scalp electrodes. In addition, in seizures with severe motor dysfunction (e.g., hypermotor seizures; Lüders et al., 1998, 2019), such as those occurring in frontal lobe

EEG seizure pattern, generalized; bilateral tonic seizure

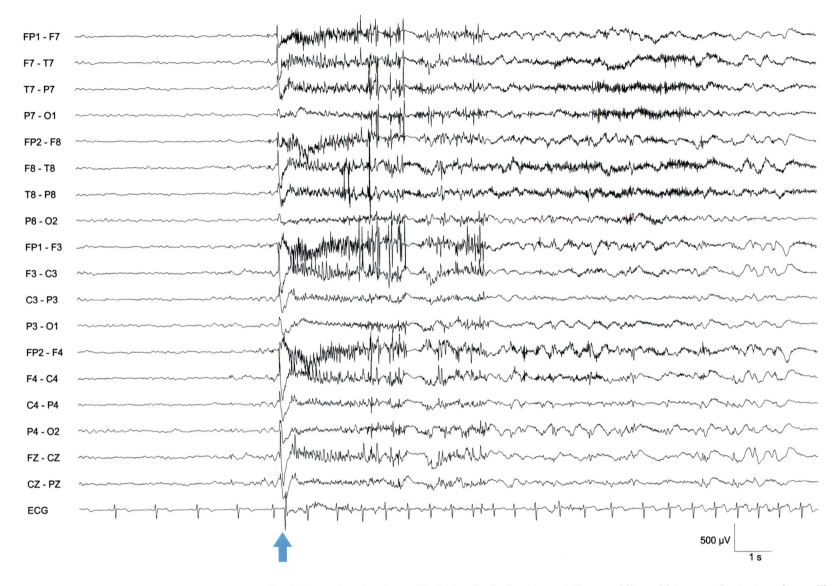

FP1 - F7
F7 - T7
T7 - P7
P7 - O1
FP2 - F8
F8 - T8
T8 - P8
P8 - O2
FP1 - F3
F3 - C3
C3 - P3
P3 - O1
FP2 - F4
F4 - C4
C4 - P4
P4 - O2
FZ - CZ
CZ - PZ
ECG

500 µV

1 s

▶ **Figure 3.169** **EEG seizure pattern, generalized; bilateral tonic seizure.** Bipolar longitudinal montage. A 12-year-old boy with Lennox–Gastaut syndrome. The generalized EEG seizure pattern with frontal maximum (blue arrow) was typically associated with bilateral tonic seizures if it lasted longer than 2 s. After the tonic seizure, a generalized slow spike–wave burst is seen.

EEG classification: Abnormal III (awake)

Seizure: EEG seizure pattern, generalized (paroxysmal beta)
Bilateral tonic seizure

EEG report: This EEG documents a bilateral tonic seizure in a patient with Lennox–Gastaut syndrome.

EEG seizure pattern, generalized; bilateral tonic seizure

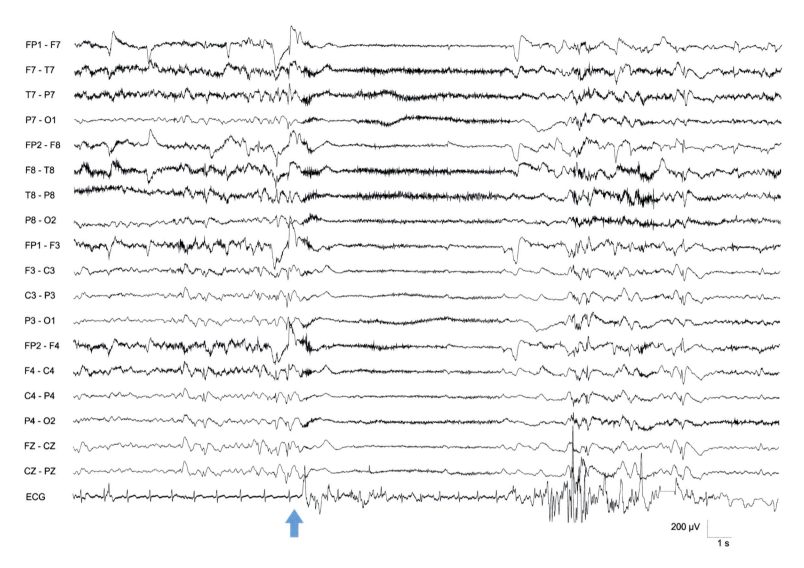

200 μV

1 s

▶ **Figure 3.170** **EEG seizure pattern, generalized; bilateral tonic seizure.** Bipolar longitudinal montage. A 21-year-old patient with Lennox–Gastaut syndrome. There is a slow background rhythm. A 1- or 2-s burst of generalized slow spike–wave is abruptly flattened with a superimposed relatively low-amplitude paroxysmal fast or EMG artifact. This artifact is most prominent in frontotemporal derivations. The electrodecremental episode lasts approximately 6 s. Approximately 1 s before the electrodecremental episode, the patient closed the eyes, and 400–450 ms before the initiation of the tonic seizure, the patient opened the eyes again. Immediately after the electrodecremental episode is over, there is a blink, and the slow background activity and slow interictal spike–wave pattern resumes.

EEG classification: Abnormal III (awake)
1. Seizure: EEG seizure pattern, generalized (electrodecremental)
   Bilateral tonic seizure
2. Slow spike–wave, generalized
3. Background slow

EEG report: This EEG documents a bilateral tonic seizure in a patient with Lennox–Gastaut syndrome.

Ictal apnea

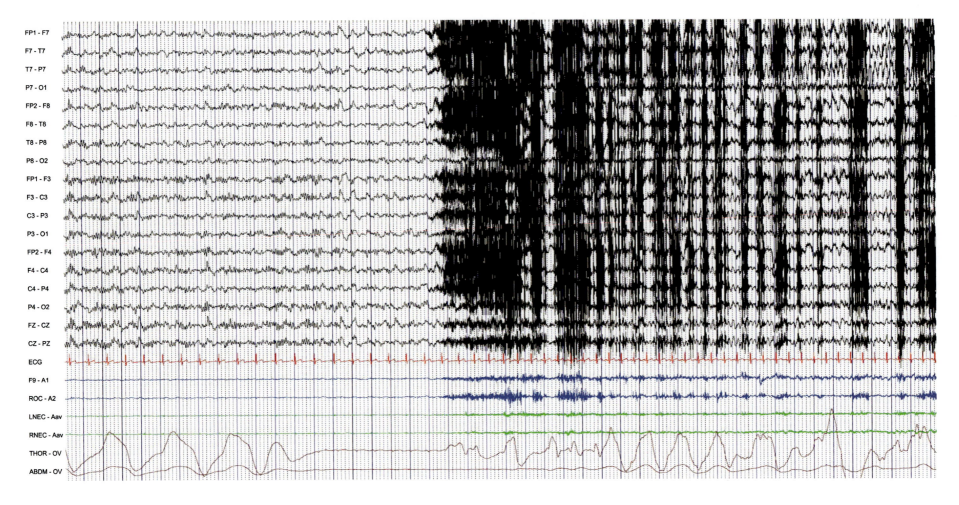

▶ **Figure 3.171 Ictal apnea.** Bipolar longitudinal derivation. A 43-year-old patient with a small left temporoparietal infarct of unknown origin. The first sign of this seizure was a central apnea that lasted 7 s and was accompanied by a slight desaturation of 88% approximately 45 s later (baseline, 92–95%). This was not associated with any significant change in heart rate, and there were no changes in the EEG throughout the period of apnea. During the apnea, the EEG continues to show the same sleep pattern, and there are no muscle or movement artifacts. The patient then had oro-alimentary automatisms and with it she started breathing again. Muscle obscured the EEG seizure onset, but later during the seizure, a clear epileptiform discharge is seen in the left temporal region.

A2, right ear electrode; Aav, average reference; ABDM, abdominal band; LNEC, left neck; OV, average of the two machine references; RNEC, right neck; ROC, right outer cantus; THOR, thoracic band.

EEG classification: Abnormal III (sleep)

Seizure: EEG seizure pattern, left temporal (paroxysmal theta)
Vegetative seizure (apnea)

EEG report: This EEG documents ictal apnea associated with a left temporal seizure pattern in a patient with a small left temporoparietal infarct.

EEG seizure pattern, generalized; generalized myoclonic seizure

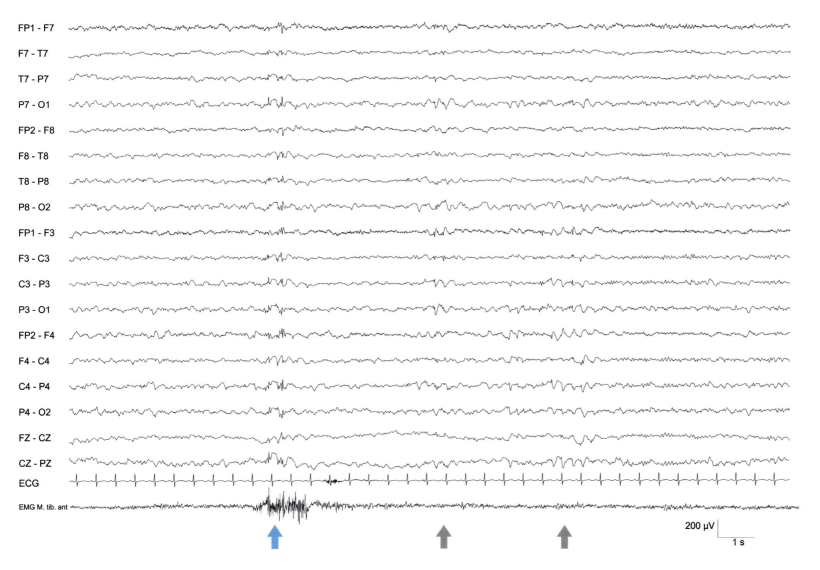

▶ **Figure 3.172** **EEG seizure pattern, generalized; generalized myoclonic seizure.** Bipolar longitudinal derivation. In this 25-year-old patient with MERFF syndrome, generalized poly-spikes were associated with myoclonic seizures (blue arrow), whereas single spikes remained subclinical (gray arrows). The patient was asleep during this EEG example.

EEG classification: Abnormal III (sleep)
1. Seizure: EEG, pattern (polyspikes), generalized
   Myoclonic seizure, generalized
2. Spikes, generalized

EEG report: This EEG documents a generalized myoclonic seizure.

EEG seizure pattern, generalized; generalized tonic–clonic seizure

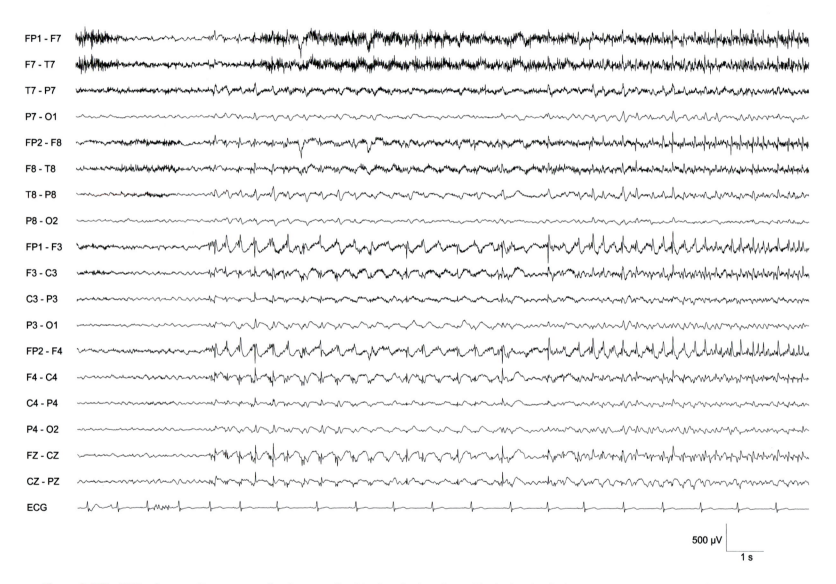

FP1 - F7

F7 - T7

T7 - P7

P7 - O1

FP2 - F8

F8 - T8

T8 - P8

P8 - O2

FP1 - F3

F3 - C3

C3 - P3

P3 - O1

FP2 - F4

F4 - C4

C4 - P4

P4 - O2

FZ - CZ

CZ - PZ

ECG

500 μV

1 s

▶ **Figure 3.173** **EEG seizure pattern, generalized; generalized tonic–clonic seizure.** Bipolar longitudinal montage. A 31-year-old patient with generalized epilepsy with febrile seizures (GEFS). The patient was staring and lost consciousness at seizure onset. EEG shows generalized polyspike–waves that vary in morphology, distribution, and amplitude. The EEG evolution of a generalized tonic–clonic seizure is shown in ▶ **Figures 3.174–3.175**. EEG classification is shown in ▶ **Figure 3.175**.

EEG seizure pattern, generalized (continued 1); generalized tonic–clonic seizure

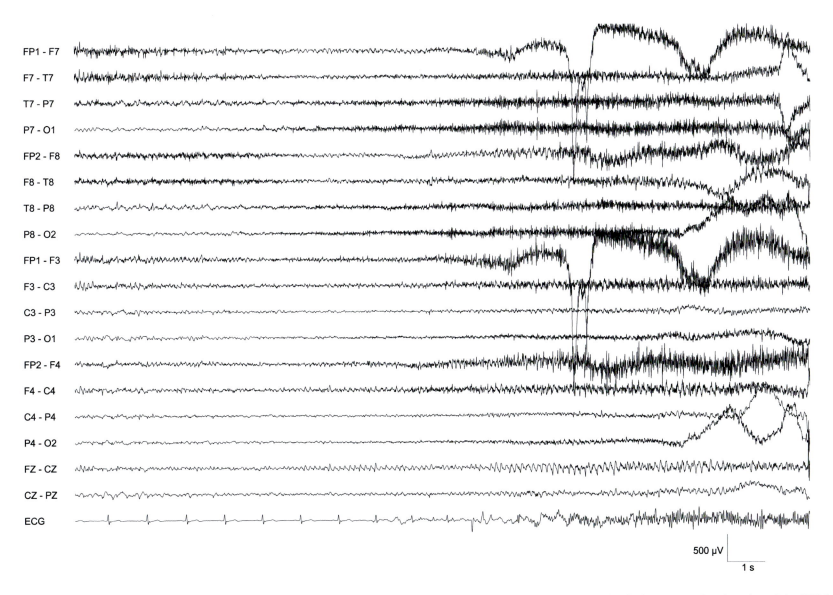

FP1 - F7

F7 - T7

T7 - P7

P7 - O1

FP2 - F8

F8 - T8

T8 - P8

P8 - O2

FP1 - F3

F3 - C3

C3 - P3

P3 - O1

FP2 - F4

F4 - C4

C4 - P4

P4 - O2

FZ - CZ

CZ - PZ

ECG

500 µV

1 s

▶ **Figure 3.174**   **EEG seizure pattern, generalized (continued 1); generalized tonic–clonic seizure.** Bipolar longitudinal montage. Continuation of the EEG from ▶ **Figure 3.173**. The generalized, frontal maximum spike–wave and polyspike–wave pattern evolves into a diffuse, low-amplitude rhythmic fast EEG seizure pattern. In addition, in the last 10 s, there is high-amplitude muscle artifact, which partially obscures the underlying EEG seizure pattern. EEG classification is shown in ▶ **Figure 3.175**.

EEG seizure pattern, generalized (continued 2); generalized tonic–clonic seizure

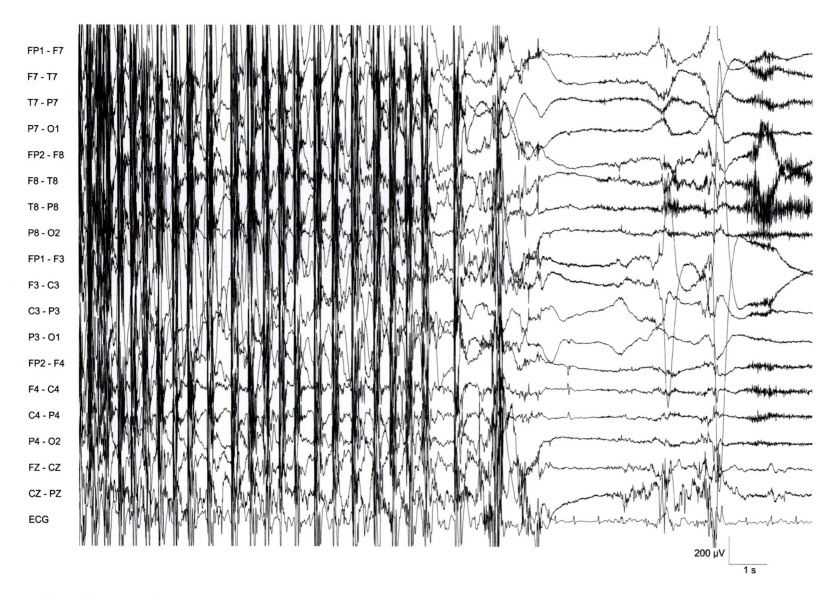

▶ **Figure 3.175** **EEG seizure pattern, generalized (continued 2); generalized tonic–clonic seizure.** Bipolar longitudinal montage. Continuation of the EEG from ▶ **Figures 3.173** and **3.174** approximately 30 s after the end of the EEG shown in ▶ **Figure 3.174**. Rhythmic muscle artifacts with gradually longer intervals dominate the EEG. Postictally, there is a considerable flattening of the background activity.

EEG classification: Abnormal III (awake)

Seizure: EEG seizure pattern, generalized (tonic–clonic seizure)
Generalized tonic–clonic seizure

EEG report: This EEG documents a generalized tonic–clonic seizure.

Subclinical rhythmic electrographic discharge of adults (SREDA)

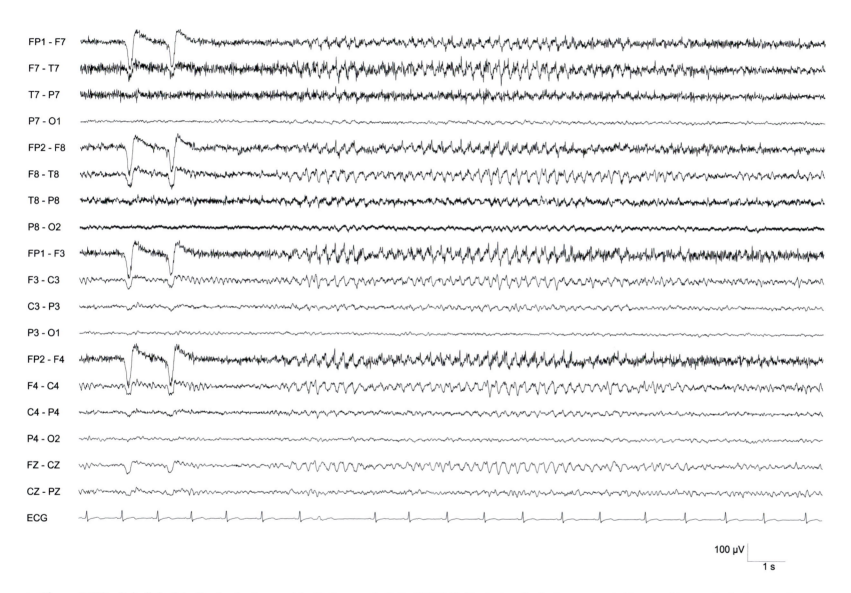

FP1 - F7
F7 - T7
T7 - P7
P7 - O1
FP2 - F8
F8 - T8
T8 - P8
P8 - O2
FP1 - F3
F3 - C3
C3 - P3
P3 - O1
FP2 - F4
F4 - C4
C4 - P4
P4 - O2
FZ - CZ
CZ - PZ
ECG

100 µV

1 s

▶ **Figure 3.176** **Subclinical rhythmic electrographic discharge of adults (SREDA).** Bipolar longitudinal montage. A 42-year-old, neurologically normal patient in whom this EEG pattern had repeatedly led to anti-seizure medication. Rhythmic, spindle-modulated, high-amplitude delta waves begin abruptly and subside rapidly. SREDA is a rare adult EEG pattern that has no clinical significance. The patient was fully responsive throughout this EEG pattern, and no clinical symptoms occurred. Note the ECG, which documents an atrioventricular block.

EEG classification: Normal (awake)

EEG report: Normal EEG.

EEG seizure pattern, left mesial frontal; bilateral tonic seizure

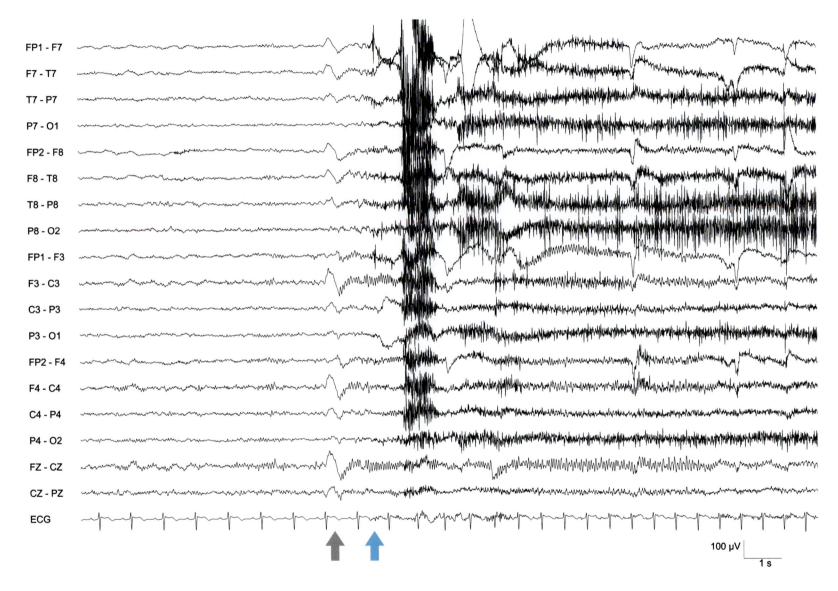

▶ **Figure 3.177   EEG seizure pattern, left mesial frontal; bilateral tonic seizure.** Bipolar longitudinal montage. A 29-year-old female patient with drug-resistant left frontal lobe epilepsy. A high-frequency seizure pattern on the left mesial frontal (electrodes F3 and FZ; blue arrow) develops out of a K-complex (gray arrow). The high-amplitude muscle artifact marks the beginning of a bilateral tonic seizure.

EEG classification: Abnormal III (awake)

Seizure: EEG seizure pattern, F3 = FZ > FP1
Bilateral tonic seizure

EEG report: This EEG documents a bilateral tonic seizure arising from a left mesial frontal lobe epilepsy.

EEG seizure pattern, right frontopolar

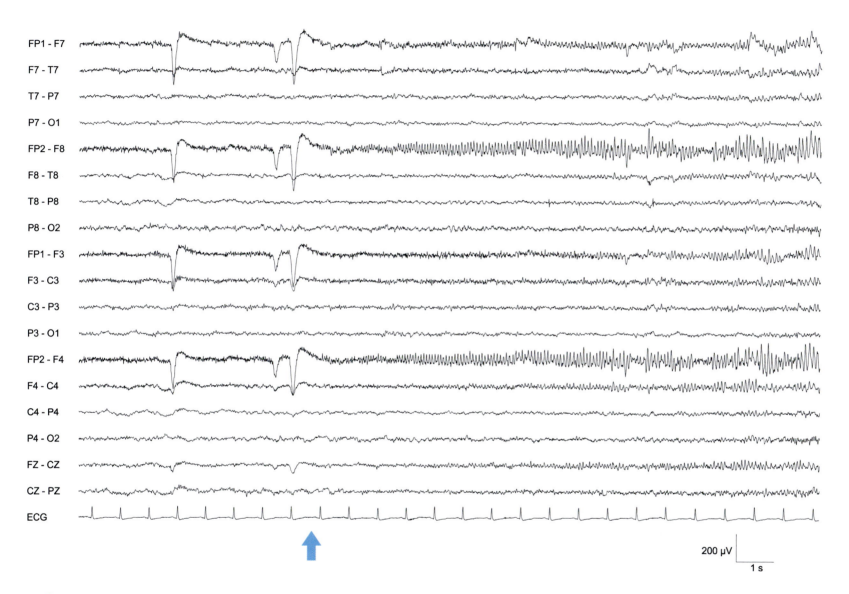

▶ **Figure 3.178** **EEG seizure pattern, right frontopolar.** Continuous slow, generalized. Bipolar longitudinal montage. A 79-year-old patient with right frontal meningioma who had suffered a first generalized convulsive seizure the day before. Clinically, the patient was inconspicuous during this EEG. The blue arrow marks the onset of the right frontopolar EEG seizure pattern. The occipital background rhythm was more pronounced at other sites of the EEG. There is a continuous generalized slow.

EEG classification: Abnormal III (awake)
1. Continuous slow, generalized
2. Seizure: EEG seizure pattern, FP2
   No clinical symptoms

EEG report: This EEG documents a right frontopolar subclinical seizure in frontal lobe epilepsy secondary to a right frontal meningioma and a mild diffuse encephalopathy.

EEG seizure pattern, right frontal

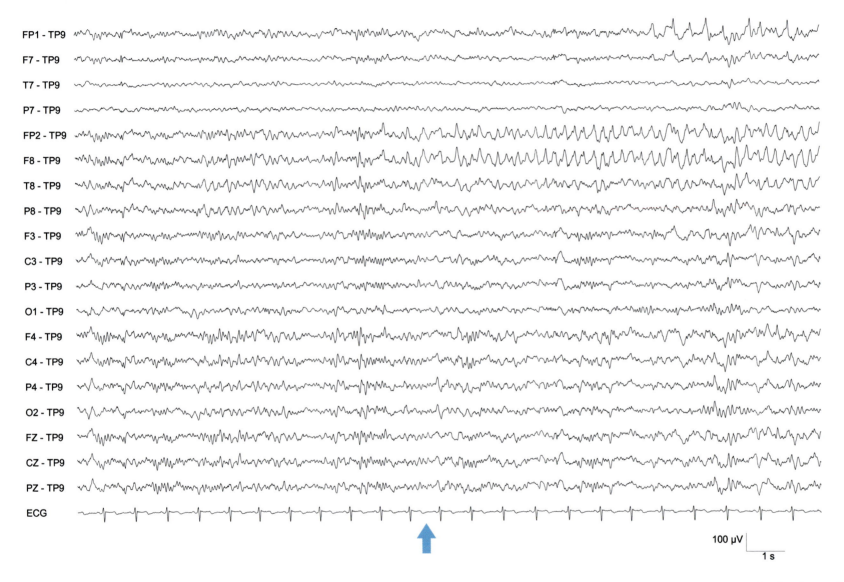

▶ **Figure 3.179** **EEG seizure pattern, right frontal.** Reference montage to left mastoid (electrode TP9). A 22-year-old patient with bilateral focal epilepsy after encephalitis at age 10 years. Out of sleep, rhythmic theta waves (blue arrow) occur at the right frontal region. This seizure activity progressively increases in amplitude and spreads to involve FP1. This seizure pattern remained without clinical correlate.

EEG classification: Abnormal III (sleep)

Seizure: EEG seizure pattern, FP2 = F8
No clinical symptoms

EEG report: This EEG documents a right frontal subclinical seizure.

EEG seizure pattern, right frontal

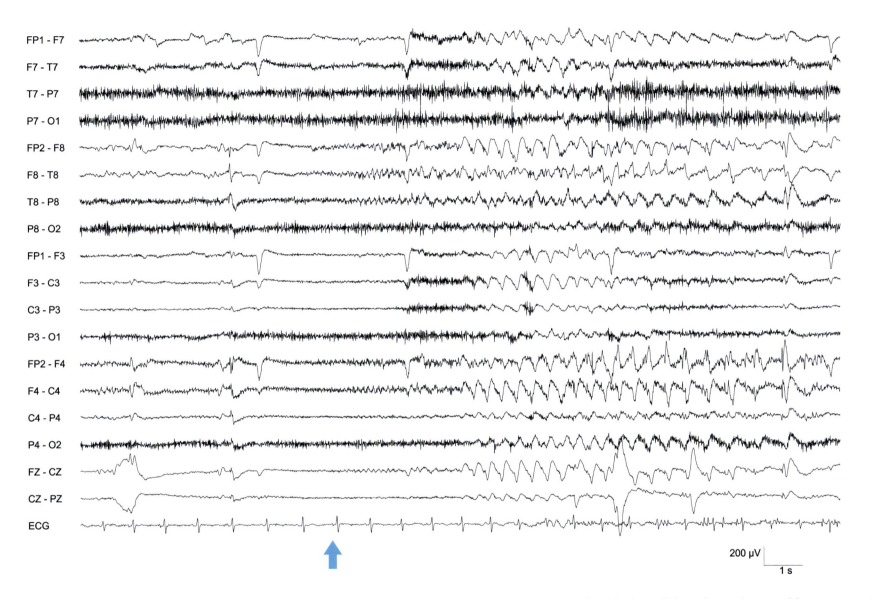

▶ **Figure 3.180** **EEG seizure pattern, right frontal.** Bipolar longitudinal montage. A 26-year-old patient with right frontal lobe epilepsy since age 23 years secondary to subarachnoid hemorrhage due to aneurysm of the anterior communicant artery, which has been surgically clipped. A low-amplitude 7 or 8 Hz paroxysmal activity arises from FP2, F8, T8, and F4 (blue arrow). Within 2 or 3 s, the paroxysmal activity changes in waveform and in frequency and spreads to involve both hemispheres. Clinically, the head and eyes turned to the left (versive seizure).

EEG classification: Abnormal III (awake)

Seizure: EEG seizure pattern, FP2 = F4 = F8
Left versive seizure

EEG report: This EEG documents the right frontal onset of a left versive seizure in right frontal lobe epilepsy.

EEG seizure pattern, left temporal

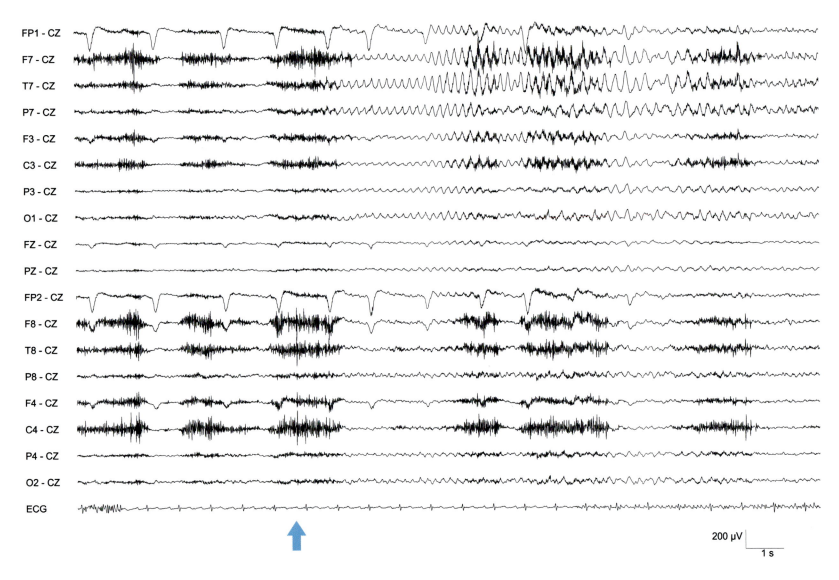

▶ Figure 3.181 **EEG seizure pattern, left temporal.** Vertex reference montage. A 53-year-old female patient with left temporal lobe epilepsy since the age of 24 years due to a dermoid tumor in the left temporal lobe. The repetitive EMG artifacts are caused by chewing movements (chewing gum). Left temporal rhythmic theta waves (blue arrow) occur during wakefulness, which first increase in amplitude, then slow down, become more irregular, and again become lower in amplitude. Clinically, an abdominal aura was followed by blank stare with loss of consciousness and manual automatisms.

EEG classification: Abnormal III (awake)

Seizure: EEG seizure pattern, T7 > F7 > P7
Abdominal aura → automotor seizure

EEG report: This EEG documents a seizure arising from the left temporal lobe.

EEG seizure pattern, left mesial temporal

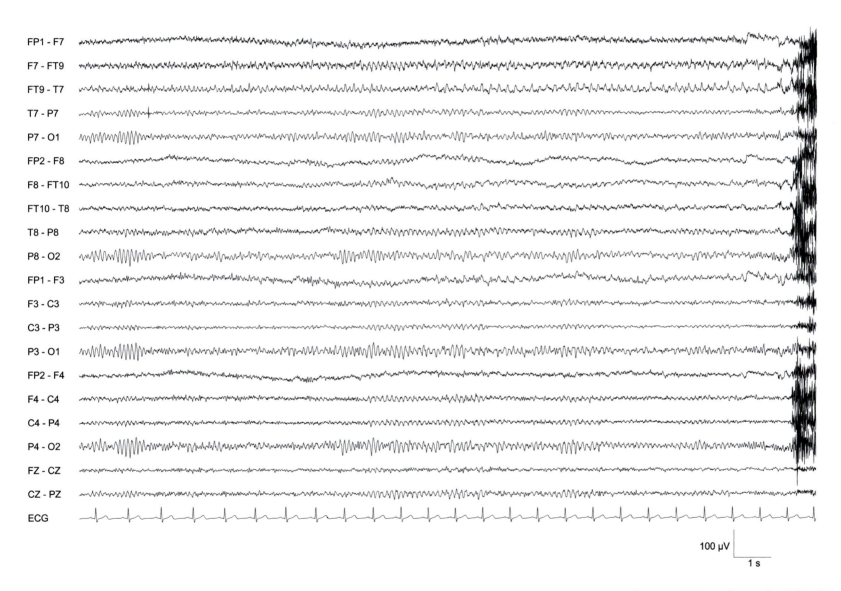

FP1 - F7
F7 - FT9
FT9 - T7
T7 - P7
P7 - O1
FP2 - F8
F8 - FT10
FT10 - T8
T8 - P8
P8 - O2
FP1 - F3
F3 - C3
C3 - P3
P3 - O1
FP2 - F4
F4 - C4
C4 - P4
P4 - O2
FZ - CZ
CZ - PZ
ECG

100 μV

1 s

▶ **Figure 3.182**   **EEG seizure pattern, left mesial temporal.** Bipolar longitudinal montage. A 43-year-old patient with left temporal lobe epilepsy. The EEG seizure shows first paroxysmal theta activity very localized to the electrode FT9. For EEG classification and report, see ▶ **Figure 3.183**.

EEG seizure pattern, left mesial temporal (continued)

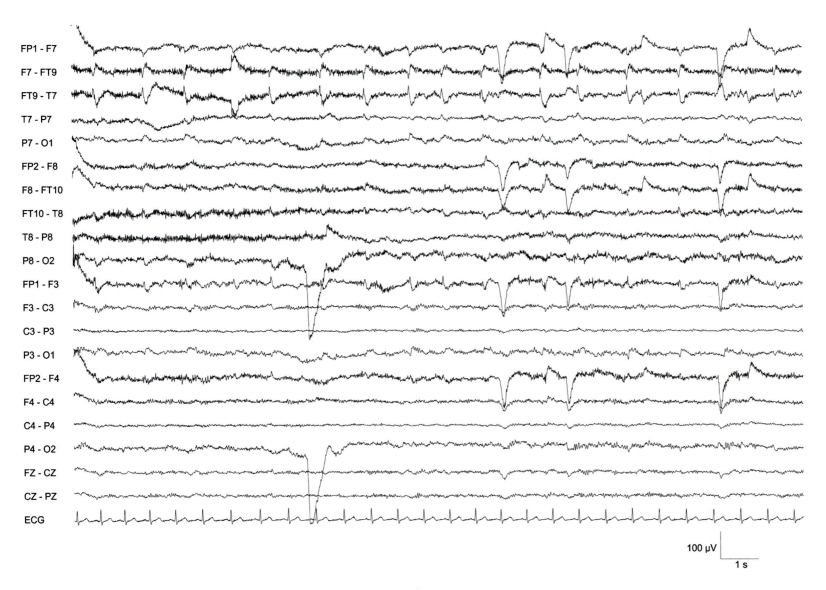

FP1 - F7
F7 - FT9
FT9 - T7
T7 - P7
P7 - O1
FP2 - F8
F8 - FT10
FT10 - T8
T8 - P8
P8 - O2
FP1 - F3
F3 - C3
C3 - P3
P3 - O1
FP2 - F4
F4 - C4
C4 - P4
P4 - O2
FZ - CZ
CZ - PZ
ECG

100 μV

1 s

▶ **Figure 3.183** **EEG seizure pattern, left mesial temporal (continued).** Bipolar longitudinal montage. Same patient as in ▶ **Figure 3.182**. After the paroxysmal theta of ▶ **Figure 3.182**, the EEG showed paroxysmal repetitive epileptiform discharges at FT9. The EEG seizure pattern was accompanied by repetitive manual automatisms and loss of consciousness (automotor seizure).

EEG classification: Abnormal III (awake)

Seizure: EEG seizure pattern, FT9
Automotor seizure

EEG report: This EEG documents a left temporal lobe seizure in left temporal lobe epilepsy.

EEG seizure pattern, right mesial temporal

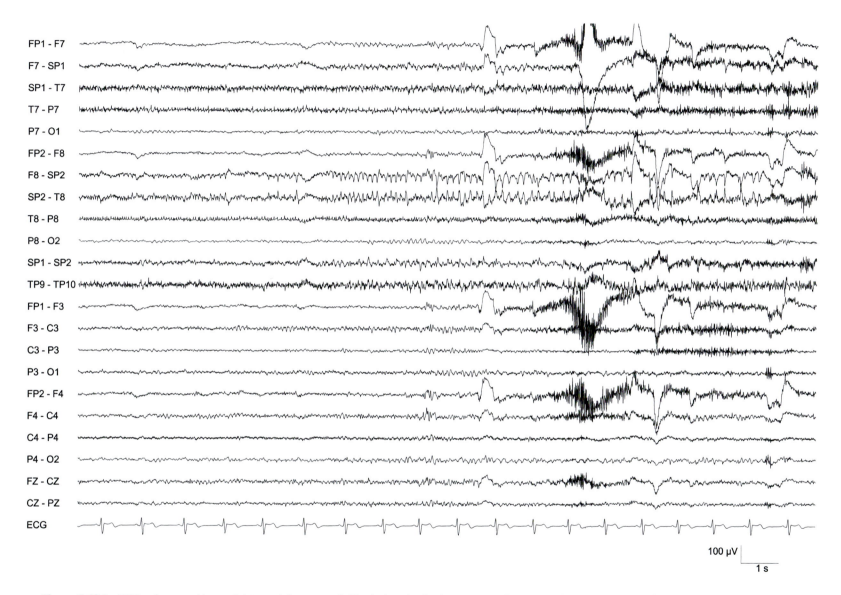

100 μV

1 s

▶ **Figure 3.184** **EEG seizure pattern, right mesial temporal.** Bipolar longitudinal montage. A 34-year-old patient with right focal epilepsy of unknown etiology. At EEG seizure onset, SP2 rhythmic theta waves are recorded. Clinically, loss of consciousness with manual and oral automatisms occurred (automotor seizures).

EEG classification: Abnormal III (awake)

Seizure: EEG seizure pattern, SP2
Automotor seizure

EEG report: This EEG documents a right mesial temporal seizure.

EEG seizure pattern, right mesial temporal

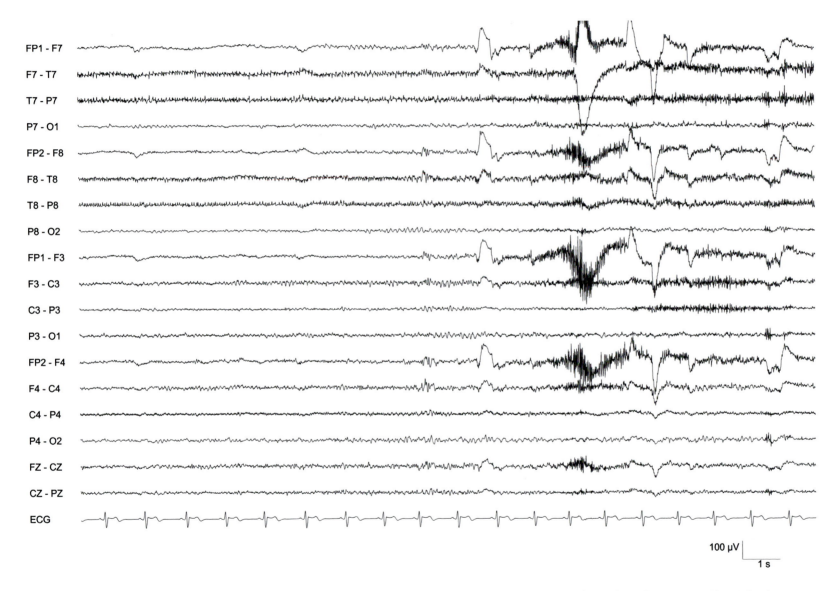

FP1 - F7

F7 - T7

T7 - P7

P7 - O1

FP2 - F8

F8 - T8

T8 - P8

P8 - O2

FP1 - F3

F3 - C3

C3 - P3

P3 - O1

FP2 - F4

F4 - C4

C4 - P4

P4 - O2

FZ - CZ

CZ - PZ

ECG

100 µV

1 s

▶ **Figure 3.185**   **EEG seizure pattern, right mesial temporal.** Bipolar longitudinal montage. Same EEG section as in ▶ **Figure 3.184**. The EEG seizure pattern shown in ▶ **Figure 3.184** cannot be appreciated without the right sphenoidal electrode (SP2).

EEG seizure pattern, frontal nonlateralized; propagation to the right temporal

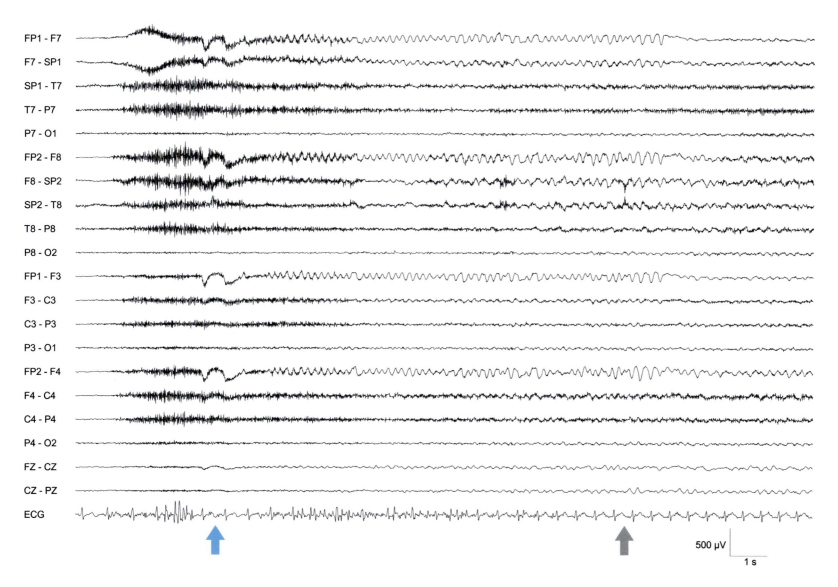

▶ **Figure 3.186** **EEG seizure pattern, frontal nonlateralized; propagation to the right temporal.** Bipolar longitudinal montage. A 34-year-old patient with right focal epilepsy of unknown etiology. After a 4-s burst of muscle artifacts, rhythmic theta waves (blue arrow) appeared bilaterally in the frontopolar regions and then spread into the right mesial temporal region (maximum in electrode SP2; gray arrow). Clinically, there was loss of consciousness with manual and oral automatisms (automotor seizure).

EEG classification: Abnormal III (awake)

Seizure: EEG seizure pattern, FP2 = FP1
Automotor seizure

EEG report: This EEG documents a bilateral frontal onset seizure. The seizure then spreads into the right mesial temporal region, suggesting a right hemispheric epileptogenic zone.

Invasive EEG seizure pattern, left mesial temporal; propagation to left frontal

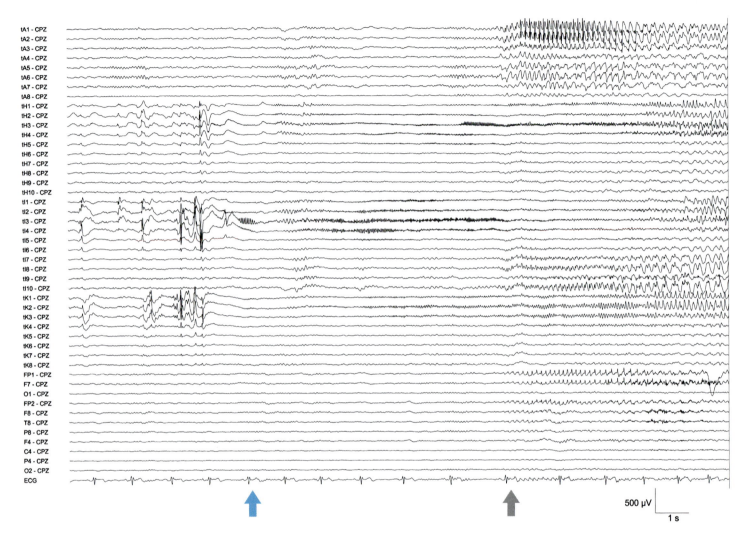

▶ **Figure 3.187** **Invasive EEG seizure pattern, left mesial temporal; propagation to left frontal.** Selection (from a 128-channel recording) of a combination of surface EEG and invasive EEG montage with left frontal, temporal, and insular stereotactically implanted depth electrodes. The location of the invasive electrodes is shown in ▶ **Figure 3.188**. Above the ECG, there are 11 EEG channels recording the activity with scalp electrodes. All the depth electrodes are identified by an initial "t," followed by the letter that identifies one of the depth electrode.

A 35-year-old patient with seizures since the age of 28 years. His MRI was negative. The noninvasive ictal and interictal EEG, the semiology of the seizures, and ictal single-photon emission computed tomography suggested a left frontal, temporal, or insular seizure onset. At seizure onset, a high-frequency EEG seizure pattern arose from the left mesial temporal region (blue arrow) and within 7 s spread to the left frontal region. The surface electrodes did not show any EEG seizure pattern corresponding to the left mesial temporal origin of the seizure recorded with depth electrodes and only reflected the propagation to the left frontal region (gray arrow).

EEG classification: Abnormal III (depth and surface electrodes—awake)

Seizure: EEG seizure pattern, left mesial temporal (paroxysmal beta, tI3>tI4)
Automotor seizure

EEG report: This invasive EEG documents a left mesial temporal seizure origin and supports the diagnosis of a left mesial temporal lobe epilepsy.

Invasive electrode position

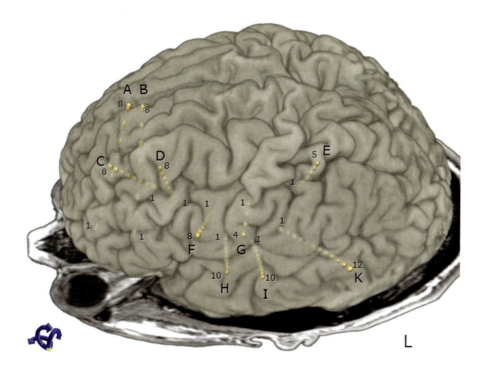

▶ **Figure 3.188** **Invasive electrode position.** Position of the stereotactically implanted depth electrodes of the patient in ▶ **Figure 3.187** (image fusion by Dr. C. Vollmar). View of the left brain hemisphere from diagonally above. Electrodes A–D are located in the frontal lobe, electrodes E–G in the insula, and electrodes H–K in the temporal lobe of the left hemisphere.

epilepsies, the ictal surface EEG is often obscured by movement and muscle artifacts (Salanova et al., 1995).

The rhythmical temporal theta bursts of drowsiness (psychomotor variant) must be distinguished from EEG seizure patterns (▶ **Figure 3.194**) (Klass & Westmoreland, 1985).The amplitude of this EEG pattern is spindle modulated but has no further evolution in frequency or morphology. This pattern has no pathological significance (▶ **Table 3.11**).

Negative myoclonic seizures sometimes are difficult to distinguish from positive myoclonic seizures. In these instances, polygraphic recordings can

document that negative myoclonus consistently is accompanied by muscle atonia (▶ **Figure 3.195**) (Noachtar et al., 1997).

It is also important to remember that sometimes clinical semiology may be subtle and will only be detected if detailed ictal and postictal testing is done (Beniczky et al., 2016). For example, we use a reaction time measurement (clicker test) to detect prolonged reaction times during short bursts of EEG slow (▶ **Figures 3.13** and **3.147–3.149**) (Browne et al., 1974). Slow spike–waves (▶ **Figures 3.154–3.156**) do not correlate well with clinical symptoms ("atypical absences"; Holmes et al., 1987).

Intense clinical testing should be performed during and immediately after recording a clinical seizure following a systematic procedure (Beniczky et al., 2016):

- Presentation of a test word for later testing of memory. This is of limited value if the EEG seizure pattern is of short duration. The result of this test is only of value if it can be documented objectively that the word to remember was given to the patient *during* the seizure and not postictally (▶ **Figures 3.147, 3.148,** and **3.153**).
- Have the patient describe the aura if the patient is able to talk.
- "Tell me your first name."
- "Please extend your arms."
- Have the patient name objects.
- If this is not possible, have the patient name the use of the objects or have them demonstrate the use of the object.
- Appropriate testing should be done in the immediate postictal period to detect postictal semiology (e.g., postictal Todd's paralysis, postictal aphasia, postictal neglect, etc.).
- After the attack, the examiner should ask the patient, "When was your last seizure?" The patient should be asked to describe in detail the seizure that just occurred if the patient remembers the current seizure. On the other hand, if the patient says that "the seizure was some time ago," appropriate testing must be done to ensure the patient does not assume that "we all know he had a seizure now" and the examiner is asking for the last seizure before the current seizure.

Both interictal and ictal information are classified independently of each other so that it is clear on which information the classification is based (Lüders et al., 2019). Seizure-like events during the recordings that are not accompanied

EEG seizure pattern, left; flattening on the left

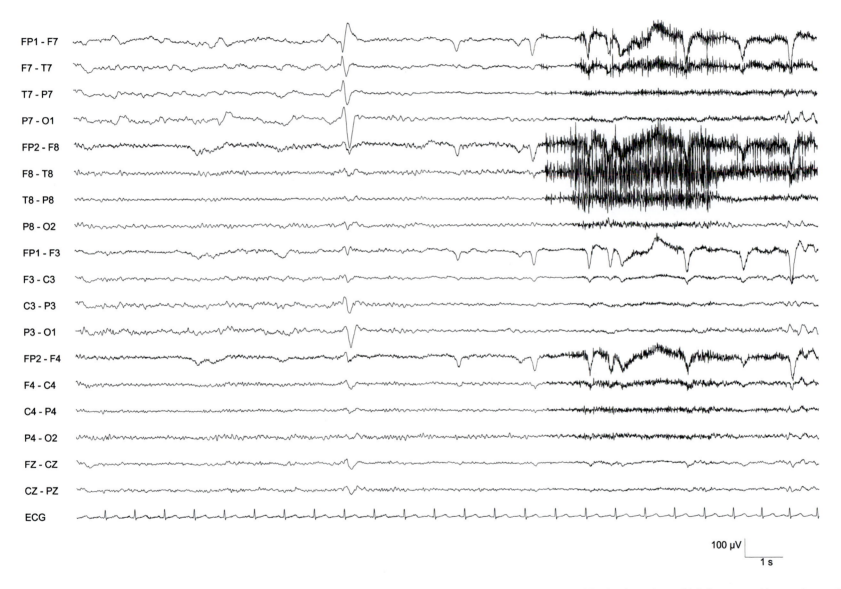

100 µV

1 s

▶ **Figure 3.189** **EEG seizure pattern, left; flattening on the left.** Bipolar longitudinal montage. An 80-year-old aphasic patient with left temporal hemorrhage after left middle cerebral artery infarction. The EEG flattened on the left hemisphere following a left temporal spike. During the seizure, the aphasic patient no longer responded to various stimuli. See ▶ **Figure 3.193** for EEG classification and report.

EEG seizure pattern, left; continuation of Figure 3.189

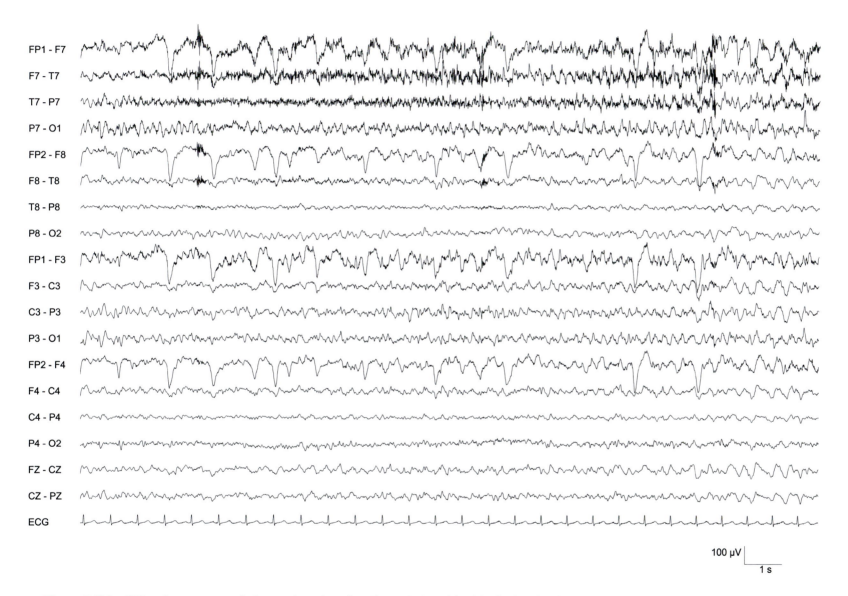

100 µV

1 s

▶ **Figure 3.190** **EEG seizure pattern, left; continuation of** ▶ **Figure 3.189 with a bipolar longitudinal montage.** A rhythmic theta activity developed over the left hemisphere. The left temporal EEG seizure pattern gradually slowed down and increased in amplitude. See ▶ **Figure 3.193** for EEG classification and report.

EEG seizure pattern, left; continuation of Figure 3.190

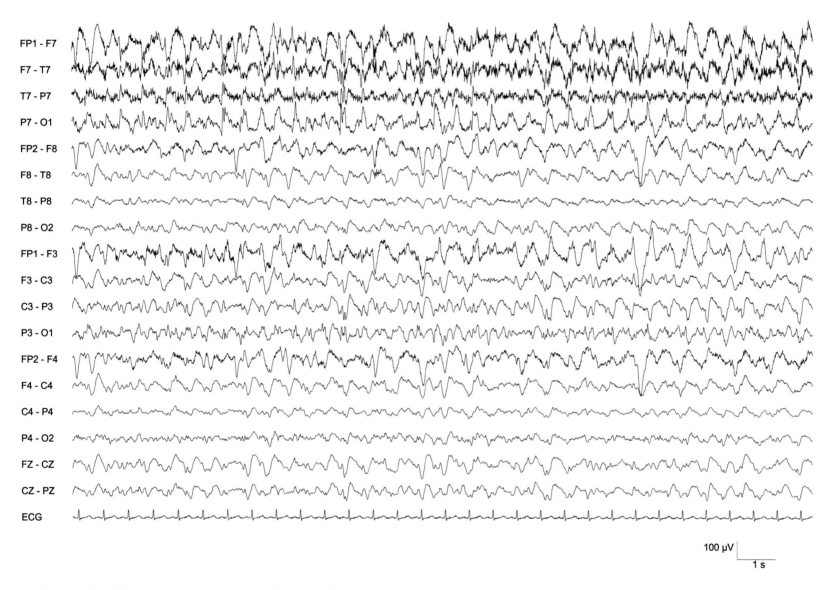

100 µV

1 s

▶ **Figure 3.191** **EEG seizure pattern, left; continuation of** ▶ **Figure 3.190 with bipolar longitudinal montage.** The rhythmic delta activity on the left continues to slow down, with a slight decrease in amplitude. See ▶ **Figure 3.193** for EEG classification and report.

EEG seizure pattern, left; continuation of Figure 3.191

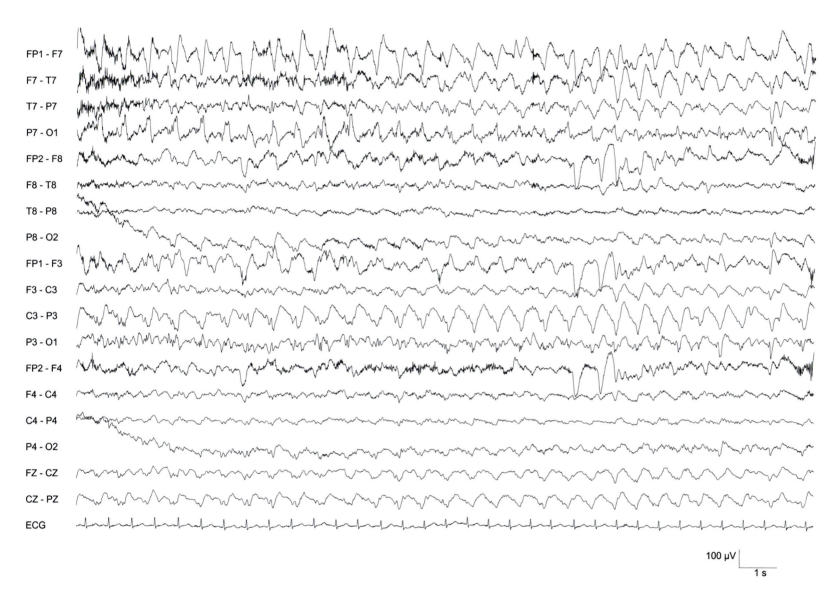

FP1 - F7
F7 - T7
T7 - P7
P7 - O1
FP2 - F8
F8 - T8
T8 - P8
P8 - O2
FP1 - F3
F3 - C3
C3 - P3
P3 - O1
FP2 - F4
F4 - C4
C4 - P4
P4 - O2
FZ - CZ
CZ - PZ
ECG

100 µV
1 s

▶ **Figure 3.192** **EEG seizure pattern, left; continuation of** ▶ **Figure 3.191 with a bipolar longitudinal montage.** The rhythmic delta activity on the left slows down and less theta waves are present. See ▶ **Figure 3.193** for EEG classification and report.

EEG seizure pattern, left; continuation of Figure 3.192

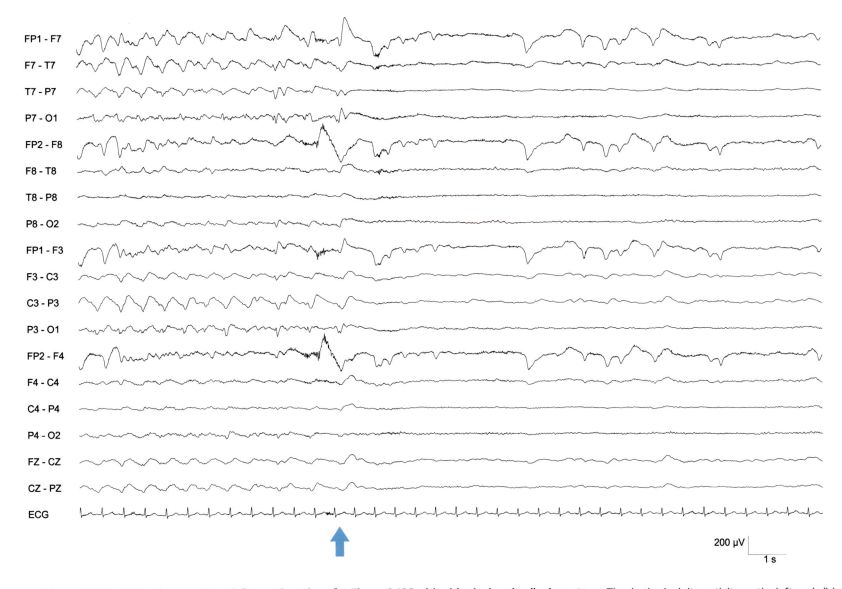

FP1 - F7
F7 - T7
T7 - P7
P7 - O1
FP2 - F8
F8 - T8
T8 - P8
P8 - O2
FP1 - F3
F3 - C3
C3 - P3
P3 - O1
FP2 - F4
F4 - C4
C4 - P4
P4 - O2
FZ - CZ
CZ - PZ
ECG

200 μV
1 s

▶ **Figure 3.193** EEG seizure pattern, left; continuation of ▶ Figure 3.192 with a bipolar longitudinal montage. The rhythmic delta activity on the left ends (blue arrow) and is followed by left hemisphere irregular delta waves with frontal maximum.

EEG classification: Abnormal III (awake)
1. Spikes, F7 > T7
2. Continuous slow, left temporal
3. Asymmetry, decreased alpha activity left
4. Seizure: EEG seizure pattern, F7 > T7
   Dialeptic seizure

EEG report: This EEG documents a dialeptic seizure arising from the left temporal region.

Rhythmic temporal theta burst of drowsiness

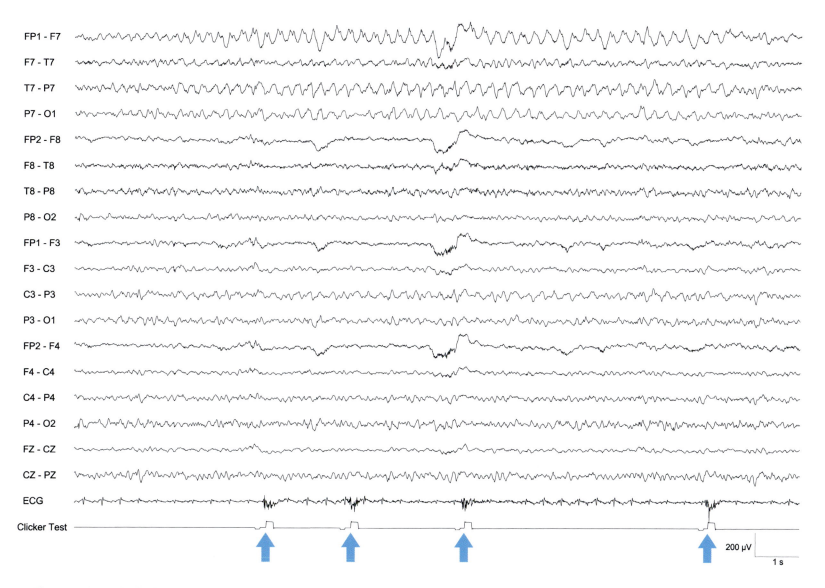

FP1 - F7
F7 - T7
T7 - P7
P7 - O1
FP2 - F8
F8 - T8
T8 - P8
P8 - O2
FP1 - F3
F3 - C3
C3 - P3
P3 - O1
FP2 - F4
F4 - C4
C4 - P4
P4 - O2
FZ - CZ
CZ - PZ
ECG
Clicker Test

200 µV

1 s

▶ **Figure 3.194** **Rhythmic temporal theta burst of drowsiness.** Bipolar longitudinal montage. A 25-year-old with vasovagal syncope. The patient responded adequately to acoustic stimuli (blue arrows) while the EEG showed the burst of left temporal rhythmical theta activity. This EEG pattern has no pathological significance.

EEG classification: Normal (awake)

EEG report: Normal EEG.

EEG seizure pattern, left central; negative myoclonic seizure, right arm

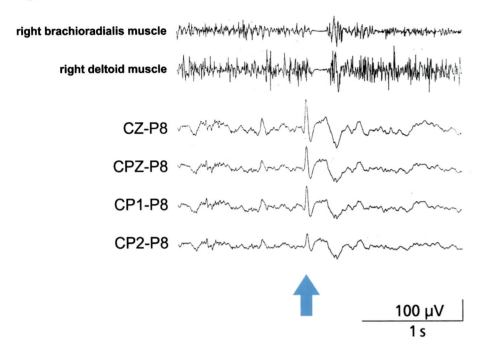

right brachioradialis muscle

right deltoid muscle

CZ-P8

CPZ-P8

CP1-P8

CP2-P8

100 µV

1 s

▶ **Figure 3.195** **EEG seizure pattern, left central; negative myoclonic seizure, right arm.** Detail of a 32-channel polygraphic derivation. To illustrate the relationship between the left centroparietal spike (blue arrow) and the subsequent short muscular atonia (silent period) in the right brachioradial and the deltoid muscle, only four centroparietal electrodes are shown.

This 28-year-old patient with extensive perinatal left-brain damage has a left focal epilepsy, a mild spastic hemiparesis on the right side, and a mild cognitive impairment since early childhood. The negative myoclonus is only detectable with muscle activation. In this example, the patient held his arms outstretched during the recording.

EEG classification: Abnormal III (awake)

Seizure: EEG seizure pattern, left centroparietal (CZ > CPZ > CP1)

Negative myoclonic seizure, right arm

EEG report: This EEG documents a left centroparietal epileptic origin of a negative myoclonic seizure of the right arm.

by an EEG change and cannot reliably be diagnosed clinically as epileptic should be classified as "paroxysmal events." The recording of non-epileptic seizures in EEG video monitoring is relatively common; non-epileptic attacks not infrequently are misdiagnosed as epileptic seizures (Benbadis, 2005). The differential diagnosis of epileptic seizures includes a long list of etiologies, but the most frequent non-epileptic paroxysmal events are syncope in elderly people and dissociative disorders in younger people. In the differential diagnosis between epileptic and non-epileptic paroxysmal events, the recording of a normal physiological occipital background rhythm in a nonresponsive patient strongly suggests that the paroxysmal event is a non-epileptic functional event (psychogenic spell) (Lüders & Noachtar, 2000b).

EEG Seizure Patterns

EEG seizure patterns in generalized epilepsies frequently are identical or very similar to interictal patterns, except that their duration is more prolonged. EEG seizure patterns in focal epilepsies are extremely variable, but consistently the epileptic discharges show major changes in frequency, amplitude, morphology, and distribution. The distribution of the EEG seizure pattern at the beginning of the EEG seizure reliably lateralizes the epileptogenic zone.

Ictal EEG changes are classified as EEG seizure pattern or EEG status pattern depending on whether the patient had an epileptic seizure or status epilepticus. The localization of the EEG seizure (status) pattern is indicated in each case. In the four-dimensional epilepsy classification that we use in our laboratories, the classification of the clinical epileptic seizure (status) is based exclusively on the semiological characteristics of the seizure and should be defined independently of the EEG seizure (status) pattern (Lüders et al., 2019).

The EEG seizure pattern of patients with focal epilepsy contains only one clinically significant piece of information, namely the *initial lateralization* of the EEG seizure pattern that with few exceptions lateralizes correctly the epileptogenic zone. On the other hand, the *initial location* of the scalp EEG seizure pattern not infrequently is misleading because with scalp electrodes, the EEG seizure pattern can only be recorded after it has spread outside the epileptogenic zone (Rémi et al., 2011a). This is particularly true in extratemporal epilepsies (Rémi et al., 2011a).

The classification of regional epileptic seizure patterns lists first the expression "EEG seizure pattern" followed by a comma and a somatotopic modifier (a specific electrode[s], left or right hemisphere, or unlocalizable). The localization should be defined ideally by listing the one to three electrodes of the highest amplitude at the beginning of the seizure. These electrodes should be listed in decreasing order of amplitude. The ">"symbol should be used if the preceding electrode was of higher amplitude, and the "="symbol should be used if the preceding electrode was of equal amplitude. The following are examples:

EEG seizure pattern, F4 = FZ > CZ (▶ **Figure 3.196**)
EEG seizure pattern, F4 = FZ = CZ (▶ **Figure 3.197**)

Special phenomena are the periodic regional or lateralized discharges that are related to a relatively characteristic clinical picture, namely an acute cerebral lesion and/or a highly epileptogenic focal epilepsy.

The EEG seizure pattern of generalized epilepsies contains two parameters of clinical significance:

1. The generalized distribution of the EEG seizure pattern indicates that the epileptogenic zone is *generalized*.
2. The EEG seizure pattern of generalized epilepsies usually, but not always, consists of prolonged interictal EEG discharges. The EEG characteristics of the ictal pattern frequently are closely related to the symptomatology of the generalized seizures. The following ictal EEG patterns are related to relatively specific generalized clinical seizures:
   a. Spike–wave → dialeptic seizure
   b. Polyspike–wave → dialeptic status
   c. 3 Hz spike–wave → dialeptic status
   d. Paroxysmal fast (relatively shorter duration) → myoclonic seizures
   e. Paroxysmal fast (relatively longer duration) → generalized tonic seizure
   f. Electrodecremental → epileptic spasm

In the classification of generalized EEG seizure patterns, we specify (a) the initial distribution of the epileptic EEG pattern and(b) the characteristic of the initial EEG discharge if it is related to a relatively specific type of generalized epileptic seizures—for example,

EEG seizure pattern (3 Hz spike–wave), generalized

EEGs that do not include an epileptic seizure or status are classified by indicating the degree of abnormality (I, II, or III), followed by the clinical level of consciousness (awake, sleep, etc.) listed in parenthesis. After an indentation, the different EEG abnormalities are listed.

EEGs that include an EEG seizure/status (without clinical manifestations) are classified as follows:

Example (▶ **Figure 3.198**)
    EEG classification: Abnormal III (awake)
    1. Continuous slow, right frontopolar
    2. Asymmetry, increased beta, reight frontal
    3. Status: EEG status pattern, FP2 > F8 > F4
            No clinical symptoms

Example (▶ **Figure 3.196**)
    EEG classification: Abnormal III (awake)
    1. Continuous slow, right frontopolar
    2. Seizure: EEG seizure pattern, F4 = FZ > CZ
            No clinical symptoms

EEGs that include an EEG and clinical seizure are classified as follows:

Example (▶ **Figures 3.189–3.193**)
    EEG classification: Abnormal III (awake)
    1. Spikes, F7 > T7
    2. Continuous slow, left temporal
    3. Asymmetry, decreased alpha activity left
    4. Seizure: EEG seizure pattern, F7 > T7
            Dialeptic seizure

Example (▶ **Figure 3.159**)
    EEG classification: Abnormal III (awake and sleep)
    1. Hypsarrhythmia
    2. Seizure: EEG seizure pattern (electrodecremental), generalized
            Epileptic spasms

EEGs that include a status epilepticus are classified as follows, with the percentage of the recording (or, as discussed below, the percentage of the EEG pattern) that is occupied by the status listed in parentheses after the expression EEG status:

EEG seizure pattern, right mesial frontal. Left ear reference montage

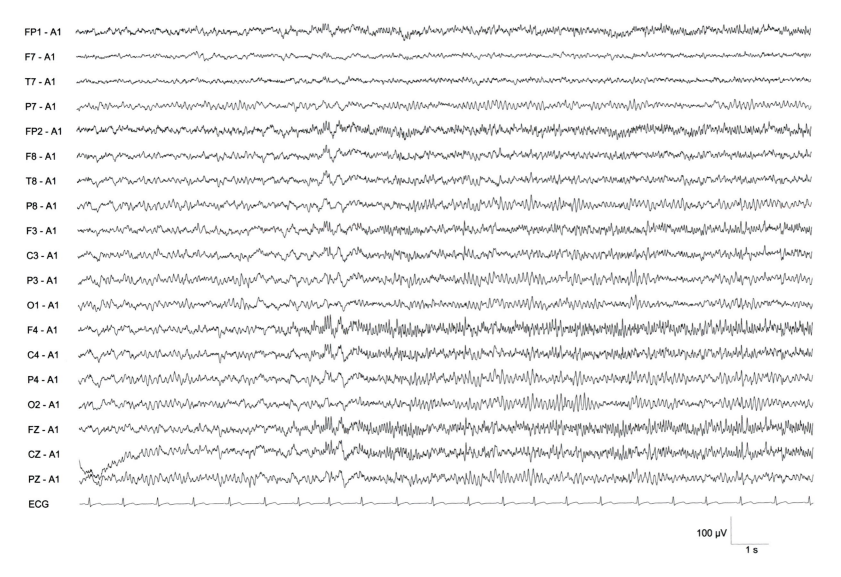

100 μV

1 s

▶ **Figure 3.196** **EEG seizure pattern, right mesial frontal.** Left ear reference montage. An 18-year-old female patient with right frontal lobe epilepsy of unknown etiology. The EEG shows a right mesial frontal seizure pattern consisting of rhythmical beta frequency with a maximum in the electrodes F4 and FZ. Clinically, the patient was inconspicuous during this EEG seizure pattern. Note the slow artifact in electrode CZ at the beginning of the EEG trace.

EEG classification: Abnormal III (awake)

Seizure: EEG classification: Abnormal III (awake)
 1. Continuous slow, right frontopolar
 2. Seizure: EEG seizure pattern, F4 = FZ > CZ
   No clinical symptoms

EEG report: This EEG documents a right mesial frontal subclinical seizure.

EEG seizure pattern, right mesial frontal. Left ear reference montage

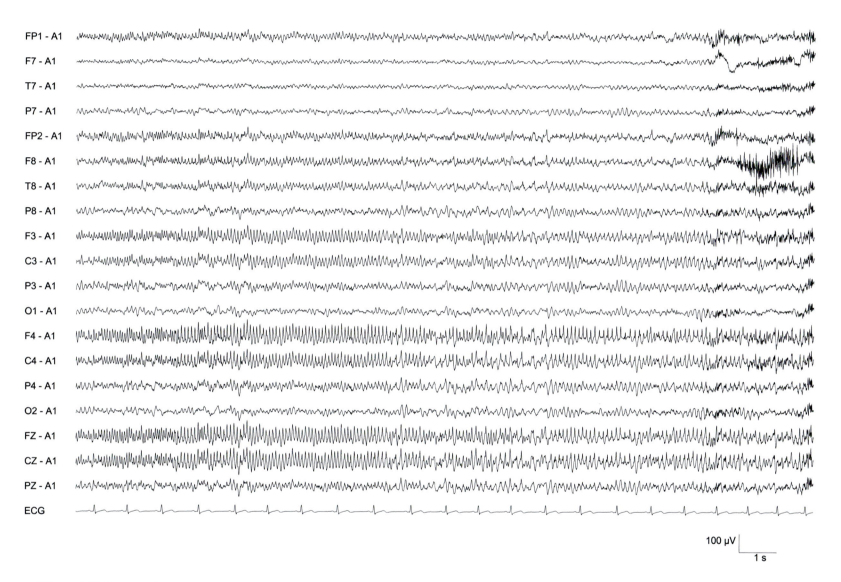

100 µV

1 s

▶ **Figure 3.197** **EEG seizure pattern, right mesial frontal.** Left ear reference montage. Continuation of ▶ **Figure 3.196**. The seizure spreads to include electrode C4 and, to a lesser extent, the contralateral electrode F3. In the last few seconds of the EEG trace, there is an EMG artifact due to movement. No clinical symptoms of the seizure were observed during this period of the EEG video monitoring.

EEG classification: Abnormal III (sleep)

Seizure: EEG seizure pattern, F4 = FZ = CZ
No clinical symptoms

EEG report: See ▶ **Figure 3.196**.

EEG status pattern, right frontopolar

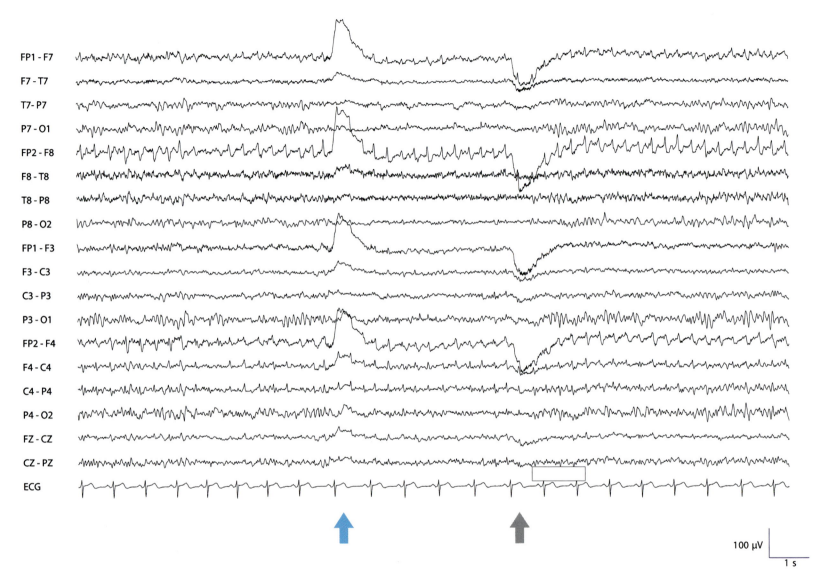

FP1 - F7
F7 - T7
T7 - P7
P7 - O1
FP2 - F8
F8 - T8
T8 - P8
P8 - O2
FP1 - F3
F3 - C3
C3 - P3
P3 - O1
FP2 - F4
F4 - C4
C4 - P4
P4 - O2
FZ - CZ
CZ - PZ
ECG

100 µV

1 s

▶ **Figure 3.198** **EEG status pattern, right frontopolar.** Bipolar longitudinal montage. A 23-year-old patient who suffered a right frontopolar concussion at age 20 years. Clinically, there was a mild frontal brain syndrome and rare nocturnal tonic seizures, which could be controlled with medication. Repeated EEGs showed continuous spikes at a repetition of 2–3.5 Hz. The occipital region shows a well-developed alpha background rhythm on both hemispheres. Eye opening (blue arrow) and eye closure (gray arrow) as well as various anti-seizure drugs (intravenous and oral) had no influence on the right frontopolar EEG status pattern. During EEG recording, the patient was fully responsive and clinically inconspicuous.

EEG classification: Abnormal III (awake)
   1. Continuous slow, right frontopolar
   2. Asymmetry, increased beta, right frontal
   3. Status: EEG status pattern, FP2 > F8 >F4
           No clinical symptoms

EEG report: This EEG documents a subclinical right frontopolar epileptic status as an expression of post-traumatic right frontal lobe epilepsy.

Example (▶ **Figure 3.199**)

EEG classification: Abnormal III (delirious)
1. Continuous slow, left hemisphere
2. Asymmetry, decreased alpha activity left
3. Status (90%): EEG seizure pattern, T7 > P7 = F7
   Delirious status

Example (▶ **Figures 3.200–3.205**)

EEG classification: Abnormal III (awake)
1. Continuous slow, left hemisphere
2. Seizure: Periodic EEG seizure pattern, F7
   Aphasic seizure

Example (▶ **Figure 3.167**)

EEG classification: Abnormal III (awake)
Seizure: EEG seizure pattern (spike–wave), generalized
   Dialeptic seizure

Example (▶ **Figure 3.172**)

1. Seizure: EEG, pattern (polyspikes), generalized
   Myoclonic seizure, generalized
2. Spikes, generalized

Example (▶ **Figure 3.181**)

Seizure: EEG seizure pattern, T7 > F7 > P7
   Abdominal aura → automotor seizure

Example (▶ **Figure 3.195**)

Seizure: EEG seizure pattern, CZ > CPZ = CP1
   Negative myoclonic seizure, right arm

3.4.2.4.10.1 Semiological Seizure Classification

The semiological seizure classification classifies seizures exclusively based on their clinical symptomatology, including the subjective symptoms the patient may report (Lüders et al., 1998, 2019. The latest version of the semiological seizure classification is presented in **Appendix 2**.

3.4.2.4.11 Status Patterns (STP)

Status epilepticus is defined as a sequence of at least two consecutive epileptic seizures without regaining consciousness (or the patient's baseline) or as an epileptic seizure lasting more than 5 min (Trinka et al., 2015). EEG status patterns are very similar to EEG seizure patterns (Feddersen & Trinka, 2012) but are of longer duration. Status epilepticus occurs in generalized and focal epilepsies. Convulsive status epilepticus is easy to detect clinically. This also includes the unilateral clonic status epilepticus (epilepsia partialis continua) (Thomas et al., 1977). In approximately half of the cases, status epilepticus cannot be detected in scalp recordings because the epileptogenic zone is too small or lies in the depth of a sulcus. In the case of seizures with a disturbance of consciousness, however, an EEG status pattern almost invariably can be detected with scalp electrodes. The exception is patients suffering from dialeptic status and the EEG is obscured by EMG and other artifacts. In other words, if the routine scalp EEG shows no EEG status pattern and the EEG is not obscured by artifacts, patients most likely do not suffer from status epilepticus, and another explanation for the clinical behavior must be found (e.g., psychogenic paroxysmal events). Clinically, nonconvulsive status epilepticus may be difficult to distinguish from non-epileptic states of confusion or encephalopathies (see Section 3.4.2.6). Frequently, only EEG recordings can distinguish these conditions.

In patients with Lennox–Gastaut syndrome, the generalized slow spike–waves are sometimes referred to as petit mal status, although in these mentally challenged patients it is often not possible to distinguish between interictal and ictal states (▶ **Figure 3.206**) (Holmes et al., 1987). Also, in patients suffering from dialeptic status epilepticus, the spike components of the generalized spike–wave complexes frequently appear "truncated" (▶ **Figures 3.207** and **3.208**), making it difficult to make the correct diagnosis even when an EEG is obtained. Occasionally, between the spike–wave bursts, a diffuse 8 Hz alpha activity can be seen (▶ **Figures 3.207** and **3.208**). Dialeptic status with spike–wave EEG status pattern often can be "broken" by a single injection of benzodiazepine (▶ **Figure 3.209**). The EEG status patterns in juvenile absence epilepsy may consist of long bursts of generalized spike– and polyspike–waves (▶ **Figure 3.210**) or, more rarely, long runs of paroxysmal fast (▶ **Figure 3.211**). Bursts of generalized spikes and polyspike–waves also characterize the generalized myoclonic status.

EEG status pattern, left temporal

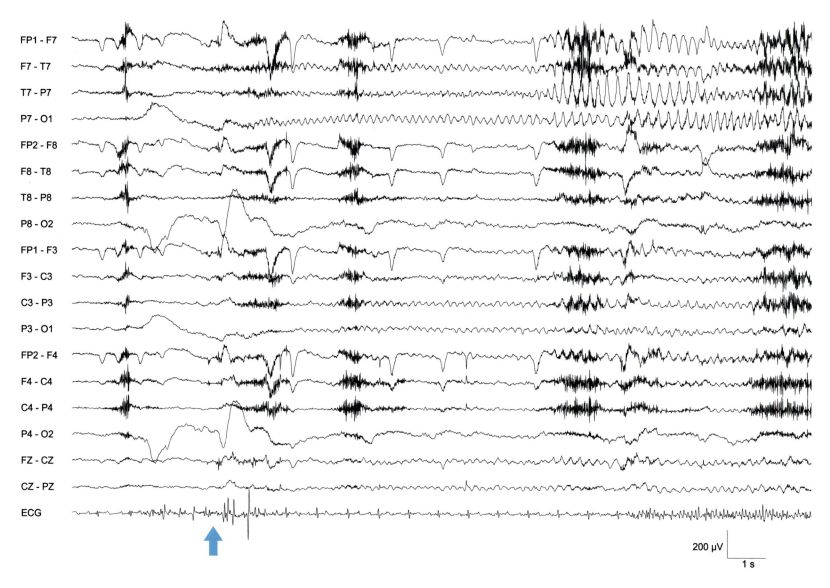

▶ **Figure 3.199** **EEG status pattern, left temporal.** Bipolar longitudinal montage. A 53-year-old female patient with focal epilepsy due to a left temporo-occipital dermoid tumor. Discontinuation of the anti-seizure medication led to the EEG status pattern seen in this figure. This EEG pattern recurred every few minutes. The EEG status pattern initially was characterized by rhythmic, approximately 8 Hz theta activity at electrodes T7 = P7 (blue arrow). During the status, the patient was confused and aphasic.

EEG classification: Abnormal III (awake)
  1. Continuous slow, left hemisphere
  2. Asymmetry, decreased alpha activity left
  3. Status (90%): EEG seizure pattern, T7 > P7 = F7
           Delirious status

EEG report: This EEG documents a left temporally generated delirious status epilepticus.

Periodic epileptiform discharges, left

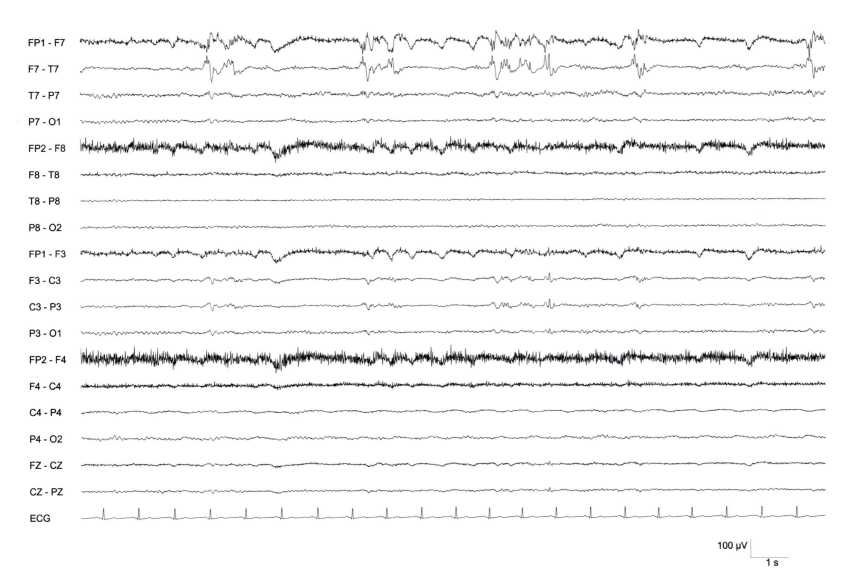

FP1 - F7

F7 - T7

T7 - P7

P7 - O1

FP2 - F8

F8 - T8

T8 - P8

P8 - O2

FP1 - F3

F3 - C3

C3 - P3

P3 - O1

FP2 - F4

F4 - C4

C4 - P4

P4 - O2

FZ - CZ

CZ - PZ

ECG

100 µV

1 s

▶ **Figure 3.200** **Periodic epileptiform discharges, left.** Bipolar longitudinal montage. A 48-year-old female with focal epilepsy due to a biopsy-proven left frontal oligodendroglioma. The anti-seizure medication had been reduced a few days before due to side effects. The patient had been aphasic for a few hours before the EEG was recorded. The EEG shows periodic epileptiform discharges localized to electrode F7. Note the symmetrical, physiological occipital 9 Hz background rhythm and the frequent blinking. The EEG pattern shown in this figure and in ▶ Figures 3.201–2.205 was repeated three times during the 20-min EEG recording. For EEG classification and report, see ▶ Figure 3.205.

EEG status pattern, left frontal; Continuation of Figure 3.200

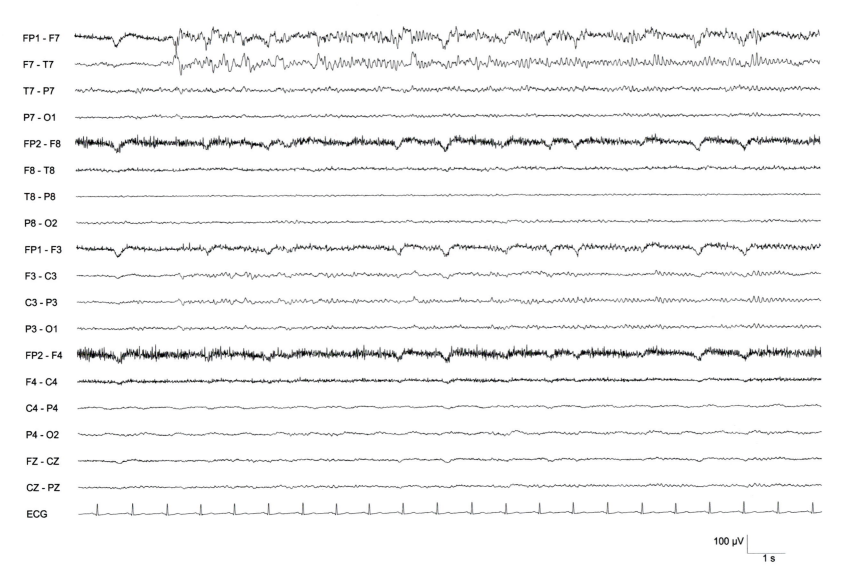

100 µV

1 s

▶ **Figure 3.201**   **EEG status pattern, left frontal.** Bipolar longitudinal montage. Continuation of ▶ **Figure 3.200**. The left-sided periodic epileptiform discharges evolve into a paroxysmal alpha activity at electrode F7. There is still frequent blinking. For EEG classification and report, see ▶ **Figure 3.205**.

EEG status pattern, left frontal; Continuation of Figure 3.201

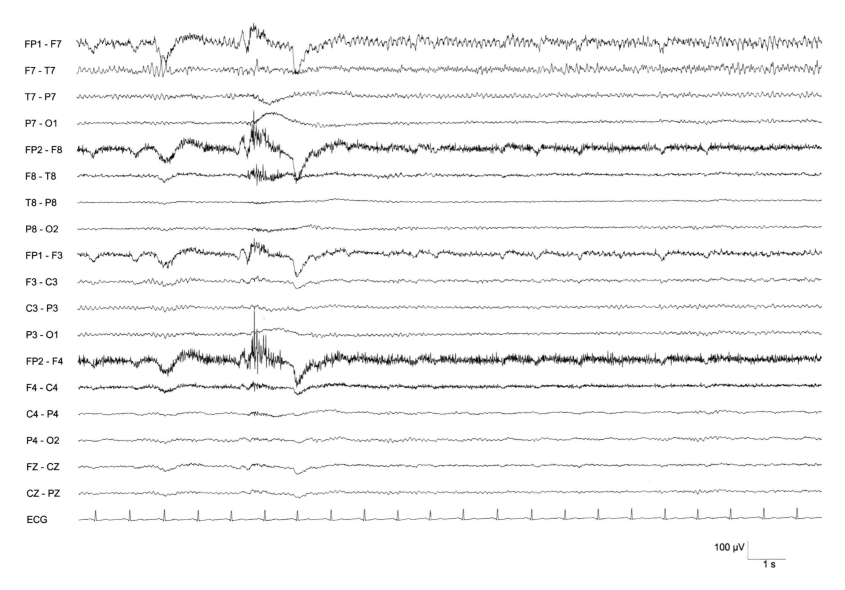

100 µV

1 s

▶ **Figure 3.202** **EEG status pattern, left frontal.** Bipolar longitudinal montage. Continuation of ▶ **Figure 3.201**. The paroxysmal alpha activity with maximum at electrode F7 continues, and paroxysmal beta activity of a similar distribution is now intermingled with the paroxysmal alpha activity.

EEG status pattern, left frontal; Continuation of Figure 3.202

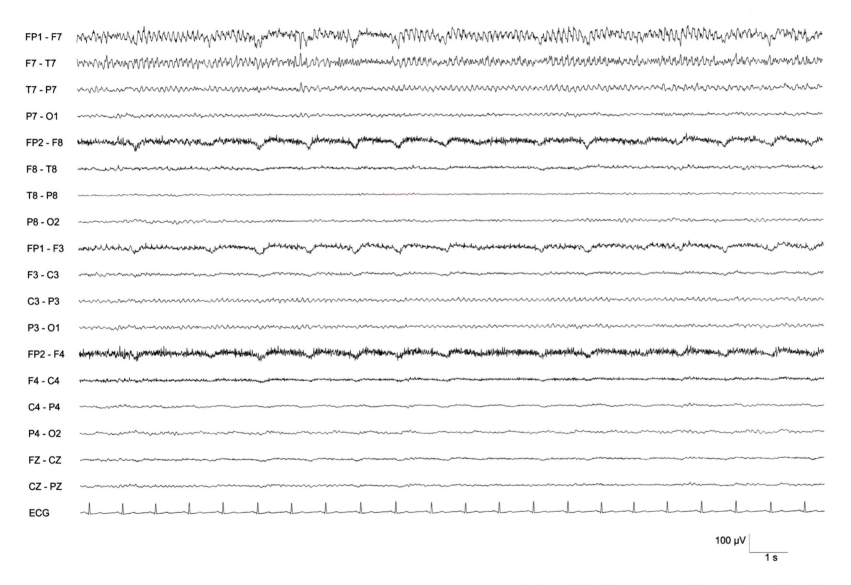

FP1 - F7

F7 - T7

T7 - P7

P7 - O1

FP2 - F8

F8 - T8

T8 - P8

P8 - O2

FP1 - F3

F3 - C3

C3 - P3

P3 - O1

FP2 - F4

F4 - C4

C4 - P4

P4 - O2

FZ - CZ

CZ - PZ

ECG

100 μV

1 s

▶ **Figure 3.203** **EEG status pattern, left frontal.** Bipolar longitudinal montage. Continuation of **Figure 3.202**. The paroxysmal alpha and beta activity with maximum at electrode F7 increases slightly in amplitude, and there is some spread to involve also electrode T7. The blinking increases in frequency and becomes more or less regular at one blink per second. For EEG classification and report, see ▶ **Figure 3.205**.

EEG status pattern, left frontal; Continuation of Figure 3.203

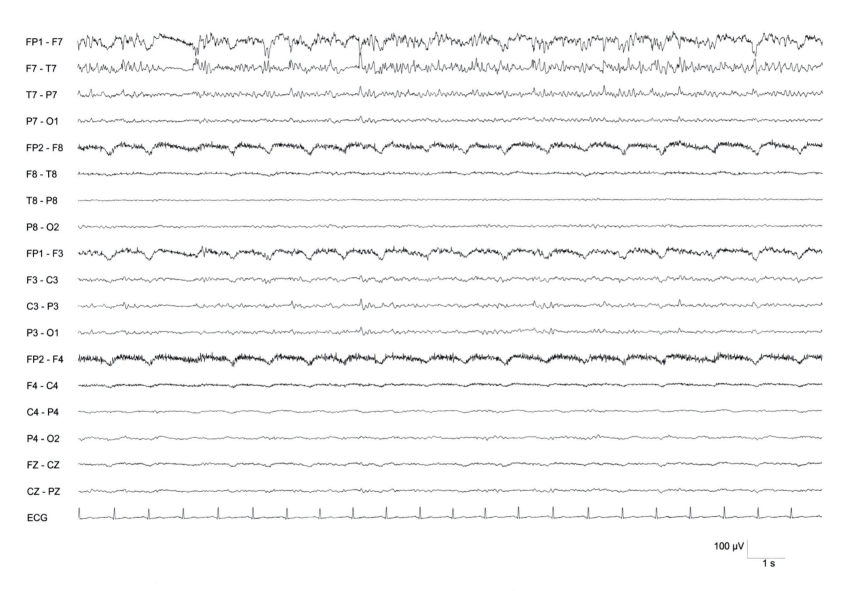

FP1 - F7
F7 - T7
T7 - P7
P7 - O1
FP2 - F8
F8 - T8
T8 - P8
P8 - O2
FP1 - F3
F3 - C3
C3 - P3
P3 - O1
FP2 - F4
F4 - C4
C4 - P4
P4 - O2
FZ - CZ
CZ - PZ
ECG

100 µV

1 s

▶ **Figure 3.204**   **EEG status pattern, left frontal.** Bipolar longitudinal montage. Continuation of ▶ **Figure 3.203**. The paroxysmal alpha and beta activity tends to group itself in a periodic pattern. The paroxysms are still very localized to F7 > T7. For EEG classification and report, see ▶ **Figure 3.205**.

EEG status pattern, left frontal

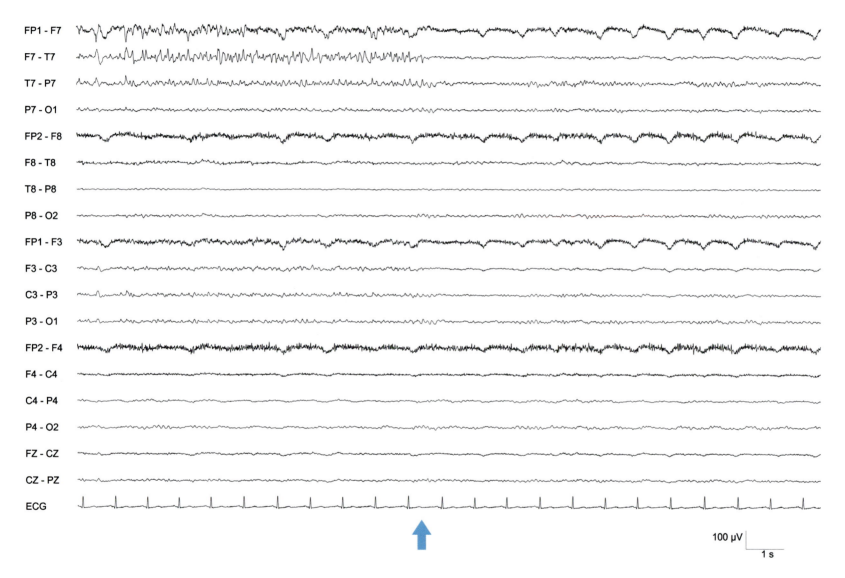

▶ **Figure 3.205** **EEG status pattern, left frontal.** Continuation of ▶ **Figure 3.204**. Bipolar longitudinal montage. The EEG status pattern ends (blue arrow). The aphasic status subsided within a few days following lorazepam administration and adjustment of the anti-seizure medication. Notice the normal alpha rhythm. The frequent blinking continues. The EEG classification and report refer to this figure and ▶ **Figures 3.200–3.204**.

EEG classification: Abnormal III (awake)
1. Continuous slow, left hemisphere
2. Seizure: Periodic EEG seizure pattern, F7
    Aphasic status

EEG report: This EEG documents a left frontal status epilepticus associated with an aphasic status epilepticus.

Slow spike–waves, generalized

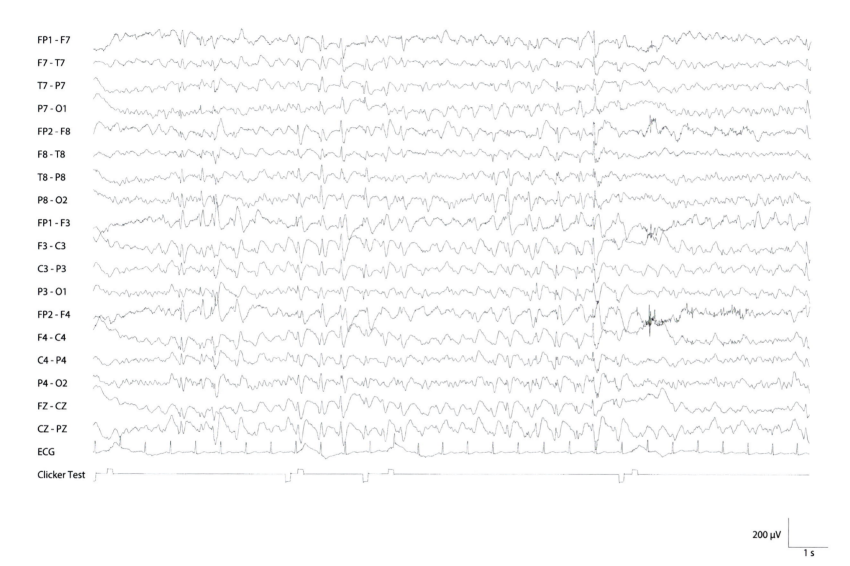

200 µV

1 s

▶ **Figure 3.206** **Slow spike–waves, generalized.** Bipolar longitudinal montage. A 21-year-old patient with Lennox–Gastaut syndrome since age 3 years. The responsiveness to acoustic stimuli (clicker) did not change during or in between the presence of bursts of generalized slow spike–wave. The patient responded consistently to acoustic stimuli (clicker test). The background occipital rhythm was 7 Hz. The EEG also showed a generalized slow.

EEG classification: Abnormal III (awake)
1. Slow spike–waves, generalized
2. Continuous slow, generalized
3. Background slow

EEG report: This EEG supports the diagnosis of Lennox–Gastaut syndrome.

EEG status epilepticus, generalized; de novo dialeptic status in pregnancy

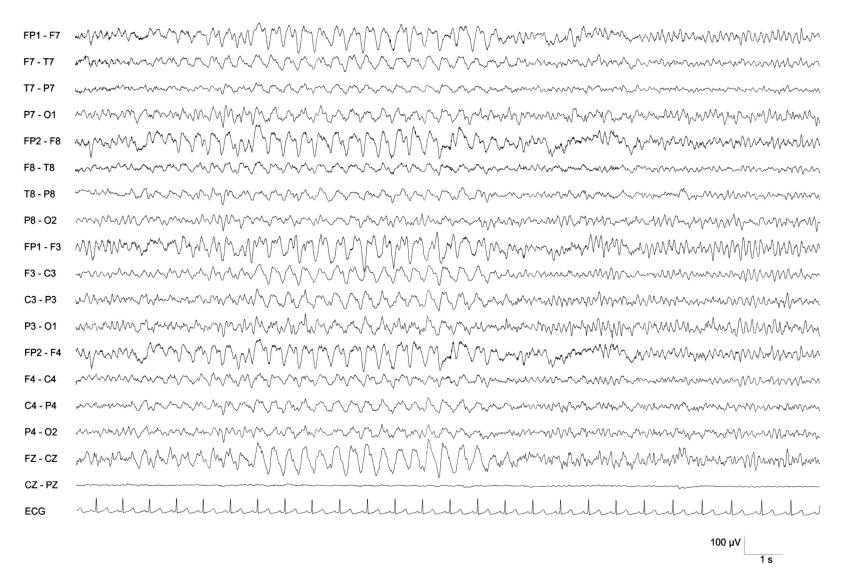

FP1 - F7

F7 - T7

T7 - P7

P7 - O1

FP2 - F8

F8 - T8

T8 - P8

P8 - O2

FP1 - F3

F3 - C3

C3 - P3

P3 - O1

FP2 - F4

F4 - C4

C4 - P4

P4 - O2

FZ - CZ

CZ - PZ

ECG

100 µV

1 s

▶ **Figure 3.207** **EEG status epilepticus, generalized; de novo dialeptic status in pregnancy.** Bipolar longitudinal montage. This 29-year-old female patient suffered a dialeptic status characterized by confusion and mutism for the first time in her life during her first pregnancy. High-amplitude 2.5 Hz delta waves occur in bursts and alternate with diffuse 8 Hz alpha waves. This diffuse alpha rhythm with maximum in the bilateral frontocentral region represents an EEG seizure pattern. It is not an occipital background rhythm. Channel CZ–PZ is defective. See ▶ **Figure 3.208** for EEG classification and report.

EEG status epilepticus, generalized; de novo dialeptic status epilepticus in pregnancy

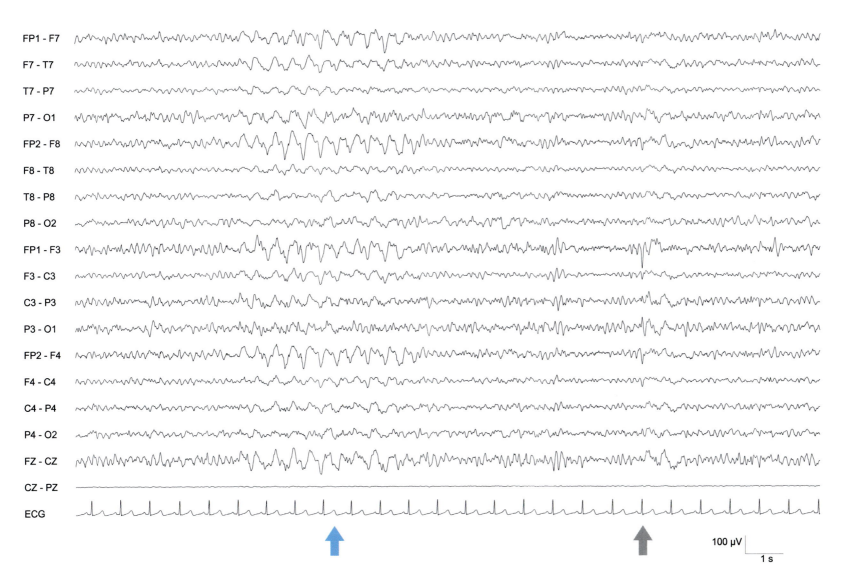

▶ **Figure 3.208**   **EEG status epilepticus, generalized; de novo dialeptic status epilepticus in pregnancy.** Bipolar longitudinal montage. EEG sample from the same EEG as in ▶ **Figure 3.207**. In this EEG sample, the delta burst (blue arrow) is shorter than in ▶ **Figure 3.207**. Alpha activity is diffusely distributed. The patient is not responsive. Note a small left central sharp transient followed by a slow wave (gray arrow) of uncertain clinical significance.

EEG classification: Abnormal III (awake)

        Status: EEG-status pattern (slow spike-waves), generalized
                   Dialeptic status epilepticus

EEG report: This EEG supports the diagnosis of a generalized dialeptic status epilepticus.

EEG status epilepticus, generalized; de novo dialeptic status in pregnancy after lorazepam medication

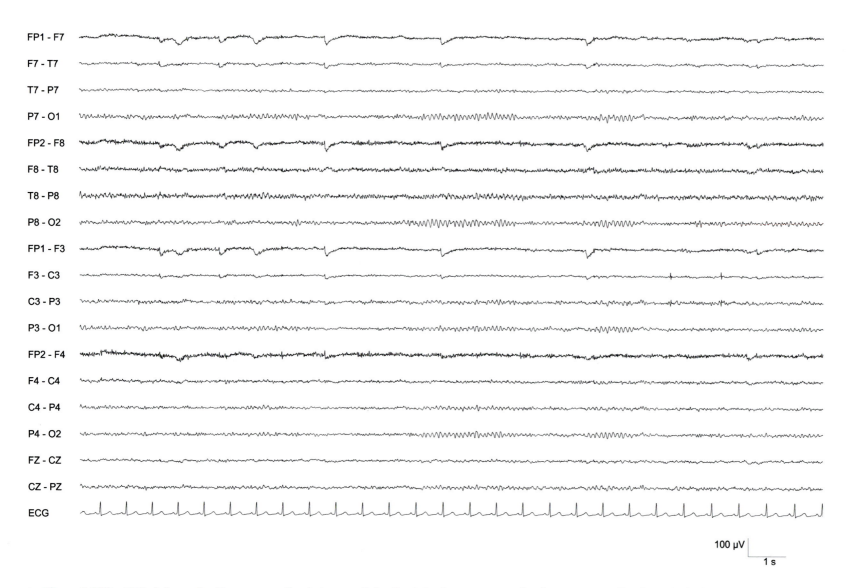

100 μV

1 s

▶ **Figure 3.209**   **EEG status epilepticus, generalized; de novo dialeptic status in pregnancy after lorazepam medication.** Bipolar longitudinal montage. Same patient as in ▶ **Figures 3.207** and **3.208**. The status was broken after intravenous administration of 4 mg lorazepam. Once the EEG status epilepticus subsided, a well-developed, spindle modulated, 11 Hz alpha occipital background activity was recorded the next day. Together with the normalization of the EEG, the patient was back to baseline and again fully conscious and responsive. Note the difference of the occipital alpha rhythm of ▶ **Figure 3.209** and the EEG seizure pattern with diffuse alpha activity of ▶ **Figures 3.207** and **3.208**.

EEG classification: Normal (awake)

EEG report: This EEG shows a normal finding. The generalized dialeptic status epilepticus documented the day before stopped.

EEG status epilepticus; dialeptic status epilepticus

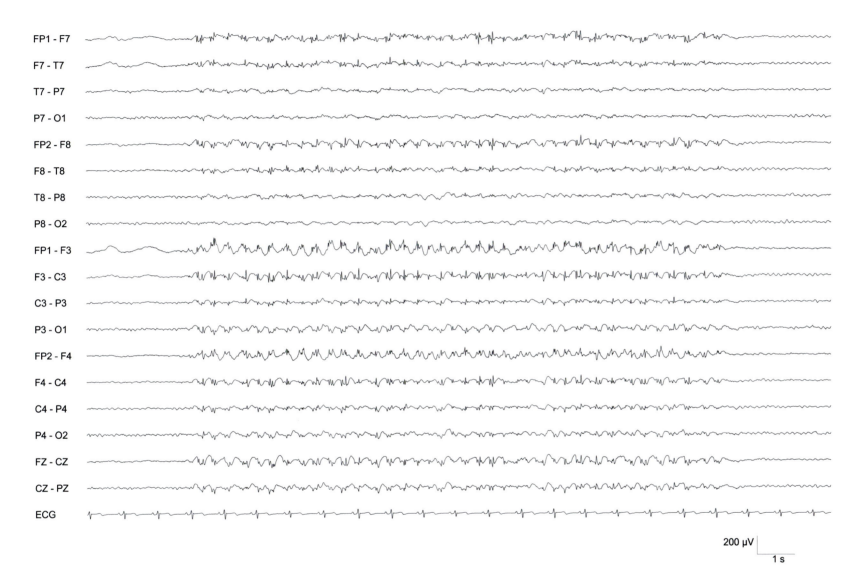

200 μV

1 s

▶ **Figure 3.210** **EEG status epilepticus; dialeptic status epilepticus.** Bipolar longitudinal montage. A 29-year-old patient with juvenile absence epilepsy. The patient was unresponsive while the EEG recordings showed 10- to 15-s bursts of generalized polyspike–waves.

EEG classification: Abnormal III (stupor)

　　　　Status: EEG status pattern, generalized
　　　　　　　Dialeptic status epilepticus

EEG report: This EEG supports the diagnosis of a generalized dialeptic status epilepticus.

EEG status epilepticus; dialeptic status

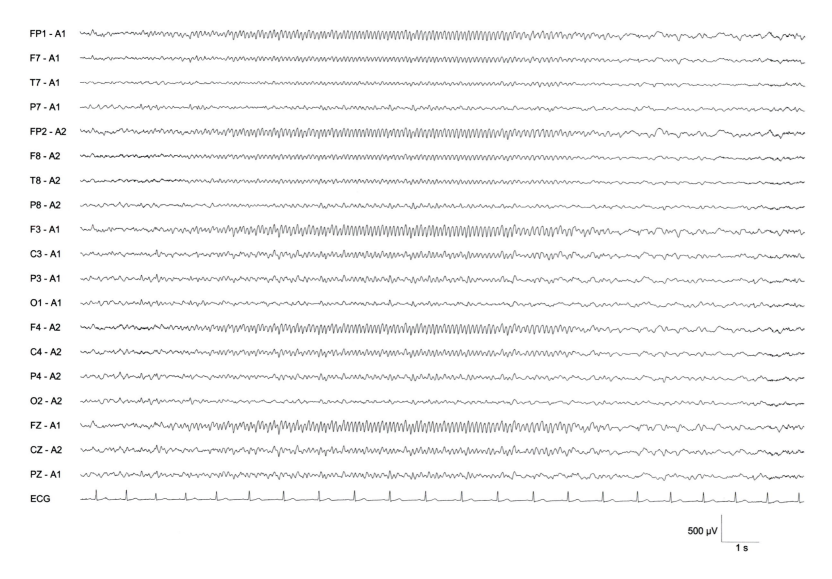

FP1 - A1

F7 - A1

T7 - A1

P7 - A1

FP2 - A2

F8 - A2

T8 - A2

P8 - A2

F3 - A1

C3 - A1

P3 - A1

O1 - A1

F4 - A2

C4 - A2

P4 - A2

O2 - A2

FZ - A1

CZ - A2

PZ - A1

ECG

500 µV

1 s

▶ **Figure 3.211** **EEG status epilepticus; dialeptic status.** Ear reference derivation. A 64-year-old patient with juvenile absence epilepsy. A dialeptic status occurred following a basal ganglion infarction. The patient had been seizure-free for many years while on valproate. The EEG status pattern consisted of recurrent periods of 10 Hz generalized frontal maximum alpha waves. These bursts were followed by generalized, irregular delta activity. The patient was unresponsive during and after the burst of paroxysmal alpha.

EEG classification: Abnormal III (stupor)

Status: EEG status pattern, generalized
Dialeptic status epilepticus

EEG report: This EEG supports the diagnosis of a generalized dialeptic status epilepticus.

In focal epilepsies, the EEG during status epilepticus usually consists of regional epileptic seizures that recur before the patient has an opportunity to recover completely (▶ Figure 3.212). Benzodiazepines also lead to cessation of the focal status epilepticus. As the focal EEG status pattern subsides, slow waves dominate in the region where the status occurred ▶ Figure 3.213). There are different focal status EEG patterns (▶ Figures 3.212–3.233). The regional clinical and EEG seizures, which constitute the nucleus of the focal status epilepticus, tend to change over time, becoming progressively "blander" and, at the same time, the repetition rate of the seizures, if untreated, increases. A similar evolution can be observed when patients experience a generalized tonic–clonic status epilepticus. Initially, they experience frequent generalized tonic–clonic seizures, followed by postictal coma. This pattern, however, progresses until the patients have a generalized (nonconvulsive) dialeptic status.

The clinical classification of status epilepticus is a modification of the classification of epileptic seizures (Rona et al., 2005). However, there is also subclinical status epilepticus, in which the EEG is similar to the EEG of a patient with clinical status epilepticus but the patient has no symptoms that can be related to the EEG abnormality (▶ Figures 3.198 and 3.214).

In some cases, regional periodic discharges trigger epileptic seizures (usually focal clonic seizures) (▶ Figure 3.233). In approximately 30% of patients with regional periodic discharges, no symptoms occur. This is particularly frequent in patients with an acute lesion due to strokes or herpes encephalitis (see ▶ Figure 3.249) (Chatrian et al., 1964).

3.4.2.4.12 Differential Diagnoses of Interictal Epileptiform Discharges

Some physiological "spiky" potentials (vertex waves, POSTS, etc.) must be distinguished from epileptiform discharges (see Section 3.4.1.2). In addition, there are the so-called variants listed below, which are also "pointed" but do not indicate epilepsy (14 & 6 Hz positive spikes, small sharp spike of sleep, wicket spikes, etc.; ▶ Table 3.11) (Benbadis & Lin, 2008; Westmoreland & Klass, 1990).

3.4.2.4.12.1 Wicket Spikes

Wicket spikes consist of intermittent groups of monophasic, arcade-shaped waves approximately 6–11 Hz with a spindle-shaped maximum from which a negative spike typically protrudes (▶ Figures 3.234 and 3.235) (Reiher & Lebel, 1977). The name refers to the shape of the arched goals in cricket. In contrast to epileptiform discharges, the spike is not followed by a slow wave—that is, the background

rhythm is not suppressed. The "wicket spike" is actually one wave within the burst that stands out more than usual but has the same waveform, distribution, and duration as all the other waves of the burst. Because this pattern can also occur during light sleep, slow waves can mix with the wicket spikes by chance, which can make it more difficult to identify the wicket spikes. The amplitude is approximately 60–200 μV, and the duration of the groups is 0.5–2 s. Occasionally, the burst is of longer duration and then may include several wicket spikes. In this case ony may consider to label the pattern as rhythmic temporal theta bursts of drowsiness (▶ Figure 3.236). The localization is temporal, and not uncommonly, wicket spikes occur alternating in the two temporal lobes. Wicket spikes occur in approximately 1% of adults during relaxed waking EEG recordings and also in sleep EEGs. Wicket spikes decrease with increasing sleep depth.

3.4.2.4.12.2 Asymmetry, Increased Background

Regional asymmetries with increased physiological beta, alpha, or theta frequencies, depending on the brain region, are the typical finding of an EEG of a patient with a bone defect ("breach rhythm"; ▶ Figure 3.237) (Cobb et al., 1979). The bone defect remains more permeable to higher frequencies than the intact bone, even if the gap has healed and closed. As a result, particularly fast frequencies have a higher amplitude over the skull defect. Not infrequently, the EEG activity recorded with scalp electrodes placed over or in close proximity to the skull defect may include sharp transients that may be confused with epileptiform discharges. The breach rhythm frequently includes wicket spikes. The location of the bone defect (i.e., the localization of physiological rhythms) determines which brain waves will be increased in amplitude. Beta frequencies dominate in the frontal region, alpha in the occipital region, theta in the temporal region, and mu rhythm in the central region. The localization of the slow and the bone defect does not have to coincide within a hemisphere and depends on the localization of the trepanation and, among other things, on the vectors of the generators (▶ Figure 3.237). Such EEG changes are typical after biopsies, abscess drainage, tumor resections, or removal of intracerebral bleeding (▶ Figure 3.238). In these settings, caution is required not to misjudge such asymmetries as epileptiform discharges. Occasionally, the term breach rhythm is used for this phenomenon. Of course, the breach (i.e., the bone defect) itself does not generate a rhythm, but it leads to an increase in the amplitude of the potentials generated by the brain due to the altered filter properties of the calotte.

EEG status epilepticus, mid-central; dialeptic status epilepticus

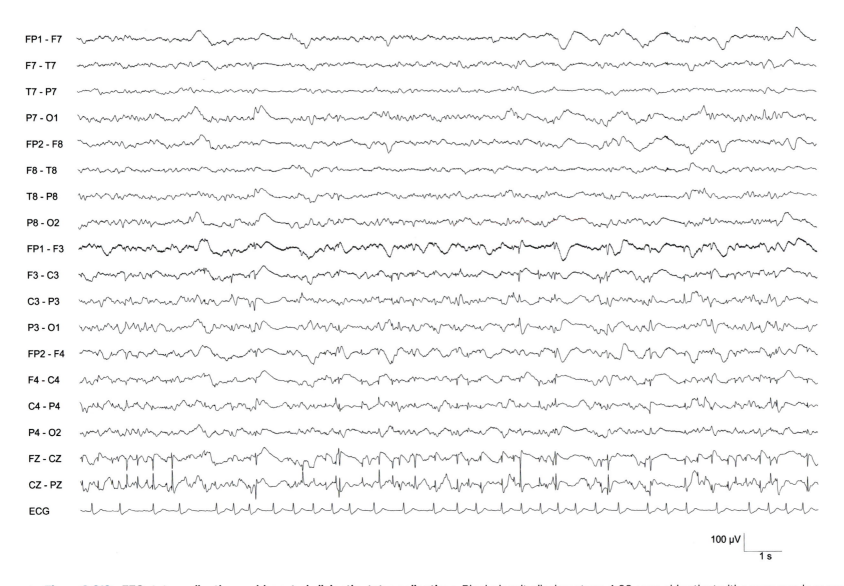

▶ **Figure 3.212**   **EEG status epilepticus, mid-central; dialeptic status epilepticus.** Bipolar longitudinal montage. A 66-year-old patient with severe anoxic encephalopathy after cardiac resuscitation.

EEG classification: Abnormal III (stupor)

Status: EEG status pattern, mid-central
Dialeptic status epilepticus

EEG report: This EEG shows a dialeptic status epilepticus associated with a mid-central epileptogenic zone in a patient with severe anoxic encephalopathy.

Delta coma; mid-central epileptic status terminated by lorazepam administration

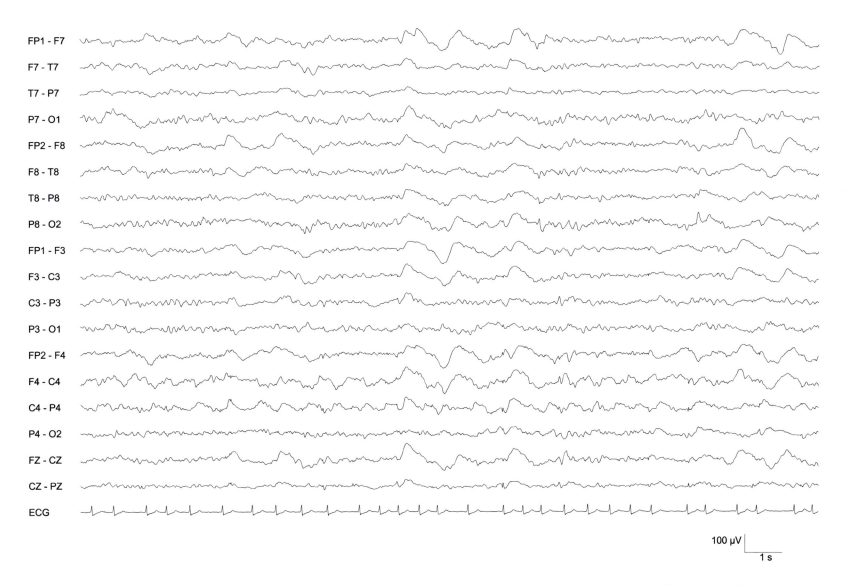

▶ **Figure 3.213** **Delta coma; mid-central epileptic status terminated by lorazepam administration.** Same patient as in ▶ **Figure 3.212**. Bipolar longitudinal montage. The EEG status pattern subsided after intravenous administration of lorazepam. The patient was then comatose, while the EEG is dominated by delta waves in the region where the seizure pattern occurred.

EEG classification: Abnormal III (coma)

1. Delta Coma
2. Continuous slow, right central

EEG report: Severe diffuse encephalopathy after termination of dialeptic–myoclonic status epilepticus by intravenous administration of lorazepam and valproate.

EEG status pattern, left frontopolar

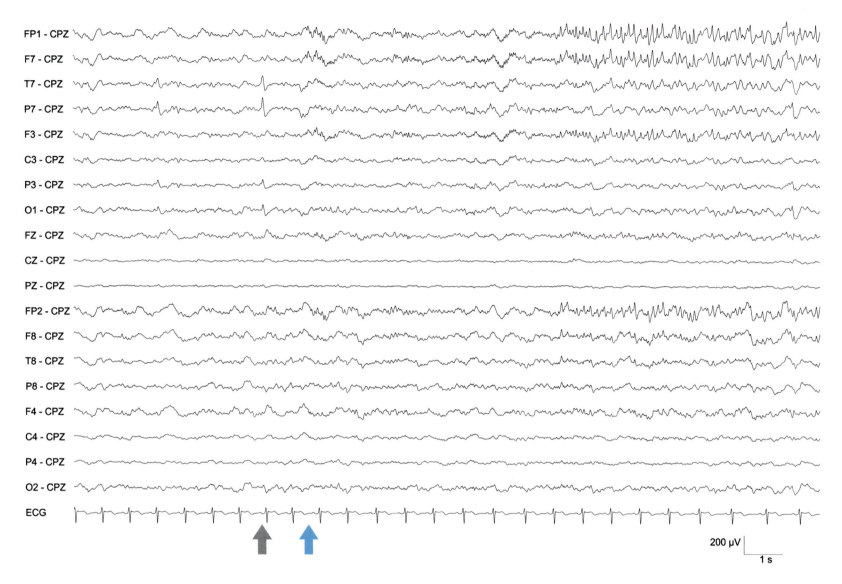

▶ **Figure 3.214** **EEG status pattern, left frontopolar; reference derivation to CPZ.** A 27-year-old female patient with mild spastic right hemiparesis who has had a left parietal empyema surgically removed after purulent meningitis at age 18 months. She had a left ventriculoperitoneal shunt. The MRI shows an extensive lesion in the left frontal and parietal regions.

The EEG status pattern occurs during slow wave sleep and consists of bursts of 8 Hz alpha activity arising in the left frontopolar region (maximum at electrodes FP1 and F7; blue arrow). Clinically, the patient was inconspicuous and continued to sleep. This EEG status pattern was repeated at intervals of a few minutes. In addition, there are left posterior temporal spikes (gray arrow).

EEG classification: Abnormal III (sleep)
1. Status (70%): EEG status pattern, FP1 > F7
    No clinical symptoms
2. Spikes, P7 > T7

EEG report: This EEG supports the diagnosis of an extensive left hemispheric epileptogenic lesion.

EEG status pattern, left

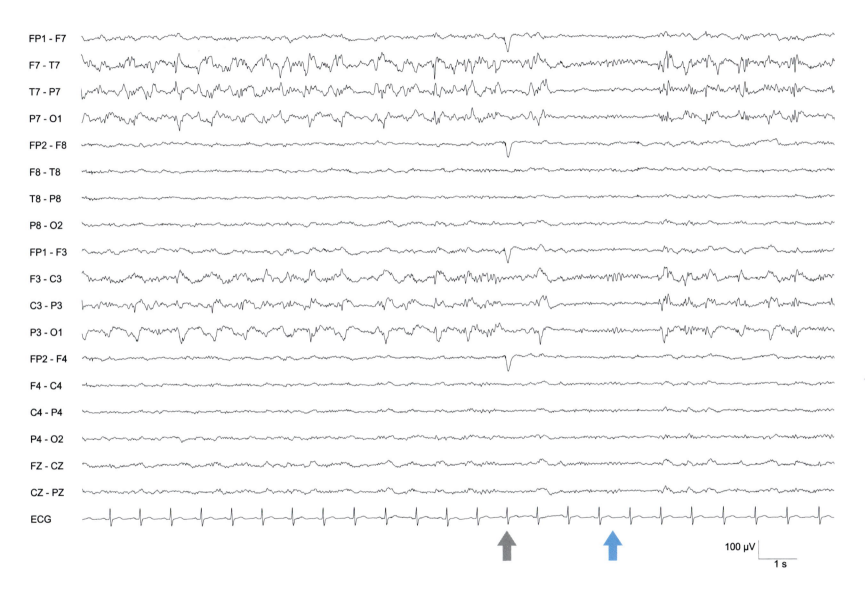

▶ **Figure 3.215** **EEG status pattern, left.** Delta stupor. Bipolar longitudinal montage. A 41-year-old patient with focal epilepsy due to a space-occupying left temporoparietal anaplastic astrocytoma (WHO grade III). The patient was not responsive during the EEG. There is no occipital background rhythm, and the EEG is dominated by relatively low-amplitude delta waves over the right hemisphere. On the left, spikes and polyspikes complexes recur at a rate of approximately 1 Hz. This activity is interrupted by a flat EEG period with low-amplitude beta and alpha frequencies for a few seconds (blue arrow). Shortly before this, an eye blink has been recorded (gray arrow).

EEG classification: Abnormal III (stupor)
1. Delta stupor
2. Periodic epileptiform discharges, C3 = P3 = P7 = T7

EEG report: This EEG reflects a left hemispheric status epilepticus. There is also evidence of a severe diffuse encephalopathy.

EEG status pattern, left frontal; delta coma

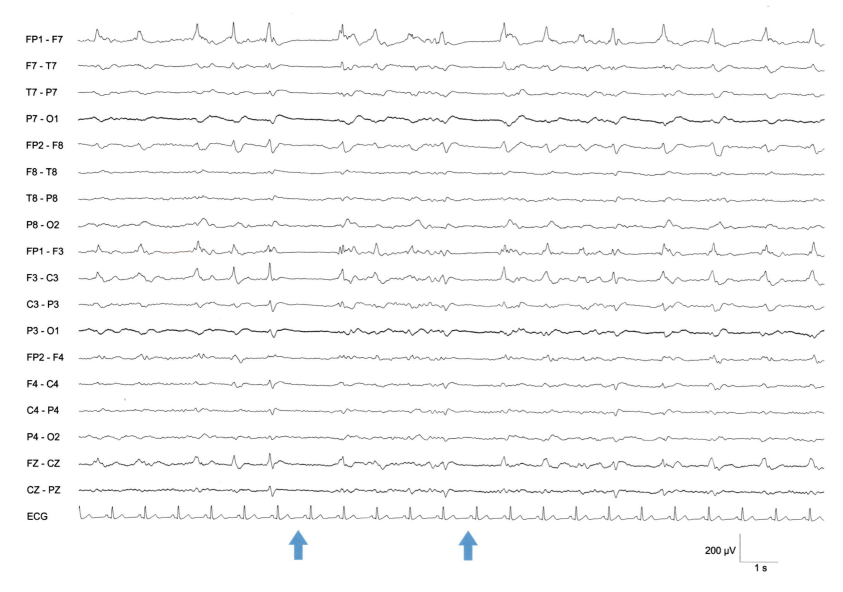

▶ **Figure 3.216** **EEG status pattern, left frontal; delta coma.** Bipolar longitudinal montage. This 86-year-old patient suffered from septic encephalopathy and multiple complications secondary to an infected hip endoprosthesis. He had initially suffered some generalized convulsive seizures and had been comatose for weeks before this EEG. This EEG shows diffuse slow and repetitive left frontopolar spikes that could only be temporarily broken by high doses of benzodiazepines and narcotics. At lower anti-seizure doses, motor seizures occurred on the right side. Note the flattening of the EEG (blue arrows) as a typical sign of encephalopathies in adults.

EEG classification: Abnormal III (coma)
 1. Delta coma
 2. Status: Periodic epileptiform discharges, FP1 > F3
       Motor seizure, right

EEG report: This EEG documents a left frontopolar epileptic status and a severe diffuse encephalopathy.

EEG status pattern, right central

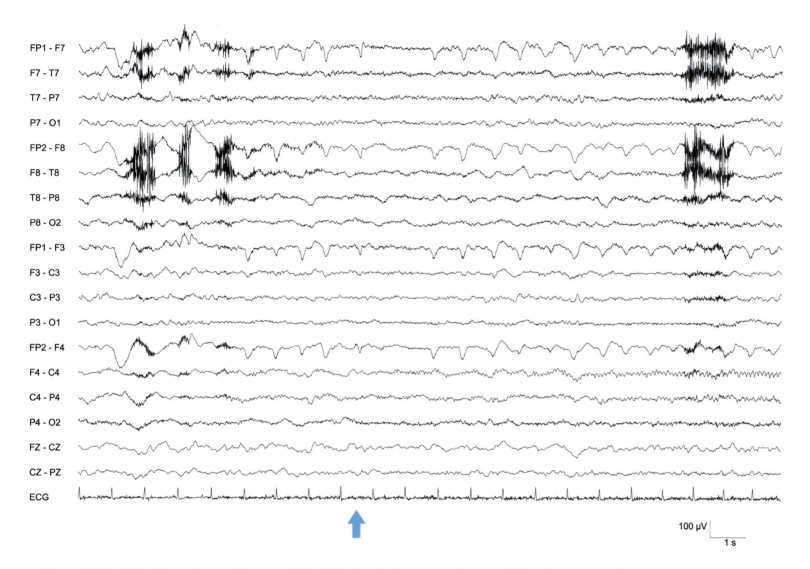

▶ **Figure 3.217** **EEG status pattern, right central.** Bipolar longitudinal montage. A 58-year-old female patient with focal epilepsy due to a space-occupying right frontoparietal astrocytoma. There is continuous slow in the right hemisphere, maximum T8 and P8. The right hemisphere shows a run of relatively low-amplitude 10 Hz activity that slowly increases in amplitude while the frequency slows down (onset at the blue arrow). In addition, the left hemisphere also shows low-amplitude, irregular delta activity. The patient was restless and confused during this time. The EEG classification and report refer to this figure and ▶ **Figures 3.218–3.220**.

EEG classification: Abnormal III (awake)
1. Status: EEG status pattern, C4
          Delirium status
2. Continuous slow, generalized
3. Continuous slow right

EEG report: This EEG documents a right central epileptic status due to a right frontoparietal astrocytoma and a mild to moderate diffuse encephalopathy.

EEG status pattern, right central

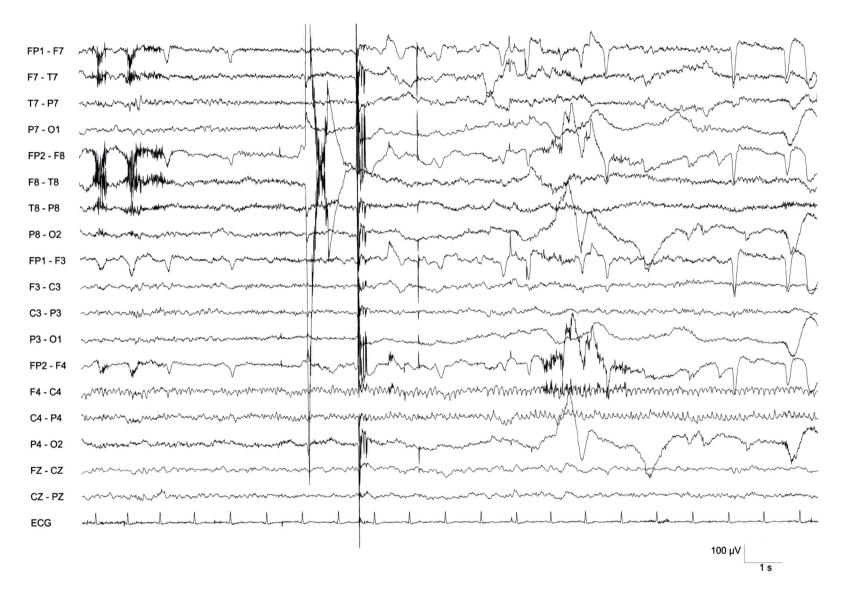

▶ **Figure 3.218** **EEG status pattern, right central; bipolar longitudinal montage.** Continuation of the EEG of ▶ **Figure 3.217**. The right central EEG status pattern develops further, with the amplitude of the status pattern increasing as the frequency deceases. For EEG classification and report, see ▶ **Figure 3.217**.

EEG status pattern, right central

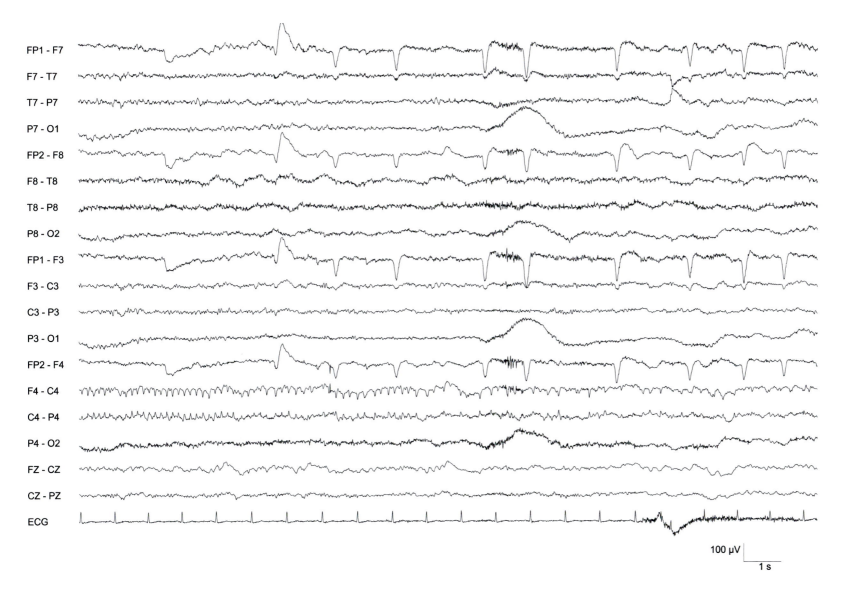

FP1 - F7
F7 - T7
T7 - P7
P7 - O1
FP2 - F8
F8 - T8
T8 - P8
P8 - O2
FP1 - F3
F3 - C3
C3 - P3
P3 - O1
FP2 - F4
F4 - C4
C4 - P4
P4 - O2
FZ - CZ
CZ - PZ
ECG

100 µV
1 s

▶ **Figure 3.219** **EEG status pattern, right central; bipolar longitudinal montage.** Continuation of the EEG of ▶ **Figure 3.218**. At the end of the page, the right central EEG status pattern decreases further in frequency and has almost completely stopped. For the EEG classification and report, see ▶ **Figure 3.217**.

EEG status pattern, right central

FP1 - F7

F7 - T7

T7 - P7

P7 - O1

FP2 - F8

F8 - T8

T8 - P8

P8 - O2

FP1 - F3

F3 - C3

C3 - P3

P3 - O1

FP2 - F4

F4 - C4

C4 - P4

P4 - O2

FZ - CZ

CZ - PZ

ECG

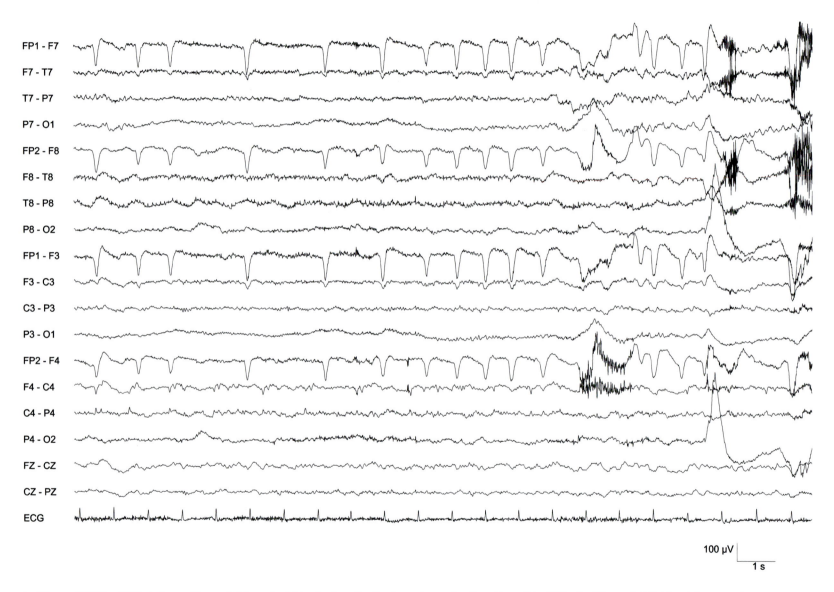

100 µV

1 s

▶ **Figure 3.220** **EEG status pattern, right central; bipolar longitudinal montage.** Continuation of the EEG of ▶ **Figure 3.219**. The right central EEG status pattern becomes increasingly irregular and evolves into a slow. For EEG classification and report, see ▶ **Figure 3.217**.

EEG status pattern, left occipital

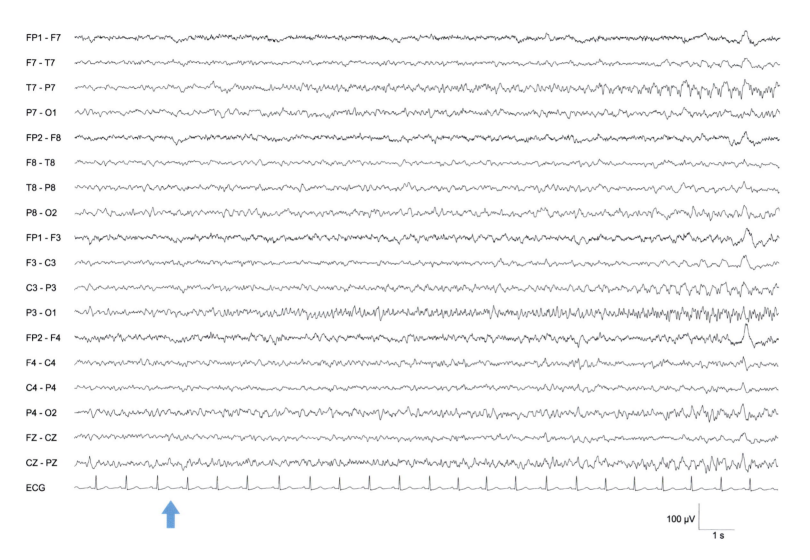

▶ **Figure 3.221** **EEG status pattern, left occipital; bipolar longitudinal montage.** This 26-year-old female patient with Rasmussen's encephalitis, which started late at age 22 years, suffered from many aphasic and right arm motor seizures. The MRI showed a slowly progressive left-brain atrophy. Medication with several anti-seizure drugs had led to background slow and generalized continuous slow. The EEG status pattern consists of rhythmic beta activity that gradually increased in amplitude on the left occipital side (blue arrow). The patient had a visual aura that she could not lateralize. The EEG status pattern was repeated at intervals of a few minutes. The EEG classification and report refer to this figure and ▶ **Figures 3.222** and **3.223**.

EEG classification: Abnormal III (awake)
  1. Status: EEG status pattern, O1 = P7
        Visual aura status
  2. Continuous slow, left and generalized
  3. Background slow

EEG report: This EEG documents a left occipital status epilepticus with visual auras and a mild diffuse encephalopathy.

EEG status pattern, left occipital

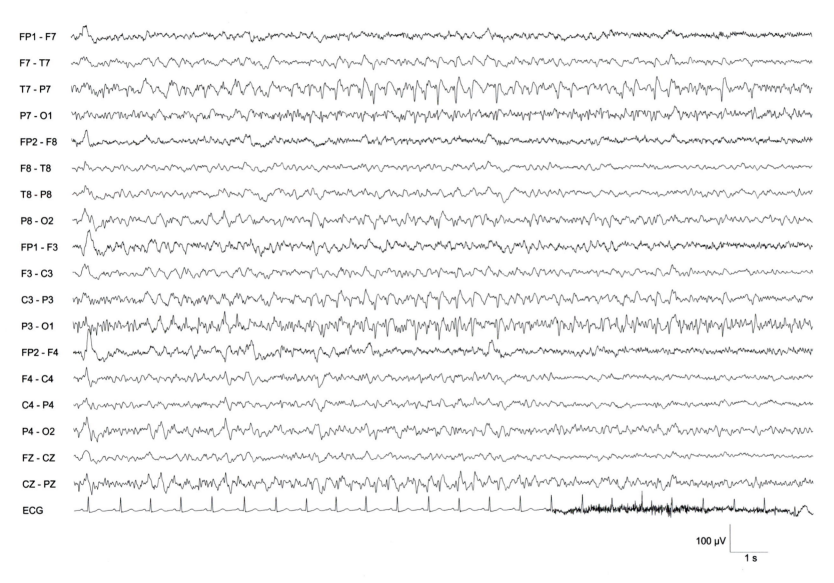

FP1 - F7

F7 - T7

T7 - P7

P7 - O1

FP2 - F8

F8 - T8

T8 - P8

P8 - O2

FP1 - F3

F3 - C3

C3 - P3

P3 - O1

FP2 - F4

F4 - C4

C4 - P4

P4 - O2

FZ - CZ

CZ - PZ

ECG

100 µV

1 s

▶ **Figure 3.222**   **EEG status pattern, left occipital; bipolar longitudinal montage.** Continuation of the EEG of ▶ **Figure 3.221**. The amplitude of the left occipital EEG status pattern gradually increased while its frequency decreased. See ▶ **Figure 3.221** for EEG classification and report.

EEG status pattern, left occipital

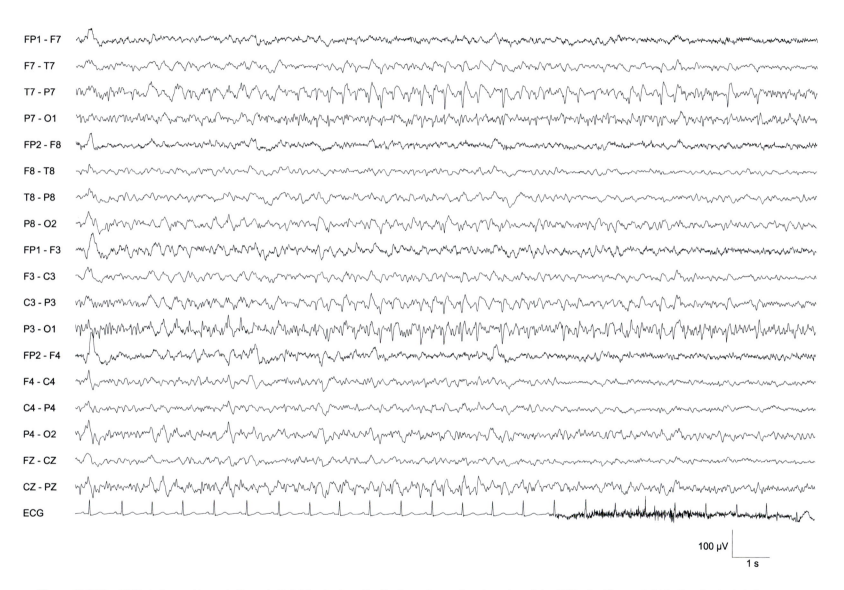

FP1 - F7

F7 - T7

T7 - P7

P7 - O1

FP2 - F8

F8 - T8

T8 - P8

P8 - O2

FP1 - F3

F3 - C3

C3 - P3

P3 - O1

FP2 - F4

F4 - C4

C4 - P4

P4 - O2

FZ - CZ

CZ - PZ

ECG

100 μV

1 s

3 Clinical Electroencephalography

▶ **Figure 3.223** **EEG status pattern, left occipital, bipolar longitudinal montage.** Continuation of the EEG of ▶ **Figure 3.222**. The rhythmic left occipital EEG status pattern broke off and evolved into irregular repetitive left occipital spikes. See ▶ **Figure 3.221** for EEG classification and report.

EEG status pattern, left temporo-occipital; delta coma

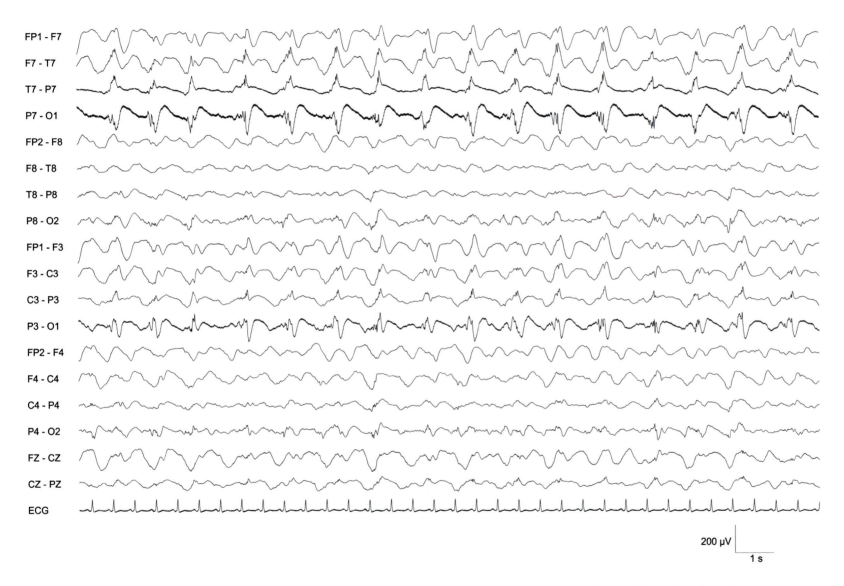

200 µV

1 s

▶ **Figure 3.224** **EEG status pattern, left temporo-occipital: delta coma.** Bipolar longitudinal montage. A 27-year-old female patient with posterior reversible encephalopathy syndrome (PRES) during pregnancy. The EEG delta coma reflects the comatose condition of the patient. There are periodic epileptiform discharges in the left posterior hemisphere maximum at P7 > T7. The periodic epileptiform discharges recur at intervals of approximately 1 s. The further evolution of the EEG status pattern is shown in ▶ **Figures 3.225–3.230**. Note the evolution of the periodic epileptiform discharges and fast frequencies. This EEG status pattern was repeated in intervals of 12–20 min. For EEG classification and report, see ▶ **Figure 3.230**.

EEG status pattern, left temporo-occipital; periodic epileptiform discharges, right temporo-parietal; delta coma

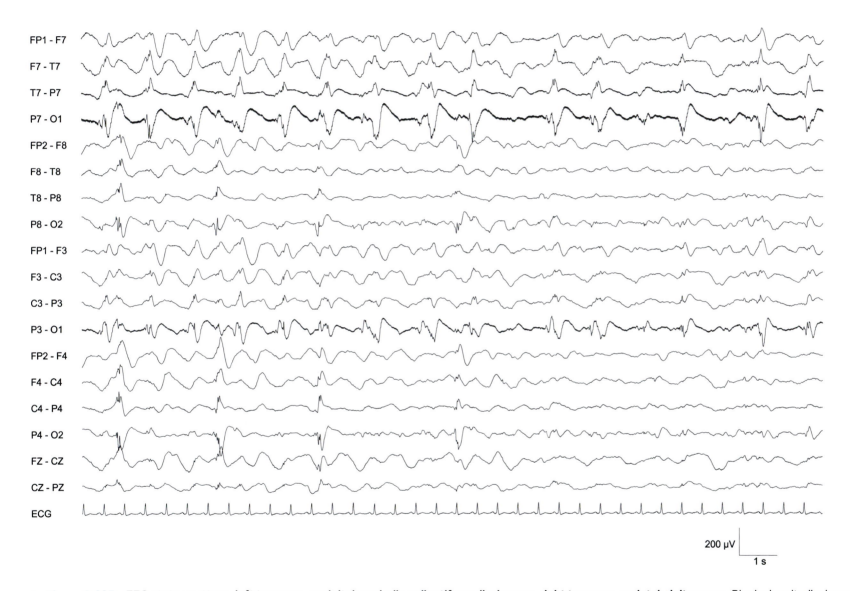

FP1 - F7
F7 - T7
T7 - P7
P7 - O1
FP2 - F8
F8 - T8
T8 - P8
P8 - O2
FP1 - F3
F3 - C3
C3 - P3
P3 - O1
FP2 - F4
F4 - C4
C4 - P4
P4 - O2
FZ - CZ
CZ - PZ
ECG

200 μV

1 s

▶ **Figure 3.225** **EEG status pattern, left temporo-occipital; periodic epileptiform discharges, right temporo-parietal; delta coma.** Bipolar longitudinal montage. Continuation of
▶ **Figure 3.224**. While the left periodic epileptiform discharges show longer intervals, less frequent periodic epileptiform discharges appear on the right side (frequency: one discharge every 3 s). For EEG classification and report, see ▶ **Figure 3.230**.

EEG status pattern, right temporo-occipital and left temporo-parietal; delta coma

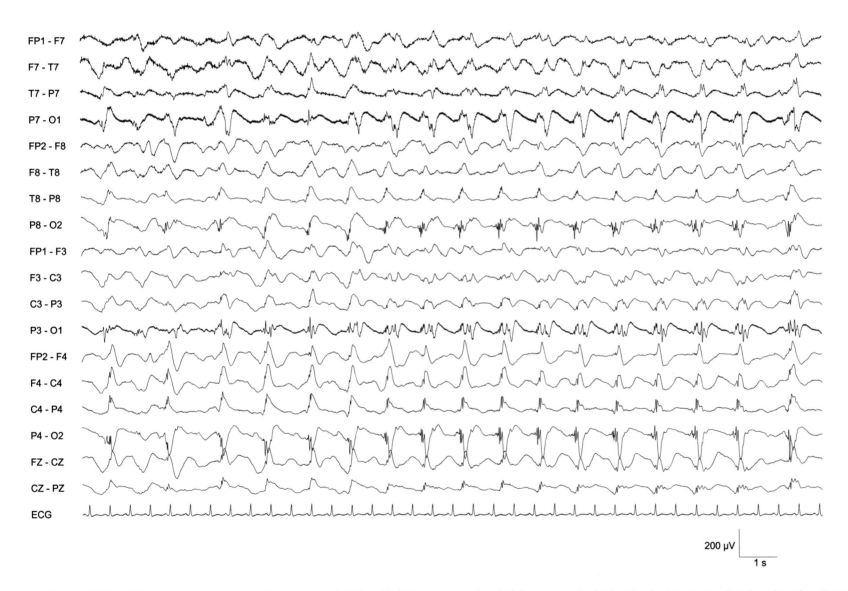

200 µV

1 s

▶ **Figure 3.226** **EEG status pattern, right temporo-occipital and left temporo-parietal; delta coma.** Bipolar longitudinal montage. Continuation of ▶ **Figure 3.225**. Now the right periodic epileptiform discharges are more prominent than the left-sided ones. In addition, the right and left periodic epileptiform discharges are synchronized. For EEG classification and report, see ▶ **Figure 3.230**.

EEG status pattern, right occipital and left occipito-temporal; delta coma

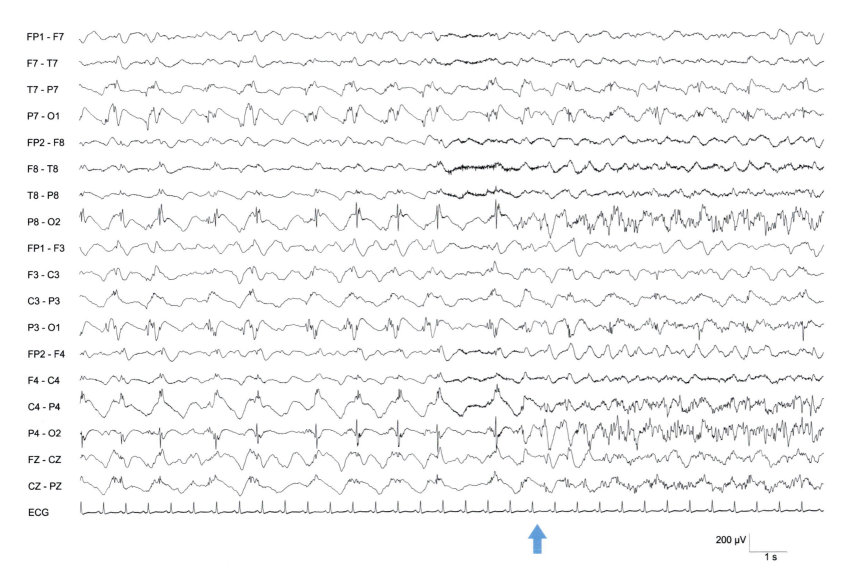

▶ **Figure 3.227** **EEG status pattern, right occipital and left occipito-temporal; delta coma.** Bipolar longitudinal montage. Continuation of ▶ **Figure 3.226**. The periodic epileptiform discharges on the right became less prominent and suddenly are replaced by high-frequency activity (blue arrow). For EEG classification and report, see ▶ **Figure 3.230**.

EEG status pattern, right temporo-occipital and left temporo-parietal; delta coma

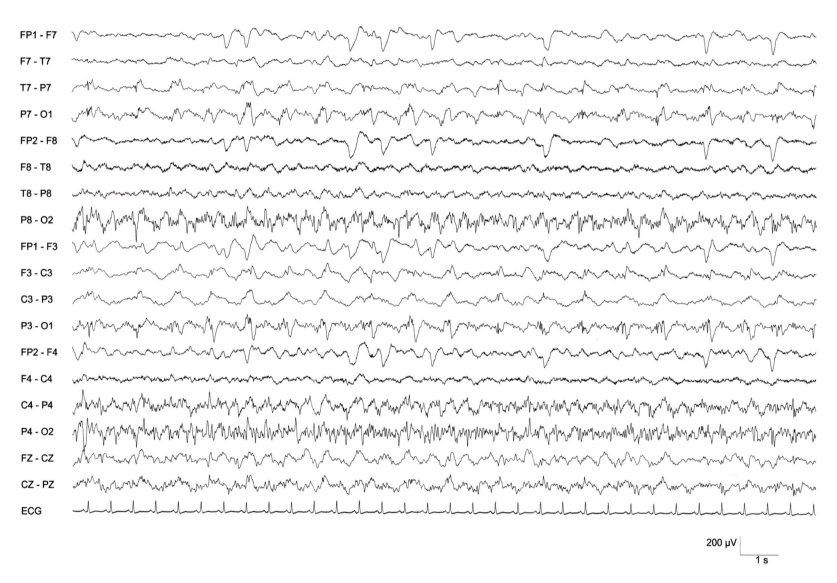

FP1 - F7

F7 - T7

T7 - P7

P7 - O1

FP2 - F8

F8 - T8

T8 - P8

P8 - O2

FP1 - F3

F3 - C3

C3 - P3

P3 - O1

FP2 - F4

F4 - C4

C4 - P4

P4 - O2

FZ - CZ

CZ - PZ

ECG

200 µV

1 s

▶ **Figure 3.228** **EEG status pattern, right temporo-occipital and left temporo-parietal; delta coma.** Bipolar longitudinal montage. Continuation of ▶ **Figure** 3.227. Bipolar longitudinal montage. The right occipital high-frequency activity and also the left periodic epileptiform discharges continue. For EEG classification and report, see ▶ **Figure** 3.230.

EEG status pattern, right temporo-occipital and left temporo-parietal; delta coma

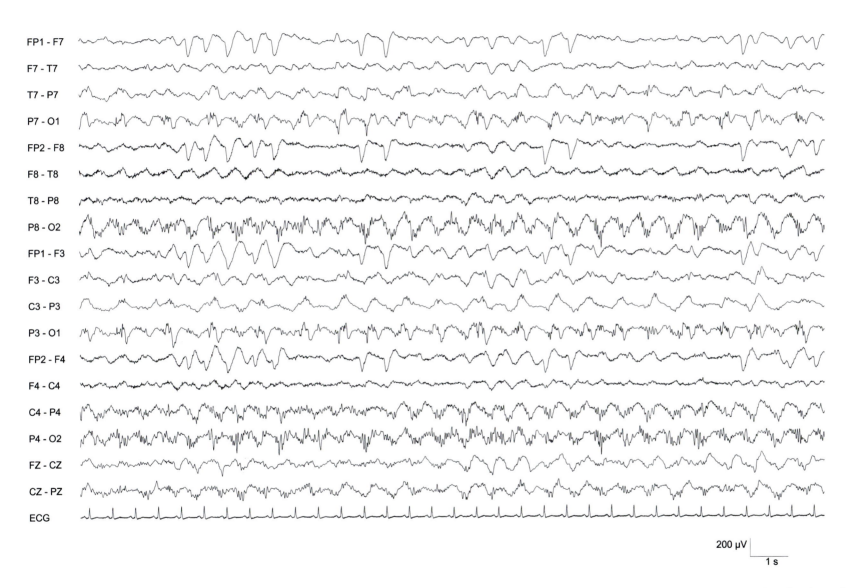

FP1 - F7
F7 - T7
T7 - P7
P7 - O1
FP2 - F8
F8 - T8
T8 - P8
P8 - O2
FP1 - F3
F3 - C3
C3 - P3
P3 - O1
FP2 - F4
F4 - C4
C4 - P4
P4 - O2
FZ - CZ
CZ - PZ
ECG

200 μV
1 s

▶ **Figure 3.229** **EEG status pattern, right temporo-occipital and left temporo-parietal; delta coma.** Bipolar longitudinal montage. Continuation of ▶ **Figure 3.228**. The more or less continuous right occipital paroxysmal fast is now progressively replaced by periodic polyspike–wave discharges at a frequency of approximately 1 Hz. For EEG classification and report, see ▶ **Figure 3.230**.

EEG status pattern, right temporo-occipital and left temporo-parietal; delta coma

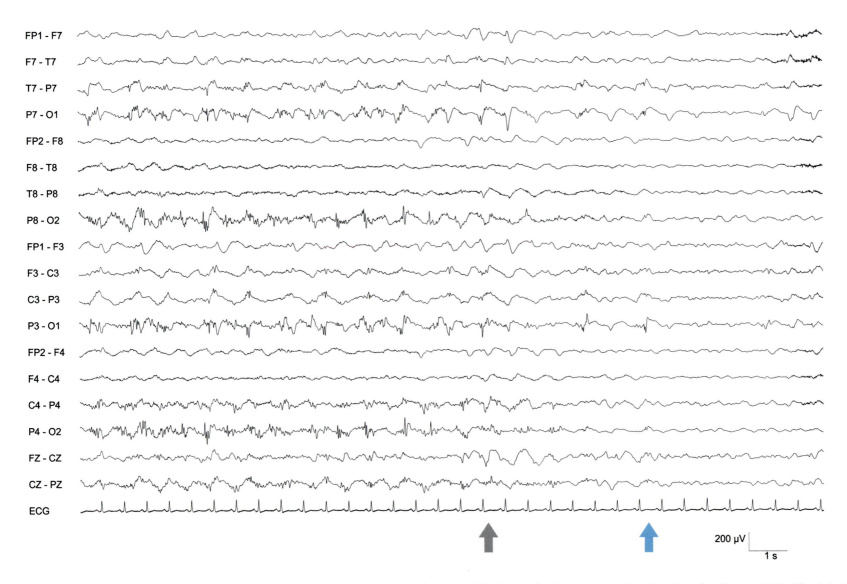

▶ **Figure 3.230**   **EEG status pattern, right and left temporo-occipital; delta coma.** Bipolar longitudinal montage. Continuation of ▶ **Figure 3.229**. The right temporo-occipital EEG status pattern ends (gray arrow). Only isolated spikes remain in the left temporo-parietal region (blue arrow). The EEG classification and report refer to ▶ **Figures 3.224–3.230**.

EEG classification: Abnormal III (awake)
  1. Delta coma
  2. Status: EEG status pattern, O2 and O1 = P7
          Coma

EEG report: This EEG documents right occipital and left temporo-occipital epileptic status. In addition, there is evidence of a severe diffuse encephalopathy.

EEG status pattern, generalized, maximum occipital.

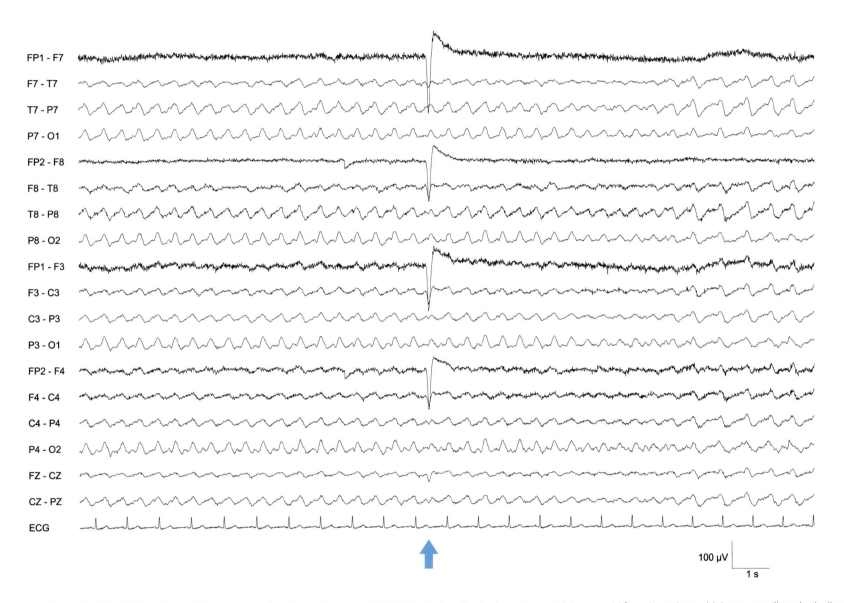

100 μV

1 s

▶ **Figure 3.231** **EEG status pattern, generalized, maximum occipital.** Bipolar longitudinal montage. A 54-year-old female patient with long-standing alcoholism (Korsakov syndrome), after liver transplantation secondary to alcoholic cirrhosis, and encephalitis due to immunosuppression. The EEG is dominated by occipital rhythmic delta waves. The patient was stuporous during this EEG. A physiological background activity cannot be identified. Note the blink artifact (blue arrow).

EEG classification: Abnormal III (stupor)

      Satus: EEG status pattern, generalized, maximum occipital

                Stupor

EEG report: This EEG of a stuporous patient documents a generalized epileptic status.

Background slow; continuous slow, generalized

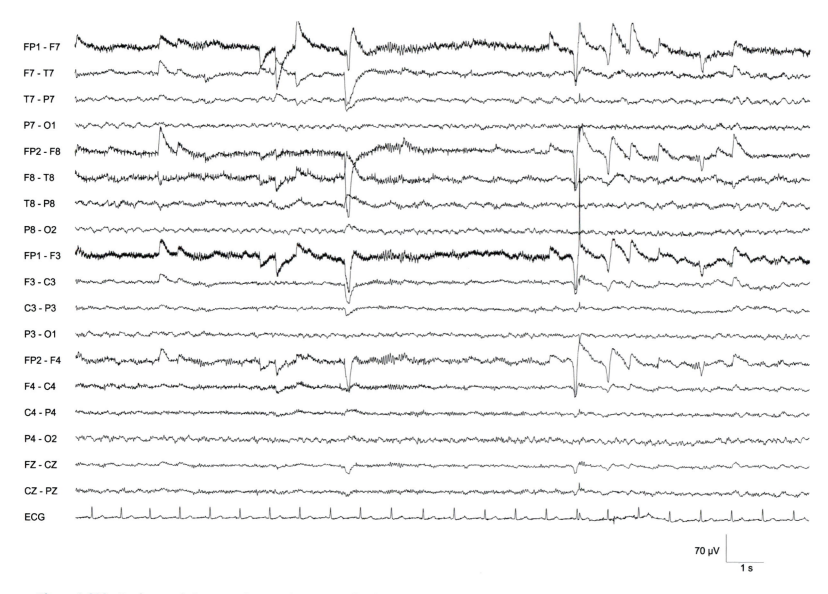

FP1 - F7

F7 - T7

T7 - P7

P7 - O1

FP2 - F8

F8 - T8

T8 - P8

P8 - O2

FP1 - F3

F3 - C3

C3 - P3

P3 - O1

FP2 - F4

F4 - C4

C4 - P4

P4 - O2

FZ - CZ

CZ - PZ

ECG

70 μV

1 s

▶ **Figure 3.232** **Background slow; continuous slow, generalized.** Bipolar longitudinal montage. Lorazepam administration ends the status epilepticus shown in ▶ **Figure 3.231.**
Intravenous administration of lorazepam has ended the status epilepticus. The background occipital rhythm is slowed to 5 Hz.

EEG classification: Abnormal II (awake)
  1. Background slow
  2. Continuous slow, generalized

EEG report: This EEG documents a moderate diffuse encephalopathy. The generalized epileptic status documented in the last EEG has subsided.

EEG seizure pattern, left central; clonic status, left lower leg

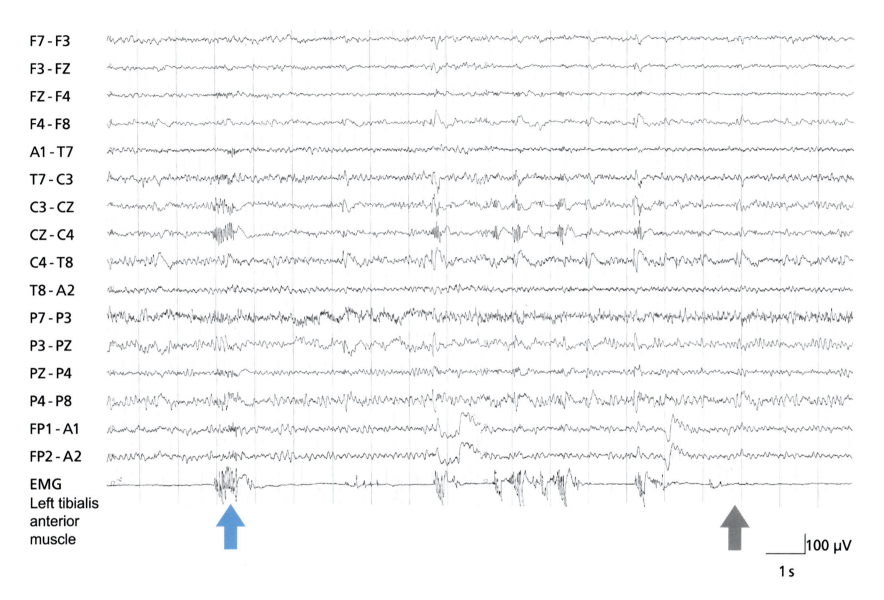

▶ **Figure 3.233** **EEG seizure pattern, left central; clonic status, left lower leg.** Bipolar transverse montage. A 69-year-old patient with 6 weeks of clonic status of the left lower leg (epilepsia partialis continua). Whereas polyspikes (blue arrow) are regularly accompanied by clonic twitching of the left lower leg, single spikes are not (gray arrow). The maximum of the interictal spikes is at CZ = C4, and the maximum of some of the polyspikes is at CZ > C3. The lateralization of the polyspikes to the left hemisphere is most probably due to the rare phenomenon of paradoxical lateralization (Catarino et al., 2012). It is also known that cortical evoked potentials generated by stimulation of the anterior tibialis nerve can have a paradoxical lateralization.

EEG classification: Abnormal III (awake)
1. Spikes, C4 = CZ
2. Status: EEG status pattern, (periodic polyspikes) C3 > CZ
   Clonic status, left lower leg

EEG report: This EEG documents a left leg clonic epileptic status.

▶ **Table 3.11** **Sharp Transients Mimicking Epileptiform Discharges**

Pattern	Frequency (Hz)	Localization	Form	Age	Duration	Level of Consciousness	Comments	References	Figures
Rhythmical temporal theta of drowsiness	4–7	Uni- or bitemporal	Rhythmical; top-notched, sharp negativity	Young adults	2–10 s	Relaxed wake, drowsiness, sleep N1	Synonymous: psychomotor variant	F. Gibbs et al. (1963)	3.48, 3.95–3.98, 3.194, 3.236
Rhythmical midline theta	4–7	Mid-frontocentral	Higher amplitude than background activity	Adults	4–60 s	Relaxed wake	Association with frontal lobe epilepsy	Beleza et al. (2009), Cigánek (1961)	3.99, 3.100
Wicket spike	6–12	Temporal	Monophasic negative polarity, arcade/spindle-shaped, mu-shaped	Adults	0.5–2 s	Wake, sleep N1	Wave form similar to the wickets used in cricket game	Reiher & Lebel (1977)	3.234, 3.235
Small sharp spike (SSS)	Single waves	Temporal > frontal	<50 ms <50 µV	Adults	50 ms	Relaxed wake, sleep N1 and N2	Synonymous: benign epileptiform transience of sleep (BETS)	F. Gibbs & Gibbs (1952), Klass & Westmoreland (1985)	3.239–3.240
14 and 6 Hz positive spikes	14 and 6 Hz	Lateral, posterior temporal	Monophasic, spiky positive polarity	Teenagers, adults	<1 s	Wake, sleep N1 and N2	Synonymous: ctenoids; 20–60% of teenagers; 14 and 6 Hz components may occur separately	F. Gibbs & Gibbs (1952), Lombroso et al. (1966)	3.241–3.243
6 Hz phantom spike and waves	5–7 Hz	Generalized	Biphasic, small spike and large wave	Teenagers, adults	<1 s	Relaxed wake, sleep N1	Synonymous: phantom spike and wave (FOLD & WHAM) (see text)	F. Gibbs & Gibbs (1952), Hughes (1980), C. Marshall, (1955)	3.244
Subclinical rhythmic electrographic discharge of adults (SREDA)	5–6	Generalized	Abrupt onset and end	Adults >40 years	10–80 s	Wake, sleep N1	Synonymous: decharges paroxystique	Westmoreland & Klass (1981)	3.176

Wicket spikes

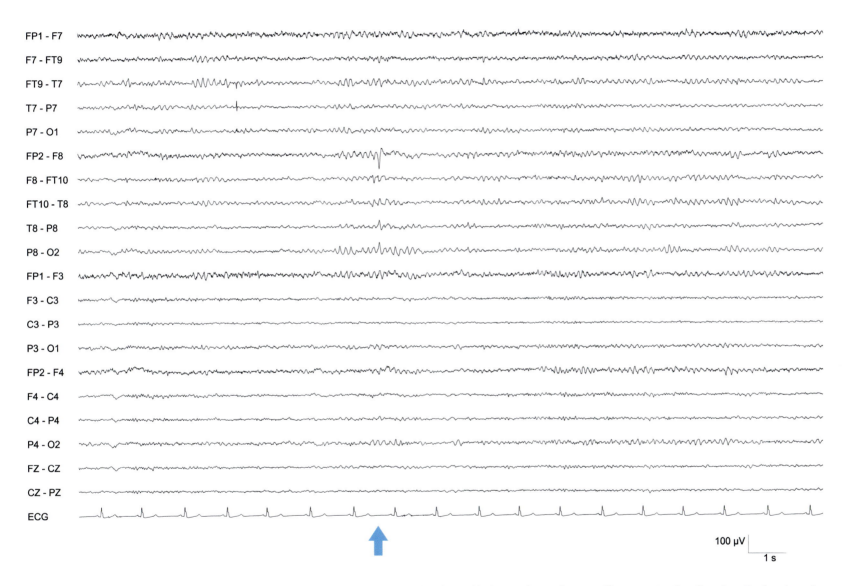

| FP1 - F7 |
| F7 - FT9 |
| FT9 - T7 |
| T7 - P7 |
| P7 - O1 |
| FP2 - F8 |
| F8 - FT10 |
| FT10 - T8 |
| T8 - P8 |
| P8 - O2 |
| FP1 - F3 |
| F3 - C3 |
| C3 - P3 |
| P3 - O1 |
| FP2 - F4 |
| F4 - C4 |
| C4 - P4 |
| P4 - O2 |
| FZ - CZ |
| CZ - PZ |
| ECG |

100 µV

1 s

▶ **Figure 3.234** **Wicket spikes.** Bipolar longitudinal montage. A 37-year-old patient with depression and unspecific concentration disorders. During drowsiness, a spindle-like rhythmic theta burst is seen. There is a sharp transient (wicket spike) at FT10 = F8 = T8 that has the same waveform and distribution as the waves of the theta burst (blue arrow). In addition, the sharp transient is not followed by a slow wave as it is typical for epileptiform spikes.

EEG classification: Normal (awake)

EEG report: Normal EEG.

Wicket spikes

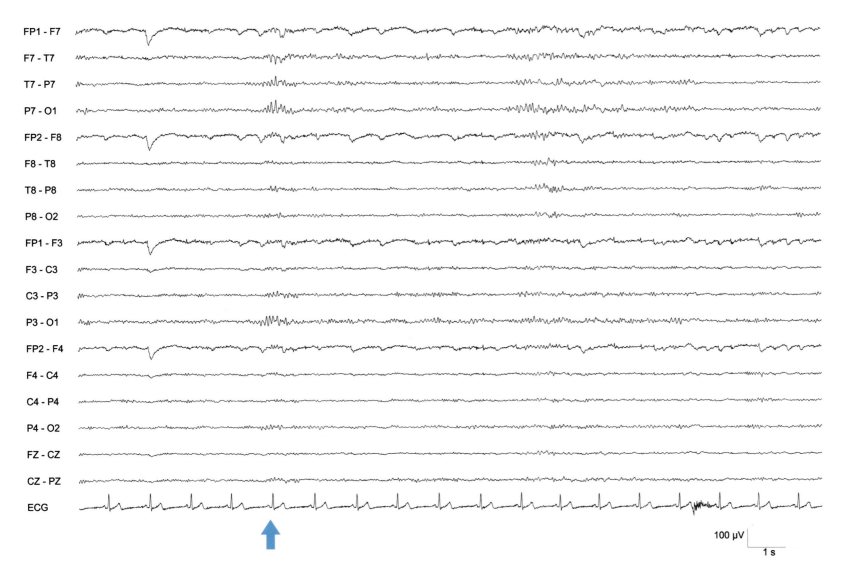

► **Figure 3.235** **Wicket spikes.** Bipolar longitudinal montage. A 30-year-old patient with tension headache. During wakefulness, a theta group spindles up. The maximum of the negative peak is in the left temporal region (blue arrow). The occipital background rhythm is approximately 13 Hz.

EEG classification: Normal (awake)

EEG report: Normal EEG.

Wicket spikes versus rhythmic temporal theta burst of drowsiness

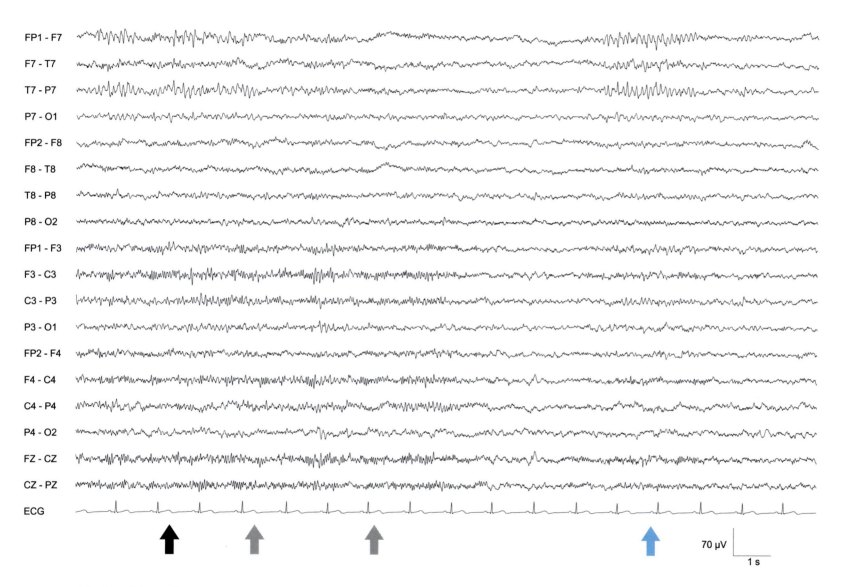

▶ **Figure 3.236   Wicket spikes versus rhythmic temporal theta burst of drowsiness.** Bipolar longitudinal montage. A 32-year-old patient with depression. The EEG shows slow horizontal eye movements (gray arrows) typical of drowsiness. There are two left temporal bursts of theta activity of 2- or 3-s duration that include several sharp transients (black and blue arrow). These sharp transients have the same characteristics as the wicket spikes illustrated in ▶ **Figure 3.235**. However, wicket spikes are usually only isolated waves that stand out from background activity. In this example, there are 2- or 3-s burst. These bursts are best classified as rhythmic temporal theta bursts of drowsiness.

EEG classification: Normal (awake)

EEG report: Normal EEG.

Asymmetry, increased background left central; continuous slow, left frontotemporal

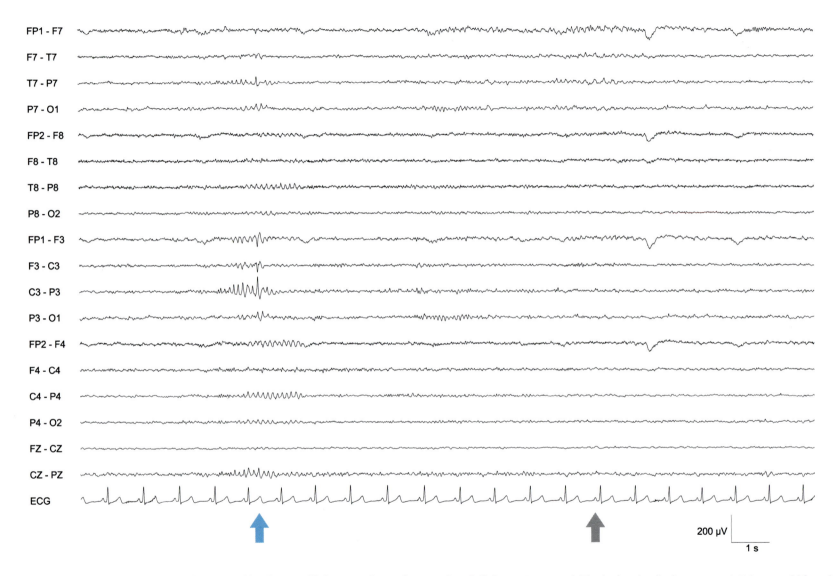

▶ **Figure 3.237** **Asymmetry, increased background left central; continuous slow, left frontotemporal.** Bipolar longitudinal montage. A 34-year-old female patient with status post partial left frontal lobe resection. The patient has had a drug-resistant left frontal lobe epilepsy since age 11 years secondary to a sinusoidal abscess and was rendered seizure-free after epilepsy surgery at age 19 years. The bone defect leads to a higher amplitude spindle-like mu activity (blue arrow). Continuous slow waves occur in the left frontal and intermittent slow waves (in this part of the EEG) in the left temporal region (gray arrow). The interpretation refers to the entire EEG.

EEG classification: Abnormal III (awake)
1. Asymmetry, increased background, left central
2. Continuous slow, left frontotemporal

EEG report: This EEG reflects a partial left frontal lobe resection.

Asymmetry, increased theta left temporal; background slow

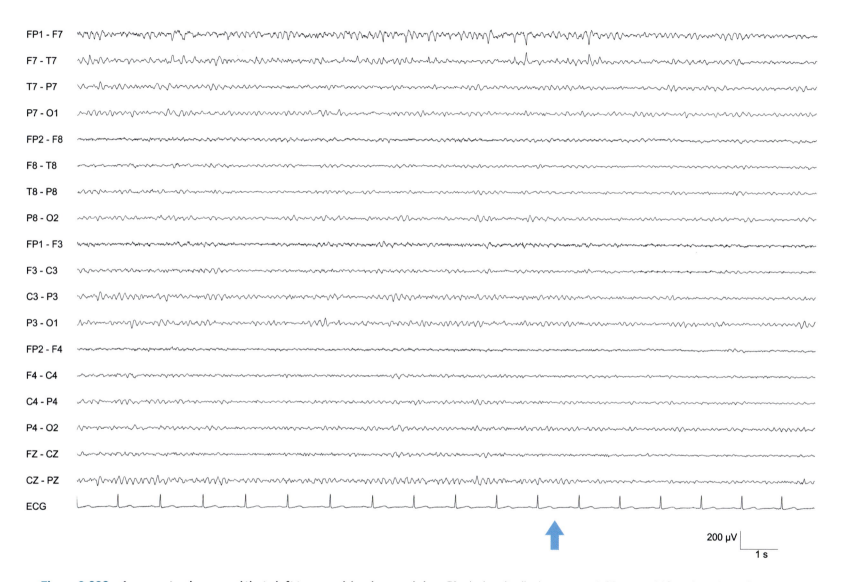

FP1 - F7

F7 - T7

T7 - P7

P7 - O1

FP2 - F8

F8 - T8

T8 - P8

P8 - O2

FP1 - F3

F3 - C3

C3 - P3

P3 - O1

FP2 - F4

F4 - C4

C4 - P4

P4 - O2

FZ - CZ

CZ - PZ

ECG

200 μV

1 s

▶ **Figure 3.238** **Asymmetry, increased theta left temporal; background slow.** Bipolar longitudinal montage. A 69-year-old female patient after several resections of a left sphenoidal meningioma. The background activity is approximately 7 Hz. In the left temporal region, there is a significant increase in amplitude of the 7 Hz activity (blue arrow), most likely due to the previous craniotomy.

EEG classification: Abnormal II (awake)
1. Asymmetry, increased theta, left temporal
2. Background slow

EEG report: This EEG reflects the partial left temporal lobe resection. There is also evidence of a mild diffuse encephalopathy.

3.4.2.4.12.3 Benign Epileptiform Transients of Sleep (BETS)

This pattern was described as "small sharp spikes" (SSS) by F. Gibbs and Gibbs (1952). The current name of the pattern emphasizes the fact that it is not an epileptiform discharge and that it occurs in adults predominantly during drowsiness and light sleep (▸ Figures 3.239 and 3.240) (White et al., 1977). The amplitude is typically below 50 μV, and the duration is usually shorter than 50 ms. The negative temporal spiky component is monophasic or biphasic, with a steep ascending and descending leg without subsequent slow wave. Occasionally, BETS (SSS) mix with individual theta waves that occur during drowsiness, giving the impression that the small spike is followed by a slow wave. BETS decrease with increasing sleep depth. BETS have a widespread potential field but are usually maximum in temporal lobe leads. The widespread distribution of BETS in temporal leads is the reason that they are of low amplitude in bipolar temporal channels and of much higher amplitude in interhemispheric derivations. BETS occur sporadically and are recorded in approximately 20% of healthy adults (White et al., 1977).

3.4.2.4.12.4 14 and 6 Hz Positive Spikes

This pattern caused confusion for a while when it was thought to be associated with asocial and aggressive behavior (Gibbs & Gibbs, 1952; Lombroso et al., 1966). It was considered an exculpating factor in U.S. courts in selected cases (see above). However, it soon turned out that this was a selection bias because this pattern was found not only in juvenile offenders but also in normal juveniles (Lombroso et al., 1966). It has also been called ctenoids because of its shape. These bursts consist of positive spikes of a repetition frequency around 14 and 6 Hz and occur predominantly in a relaxed awake state and light sleep (▸ Figure 3.241). The bursts have an arched shape with a spiky positive component and a rounded negative component. The localization is posterior temporal on one or both sides. The 6 Hz component can dominate the pattern (▸ Figures 3.242 and 3.243). The duration of the bursts of 14 and 6 positive spikes is typically less than 1 s. The 14 and 6 Hz positive spikes are found from the third year of life and are maximum in the teenage years. After that, they become less frequent. It is now unanimously agreed that this pattern has no abnormal significance.

3.4.2.4.12.5 6 Hz "Phantom" Spike and Wave

The 6 Hz phantom spike and wave are called "phantom" because the negative spikes typically have a significantly lower amplitude than the relatively high-amplitude slow waves (▸ Figure 3.244). The repetition frequency is approximately 6 Hz (range, 5–7 Hz). The duration of the bursts is 1 or 2 s, rarely 3 or 4 s. The pattern can be seen from young adulthood in approximately 2.5% of healthy adults. It has no abnormal significance. However, it has been associated with several pathologies due to selection bias. Two forms of this pattern have been described, depending on whether the pattern was of maximum amplitude in occipital or frontal derivations (WHAM: Waking, High amplitude spike, Anterior, Male; and FOLD: Female, Occipital, Low amplitude spike, Drowsy). This differentiation is of no clinical relevance. This pattern is not epileptiform. The main difference with epileptiform patterns is the greater amplitude of the spikes in actual epileptiform discharges. In addition, phantom spikes frequently have a variable time relationship with the slow waves, and it is not unusual to observe spikes that are located "on top of the slow waves" instead of immediately before the slow wave. Sometimes slow alpha variant posterior background intermixes with alpha wave, giving a similar impression (▸ Figure 3.245).

3.4.2.5 Periodic Patterns (PP)

Periodic patterns include several EEG abnormalities which consist of more or less stereotyped waveforms that are of relatively high amplitude compared to the background EEG activity and that recur at approximately constant intervals.

Periodic patterns can be subdivided as follows:
- Periodic non-epileptiform discharges (labeled "periodic discharges")
- Periodic epileptiform discharges
- Triphasic waves
- Burst attenuation
- Burst Suppression

3.4.2.5.1 Periodic Discharges

Except for lateralized periodic discharges (LPD), the periodic patterns are associated with encephalopathies. Lateralized periodic discharges (LPD) have a relatively high association with acute brain lesions, such as encephalitis and stroke (Chatrian et al., 1964). A high proportion of LPD patients have seizures but not all do, which prompted the ACNS to abandon the term epileptiform in PLED (Hirsch et al., 2021). Note that in the recommendations by the ACNS, the term LPD supplants the term PLED. The ACNS classification is at

Benign epileptiform transients of sleep (BETS)

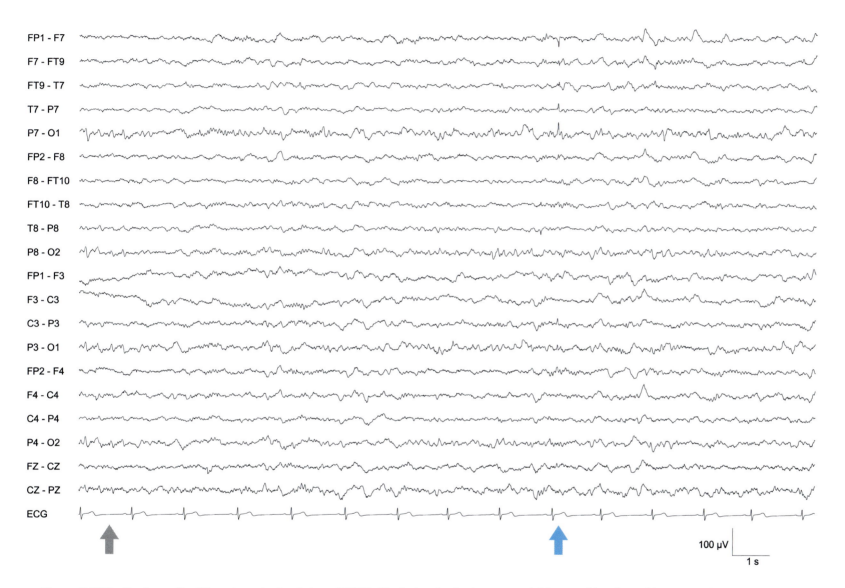

▶ **Figure 3.239   Benign epileptiform transients of sleep (BETS).** Bipolar longitudinal montage. A 23-year-old patient with vasovagal syncope. In light sleep, positive sharp transients of sleep (POSTS) (gray arrow) appear. A low-amplitude (~50 µV), short left temporal (F7, FT9, T7) sharp transient occurs without a following slow wave (blue arrow). This benign transient is also labeled small sharp spike (SSS).

EEG classification: Normal (sleep)

EEG report: Normal EEG.

Benign epileptiform transients of sleep (BETS)

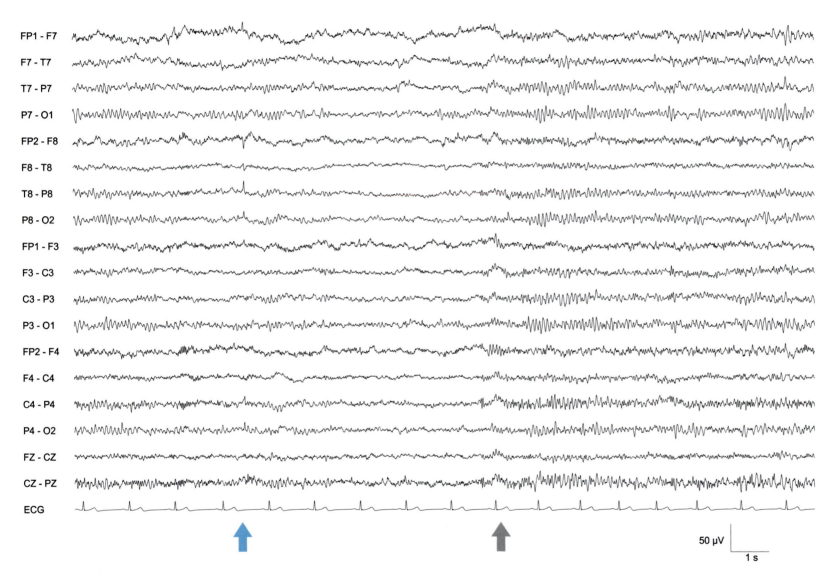

▶ **Figure 3.240** **Benign epileptiform transients of sleep (BETS).** Bipolar longitudinal montage. A 35-year-old patient with non-epileptic seizures in dissociative disorder. Low-amplitude, right temporal spike without subsequent slow wave (blue arrow). At the time of the gray arrow, the patient alerts and an occipital alpha background rhythm appears.

EEG classification: Normal (awake)

EEG report: Normal EEG.

14 and 6 Hz positive spikes

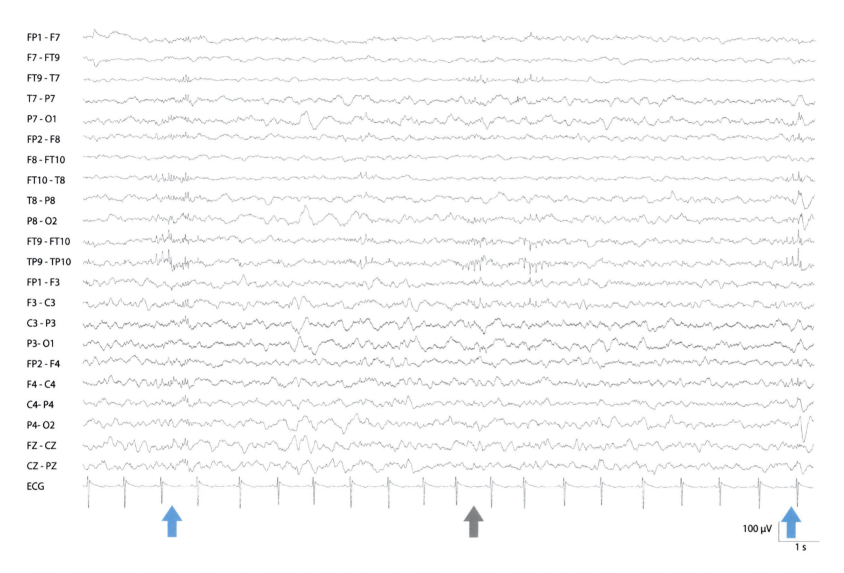

▶ **Figure 3.241** **14 and 6 Hz positive spikes.** Bipolar longitudinal montage. A 9-year-old boy with behavioral problems. During light sleep, positive spikes with a frequency of approximately 14 Hz occur in the right (blue arrows) and at other times in the left (gray arrow). These 14 Hz positive sharp transients are intermixed with positive sharp transients of approximately 6 Hz. The positive spikes are best represented in the transhemispheric channels TP10–TP9 and FT10–FT9. The 14 and 6 Hz positive sharp transients have a wide distribution maximum at posterior temporal electrodes bilaterally.

EEG classification: Normal (sleep)

EEG report: Normal EEG.

6 Hz positive spikes

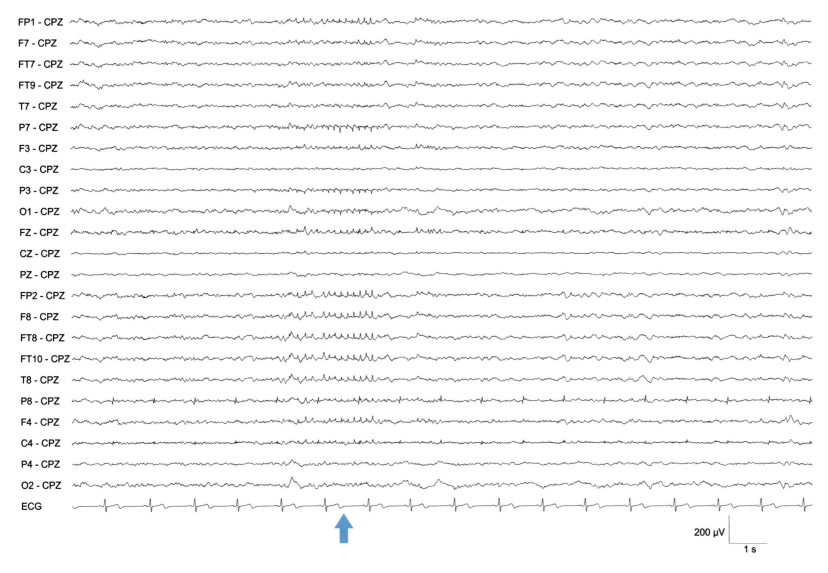

▶ **Figure 3.242** **6 Hz positive spikes.** CPZ reference derivation. A 20-year-old female patient with non-epileptic paroxysmal events and a dissociative disorder. In light sleep, rhythmic positive sharp transients occur with a frequency of approximately 6 Hz (blue arrow). The positive sharp transients show a clear phase reversal indicating that the reference electrode is active. Assuming that the 6 Hz sharp transients are positive, it can be concluded that they are maximum at P7 > P3 = O1. This is the typical distribution of these 14 and 6 Hz sharp transients. There is an ECG artifact at electrode P8 and, to a lesser degree, at electrode C4.

EEG classification: Normal (sleep)

EEG report: Normal EEG.

6 Hz positive spikes

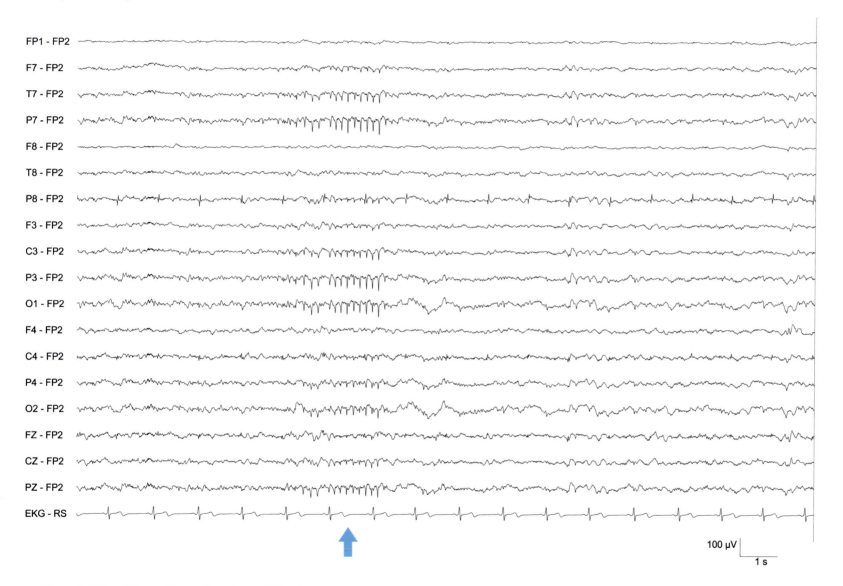

▶ **Figure 3.243** **6 Hz positive spikes.** Same EEG as in ▶ **Figure 3.242** in a FP2 reference dericvtion. With a FP2 reference, no phase reversal is present. The maximum positivity of the 6 Hz positive spikes is at P7 > O1 = P3 (blue arrow). For EEG classification and report, see ▶ **Figure 3.242**.

6 Hz "phantom" spike and wave

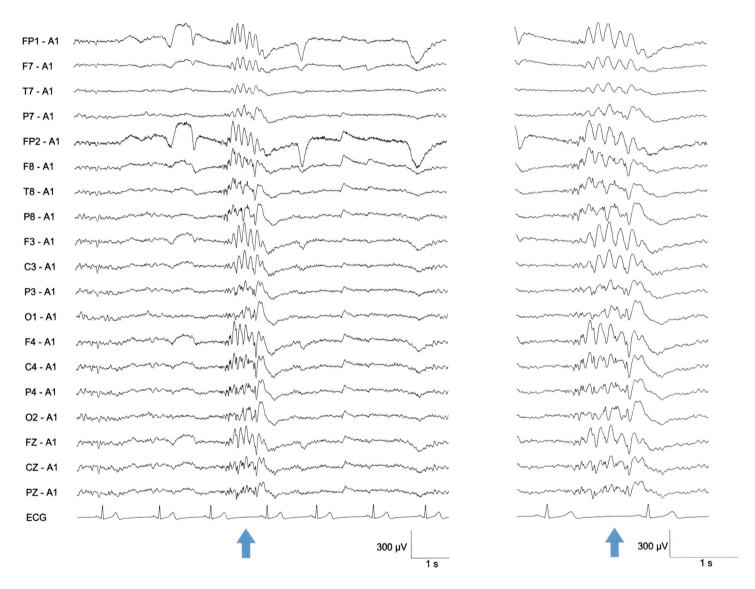

▶ **Figure 3.244** **6 Hz "phantom" spike and wave.** Left ear reference montage. A 19-year-old female patient with vasovagal syncope. Generalized 6 Hz theta waves of frontal maximum with preceding up to 130 μV sharp transients also of a widespread distribution maximum at C4 = P4 occur during wakefulness (blue arrows). The time axis is spread on the right side of the figure to better illustrate the pattern.

EEG classification: Normal (awake)

EEG report: Normal EEG.

Slow alpha variant

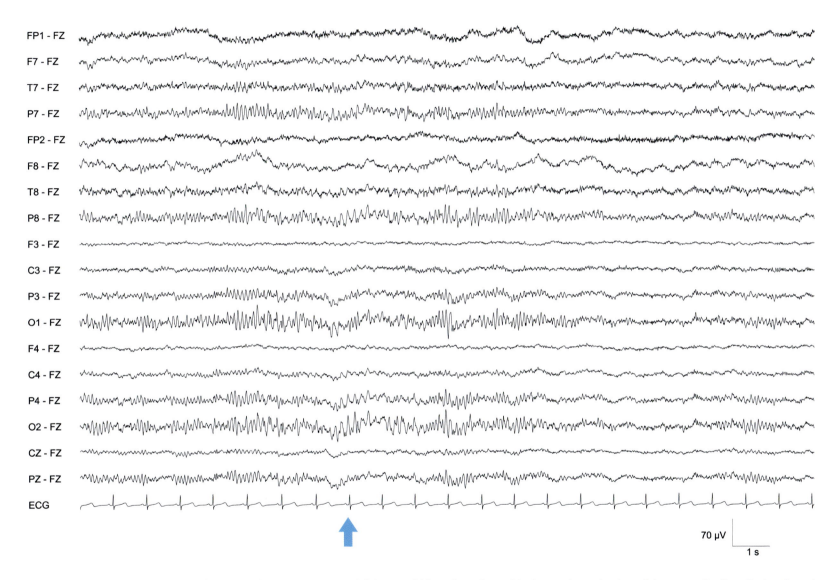

FP1 - FZ
F7 - FZ
T7 - FZ
P7 - FZ
FP2 - FZ
F8 - FZ
T8 - FZ
P8 - FZ
F3 - FZ
C3 - FZ
P3 - FZ
O1 - FZ
F4 - FZ
C4 - FZ
P4 - FZ
O2 - FZ
CZ - FZ
PZ - FZ
ECG

70 µV

1 s

▶ **Figure 3.245** **Slow alpha variant.** FZ reference montage. A 24-year-old female patient with depression episodes of depersonalization. During drowsiness (slow eye movements), occipitally pronounced 6 Hz theta waves intermix with some alpha waves (blue arrow).

EEG classification: Normal (awake)

EEG report: Normal EEG.

first a purely descriptive one, and where applicable, it should be used. Because PLED are highly associated (albeit not exclusively) with seizures, we prefer to use the term wherever applicable—that is, when the pattern is associated with epilepsy.

Periodic discharges can be modified according to their localization. The new labeling is LPD for regional discharges (▶ Figures 3.246–3.249) and GPD for generalized periodic discharges (▶ Figures 3.250 and 3.252). The same holds true for periodic epileptiform discharges (PED; ▶ Figure 3.253).

Periodic discharges of a generalized distribution (which are much more common in non-epilepsy-related clinical situations as opposed to the LPD/PLED association) occur in severe diffuse nonspecific encephalopathies (▶ Figures 3.250 and 3.251). They may consist of high-amplitude bursts separated by relatively flat EEG (▶ Figure 3.252). These rhythmical bursts do not fulfill the criteria for burst attenuation (EEG of relatively attenuated background activity has an amplitude of <20 µV; see ▶ Figure 3.271) or burst suppression (EEG of relatively attenuated background activity has an amplitude of <10 µV; see ▶ Figures 3.267–3.270). This pattern is frequently seen in patients with anoxic encephalopathy. Not infrequently, the bursts, particularly if they are epileptiform, will trigger a generalized myoclonic status, with each burst of epileptiform discharge triggering a generalized myoclonic jerk. Anti-seizure medications cannot control the myoclonic jerks, but, at least in some cases, they may prevent secondarily generalized tonic–clonic seizures (Elmer et al., 2016; Wijdicks & Rabinstein, 2016).

Sometimes the repetition rate and/or the waveform of the repetitive pattern is relatively characteristic of the etiology of the brain dysfunction. For example, periodic patterns with a repetition rate of one discharge per 4 s or slower are typical for subacute sclerosing panencephalitis secondary to measles infection. Another example is generalized triphasic waves (▶ Figures 3.260–3.266), which are a subgroup of periodic discharges with a typical triphasic morphology of the recurrent discharges, seen most frequently in patients with metabolic encephalopathies. Periodic high-amplitude slow waves indicate less severe encephalopathy (▶ Figure 3.254).

Regional periodic discharges can be seen in two clinical settings:
1. An acute brain lesion such as a cerebral hemorrhage or stroke, encephalitis, or rapidly expanding space-occupying lesion (brain metastasis and glioblastoma multiple) (▶ Figures 3.246–3.249 and 3.253) (Fitzpatrick & Lowry, 2007; Pohlmann-Eden et al., 1996). In stroke or hemorrhage patients, regional periodic discharges (RPD) evolve as follows:
   - Initially, the patients may suffer several focal seizures. An EEG obtained at that time shows EEG seizures followed by relative suppression of all background activities.
   - The seizures then become less frequent and RPDs occur.
   - One or two weeks after the stroke or hemorrhage, the EEG shows mainly RPD (no seizures occur anymore).
   - Three or four weeks after the cerebrovascular accident, the RPD become progressively less epileptiform and decrease in amplitude and eventually disappear completely.
2. Patients have a focal epilepsy that frequently has been activated by withdrawal of anti-seizure medication.

Notice that the term regional periodic discharge corresponds to the well-established term PLED and that PLED+ corresponds to the term regional periodic epileptiform discharges (RPED).

The degree of epileptogenicity of PD can be listed in decreasing order of epileptogenicity as follows:

Burst suppression (BS) → burst attenuation (BA) → periodic epileptiform discharges (PED) → periodic discharges (PD)

Bilateral independent RPD have a significantly worse prognosis than unilateral RPED and are often associated with anoxic encephalopathy and less frequently an expression of status epilepticus (Brenner, 2002) (▶ Figure 3.253).

PD are classified as abnormal EEG III because they indicate (a) if they have a regional distribution, an acute or subacute structural lesion or an active epileptogenic focus; and (b) if they have a generalized distribution, GPD are indicative of a severe diffuse encephalopathy. Anti-seizure medications are relatively ineffective in regional and also in generalized PED, and it is of no value to try to control PED or PD with these drugs.

Periodic discharges, right, continuous slow, left hemisphere; asymmetry, decreased backgound rhythm right hemisphere

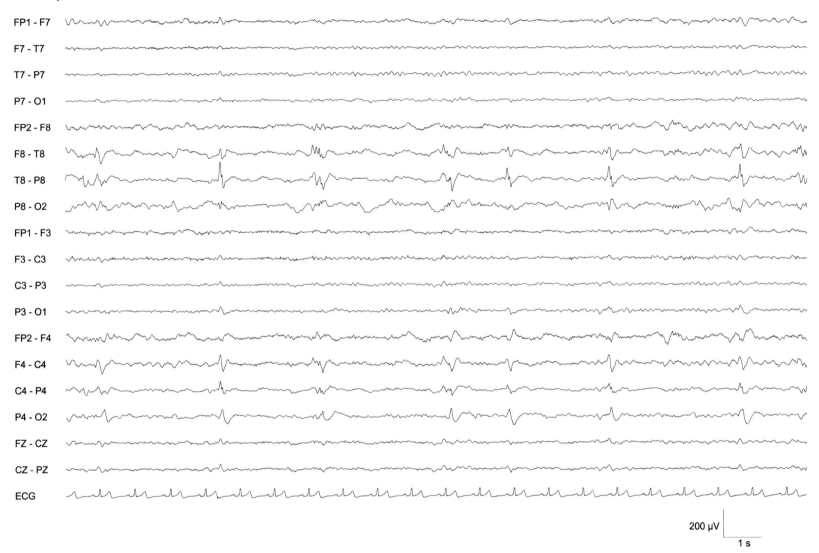

200 µV

1 s

▶ **Figure 3.246** **Periodic discharges, right.** Bipolar longitudinal montage. A 64-year-old patient with acute left sensorimotor hemisyndrome due to right middle cerebral artery (MCI) infarction. Periodic discharges with intervals of 1–2.5 s are seen in the right hemisphere. Note the typical variable morphology of the periodic epileptiform discharges. There is also a left hemisphere continuous slow, and the alpha rhythm is absent in the right hemisphere.

EEG classification: Abnormal III (awake)
1. Periodic discharges, right
2. Continuous slow, left hemisphere
3. Asymmetry, decreased alpha rhythm right hemisphere

EEG report: This EEG reflects the right MCI infarction.

Periodic discharges, right; asymmetry, decreased background, right

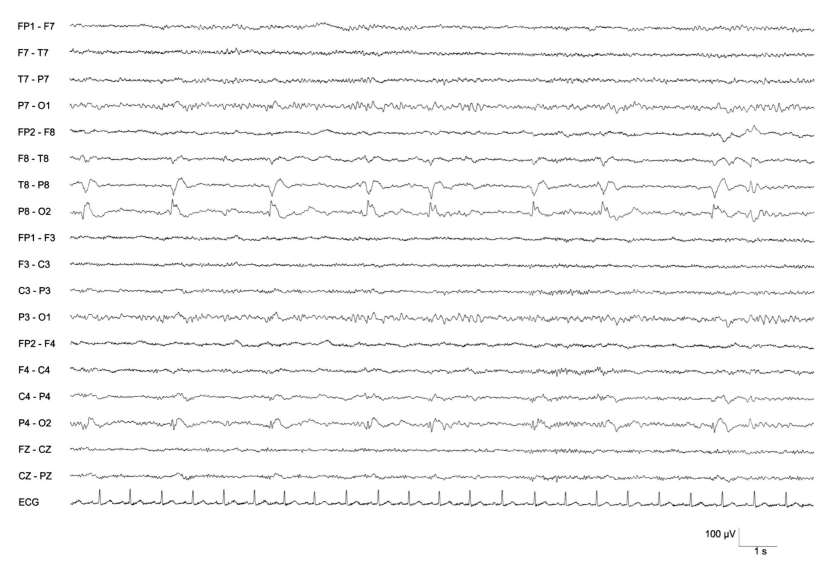

Figure 3.247 Periodic discharges, right; asymmetry, decreased right background. Bipolar longitudinal montage. A 74-year-old female patient with homonymous hemianopsia to the left due to acute right posterior infarction. Right posterior temporal periodic epileptiform discharges occur at intervals of 2 or 3 s. Beta and alpha frequencies are reduced in amplitude on the right.

EEG classification: Abnormal III (awake)
1. Periodic discharges, P8 > T8 = O2
2. Asymmetry, decreased background, right

EEG report: This EEG shows an acute right posterior temporal epileptogenic lesion.

Periodic discharges, left; asymmetry, decreased alpha activity, left

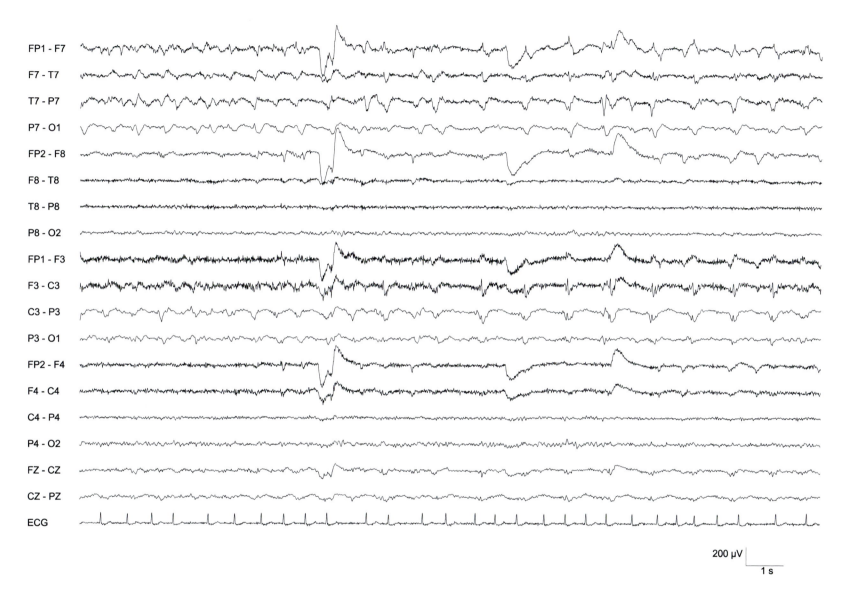

FP1 - F7
F7 - T7
T7 - P7
P7 - O1
FP2 - F8
F8 - T8
T8 - P8
P8 - O2
FP1 - F3
F3 - C3
C3 - P3
P3 - O1
FP2 - F4
F4 - C4
C4 - P4
P4 - O2
FZ - CZ
CZ - PZ
ECG

200 μV

1 s

▶ **Figure 3.248   Periodic discharges, left; continuous slow, left.** Bipolar longitudinal montage. A 72-year-old aphasic patient with embolic left middle cerebral artery infarction due to atrial fibrillation. There are periodic discharges in the left hemisphere maximum midhemispheric. There is a poorly developed alpha background activity of significantly lower amplitude on the left side. Following each periodic discharge, there is an approximately 1-s slow wave. It is unclear if that slow wave is part of the periodic discharge or represents a pathological background activity on the left hemisphere.

EEG classification: Abnormal III (awake)
1. Periodic discharges, left
2. Asymmetry, decreased alpha activity, left

EEG report: This EEG reflects the left-sided thromboembolic middle cerebral artery infarction.

Periodic discharges, right

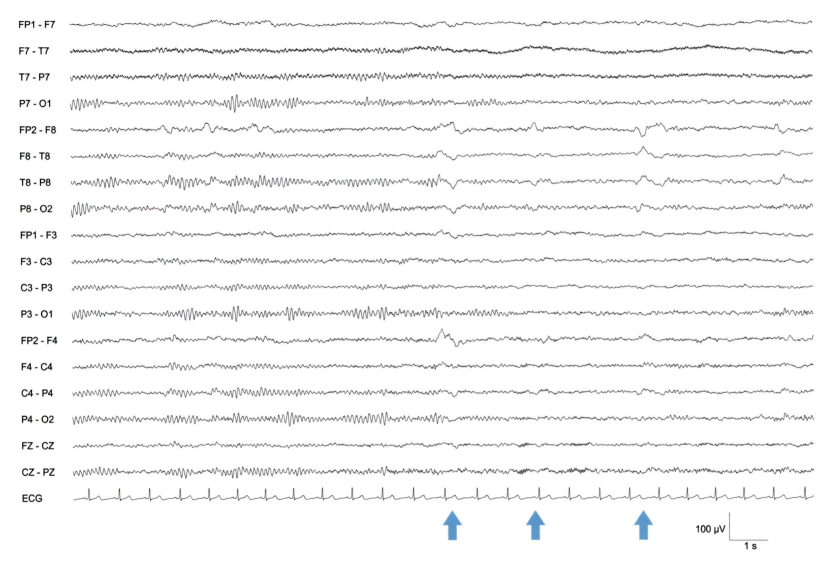

▶ **Figure 3.249** **Periodic discharges, right.** Bipolar longitudinal montage. A 31-year-old patient with cardioembolic right middle cerebral artery infarction. No epileptic seizures. The occipital background rhythm is well-developed bilaterally. The periodic discharges are maximum at F8 and become clearer (blue arrows) as the background alpha disappears with drowsiness.

EEG classification: Abnormal III (awake)
Periodic discharges, right

EEG report: This EEG reflects the right middle cerebral artery infarction.

Periodic discharges, generalized; anoxic encephalopathy

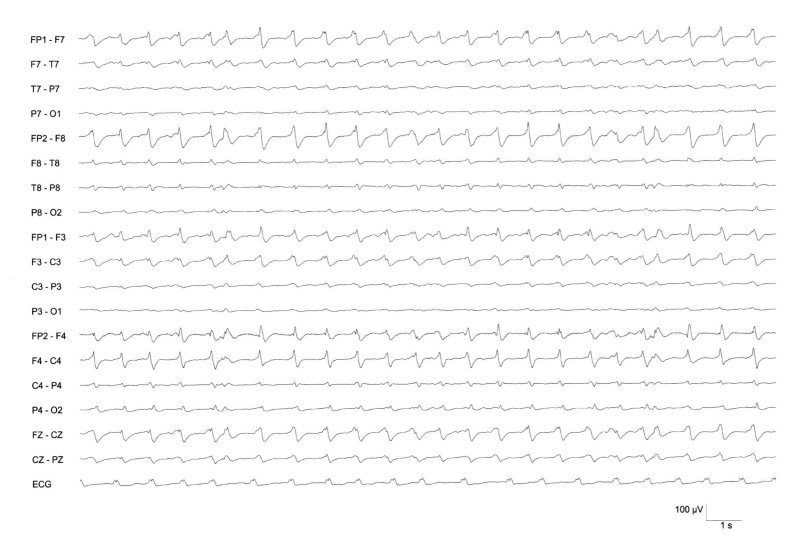

100 μV

1 s

▶ **Figure 3.250** **Periodic discharges, generalized; anoxic encephalopathy.** Bipolar longitudinal montage. A 76-year-old comatose patient with anoxic encephalopathy after acute cardiovascular arrest with resuscitation. There was a report of mild myoclonias in the face and limbs. This EEG sample, however, shows no evidence of myoclonias. The recording shows generalized periodic discharges repeating at intervals of 0.5–1.5 s. No other brain activity is seen.

EEG classification: Abnormal III (coma)
   Periodic discharges, generalized

EEG report: This EEG shows generalized periodic discharges. This EEG pattern is of guarded prognosis in patients who suffered an anoxic encephalopathy and are not on sedative medication or hypothermia.

Periodic discharges, generalized; anoxic encephalopathy (myoclonic status)

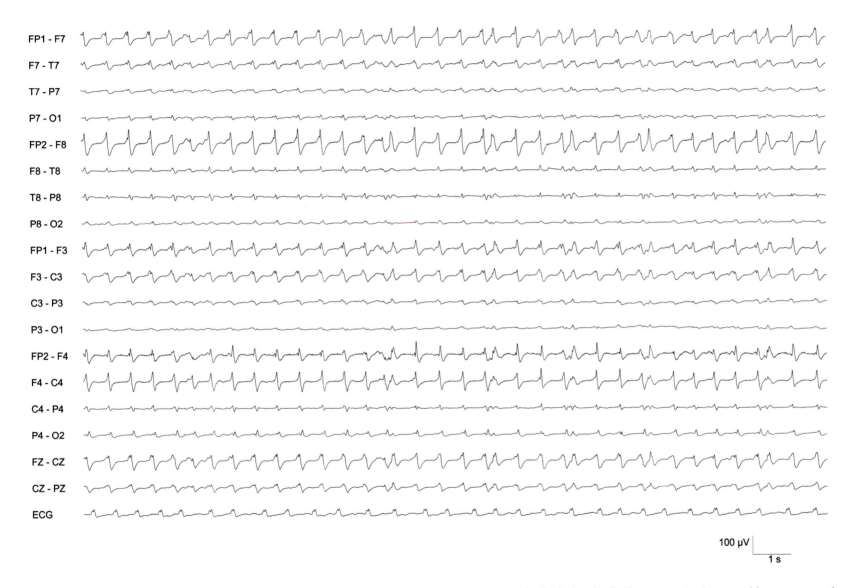

▶ **Figure 3.251** **Periodic discharges, generalized; anoxic encephalopathy (myoclonic status).** Bipolar longitudinal montage. An 81-year-old comatose patient with anoxic encephalopathy after acute cardiovascular arrest with resuscitation. Mild myoclonias were present in the face and limbs. Note the generalized periodic epileptiform discharges repeating at intervals of 1.5–2 s. No other brain activity is seen.

EEG classification: Abnormal III (coma)
    Periodic discharges, generalized

EEG report: This EEG shows generalized periodic discharges. This EEG pattern is of guarded prognosis in patients who suffered an anoxic encephalopathy and are not on sedative medication or hypothermia.

Periodic discharges, generalized; anoxic encephalopathy (myoclonic status)

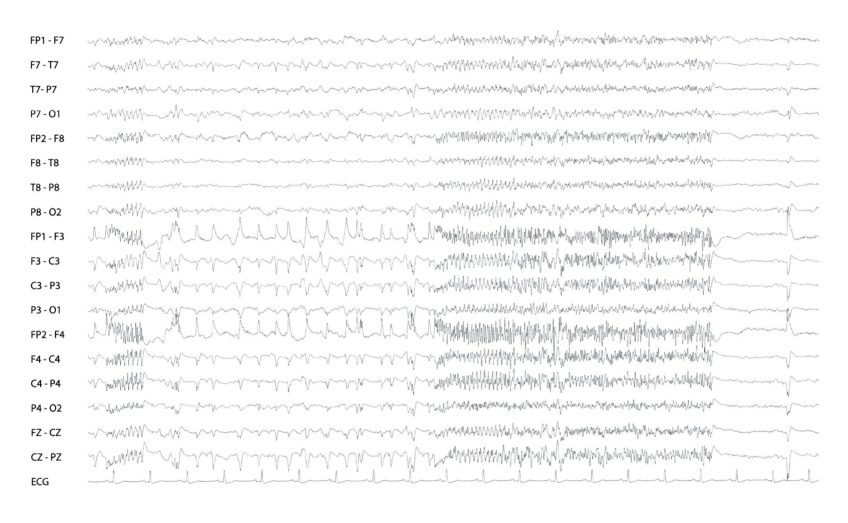

100 µV

1 s

▶ **Figure 3.252** **Periodic discharges, generalized; anoxic encephalopathy (myoclonic status).** Bipolar longitudinal montage. An 81-year-old comatose patient with right basal ganglia hemorrhage and anoxic encephalopathy after myocardial infarction with acute cardiovascular arrest and resuscitation. This EEG sample shows a 6- or 7-s burst of generalized paroxysmal fast and another 7-s burst of generalized, positive polarity periodic epileptiform discharges. In addition, there were also episodes of background suppression on other EEG samples producing an EEG pattern of burst suppression. Mild myoclonia was present in the face and limbs.

EEG classification: Abnormal III (coma)
  1. Periodic discharges, generalized
  2. Myoclonic status

EEG report: This EEG reflects status myoclonus due to severe anoxic encephalopathy. This EEG shows generalized periodic discharges and burst-attenuation pattern (in other EEG samples). These EEG patterns are of guarded prognosis in patients who suffered an anoxic encephalopathy and are not on sedative medication or hypothermia.

Periodic epileptiform discharges, right and left

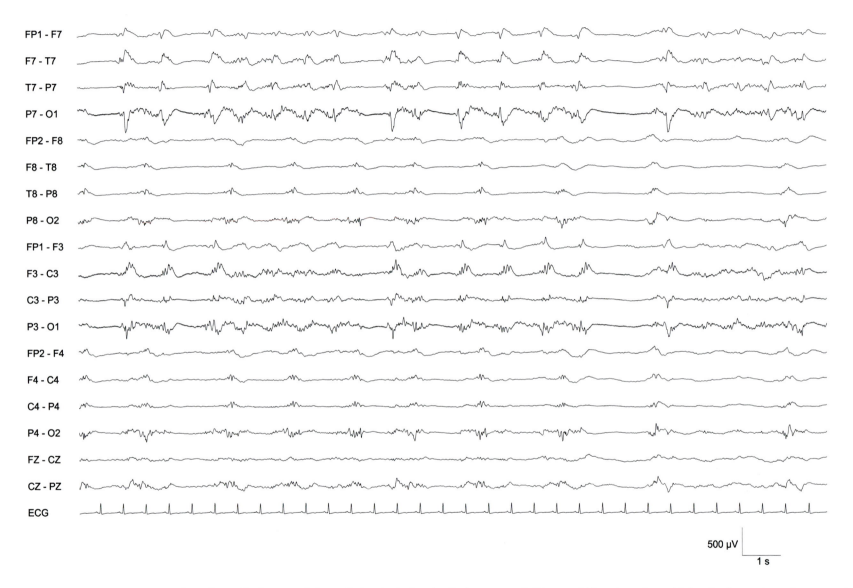

FP1 - F7

F7 - T7

T7 - P7

P7 - O1

FP2 - F8

F8 - T8

T8 - P8

P8 - O2

FP1 - F3

F3 - C3

C3 - P3

P3 - O1

FP2 - F4

F4 - C4

C4 - P4

P4 - O2

FZ - CZ

CZ - PZ

ECG

500 μV

1 s

▶ **Figure 3.253**   **Periodic epileptiform discharges, right and left.** Bipolar longitudinal montage. A 27-year-old female patient with focal epilepsy due to hypertensive posterior reversible encephalopathy syndrome (PRES). The right and left side show nonsynchronized independent periodic epileptiform discharges.

EEG classification: Abnormal EEG III (awake)
      Periodic epileptiform discharges, right and left

EEG report: This EEG supports the diagnosis of bilateral independent highly epileptogenic foci.

Periodic discharges, generalized; background slow

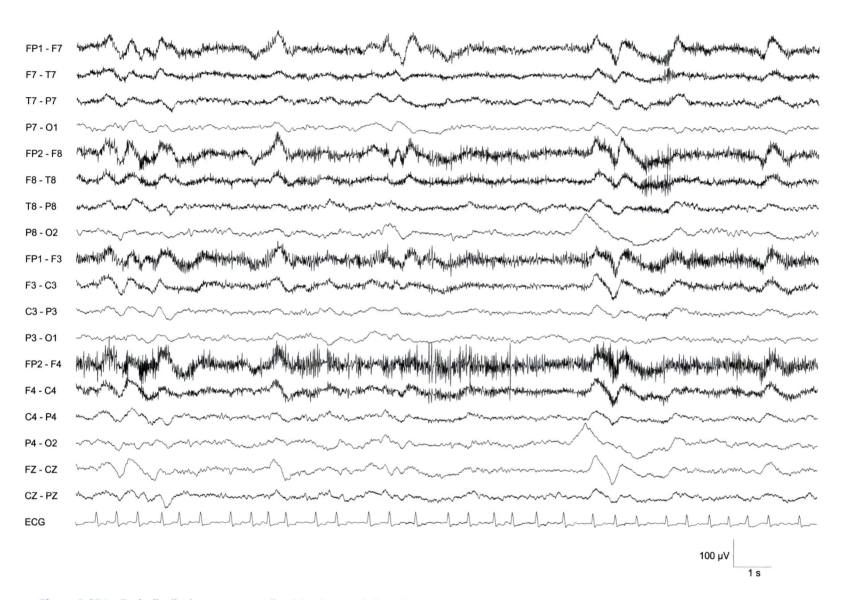

100 µV

1 s

▶ **Figure 3.254** **Periodic discharges, generalized; background slow.** Bipolar longitudinal montage. This 70-year-old diabetic patient suffered from metabolic encephalopathy due to renal insufficiency. The predominant background occipital rhythm is slowed to 7 Hz. At intervals of 1.5–3 s, bursts of 1–4 Hz high-amplitude generalized delta waves occur.

EEG classification: Abnormal III (awake)
1. Periodic discharges, generalized
2. Background slow

EEG report: This EEG shows a moderate diffuse encephalopathy.

3.4.2.5.2 Periodic Epileptiform Discharges (PED)

Periodic epileptiform discharges are a subgroup of PD in which the periodic burst includes epileptiform discharges (spikes, polyspikes, etc.; (▶ **Figures 3.253, 3.255,** and **3.256**). PED may have a generalized or regional distribution.

RPED are often better displayed in a bipolar longitudinal montage (▶ **Figure 3.255**) than in a vertex reference montage (**Figure 3.256**). because the vertex reference often lies in the RPED field and RPED can be either lateralized on one hemisphere (▶ **Figures 3.255–3.257**) or occur independently over both hemispheres (▶ **Figure 3.253**). The periodic burst frequently has a multiphasic, complex morphology. When the periodic bursts include epileptiform components, we use the term PED. If the periodic bursts do not include epileptiform discharges, we call them just PD.

RPED can—although rarely—occur in the midline; thus, it may be difficult to localize or even lateralize the PD (Hartl et al., 2017). In these cases, analysis of only the EEG may not allow one to determine if the patient has regional or generalized PED (i.e., if the pathology causing the PD is generalized or regional). In patients with PD, the occipital background rhythm may be preserved (▶ **Figures 3.248** and **3.249**), or in some patients, a significant slowing of background rhythms may occur depending on whether an encephalopathy is also present (▶ **Figures 3.254** and **3.257**).

Periodic discharges, and particularly PED, are frequently seen in patients who have both PED and epileptic seizures. In many cases, the bursts of PED do not trigger epileptic seizures, but the PD progressively increase in frequency and amplitude and eventually a seizure discharge occurs. The seizure discharge tends to spread, and together with the development of an EEG seizure pattern, the epileptiform discharge may become symptomatic. In these cases, we must classify the EEG as shown in the following example:

EEG classification: Abnormal III (awake)
1. Continuous slow, right mesial central
2. PED, CZ = C4
3. Seizure: EEG seizure pattern, CZ = C4
   Clonic status, left leg

On other occasions, each burst of the PD triggers a short seizure—for example, a myoclonic jerk. The burst of PED that trigger fast frequencies frequently include polyspikes (▶ **Figures 3.258** and **3.259**), which is often associated with seizures or status epilepticus (Feddersen & Trinka, 2012; Hirsch & Gaspard,

2013; Reiher et al., 1991). The EEG of patients in which each burst of PED triggers a clinical manifestation would be classified as follows:
EEG classification: Abnormal III (awake)
1. Continuous slow, right mesial central
2. Seizure: PED, CZ = C4.
   Clonic status, left leg

Notice the different classification strategy of the examples given above. In the first case, we classify independently the PED and the EEG seizure pattern. In the second case, the left leg clonus status is nested within the CZ = C4 PED.

3.4.2.5.3 Triphasic Waves (TW)

Triphasic waves are a subset of a periodic pattern consisting of high-amplitude (>70 μV) positive sharp transients framed by relatively low-amplitude negative waves (▶ **Figures 3.260** and **3.261**). The counting of the phases is not uniform in the literature. The first wave is negative and usually has a lower amplitude than the following positive wave. The third wave is negative again and usually is slower than both previous waves (▶ **Figure 3.260**). The distribution is generalized, and often in a bipolar fronto-occipital longitudinal row, the highest deflections occur in the anterior channels. In patients with focal lesions, surprisingly the triphasic waves may be of higher amplitude on the side of the lesion, suggesting that the abnormal waves are "generated" by the lesion. In fronto-occipital longitudinal bipolar montages, there appears to be a fronto-occipital delay of the triphasic wave. The lag is not apparent in referential montages, suggesting that it is primarily due to small changes over time of amplitude of the different components of the triphasic wave. Nevertheless, the apparent fronto-occipital delay is seen frequently and is a useful criterion when trying to differentiate between triphasic waves and epileptic discharges.

Triphasic waves tend to have a repetition rate of approximately 1 or 2 Hz and most frequently occur in patients with a metabolic encephalopathy. The diagnosis of triphasic waves is, like the diagnosis of epileptiform discharges, subjective. Some studies have tried to differentiate triphasic waves from epileptic PED (Alkhachroum et al., 2018; Boulanger et al., 2006). In many cases, the differential diagnosis is relatively clear, but even if we apply the criteria outlined above, there remains a significant percentage of borderline cases.

Periodic epileptiform discharges, right. Bipolar longitudinal montage

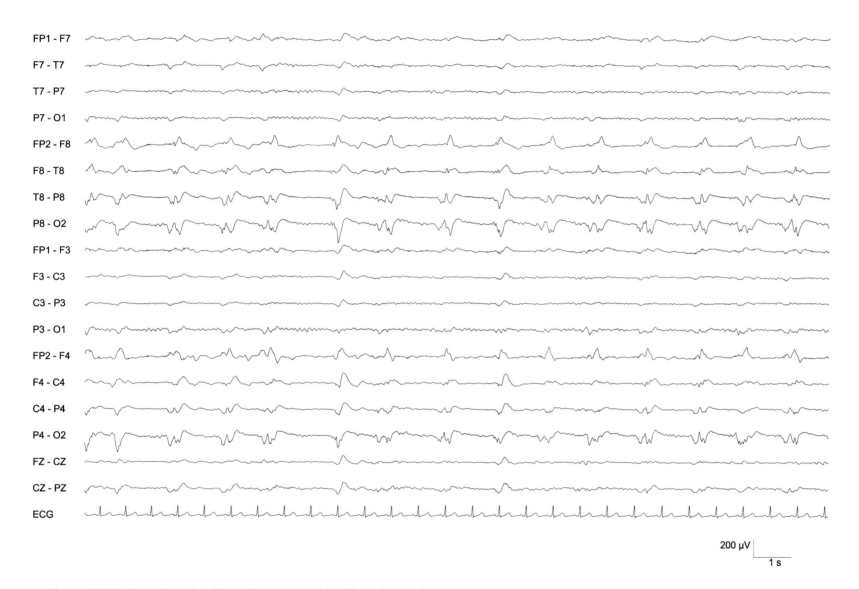

200 µV

1 s

▶ **Figure 3.255** **Periodic epileptiform discharges, right.** Bipolar longitudinal montage. A 51-year-old patient status post left clonic status epilepticus due to hypertensive posterior reversible leukoencephalopathy syndrome (PRES). The right hemisphere shows periodic epileptiform discharges at a repetition rate of approximately 1 Hz dominate the right hemisphere. Note that the occipital alpha background rhythm is well-developed bilaterally.

EEG classification: Abnormal III (awake)
    Periodic epileptiform discharges, right

EEG report: This EEG shows a highly epileptogenic abnormality in the right hemisphere.

Periodic epileptiform discharges, right

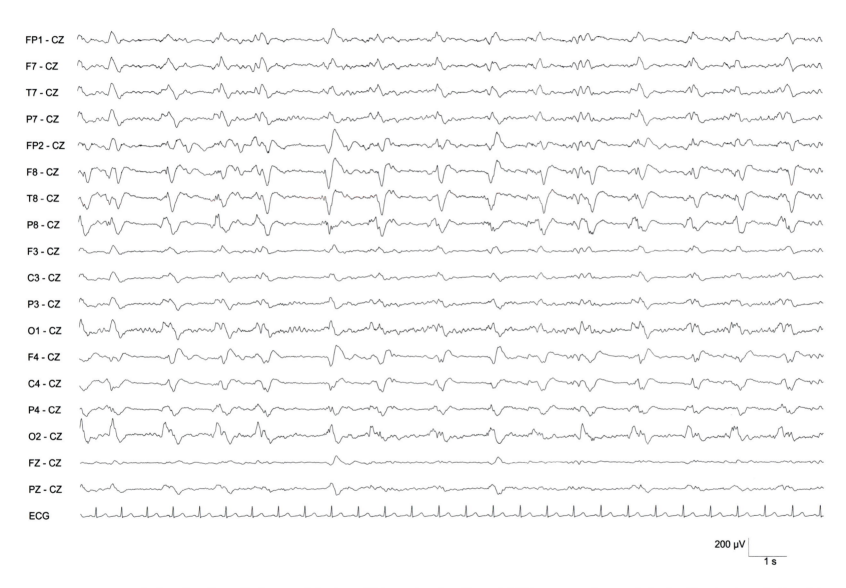

FP1 - CZ

F7 - CZ

T7 - CZ

P7 - CZ

FP2 - CZ

F8 - CZ

T8 - CZ

P8 - CZ

F3 - CZ

C3 - CZ

P3 - CZ

O1 - CZ

F4 - CZ

C4 - CZ

P4 - CZ

O2 - CZ

FZ - CZ

PZ - CZ

ECG

200 µV

1 s

▶ **Figure 3.256** **Periodic epileptiform discharges, right.** Same EEG sample as in ▶ **Figure 3.255** in a vertex reference derivation. The clear lateralization of the periodic epileptiform discharges to the right in ▶ **Figure 3.255** can hardly be appreciated in a vertex reference montage because the vertex reference lies in the electric field of the periodic epileptiform discharges and introduces phase-inverted deflections into several EEG channels.

Periodic epileptiform discharges

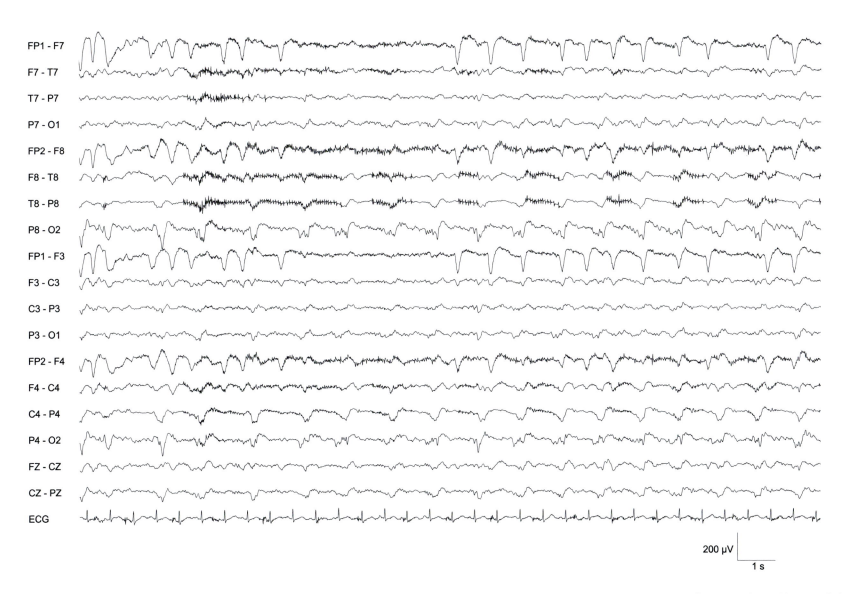

▶ **Figure 3.257** **Periodic epileptiform discharges, right occipital; background slow.** Bipolar longitudinal montage. A 67-year-old female patient with pre-existing Alzheimer's dementia and acute right occipital intracerebral hemorrhage. Right occipital (O2 = P4 > PZ) periodic epileptiform discharges occur with a repetition rate of approximately 1 Hz. The artifacts caused by frequent eye blinks outweigh the periodic epileptiform discharges in amplitude. The occipital background rhythm is slowed to approximately 6 Hz and is absent on the right side. Intensive care unit recording with an electrical artifact due to infusion pump (at electrode T8).

EEG classification: Abnormal III (awake)
1. Periodic epileptiform discharges, right parieto-occipital maximum
2. Asymmetry, decreased posterior background right
3. Background slow

EEG report: This EEG shows an acute, highly epileptogenic lesion on the right and a moderate diffuse encephalopathy.

Periodic epileptiform discharges, right; EEG status pattern, right

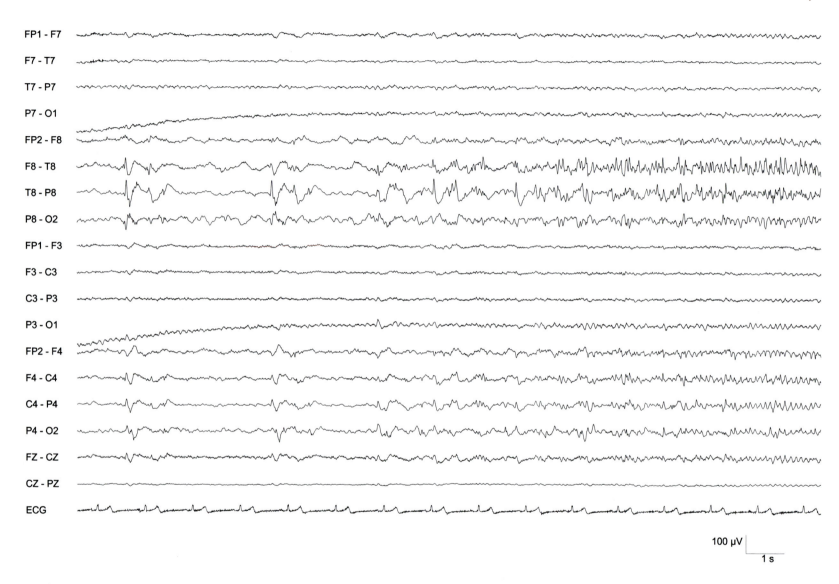

100 μV

1 s

▶ **Figure 3.258** **Periodic epileptiform discharges, right; EEG status pattern, right.** Bipolar longitudinal montage. A 45-year-old patient with status post resection of a right temporo-occipital metastasis of a gastric adenocarcinoma and frequent epileptic seizures. Right temporo-occipital periodic epileptiform discharges evolve into a fast EEG status pattern. This EEG seizure pattern was repeated several times within 20 min. Note that the main component of the discharge at electrode P8 is positive.

EEG classification: Abnormal III (awake)

Status: Periodic epileptiform discharges, P8 > O2

   Dialeptic status epilepticus

EEG report: This EEG shows a right status epilepticus.

Periodic epileptiform discharges, right; EEG status pattern, right

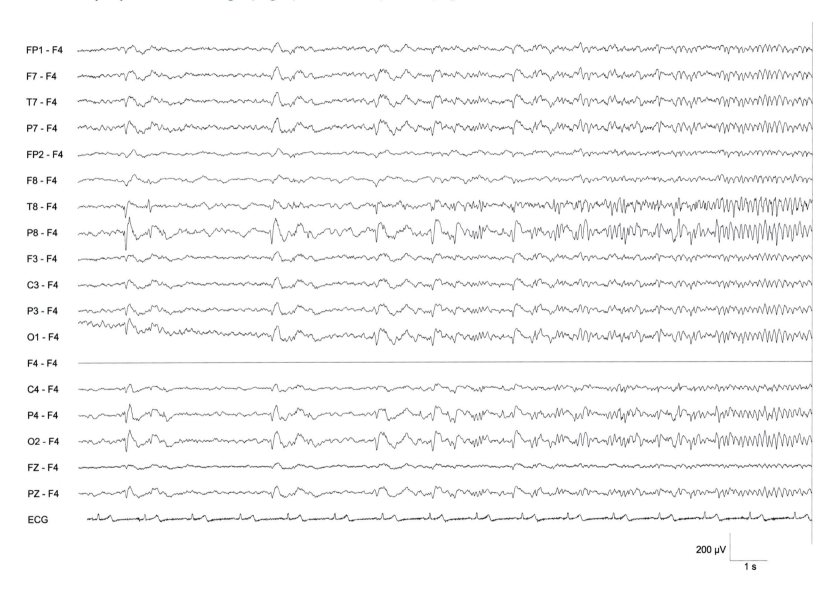

200 µV

1 s

▶ **Figure 3.259** **Periodic epileptiform discharges, right; EEG status pattern, right.** Referential montage to electrode F4. Same EEG as in ▶ **Figure 3.258**. The referential montage to electrode F4 shows best the positive discharge because there is no phase reversal in a referential montage. For EEG classification and report, see ▶ **Figure 3.258**.

The three phases of the triphasic waves

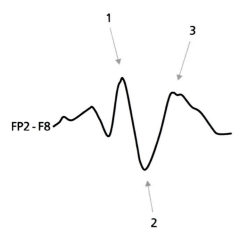

▶ **Figure 3.260** **The three phases of the triphasic waves.** Although some controversy exists, the definition of triphasic waves is as follows: A prominent positive wave (wave 2) is preceded by a somewhat lower amplitude negative wave (wave 1) and followed by a slower, low-amplitude negative wave (wave 3).

The expression of triphasic waves can vary greatly inter- and intraindividually (▶ **Figures 3.261–3.265**). The degree of slowing of the background rhythms, as usual, is a good index of the degree of encephalopathy the patient is suffering from. ▶ **Figure 3.264** illustrates that the differential diagnosis between generalized slow spike–waves and triphasic waves not infrequently is difficult, if not impossible. In addition, patients with benign focal epilepsy of childhood occasionally show bi-occipital BFED that trigger bifrontal BFED. This results in an EEG pattern that resembles generalized slow spike–waves. However, considering the clinical history (Lennox–Gastaut syndrome vs. metabolic encephalopathy vs. benign focal epilepsy of childhood), it is usually easy to differentiate the three conditions.

Benzodiazepine injections affect triphasic waves as well as epileptiform discharges (**Figure 3.262**). Therefore, the benzodiazepine response does not help distinguish a generalized EEG status pattern from triphasic waves (▶ **Figures 3.261–3.263** and **3.266**).

Triphasic waves are classified as abnormal III because of their correlation to diffuse encephalopathies, particularly metabolic encephalopathies.

3.4.2.5.4 Burst Suppression (BUS)

Burst suppression is a special form of periodic pattern in which brain activity of less than 10 μV alternates with short bursts of relatively higher amplitude (▶ **Figures 3.267** and **3.268**). Generalized burst suppression is seen in severe toxic, metabolic, or anoxic encephalopathies. Patients with burst suppression usually are stuporous or comatose.

This EEG pattern can also be caused by sedation in the treatment of status epilepticus by anesthesia (barbiturates, propofol, etc.). In these patients, the percentage of time in which there is background suppression may be used to assess the depth of anesthesia.

Generalized burst suppression, if not triggered by sedative medication or hypothermia, has a prognosis that is almost as poor as that for generalized electrocerebral inactivity.

A burst suppression pattern can also occur over only one hemisphere and then is indicative of a severe unilateral brain lesion (▶ **Figure 3.269**). Bilaterally alternating burst suppression patterns have a prognosis similar to that for a generalized burst suppression pattern (▶ **Figure 3.270**).

When performing prolonged EEG monitoring, it is important to specify what percentage of time the patient is in background suppression, background attenuation, burst attenuation pattern, or burst suppression. This information could be added to the EEG classification, but it would add excessive complexity to it. Therefore, we include this information in the description of the EEG. As mentioned previously, patients who have burst suppression or burst attenuation frequently also have seizures. The classification of these seizures should follow the same principles specified above for seizures occurring in the context of PED or PD.

Burst suppression is classified as abnormal EEG III because it is associated with severe encephalopathies or very severe hemispheric lesions.

3.4.2.5.5 Burst Attenuation (BUA)

The burst attenuation pattern is similar to the burst suppression pattern, but the interburst periods show some brain activity, although it is of relatively low amplitude (between 10 and 20 μV). It may occur in generalized (▶ **Figure 3.271**) or unilateral fashion (▶ **Figure 3.272**). Unilateral burst attenuation indicates severe hemispheric pathology.

In the burst suppression pattern, there is essentially no brain activity (<10 μV) in the interburst periods (▶ **Figures 3.267** and **3.268**). Patients in

Triphasic waves

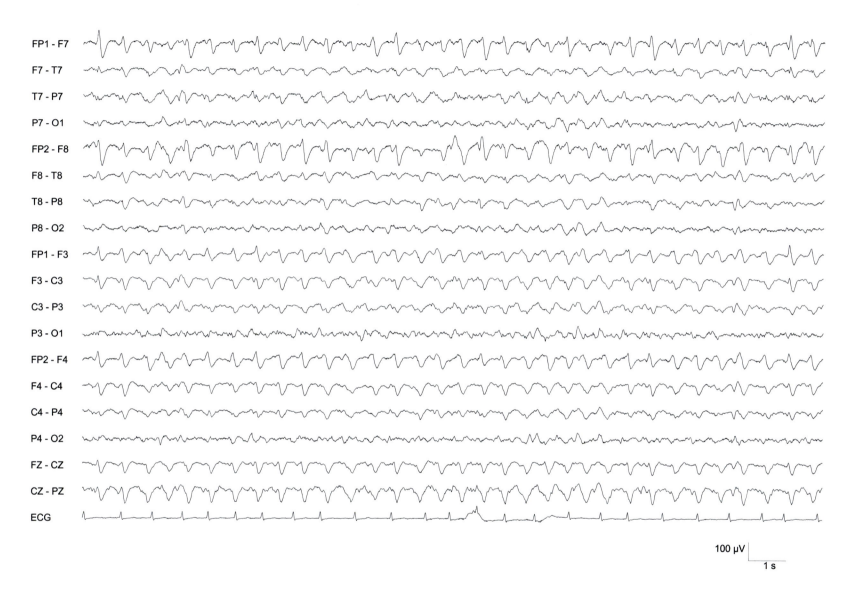

▶ **Figure 3.261** **Triphasic waves.** Bipolar longitudinal montage. An 80-year-old female patient with encephalopathy due to sepsis and renal insufficiency. The EEG shows triphasic waves in a generalized distribution and a repetition rate of 2 Hz. The high amplitude and diffuse distribution of the triphasic waves obscure the background activity. In addition, the high frequency of the triphasic waves does not permit evaluation of the brain activity in the inter-triphasic time. The degree of encephalopathy cannot be determined because of these limitations. The classification and report refer to this figure and ▶ **Figure 3.262**.

EEG classification: Abnormal III (somnolence)

Triphasic waves, generalized

EEG report: This EEG supports the diagnosis of a diffuse metabolic encephalopathy.

Triphasic waves after 1 mg lorazepam

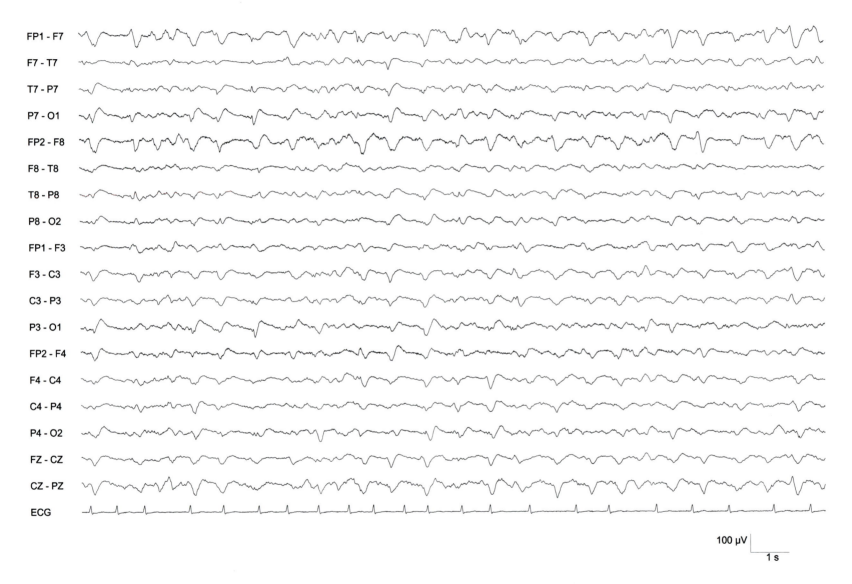

100 μV

1 s

▶ **Figure 3.262** **Triphasic waves after 1 mg lorazepam.** Bipolar longitudinal montage. Same EEG as in ▶ **Figure 3.261** after intravenous administration of 1 mg lorazepam. The initial negative sharp transient of the triphasic waves (component 1 in ▶ **Figure 3.260**) is now of significantly lower amplitude and the positive main component of the triphasic wave (component 1 in ▶ **Figure 3.260**) is now of significantly longer duration. The patient became drowsier after the injection. See ▶ **Figure 3.261** for EEG classification and report.

Triphasic waves

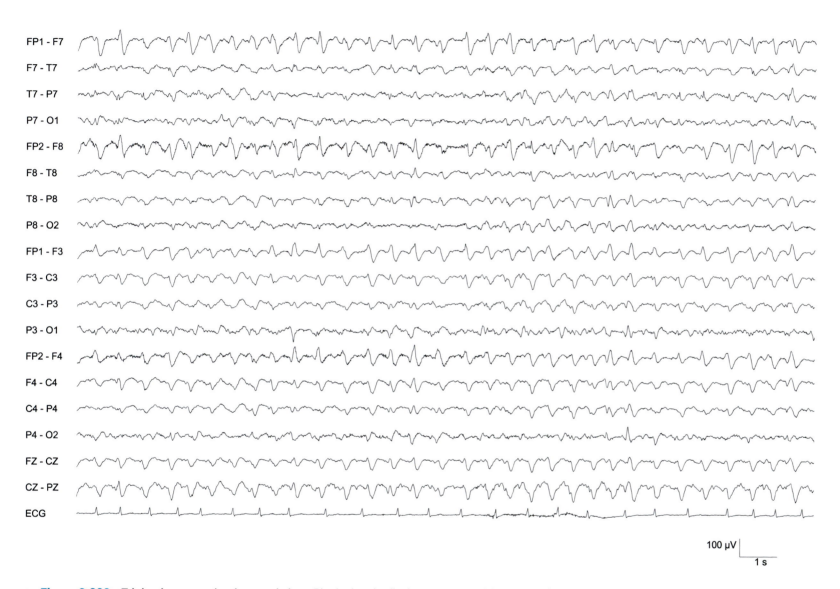

FP1 - F7

F7 - T7

T7 - P7

P7 - O1

FP2 - F8

F8 - T8

T8 - P8

P8 - O2

FP1 - F3

F3 - C3

C3 - P3

P3 - O1

FP2 - F4

F4 - C4

C4 - P4

P4 - O2

FZ - CZ

CZ - PZ

ECG

100 µV

1 s

▶ **Figure 3.263** **Triphasic waves; background slow.** Bipolar longitudinal montage. An 80-year-old female patient with metabolic encephalopathy. The EEG shows diffuse triphasic wave. The patient was somnolent but responsive to external stimuli. Generalized triphasic waves frequently make evaluation of background rhythms impossible. Therefore, in the presence of triphasic waves, it is frequently not possible to determine the degree of encephalopathy a patient is suffering from.

EEG classification: Abnormal III (awake)

Triphasic waves, generalized

EEG report: This EEG supports the diagnosis of a diffuse metabolic encephalopathy.

Triphasic waves; background slow

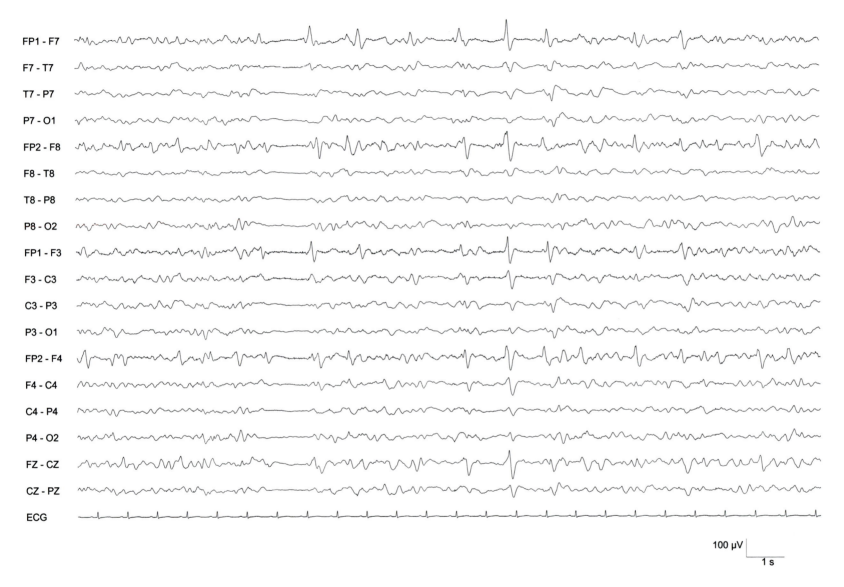

FP1 - F7

F7 - T7

T7 - P7

P7 - O1

FP2 - F8

F8 - T8

T8 - P8

P8 - O2

FP1 - F3

F3 - C3

C3 - P3

P3 - O1

FP2 - F4

F4 - C4

C4 - P4

P4 - O2

FZ - CZ

CZ - PZ

ECG

100 µV

1 s

▶ **Figure 3.264**　**Triphasic waves; background slow.** Bipolar longitudinal montage. A 66-year-old patient with metabolic encephalopathy. Triphasic waves of different amplitude occur repeatedly. Notice that in this case, component 1 (see ▶ **Figure 3.260**) of most of the triphasic waves is very prominent. In this EEG, the occipital background rhythm is slowed to approximately 5 Hz. The patient was confused and somnolent.

EEG classification:　Abnormal III (awake)
1. Triphasic waves
2. Background slow

EEG report:　This EEG supports the diagnosis of a moderate diffuse metabolic encephalopathy.

Triphasic waves; background slow

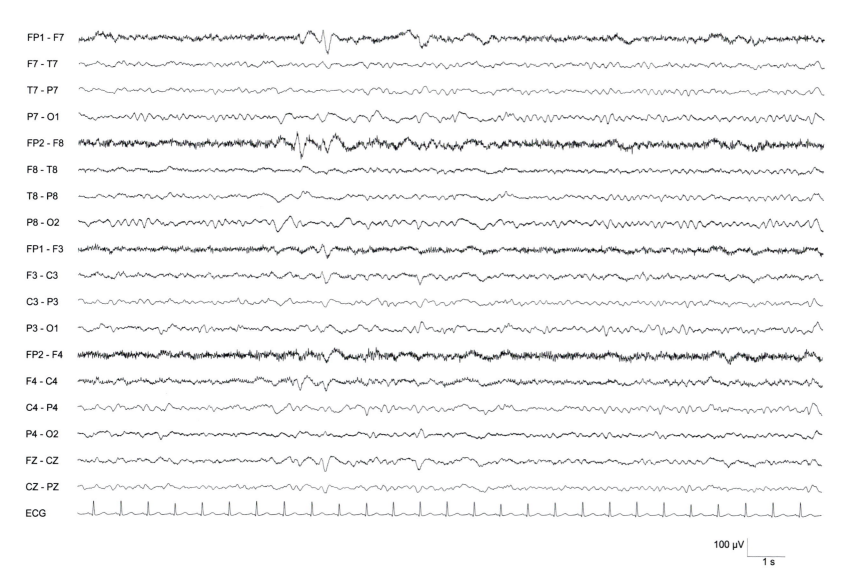

100 µV

1 s

▶ **Figure 3.265** **Triphasic waves; background slow.** Bipolar longitudinal montage. A 77-year-old female patient with metabolic encephalopathy. The occipital background rhythm is slowed to 6 Hz. The EEG showed only infrequent triphasic waves. In this case also, component 1 of the triphasic wave is relatively prominent.

EEG classification: Abnormal III (awake)
1. Triphasic waves
2. Background slow

EEG report: This EEG shows a moderate diffuse encephalopathy.

Triphasic waves after lorazepam administration

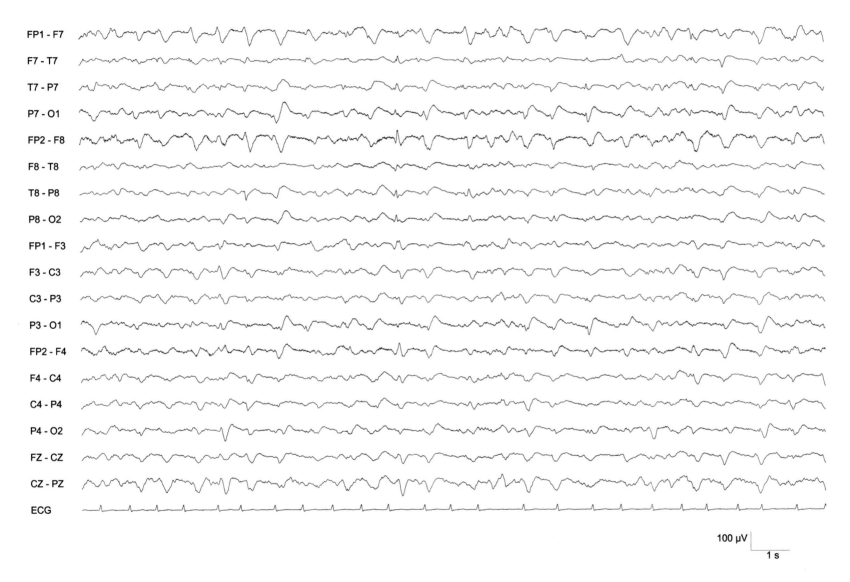

FP1 - F7

F7 - T7

T7 - P7

P7 - O1

FP2 - F8

F8 - T8

T8 - P8

P8 - O2

FP1 - F3

F3 - C3

C3 - P3

P3 - O1

FP2 - F4

F4 - C4

C4 - P4

P4 - O2

FZ - CZ

CZ - PZ

ECG

100 μV

1 s

▶ **Figure 3.266** **Triphasic waves after lorazepam administration.** Bipolar longitudinal montage. Same patient as in ▶ **Figure 3.263**. This EEG sample was recorded after intravenous administration of lorazepam. The frequency of the triphasic waves slowed down from 2 to 1 Hz. In addition, all the components, particularly component 1 (see ▶ **Figure 3.260**), are now of significantly longer duration. For EEG classification and report, see ▶ **Figure 3.263**.

Burst suppression, generalized

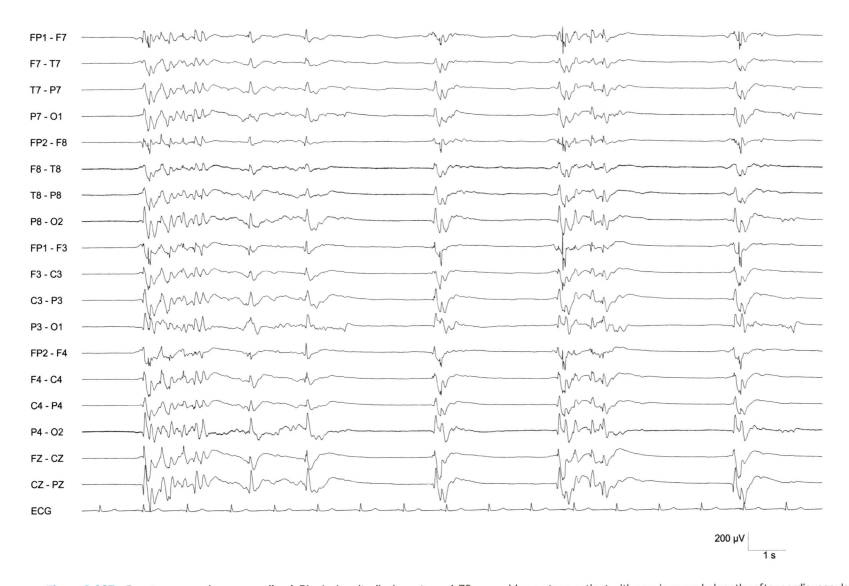

FP1 - F7
F7 - T7
T7 - P7
P7 - O1
FP2 - F8
F8 - T8
T8 - P8
P8 - O2
FP1 - F3
F3 - C3
C3 - P3
P3 - O1
FP2 - F4
F4 - C4
C4 - P4
P4 - O2
FZ - CZ
CZ - PZ
ECG

200 μV
1 s

▶ **Figure 3.267** **Burst suppression, generalized.** Bipolar longitudinal montage. A 70-year-old comatose patient with anoxic encephalopathy after cardiovascular arrest and resuscitation. The EEG is characterized by alternating high-amplitude bursts and flat sections of a few seconds' duration.

EEG classification: Abnormal III (coma)
Burst suppression, generalized

EEG report: This EEG indicates severe anoxic encephalopathy.

Burst suppression, generalized

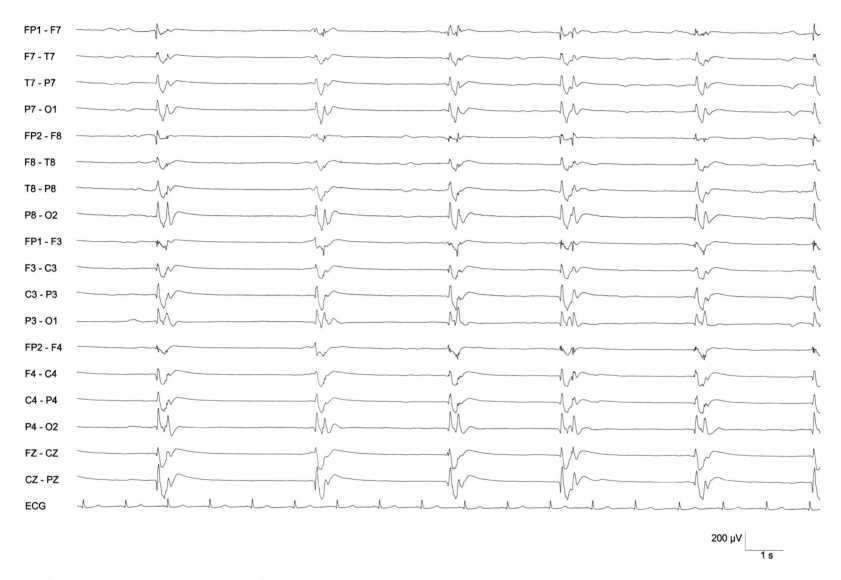

FP1 - F7
F7 - T7
T7 - P7
P7 - O1
FP2 - F8
F8 - T8
T8 - P8
P8 - O2
FP1 - F3
F3 - C3
C3 - P3
P3 - O1
FP2 - F4
F4 - C4
C4 - P4
P4 - O2
FZ - CZ
CZ - PZ
ECG

200 µV
1 s

▶ **Figure 3.268** **Burst suppression, generalized.** Bipolar longitudinal montage. A 62-year-old comatose patient with anoxic encephalopathy after cardiovascular arrest and resuscitation. The EEG shows alternating short, high-amplitude (>200 µV) bursts and flat sections of approximately 3-s duration.

EEG classification: Abnormal III (coma)
Burst suppression, generalized

EEG report: This EEG is indicative of a severe diffuse encephalopathy. A generalized burst-suppression pattern after an anoxic encephalopathy, in the absence of sedative medication or hypothermia, is of guarded prognosis.

Burst suppression, right and left

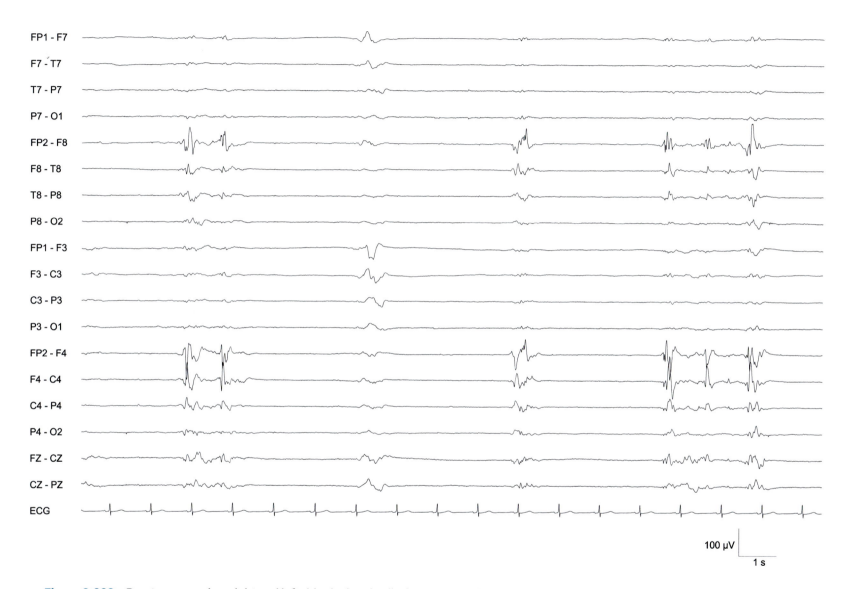

100 µV

1 s

▶ **Figure 3.269** **Burst suppression, right and left; bipolar longitudinal montage.** A 37-year-old comatose, immunosuppressed patient with severe septic–embolic encephalopathy secondary to aortic valve inflammation and multiorgan failure. High-amplitude bursts alternate with flat EEG sections in the right hemisphere. The left hemisphere is flat and occasionally shows single bursts.

EEG classification: Abnormal III (coma)

Burst suppression, right and left

EEG report: This EEG indicates severe, diffuse encephalopathy. A generalized burst-suppression pattern, in the absence of sedative medication or hypothermia, is of guarded prognosis.

Burst suppression, left and right hemisphere

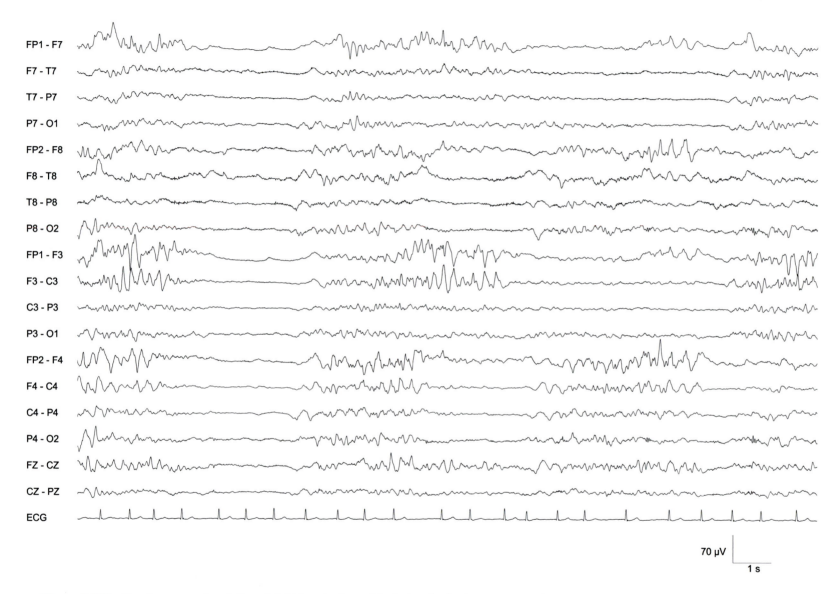

FP1 - F7
F7 - T7
T7 - P7
P7 - O1
FP2 - F8
F8 - T8
T8 - P8
P8 - O2
FP1 - F3
F3 - C3
C3 - P3
P3 - O1
FP2 - F4
F4 - C4
C4 - P4
P4 - O2
FZ - CZ
CZ - PZ
ECG

70 μV

1 s

▶ **Figure 3.270** **Burst suppression, left and right hemisphere.** Bipolar longitudinal montage. An 80-year-old comatose patient with severe encephalopathy after complications of open-heart surgery. Over both hemispheres, bursts and flat EEG segments alternate independently of each other.

EEG classification: Abnormal III (coma)

  Burst suppression, left and right hemisphere

EEG report: This EEG indicates a severe, diffuse encephalopathy.

Burst attenuation, generalized

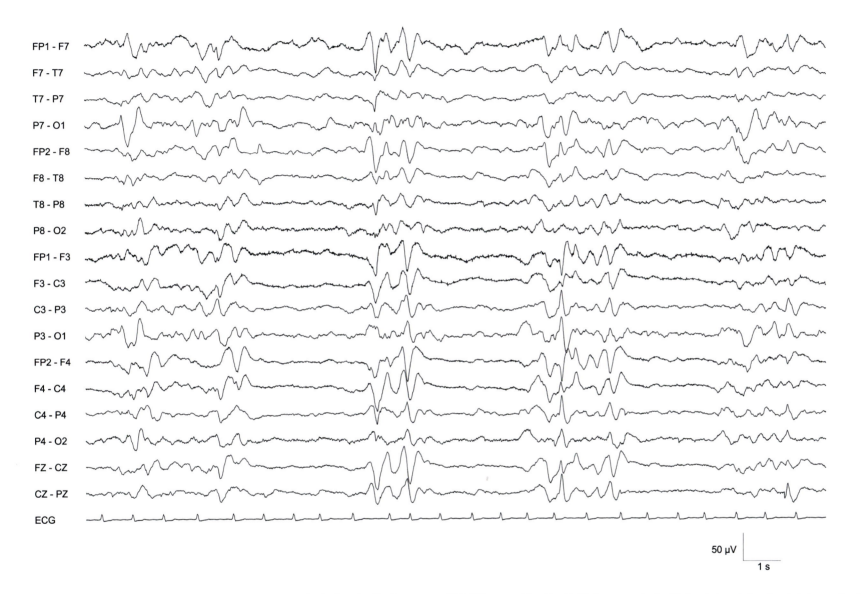

FP1 - F7
F7 - T7
T7 - P7
P7 - O1
FP2 - F8
F8 - T8
T8 - P8
P8 - O2
FP1 - F3
F3 - C3
C3 - P3
P3 - O1
FP2 - F4
F4 - C4
C4 - P4
P4 - O2
FZ - CZ
CZ - PZ
ECG

50 µV

1 s

▶ **Figure 3.271** **Burst attenuation, generalized.** Bipolar longitudinal montage. This 75-year-old patient initially presented with frontal nonlateralized status epilepticus associated with meningitis and an old left media infarction. During deep sedation, EEG showed this pattern, in which generalized high-amplitude bursts alternated with attenuated sections.

EEG classification: Abnormal III (coma)
Burst attenuation, generalized

EEG report: This EEG reflects the deep sedation.

Burst attenuation, left; continuous slow, generalized and background slow

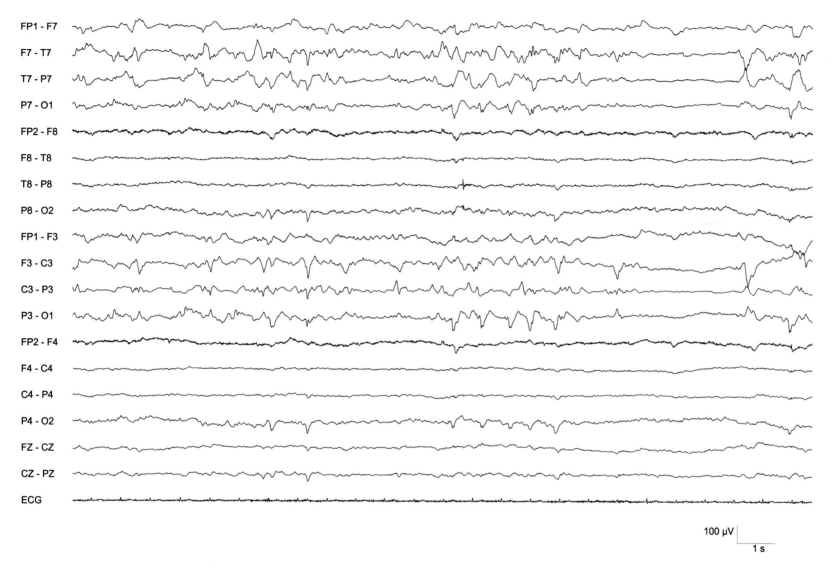

FP1 - F7	
F7 - T7	
T7 - P7	
P7 - O1	
FP2 - F8	
F8 - T8	
T8 - P8	
P8 - O2	
FP1 - F3	
F3 - C3	
C3 - P3	
P3 - O1	
FP2 - F4	
F4 - C4	
C4 - P4	
P4 - O2	
FZ - CZ	
CZ - PZ	
ECG	

100 µV
1 s

▶ **Figure 3.272   Burst attenuation, left; continuous slow, generalized and background slow.** Bipolar longitudinal montage. This 61-year-old patient has had a left hemisphere glioblastoma. He was obtandant during this EEG. The occipital background is poorly developed and approximately 4 Hz. Generalized continuous slow is also present in 90% of the recording.

EEG classification: Abnormal III (obtundant)
1. Burst attenuation, left
2. Continuous slow, generalized
3. Background slow

EEG report: This EEG reflects the left hemisphere glioblastoma and a moderate to severe diffuse encephalopathy.

generalized burst suppression are almost always comatose, and the whole recording tends to show the burst suppression pattern. That is not the case for burst attenuation. Therefore, it is essential to distinguish between burst-suppression (usually of very poor prognosis if not caused by sedative medication or hypothermia) and burst attenuation, which frequently is a reversible EEG pattern. In addition, in patients with burst suppression, the percentage of time occupied by suppression is directly related to prognosis. In prolonged recordings, it is important to specify what percentage of time the patient's EEG shows background suppression, background attenuation, burst attenuation, or burst attenuation. This is best specified in the EEG description or in the description of the different EEG patterns.

3.4.2.6 Differentiation of Nonconvulsive Status Epilepticus and Encephalopathies

The EEG can help in the differentiation of a nonconvulsive status epilepticus from encephalopathies (Boulanger et al., 2006; Kaplan et al., 2021). Diffuse encephalopathies are caused by a variety of etiologies, including metabolic disorders; intoxications; and neurodegenerative, vascular, autoimmune, or inflammatory pathologies. The EEG of patients with a mild encephalopathy shows slight slowing of the background rhythmical activity (<8 Hz to ≥ 7 Hz; ▶ **Figures 3.64** and **3.68**). Moderate diffuse encephalopathy is characterized by additional slowing of the background rhythms (<7 Hz; ▶ **Figure 3.69**). In addition, as the background rhythmic activity slows down, it also tends to increase in amplitude and to move anteriorly. Eventually, all the rhythmic slow activity is replaced by an irregular, polymorphic delta activity (severe diffuse encephalopathy). At this stage of encephalopathy, triphasic waves (▶ **Figures 3.261–3.266**) and also generalized periodic patterns (▶ **Figures 3.250** and **3.251**) may occur. Differentiation of triphasic waves and periodic patterns from epileptiform status patterns may be difficult (Boulanger et al., 2006). With deeper levels of encephalopathy, the irregular, continuous slow progressively decreases in amplitude, and eventually in deep levels of coma, generalized background attenuation occurs. At the same time, in patients suffering from drug-resistant generalized status epilepticus, the EEG initially shows the typical EEG/EMG characteristic of generalized tonic–clonic seizures. However, as the status continues, the EEG shows diffuse slowing and periodic generalized spikes. Eventually, the spikes are replaced by nonspecific slow waves, and the EEG cannot differentiate between a deep coma due to a severe encephalopathy or the diffuse background attenuation that characterizes the postictal EEG of patients suffering from a prolonged generalized status epilepticus, making it increasingly difficult to distinguish it from encephalopathy.

In some comatose patients (8%), there are recurrent EEG seizure patterns without a clinical correlate (Towne et al., 2000). This EEG pattern has been called "subclinical status." The distinction between generalized, epileptic subclinical EEG status patterns and encephalopathic EEG patterns is difficult (Benbadis & Tatum, 2000; Boulanger et al., 2006). Some EEG patterns classified as epileptic EEG status patterns can also be interpreted as triphasic waves in encephalopathic patients (Benbadis & Tatum, 2000). In these cases, the evaluation of the effect of benzodiazepine on the EEG is of little help in the differential diagnosis because benzodiazepine can suppress both EEG seizure patterns (▶ **Figures 3.212** and **3.213**) and triphasic waves (▶ **Figures 3.261** and **3.262**). In diseases associated with encephalopathies and epileptic seizures, such as Creutzfeldt–Jakob disease and Alzheimer's disease, it is particularly difficult to distinguish between encephalopathic and status patterns. Criteria for distinguishing between triphasic waves and generalized EEG status patterns were presented in Section 3.4.2.5.3 (Boulanger et al., 2006) .

3.4.2.7 Special Patterns

The following are special EEG patterns:
- Excessive beta (EB)
- Asymmetry (ASY)
- Sleep-onset REM (SOREM)

3.4.2.7.1 Excessive Beta (EB)
Excessive beta is defined as at least 50% of the wake derivation being dominated by a beta activity with an amplitude of at least 50 μV (reference derivation). Excessive beta refers exclusively to generalized EEG changes (▶ **Figure 3.273**). Regionally amplitude-increased beta activity is classified as asymmetry (▶ **Figure 3.274**).

Excessive beta

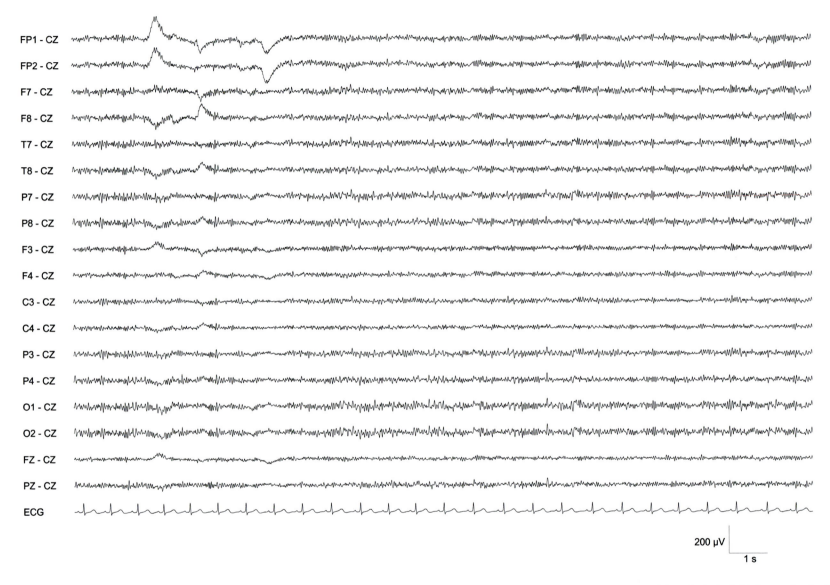

FP1 - CZ
FP2 - CZ
F7 - CZ
F8 - CZ
T7 - CZ
T8 - CZ
P7 - CZ
P8 - CZ
F3 - CZ
F4 - CZ
C3 - CZ
C4 - CZ
P3 - CZ
P4 - CZ
O1 - CZ
O2 - CZ
FZ - CZ
PZ - CZ
ECG

200 µV

1 s

▶ **Figure 3.273** **Excessive beta.** Ear reference derivation. A 24-year-old female patient with benzodiazepine abuse. Beta activity of relatively high-amplitude dominates the EEG.

EEG classification: Abnormal II (awake)
Excessive beta

EEG report: This EEG shows excessive beta activity most likely due to benzodiazepine abuse.

Asymmetry, increased beta, right

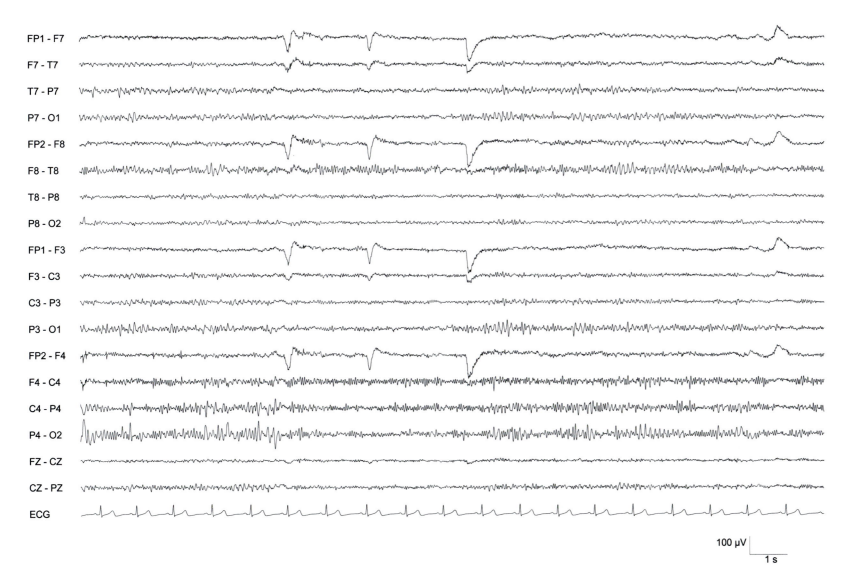

FP1 - F7

F7 - T7

T7 - P7

P7 - O1

FP2 - F8

F8 - T8

T8 - P8

P8 - O2

FP1 - F3

F3 - C3

C3 - P3

P3 - O1

FP2 - F4

F4 - C4

C4 - P4

P4 - O2

FZ - CZ

CZ - PZ

ECG

100 µV

1 s

▶ **Figure 3.274** **Asymmetry, increased beta, right.** Bipolar longitudinal montage. A 43-year-old female patient with focal epilepsy since age 5 years due to a right parieto-occipital pilocytic astrocytoma. Resective epilepsy surgery led to seizure freedom at age 34 years. Note the significantly higher amplitude of the beta activity on the right side.

EEG classification: Abnormal II (awake)

  Asymmetry, increased beta, right

EEG report: This EEG reflects the right craniotomy.

There is a familial, low-amplitude occipital beta activity (~20 μV) that occurs as a background rhythm variant in healthy individuals (▶ **Figures 3.34** and **3.35**) (Kozelka & Pedley, 1990; Vogel, 1958).

Excessive beta is most frequently the consequence of drug effects (particularly benzodiazepines and barbiturates).

Excessive beta is classified as abnormal I. If the sedative medication leads to more severe brain dysfunction, excessive beta is usually accompanied by a more or less pronounced generalized slow, which increases the degree of EEG abnormality. This should be differentiated from beta coma, in which beta frequencies dominate the EEG of a patient in stupor or coma (see Section 3.4.2.8.3). In a comatose patient, a diffuse slow in combination with excessive beta would be classified as follows if the delta activity is the highest amplitude frequency but the beta activity is still more than 50 μV:

Abnormal EEG III (coma)
1. Delta coma
2. Excessive Beta

On the other hand, if in a comatose patient the EEG shows mainly beta activity, even if of low amplitude (<50 μV), the EEG would be classified as follows:

Abnormal EEG III (coma)
1. Beta coma

3.4.2.7.2 Asymmetry (ASY)

Asymmetry refers to amplitude differences of background EEG activity between the two hemispheres or between homotopic brain regions of the two hemispheres. When classifying an asymmetry, we must define first which of the two hemispheres is the normal or more normal hemisphere. Sometimes it is obvious which hemisphere is pathological because one side has a normal background activity. In that case, we only have to determine if one or more of the physiological rhythms usually seen in normal individuals (alpha rhythm, beta activity, sleep spindles, etc.) are increased (▶ **Figures 3.275** and **3.276**) or decreased in the pathological hemisphere (▶ **Figure 3.277**). The following example illustrates how we would classify the EEG of a patient with a left temporal lesion. Because of the lesion, he has left temporal continuous slow. The extensive left temporal lesion leads to reduction of the background activity of the left hemisphere. This EEG would be classified as follows:

Abnormal III (awake and sleep) (▶ **Figure 3.277**)
1. Continuous slow, maximum left temporal
2. Asymmetry, decreased background left

Asymmetries with reduced background rhythm are a reliable sign for regional, structural, mostly cortical lesions (e.g., a porencephalic cyst) and often combine with slow of the same hemisphere (▶ **Figure 3.277**). The amplitude of the background rhythm is reduced in the region of a lesion (e.g., a porencephalic cyst). Unilateral subdural hematomas can also cause asymmetry in the sense of reduced amplitude of background activity. In this case, the reduced amplitude may be due to the increased resistance and the increased distance between the brain generator and the recording electrode. On the other hand, there is evidence that background rhythms can rarely be increased in chronic lesions with scar changes.

Asymmetries with increased background rhythm of a brain region are usually caused by bone defects due to trepanations or biopsy drill holes (so-called breach rhythm; ▶ **Figures 3.275, 3.276, 3.278,** and **3.279**). On the other hand, a decrease in background activity is usually due to an extensive lesion that, as explained in the example above, impairs the ability of the affected hemisphere to generate the background activity (▶ **Figure 3.277**).

The skull acts like a high-frequency filter. Thus, a bone defect leads to higher amplitude background activity on the side of the bone defect (▶ **Figures 3.278** and **3.279**). This involves all physiological rhythms, such as frontal beta, central mu, or posterior alpha (▶ **Figures 3.275, 3.276, 3.278,** and **3.279**).

When the patient is encephalopathic and the background rhythms are abnormal, we have to decide first which of the two hemispheres is the more normal hemisphere. Frequently, we need the clinical information to decide which side is more pathological. Once we decide which is the more abnormal hemisphere, we classify the abnormality caused by the lesion (epileptiform activity and/or regional slow). Then we pay attention to the background rhythms and decide if they are asymmetric and if they are of higher or lower amplitude on the pathological side. For example, ▶ **Figure 3.280** shows a similar situation as in ▶ **Figure 3.277**, but now the patient has a more severe lesion and, in addition to the abnormality caused by the left hemisphere, has a severe encephalopathy manifested by a delta coma. The EEG would now be classified as follows:

EEG classification: Abnormal III (coma) (▶ **Figure 3.280**)
1. Delta coma
2. Asymmetry, decreased background rhythms right

Asymmetry, increased alpha left occipital

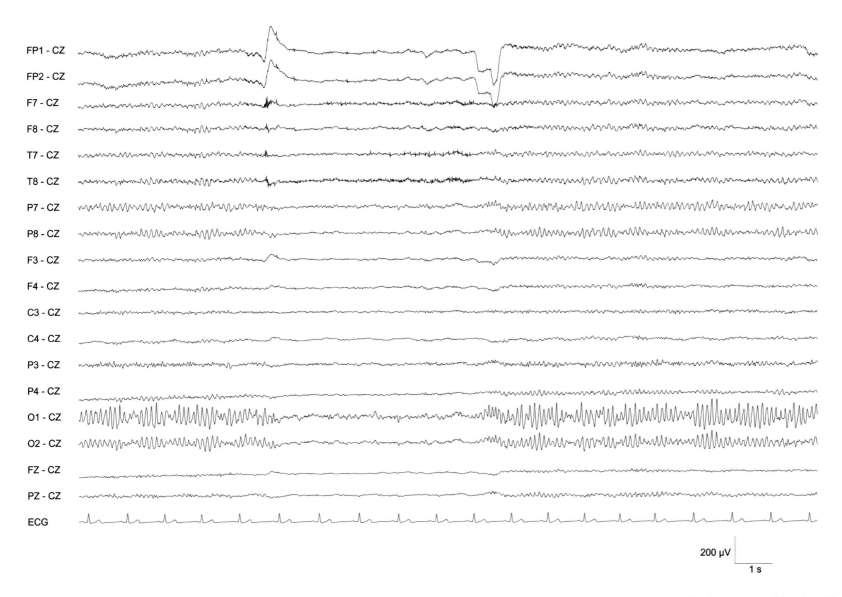

200 µV

1 s

▶ **Figure 3.275** **Asymmetry, increased alpha left occipital.** Vertex reference derivation. A left occipital meningioma was resected in this 74-year-old patient. The amplitude of the alpha activity is higher on the right. Normally, the alpha activity tends to be of higher amplitude on the right side. In this case, the degree of alpha asymmetry is definitely pathological.

EEG classification: Abnormal II (awake)

Asymmetry, increased alpha, left occipital

EEG report: This EEG reflects the right occipital craniotomy.

Asymmetry, increased alpha and beta left

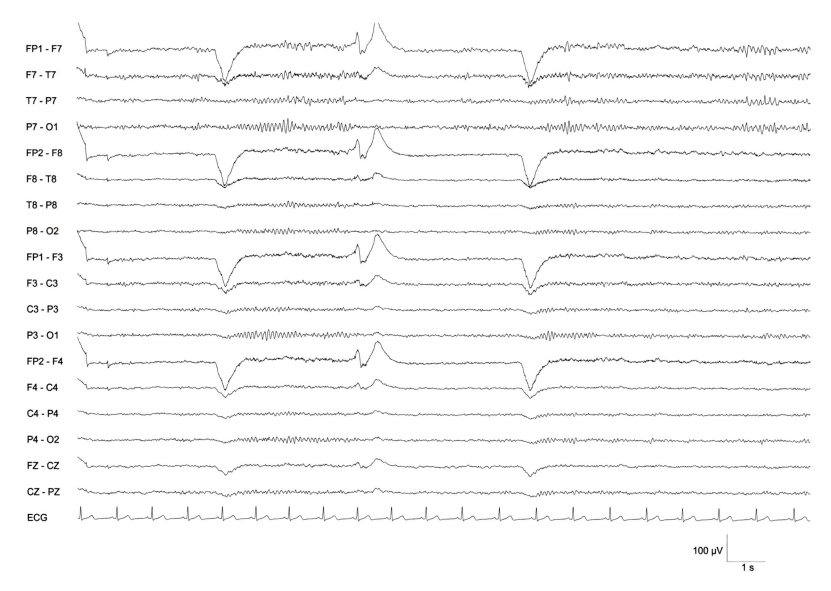

FP1 - F7
F7 - T7
T7 - P7
P7 - O1
FP2 - F8
F8 - T8
T8 - P8
P8 - O2
FP1 - F3
F3 - C3
C3 - P3
P3 - O1
FP2 - F4
F4 - C4
C4 - P4
P4 - O2
FZ - CZ
CZ - PZ
ECG

100 µV

1 s

▶ **Figure 3.276** **Asymmetry, increased alpha and beta left; bipolar longitudinal montage.** A 47-year-old patient with pharmacoresistant epilepsy caused by left temporal cavernoma. The cavernoma was surgically treated at ages 22 and 29 years. The beta and alpha activity is of higher amplitude on the left side.

EEG classification: Abnormal II (awake)

Asymmetry, increased beta and alpha left

EEG report: This EEG reflects the resection of the left temporal cavernoma.

Asymmetry, reduced background rhythm on the left; continuous slow, maximum left temporal

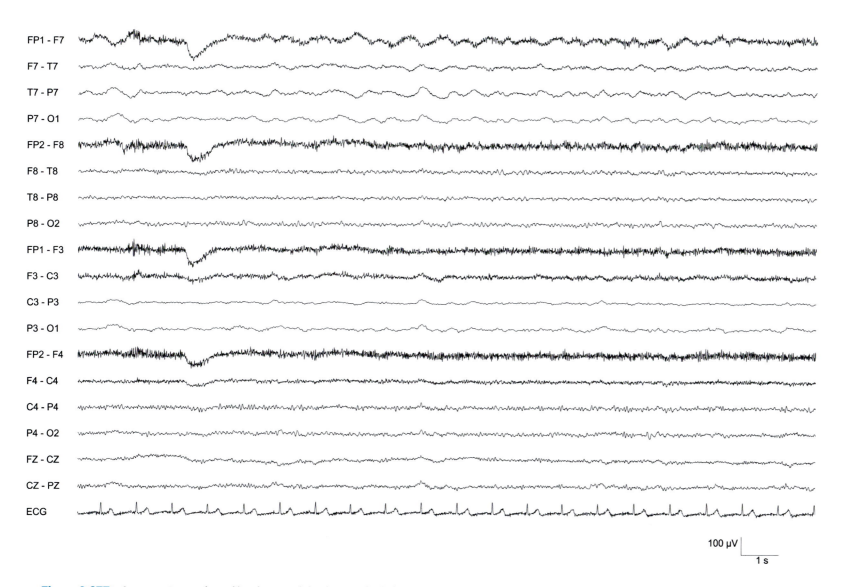

FP1 - F7

F7 - T7

T7 - P7

P7 - O1

FP2 - F8

F8 - T8

T8 - P8

P8 - O2

FP1 - F3

F3 - C3

C3 - P3

P3 - O1

FP2 - F4

F4 - C4

C4 - P4

P4 - O2

FZ - CZ

CZ - PZ

ECG

100 µV

1 s

▶ **Figure 3.277** **Asymmetry, reduced background rhythm on the left; continuous slow, maximum left temporal.** Bipolar longitudinal montage. A 58-year-old female patient with a left temporal glioblastoma. The EEG showed continuous irregular left temporal delta slow as well as a significant reduction of the background activity (beta and alpha) on the left.

EEG classification: Abnormal III (awake)
1. Continuous slow, left maximum temporal
2. Asymmetry, decreased background left

EEG report: This EEG reflects the left temporal glioblastoma.

Asymmetry, increased background, left; continuous slow, left temporal

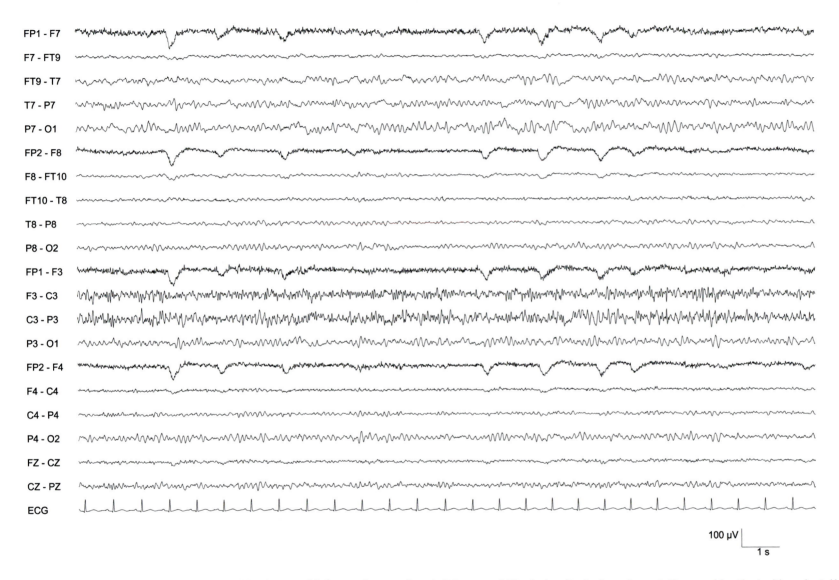

FP1 - F7
F7 - FT9
FT9 - T7
T7 - P7
P7 - O1
FP2 - F8
F8 - FT10
FT10 - T8
T8 - P8
P8 - O2
FP1 - F3
F3 - C3
C3 - P3
P3 - O1
FP2 - F4
F4 - C4
C4 - P4
P4 - O2
FZ - CZ
CZ - PZ
ECG

100 µV
1 s

▶ **Figure 3.278   Asymmetry, increased background, left; continuous slow, left temporal.** Bipolar longitudinal montage. A 41-year-old patient with perinatal brain damage on the left and ventriculoperitoneal shunt on the left. The EEG showed a continuous irregular left-sided delta and an increase in alpha and beta frequencies on the left.

EEG classification: Abnormal III (awake)
1. Continuous slow, left temporal
2. Asymmetry, increased background left

EEG report: This EEG reflects the perinatal left-sided brain lesion and the left ventriculoperitoneal shunt.

Asymmetry, increased beta and mu, left; continuous slow, left fronto-polar

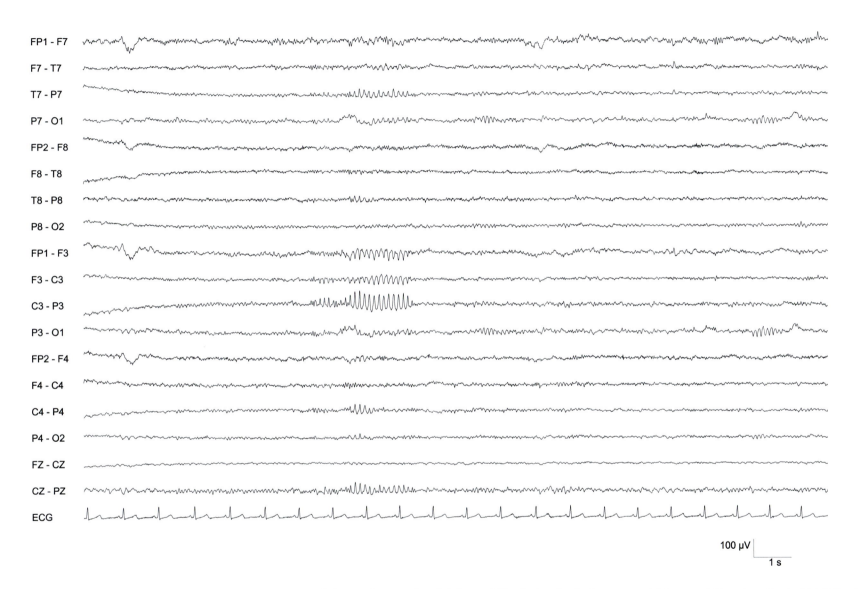

▶ **Figure 3.279** **Asymmetry, increased beta and mu, left; continuous slow, left frontal.** Bipolar longitudinal montage. A 34-year-old female patient with left frontal lobe epilepsy after left frontal sinusitis and brain abscess at age 11 years. Following partial left frontal lobe resection at age 19 years, the patient remained seizure-free off medication for more than 16 years. The amplitude of the mu activity is high in the left central and the beta activity is also of higher amplitude in the left frontal region. A continuous irregular theta–delta slow prevails in the left frontopolar area.

EEG classification: Abnormal III (awake)
1. Continuous slow, left frontopolar
2. Asymmetry, increased beta and mu, left

EEG report: This EEG reflects the status post left frontal resection.

Asymmetry, reduced background activity, right; delta coma

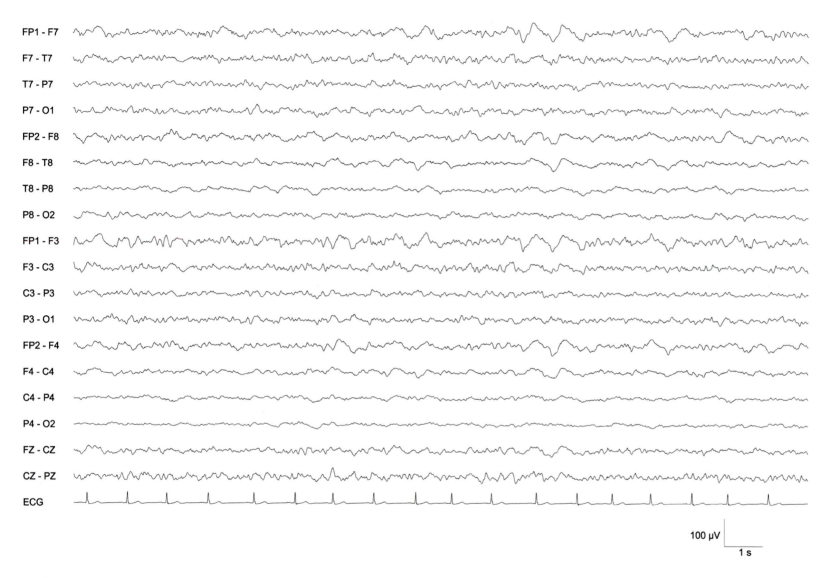

FP1 - F7

F7 - T7

T7 - P7

P7 - O1

FP2 - F8

F8 - T8

T8 - P8

P8 - O2

FP1 - F3

F3 - C3

C3 - P3

P3 - O1

FP2 - F4

F4 - C4

C4 - P4

P4 - O2

FZ - CZ

CZ - PZ

ECG

100 µV

1 s

▶ **Figure 3.280** **Asymmetry, reduced background activity, right; delta coma.** Bipolar longitudinal montage. A 74-year-old patient with severe metabolic encephalopathy and intracerebral hemorrhage associated with warfarin treatment for atrial fibrillation. The EEG is dominated by irregular delta waves. It shows lower amplitudes of the alpha and theta frequencies on the right side.

EEG classification: Abnormal III (coma)
1. Delta coma
2. Asymmetry, decreased background, right

EEG report: This EEG supports the diagnosis of a severe diffuse encephalopathy and a right cerebral lesion.

EEG report: This EEG supports the diagnosis of a severe diffuse encephalopathy and a right cerebral lesion.

The decrease in amplitude of the background rhythms is most likely because the left-sided lesion is interfering with the generation of background rhythms on the affected side. This is also true for physiological activity such arousal patterns (▶ Figures 3.281 and 3.282).

When assessing asymmetries, it should be considered that the occipital background rhythm is physiologically higher on the right. Unilateral absence of occipital alpha suppression caused by eye opening is a rare abnormality indicative of a lesion ipsilateral to the side the alpha is not attenuated by eye opening. This asymmetry is not included in the EEG classification.

The following steps must be followed when classifying an asymmetry:

STEP 1:   Define if the amplitude is "increased" or "decreased."
STEP 2:   Decide *what* brain activity is increased or decreased.
STEP 3:   Define *where* the brain activity is increased or decreased.

Examples
- Asymmetry, increased alpha left occipital (▶ **Figure 3.275**)
- Asymmetry, decreased background left (▶ **Figure 3.277**)

The degree of EEG abnormality of asymmetry as an isolated EEG change is classified as abnormal EEG II.

3.4.2.7.3   Sleep-Onset REM (SOREM)

Sleep-onset REM means the early occurrence of REM sleep (<15 min after falling asleep), as is typical for narcolepsy. However, there are also other causes for sleep-onset REM, including REM rebound due to sleep apnea or after discontinuation of monoamine oxidase inhibitors (▶ **Figure 3.283**). In newborns, sleep-onset REM is a physiological phenomenon.

Because of its high association with narcolepsy, sleep-onset REM is classified as abnormal grade III.

3.4.2.8   Special Patterns in Stupor and Comas

The EEG is an essential part of the neurological assessment of comatose patients. Coma-induced EEG changes are not specific to a cause or disorder but provide

valuable prognostic information. In comatose or stuporous patients, one of the following EEG patterns, in addition to background suppression, background attenuation, burst suppression, or burst attenuation, may be recorded:

- Alpha coma (AC)/alpha stupor (AS)
- Spindle coma (SC)/spindle stupor (SS)
- Beta coma (BC)/beta stupor (BES)
- Theta coma (TC)/theta stupor (TS)
- Delta coma (DC)/delta stupor (DS)

All these patterns indicate severe encephalopathies. In addition to one of these five abnormal EEG patterns, which represent the "background activity," each of the other abnormal EEG categories mentioned above (slow, epileptiform discharges, or special patterns) can be added to the classification.

Example (▶ **Figure 3.284**)
EEG classification: Abnormal EEG III (coma)
1. Alpha coma
2. Continuous slow, left
3. Asymmetry, increased background left

Coma is defined as a severe abnormal decrease of vigilance with unresponsiveness to external stimulation. Coma may be the result of either infratentorial damage to the ascending reticular formation (arousal system) in the region of the ponto-mesencephalic tegmentum or a supratentorial diffuse dysfunction of the cortex.

Coma due to an infratentorial process is usually due to a direct lesion of the ascending reticular formation as a result of vascular damage or pressure damage. Diffuse supratentorial encephalopathies leading to coma are mostly diffuse hypoxic, metabolic, or toxic encephalopathies.

Alpha coma and spindle coma may occur in brainstem lesions. In these cases, the prognosis depends on the coma-inducing brainstem lesion. Even with generalized hypoxic or anoxic brain damage, an alpha coma can occur without preserved response to eye opening. Here, the prognosis is usually unfavorable. In contrast, an alpha coma or beta coma induced by intoxication, usually has a good prognosis if the intoxication can recede.

Theta coma and delta coma indicate severe diffuse encephalopathies with cortical involvement. Both EEG patterns are reversible in principle; the prognosis depends on the course of the underlying disease. A rather negative sign

Asymmetry, reduced arousal, right; continuous slow, right frontotemporal

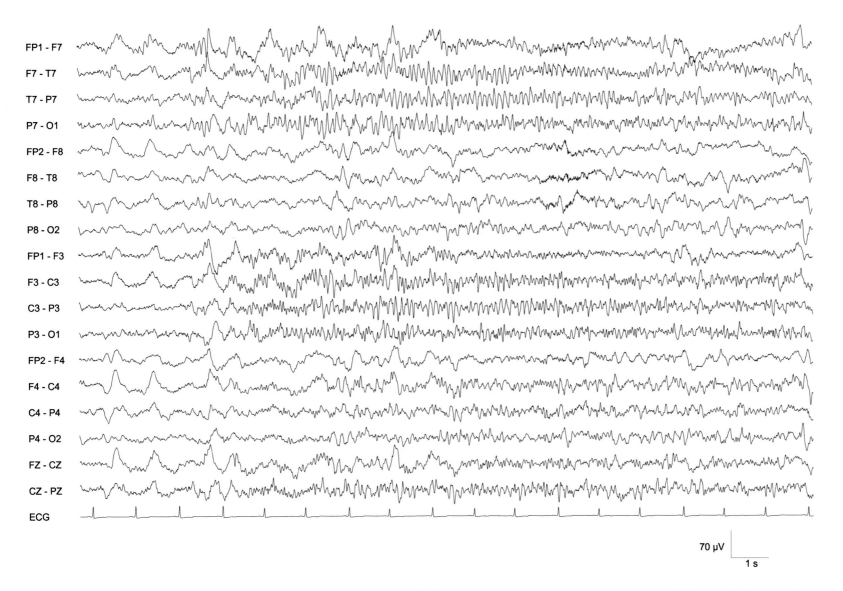

FP1 - F7
F7 - T7
T7 - P7
P7 - O1
FP2 - F8
F8 - T8
T8 - P8
P8 - O2
FP1 - F3
F3 - C3
C3 - P3
P3 - O1
FP2 - F4
F4 - C4
C4 - P4
P4 - O2
FZ - CZ
CZ - PZ
ECG

70 µV

1 s

▶ **Figure 3.281 Asymmetry, reduced arousal, right; continuous slow, right frontotemporal.** Bipolar longitudinal montage. A 70-year-old female patient with space-occupying right sphenoidal meningioma leading to brainstem compression. The arousal pattern is well-developed on the left but hardly identifiable on the right. There was a right frontotemporal continuous irregular slow.

EEG classification: Abnormal III (sleep)
   1. Continuous slow, right frontotemporal
   2. Asymmetry, reduced arousal, right

EEG report: This EEG reflects the space-occupying right sphenoidal meningioma.

Asymmetry, reduced arousal, right; continuous slow, right frontotemporal

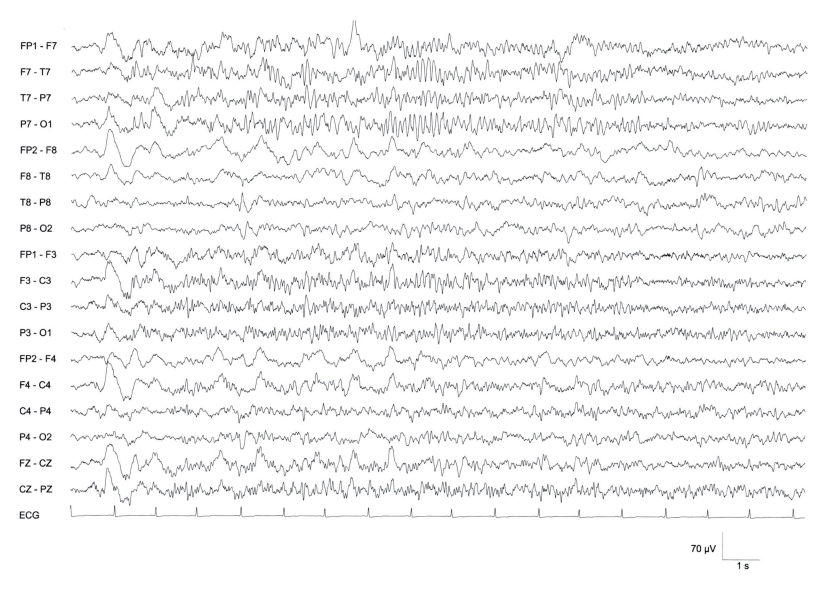

70 µV

1 s

▶ **Figure 3.282**   **Asymmetry, reduced arousal, right; continuous slow, right frontotemporal.** Bipolar longitudinal montage. EEG sample of the same patient as in ▶ **Figure 3.281** a few minutes later. The arousal pattern is well-developed on the left but hardly identifiable on the right. There was a right frontotemporal continuous irregular slow.

EEG classification: Abnormal III (sleep)
1. Continuous slow, right frontotemporal
2. Asymmetry, reduced arousal, right

EEG report: See ▶ **Figure 3.281**.

Sleep-onset REM

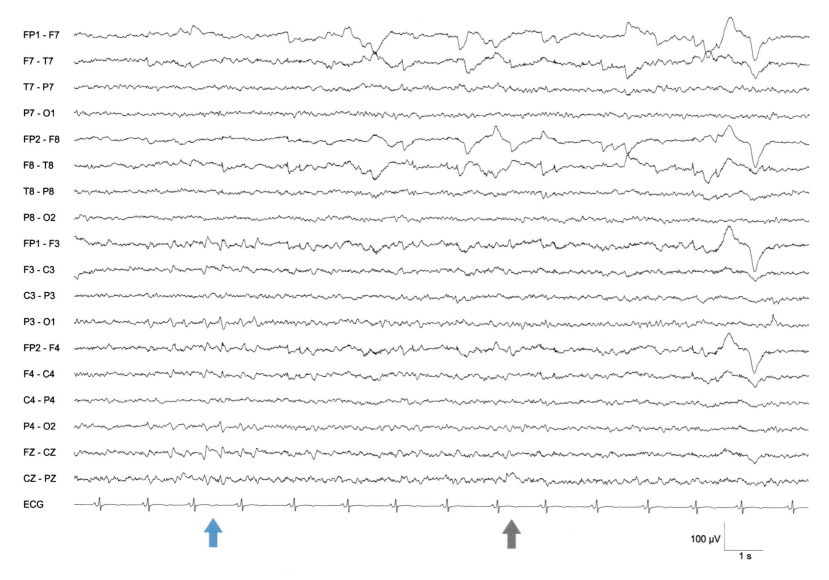

▶ **Figure 3.283** **Sleep-onset REM.** Bipolar longitudinal montage. A 40-year-old female patient with narcolepsy. This REM phase occurred within 7 min after the onset of EEG recording and 5 min after falling asleep. REM sleep is characterized by predominantly horizontal saccadic eye movements (gray arrow). Note the sawtooth waves (blue arrow) maximum bilaterally midhemispheric that are typical of REM sleep.

EEG classification: Abnormal III (sleep)
    Sleep-onset REM

EEG report: This EEG supports the diagnosis of narcolepsy.

Alpha coma; continuous slow, left; asymmetry, increased background, left

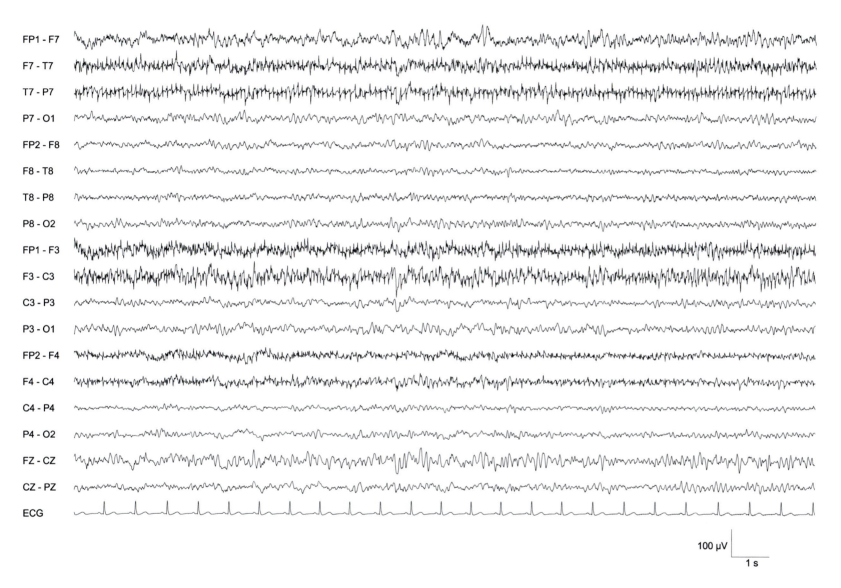

FP1 - F7

F7 - T7

T7 - P7

P7 - O1

FP2 - F8

F8 - T8

T8 - P8

P8 - O2

FP1 - F3

F3 - C3

C3 - P3

P3 - O1

FP2 - F4

F4 - C4

C4 - P4

P4 - O2

FZ - CZ

CZ - PZ

ECG

100 µV

1 s

▶ **Figure 3.284 Alpha coma; continuous slow, left; asymmetry, increased background, left.** Bipolar longitudinal montage. A 43-year-old comatose patient with cardiac embolic thrombosis of the basilar artery leading to pontine, midbrain, and left middle cerebral artery infarction. There is diffuse alpha activity that is of higher amplitude on the left hemisphere. Note the left frontotemporal more than right frontal tonic muscle artifact.

EEG classification: Abnormal III (coma)
1. Alpha coma
2. Continuous slow, left
3. Asymmetry, increased background left

EEG report: This EEG supports the diagnosis of a coma secondary to a pontine and midbrain lesion, as does the history of a left supratentorial lesion. The increased amplitude of the alpha activity on the left side may be related to the left ventricular shunt.

is when a theta coma develops into a delta coma during the disease. The EEG changes in anoxic encephalopathy due to cardiopulmonary arrest have been divided into five degrees depending on the increasing severity (Hockaday et al., 1965; Prior, 1973):

- Dominant alpha activity
- Dominant theta activity
- Diffuse delta activity with response to external stimuli
- Diffuse delta activity without response to external stimuli
- Background suppression

Responsiveness of the coma/stupor pattern to external stimuli (acoustic, sensory, and pain) is a favorable sign. The EEG then typically shows an acceleration of the background delta or theta activity (▶ **Figures 3.285** and **3.286**). However, occasionally a slowing of the background activity may also occur. This is called a "paradoxical response" (▶ **Figure 3.287**).

3.4.2.8.1   Alpha Coma (AK) and Alpha Stupor (AS)

Alpha coma and alpha stupor correspond to an EEG in comatose/stuporous patients in which alpha activity dominates (▶ **Figure 3.288**). Patients with alpha stupor may have eye blinks (▶ **Figure 3.289**). However, in contrast to the physiological alpha that consistently is blocked by eye opening, the alpha activity of comatose (stuporous) patients is not inhibited by eye opening. In addition, the distribution of the alpha activity of patients in alpha coma is diffuse and frequently of highest amplitude frontally. This is in clear contrast to the predominant occipital distribution of normal alpha activity that is suppressed by eye opening. Alpha coma (stupor) occurs most frequently in patients suffering from a severe diffuse anoxic encephalopathy. Drug intoxications can also produce alpha coma (stupor).

In patients, in whom lesions of the brainstem at the ponto-mesencephalic junction are large enough to affect consciousness but do not interfere with the mechanisms that generate the physiological waking EEG pattern, the distribution of the alpha activity may be normal, and the alpha activity may even be attenuated by eye opening. The same is true for patients with small ponto-mesencephalic junction who are suffering from a locked-in syndrome. However, these patients are not in coma but are unable to respond to external stimuli due to generalized paralysis. The prognosis of patients with alpha coma due to circumscribed ponto-mesencephalic lesions, including patients suffering from the locked-in syndrome, is extremely poor. The overwhelming majority of alpha coma cases are due to anoxia or drug intoxication.

Alpha coma (stupor) has a poor prognosis with the exception of drug-induced cases, which may be reversible (Bauer, 1993).

Alpha coma (stupor) EEGs are classified as abnormal III because they are an index of a severe, usually irreversible encephalopathy.

3.4.2.8.2   Spindle Coma (SK) and Spindle Stupor (SS)

Patients who show an EEG similar to stage 2 sleep with sleep spindles but are in coma (stupor) are classified as having spindle coma (stupor) (▶ **Figures 3.290** and **3.291**).

This EEG pattern is seen in patients with brainstem lesions that are sufficient to cloud alertness but do not interfere with normal sleep-generating mechanisms. The lesions are mostly located at the higher ponto-mesencephalic transition and, if not due to a progressive lesion, usually have a relatively good prognosis, Spindle coma (stupor) may also be seen in intoxication with sedative medications (barbiturates and benzodiazepines).

Spindle coma and spindle stupor are classified as abnormal III because of the correlation to severe disturbances of consciousness (stupor or coma).

3.4.2.8.3   Beta Coma (BK) and Beta Stupor (BES)

Beta coma and beta stupor are indicated by EEG recordings with predominant beta activity in comatose/stuporous patients (▶ **Figure 3.292**).

Beta coma and beta stupor are mostly caused by drug intoxications and are therefore reversible in most cases (Carroll & Mastaglia, 1979).

This EEG pattern is classified as abnormal III because of the association of the EEG pattern with severe encephalopathies.

3.4.2.8.4   Theta Coma (TK) and Theta Stupor (TS)

Theta coma and theta stupor are indicated by EEG recordings from comatose/stuporous patients with theta frequencies (▶ **Figure 3.293**).

Theta coma is seen in EEG of comatose/stuporous patients with severe diffuse encephalopathy. The prognosis of this pattern depends on the etiology of the encephalopathy and is potentially reversible (Synek & Synek, 1987).

This EEG pattern is classified as abnormal III because of its association with coma (stupor).

Delta coma; response to pain stimulus

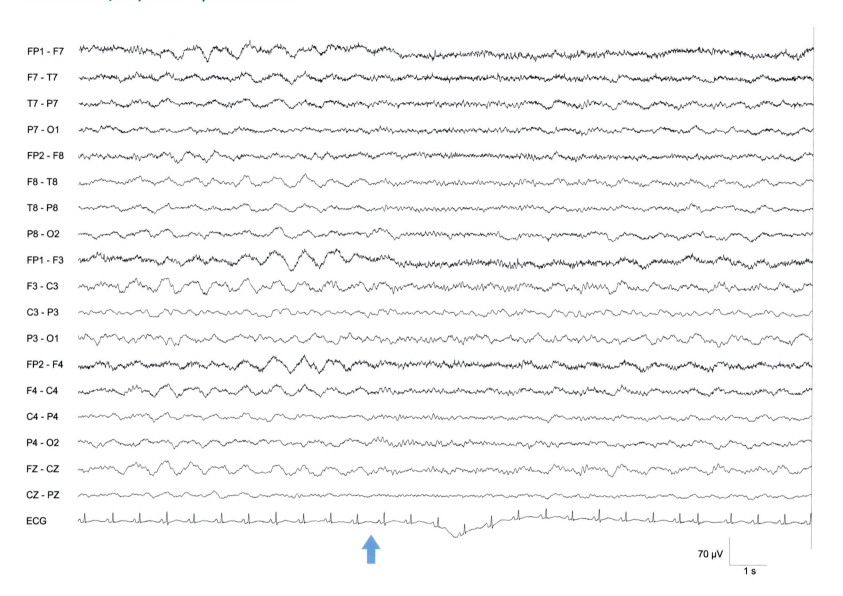

70 μV

1 s

▶ **Figure 3.285** **Delta coma; response to pain stimulus.** Bipolar longitudinal montage. A 63-year-old patient with cardiac insufficiency and acute myeloid leukemia. The EEG shows relatively high-amplitude delta waves (~100 μV) with intermixed low-amplitude (10–20 μV) 10 Hz alpha activity. With painful stimuli, the delta waves disappear and the alpha activity becomes dominant for 2 or 3 s (blue arrow).

EEG classification: Abnormal III (coma)

Delta coma

EEG report: This EEG shows a severe diffuse encephalopathy. A delta coma pattern after an anoxic encephalopathy is a completely reversible EEG pattern. In addition, the EEG response to external stimulation is associated with a good prognosis.

Delta coma; response to pain stimulus

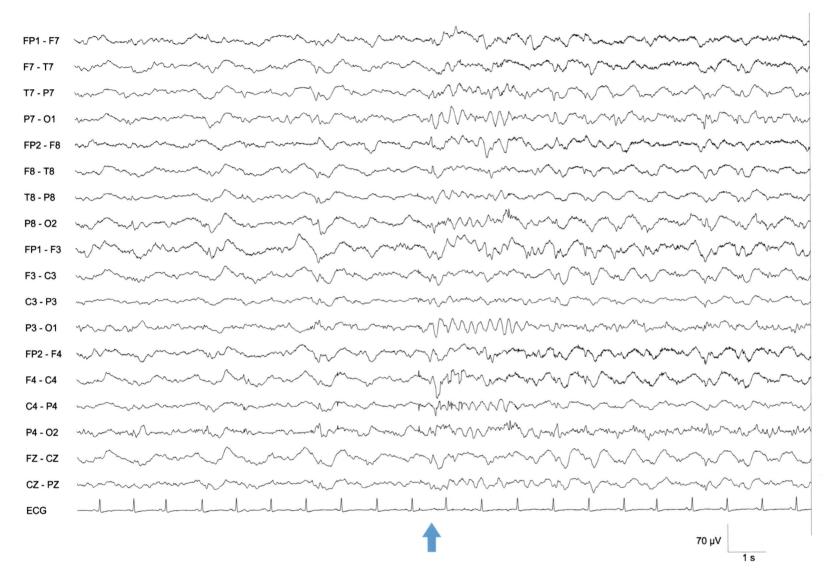

Figure 3.286 **Delta coma; response to pain stimulus.** Bipolar longitudinal montage. A 70-year-old comatose patient who had suffered cardiovascular arrest and resuscitation. The EEG shows generalized, relatively high-amplitude delta waves (-70 μV). With painful stimuli (blue arrow), a 2-s burst of generalized 4 Hz theta rhythm appears.

EEG classification: Abnormal III (coma)

      Delta coma

EEG report: This EEG supports the diagnosis of a severe diffuse encephalopathy. A delta coma pattern after an anoxic encephalopathy is a completely reversible EEG pattern. In addition, the EEG response to external stimulation is associated with a good prognosis.

Paradoxical response in alpha coma

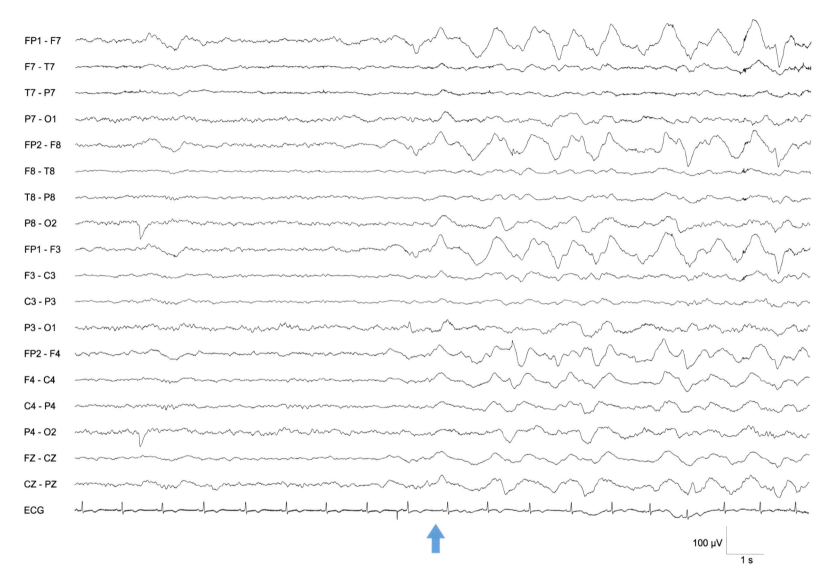

▶ **Figure 3.287** **Paradoxical response in alpha coma.** Bipolar longitudinal montage. A 69-year-old comatose patient with subarachnoid hemorrhage and ponto-mesencephalic infarcts from an aneurysm of the vertebral artery. The EEG shows a low-amplitude (10–20 μV) diffuse alpha coma. Pain stimulus (blue arrow) triggers high-amplitude (100–150 μV) 0.5–1 Hz slow waves of a general distribution maximum bifrontally.

EEG classification: Abnormal III (coma)
Alpha coma

EEG report: This EEG indicates a severe diffuse encephalopathy. Alpha coma is a reversible EEG pattern. In addition, an EEG response to external stimulation is a good prognostic sign.

Alpha coma

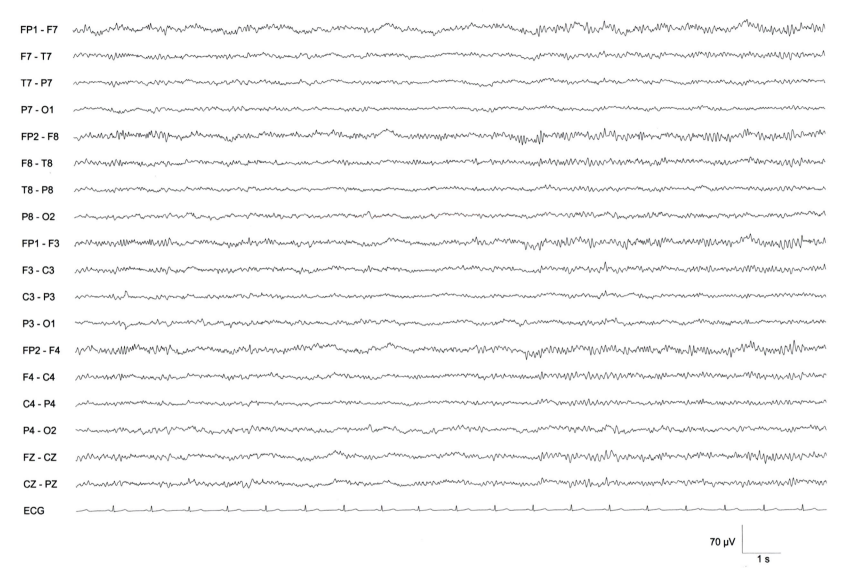

FP1 - F7

F7 - T7

T7 - P7

P7 - O1

FP2 - F8

F8 - T8

T8 - P8

P8 - O2

FP1 - F3

F3 - C3

C3 - P3

P3 - O1

FP2 - F4

F4 - C4

C4 - P4

P4 - O2

FZ - CZ

CZ - PZ

ECG

70 μV

1 s

▶ **Figure 3.288** **Alpha coma.** Bipolar longitudinal montage. A 41-year-old juvenile diabetic patient who suffered a severe cerebral anoxia due to cardiac arrest and diffuse leukoencephalopathy.

EEG classification: Abnormal III (coma)
　　Alpha coma

EEG report: This EEG indicates severe diffuse encephalopathy.

Alpha stupor

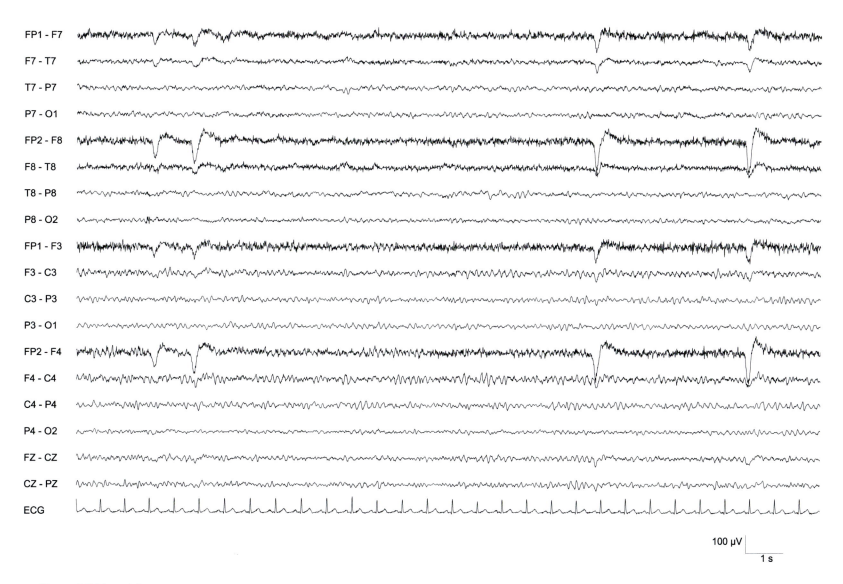

100 µV

1 s

▶ **Figure 3.289** **Alpha stupor.** Bipolar longitudinal montage. A 71-year-old stuporous patient with pontine myelinolysis after metabolic decompensation in the setting of colon carcinoma resection. The EEG shows diffusely distributed alpha activity. Note the eye blinks.

EEG classification: Abnormal III (stupor)
 Alpha stupor

EEG report: This EEG indicates severe diffuse encephalopathy. Alpha stupor is a potentially reversible EEG pattern, depending on the etiology.

Spindle coma

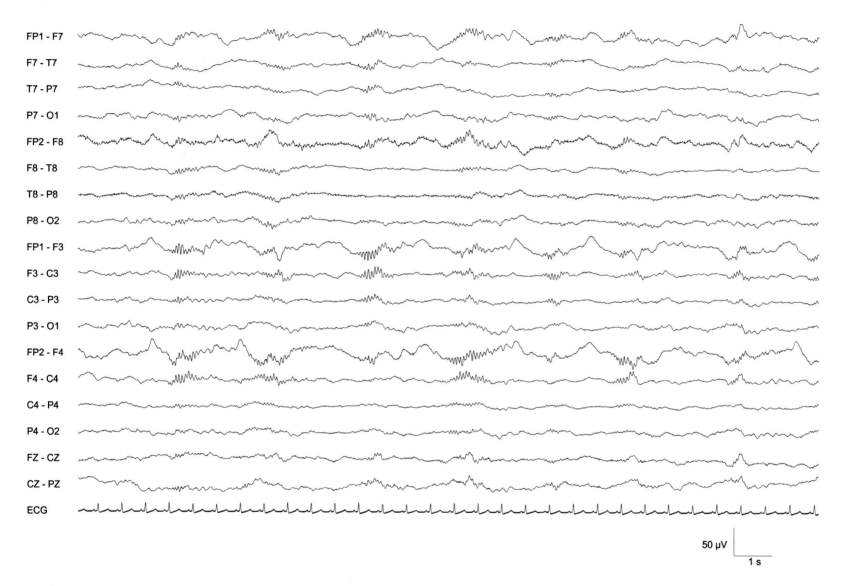

FP1 - F7

F7 - T7

T7 - P7

P7 - O1

FP2 - F8

F8 - T8

T8 - P8

P8 - O2

FP1 - F3

F3 - C3

C3 - P3

P3 - O1

FP2 - F4

F4 - C4

C4 - P4

P4 - O2

FZ - CZ

CZ - PZ

ECG

50 μV

1 s

▶ **Figure 3.290**   **Spindle coma; bipolar longitudinal montage.** A 43-year-old comatose patient with pontine myelinolysis associated with severe alcohol toxic liver cirrhosis. The EEG shows delta waves and approximately 2-s bursts of 12 Hz spindles occurring every 3 or 4 s.

EEG classification: Abnormal III (coma)

   Spindle coma

EEG report: This EEG is indicative of a severe diffuse encephalopathy. Spindle coma is a potentially reversible EEG pattern, depending on the underlying etiology.

Spindle coma, asymmetry, increased spindle, left

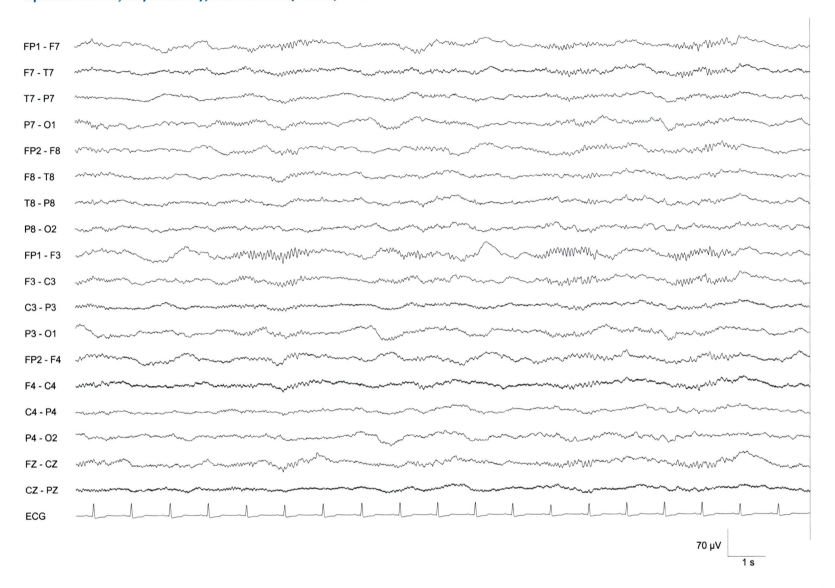

▶ **Figure 3.291** **Spindle coma; bipolar longitudinal montage.** A 56-year-old comatose patient with brainstem and ventricle hemorrhage, sepsis, and renal failure. Increased intraventricular pressure required a ventricle shunt, which was placed on the left lateral ventricle. The EEG shows slow waves and repetitive, left frontal maximum spindles of approximately 10 Hz.

EEG classification: Abnormal III (coma)
1. Spindle coma
2. Asymmetry, increased spindle, left

EEG report: This EEG is indicative of a severe diffuse encephalopathy and reflects the left ventricle shunt. Spindle coma is a potentially reversible EEG pattern.

Beta coma

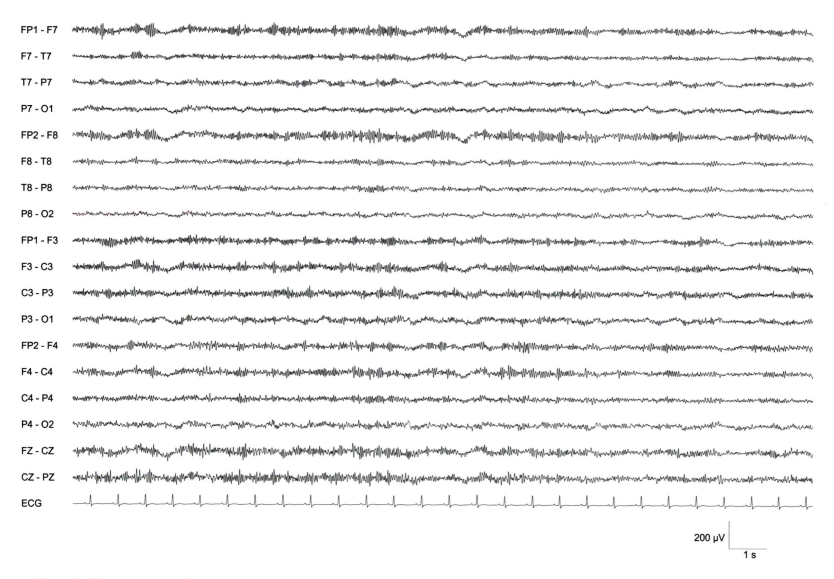

FP1 - F7
F7 - T7
T7 - P7
P7 - O1
FP2 - F8
F8 - T8
T8 - P8
P8 - O2
FP1 - F3
F3 - C3
C3 - P3
P3 - O1
FP2 - F4
F4 - C4
C4 - P4
P4 - O2
FZ - CZ
CZ - PZ
ECG

200 µV

1 s

▶ **Figure 3.292** **Beta coma.** Bipolar longitudinal montage. A 44-year-old comatose patient with intoxication by various antidepressants and sedatives. The EEG is dominated by diffusely distributed beta waves of an amplitude of 40–80 µV.

EEG classification: Abnormal III (coma)

  Beta coma

EEG report: This EEG supports the diagnosis of a severe diffuse encephalopathy due to intoxication is a potentially reversible with sedatives. Beta coma due to intoxication is a potentially reversible EEG pattern.

Theta coma

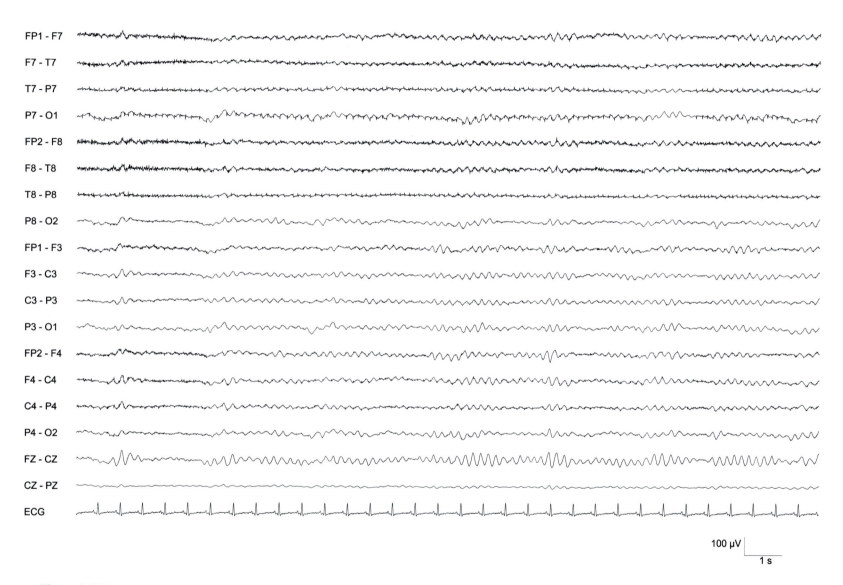

FP1 - F7

F7 - T7

T7 - P7

P7 - O1

FP2 - F8

F8 - T8

T8 - P8

P8 - O2

FP1 - F3

F3 - C3

C3 - P3

P3 - O1

FP2 - F4

F4 - C4

C4 - P4

P4 - O2

FZ - CZ

CZ - PZ

ECG

100 µV

1 s

▶ **Figure 3.293** **Theta coma.** Bipolar longitudinal montage. A 74-year-old comatose patient with encephalopathy due to anoxia (cardiorespiratory resuscitation) and sepsis. The EEG is dominated by generalized theta waves.

EEG classification: Abnormal III (coma)

Theta coma

EEG report: This EEG indicates severe diffuse encephalopathy. Theta coma is a potentially reversible EEG pattern.

Delta coma

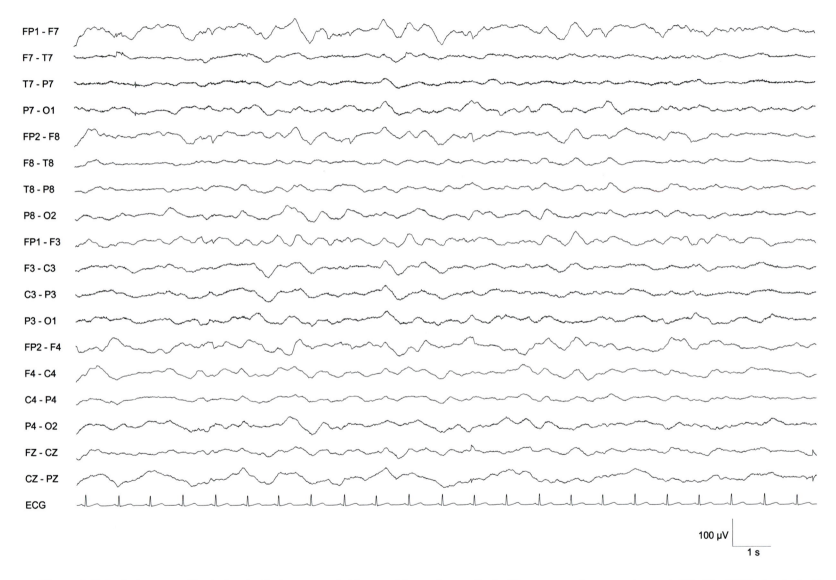

FP1 - F7
F7 - T7
T7 - P7
P7 - O1
FP2 - F8
F8 - T8
T8 - P8
P8 - O2
FP1 - F3
F3 - C3
C3 - P3
P3 - O1
FP2 - F4
F4 - C4
C4 - P4
P4 - O2
FZ - CZ
CZ - PZ
ECG

100 μV

1 s

▶ **Figure 3.294** **Delta coma.** Bipolar longitudinal montage. A 44-year-old comatose patient with severe meningococcal encephalitis. The EEG is dominated by generalized delta waves.

EEG classification: Abnormal III (coma)
Delta coma

EEG report: This EEG indicates severe diffuse encephalopathy. Delta coma is a potentially reversible EEG pattern, depending on the underlying etiology.

Delta coma

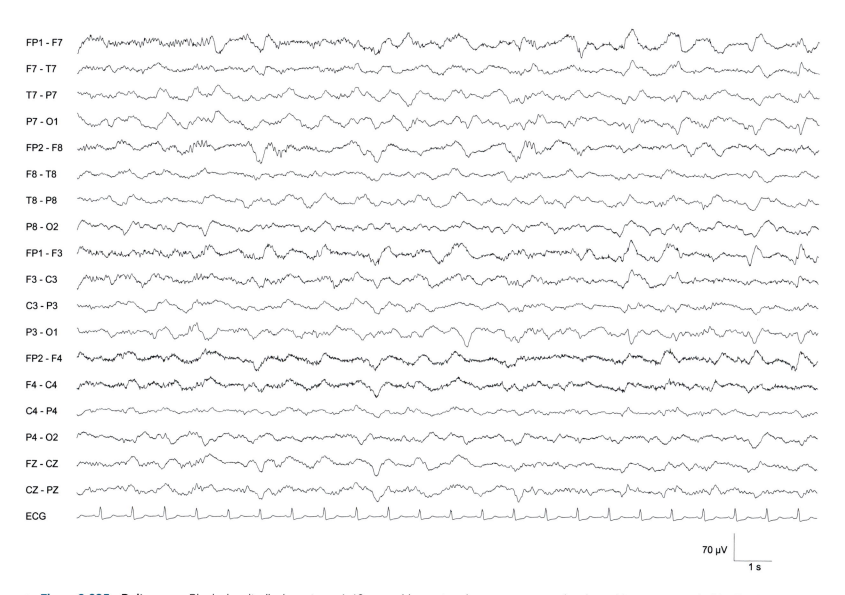

▶ **Figure 3.295** **Delta coma.** Bipolar longitudinal montage. A 48-year-old comatose immunosuppressed patient with severe encephalitis. The EEG is dominated by diffuse distributed 50–100 μV delta activity with intermingled low-amplitude (5–15 μV) alpha/beta rhythms.

EEG classification: Abnormal III (coma)
    Delta coma

EEG report: This EEG indicates severe diffuse encephalopathy. Delta coma is a potentially reversible EEG pattern, depending on the underlying etiology.

3.4.2.8.5 Delta Coma (DK) and Delta Stupor (DS)

Delta coma and delta stupor are indicated by EEG recordings from comatose/stuporous patients whose EEG shows irregular, usually relatively high-amplitude delta activity (▶ **Figures 3.294** and **3.295**). Delta coma (stupor) occurs in comatose (stuporous) patients with severe diffuse encephalopathy of different etiologies (Husain, 2006; Synek, 1988). The prognosis depends mainly on the cause of the encephalopathy. The pattern is potentially reversible. As is true for all patients in coma (stupor), a change in the EEG elicited by external stimuli is a prognostically favorable sign (▶ **Figures 3.285–3.287**).

This EEG pattern is classified as abnormal EEG III because of the patient's comatose/stuporous state of consciousness.

APPENDIX 1

EEG Guidelines of the American Clinical Neurophysiological Society

1	Minimum Technical Requirements for Performing Clinical EEG	Sinha et al. (2016)
2	Guidelines for Standard Electrode Position Nomenclature	Acharya, Hani, Cheek, et al. (2016)
3	Proposal for Standard Montages to be Used in Clinical EEG	Acharya, Hani, Thirumala, et al. (2016)
4	Guidelines for Recording Clinical EEG on Digital Media	Halford et al. (2016)
5	Minimum Technical Standards for Pediatric EEG	Kuratani et al. (2016)
6	Minimum Technical Standards for EEG Recording in Suspected Cerebral Death	Stecker et al. (2016)
7	Guidelines for EEG Reporting	Tatum et al. (2016)
12	Guidelines for Long-Term Monitoring for Epilepsy	*American Clinical Neurophysiology Society* (2008)

Source: American Clinical Neurophysiological Society (https://www.acns.org/practice/guidelines).

APPENDIX 2

Semiological Seizure Classification

The semiological seizure classification focuses on the signs and symptoms occurring during epileptic seizures. For details, the reader is referred to Lüders et al. (1998, 2019)

A.1 Seizure Type

Seizure components marked with an asterisk (★) have a somatotopic modifier.

Aura

Auditory aura*
Autonomic aura

Abdominal aura
Dipsosic aura
Fecal aura
Hunger aura
Tachycardic aura

Cephalic sensation aura

Headache aura

Choking aura
General body sensation aura
Gustatory aura
Olfactory aura
Psychic aura

Affective aura

Pleasure aura

Ecstasy aura
Religious aura
Sexual aura

Unpleasant aura

Anger aura
Depression/sadness aura
Embarrassment/guilt aura
Fear/panic aura

Experiential aura
Familiarity aura

Deja vu aura
Jamais vu aura

Forced thinking

Hallucinatory aura

Auditory hallucinatory aura
Visual hallucinatory aura

Illusional aura

Auditory illusional aura
Body illusional aura
Time illusional aura
Visual illusional aura

Somatosensory aura*

Painful somatosensory aura*
Paresthetic somatosensory aura*
Thermal somatosensory aura*

Vestibular aura
Visual aura*

Ictal blindness aura*

Autonomic seizure

    Abdominal seizure

    Anisocoric seizure*

    Bradycardic seizure

    Central apnea seizure

    Diaphoretic seizure

    Ejaculation/erection seizure

    Emetic seizure

    Fecal seizure

    Hippus seizure

    Hyperhydrosic seizure

    Hyperventilation seizure

    Lacrimatory seizure

    Miotic seizure*

    Mydriatic seizure*

    Pilomotor seizure*

    Sialorrheic seizure

    Tachycardic seizure

    Urinary seizure

    Vasomotor seizure

    Water drinking seizure

Discognitive seizure

    Amnestic seizure

    Aphasic seizure

    Akinetic seizure

    Dialeptic seizure

    Word deafness seizure

(continued on next page)

Motor seizure*

    Complex motor seizure

        Alien limb seizure

        Automotor seizure

            Gesticulatory seizure*

            Oro-alimentary seizure

        Blinking seizure*

        Dacrystic seizure

        Ear plugging seizure

        Gelastic seizure

        Hypermotor seizure

            Emotional hypermotor seizure

        Kissing seizure

        Melodious seizure

            Humming seizure

            Singing seizure

        Spitting seizure

        Verbalization seizure

        Yawning seizure

    Simple motor seizure

        Clonic seizure*

        Dystonic seizure*

        Early head turn seizure*

        Epileptic spasm seizure*

            Epileptic nod seizure

        Figure of 4 seizure*

        Grimacing seizure*

        Gyratory seizure*

        Ictal-end clonic seizure*

        Ictal-end versive seizure*

        M2e seizure*

        Myoclonic seizure*

        Nystagmoid seizure*

        Opsoclonic seizure

        Pouting seizure

        Tonic seizure*

        Tonic–clonic seizure*

        Versive seizure*

        Vocalization seizure

Special seizure	
	Atonic seizure*
	Epileptic drop seizure
	Fear facies seizure
	Hypnopompic seizure
	Hypomotor seizure
	Negative myoclonic seizure*
	Water drinking seizure

A.2 Lateralizing Signs

Seizure components marked with an asterisk (★) have a somatotopic modifier.

Automotor seizure without dialepsis

Immediate postictal speech

Postictal akinesia

Postictal aphasia

Postictal hemianopia*

Postictal hemineglect*

Postictal hemiparesis* (Todd's paralysis)

Postictal hemisensory deficit*

Postictal nose wiping*

Postictal unilateral pupillary dilation*

A.3 Diagnostic Signs

Seizure components marked with an asterisk (⋆) have a somatotopic modifier.

Forceful ictal eye closure

Forceful ictal mouth closure

Ictal cry

Ictal grasping*

Ictal tongue biting

Postictal apraxia

Postictal automatisms

Postictal blindness

Postictal bulimia

Postictal coma

Postictal coughing

Postictal dystonic posturing

Postictal headache

Postictal psychosis

Postictal stertorous breathing

Postictal tonic posturing

Postictal urinary incontinence

References

Acharya, J. N., Hani, A., Cheek, J., Thirumala, P., & Tsuchida, T. N. (2016). American Clinical Neurophysiology Society Guideline 2: Guidelines for standard electrode position nomenclature. *Journal of Clinical Neurophysiology, 33*(4), 308–311.

Acharya, J. N., Hani, A. J., Thirumala, P. D., & Tsuchida, T. N. (2016). American Clinical Neurophysiology Society Guideline 3: A proposal for standard montages to be used in clinical EEG. *Journal of Clinical Neurophysiology, 33*(4), 312–316. https://doi.org/10.1097/WNP.0000000000000317

Adelman, S., Lueders, H., Dinner, D. S., & Lesser, R. P. (1982). Paradoxical lateralization of parasagittal sharp waves in a patient with epilepsia partialis continua. *Epilepsia, 23*(3), 291–295.

Ajmone-Marsan, C. A., & Zivin, L. S. (1970). Factors related to the occurrence of typical paroxysmal abnormalities in the EEG records of epileptic patients. *Epilepsia, 11*, 361–381.

Alkhachroum, A. M., Al-Abri, H., Sachdeva, A., Maturu, S., Waldron, J., Wang, H., Rizvi, M., Fernandez-Baca Vaca, G., & Lüders, H. O. (2018). Generalized periodic discharges with and without triphasic morphology. *Journal of Clinical Neurophysiology, 35*(2), 144–150. https://doi.org/10.1097/WNP.0000000000000441

American Clinical Neurophysiology Society (2008). Guideline Twelve: Guidelines for Long-Term for Epilepsyy. *Journal of Clinical Neurophysiology*, 25, 170–180. https://www.acns.org/UserFiles/file/Guideline_Twelve__Guidelines_for_Long_Term.8.pdf

Amin, U., & Benbadis, S. R. (2019). The role of EEG in the erroneous diagnosis of epilepsy. *Journal of Clinical Neurophysiology, 36*(4), 294–297. https://doi.org/10.1097/WNP.0000000000000572

Arenas, A. M., Brenner, R. P., & Reynolds, C. F. (1986). Temporal slowing in the elderly revisited. *American Journal of EEG Technology, 26*(2), 105–114. https://doi.org/10.1080/00029238.1986.11080192

Baldin, E., Hauser, W. A., Buchhalter, J. R., Hesdorffer, D. C., & Ottman, R. (2014). Yield of epileptiform electroencephalogram abnormalities in incident unprovoked seizures: A population-based study. *Epilepsia, 55*(9), 1389–1398. https://doi.org/10.1111/epi.12720

Bauer, G. (1993). EEG, drug effects, and central nervous system poisoning. In E. Niedermeyer & F. H. Lopes da Silva (Eds.), *Electroencephalography: Basic principles, clinical applications, and related fields* (3rd ed., pp. 631–642). William & Wilkins.

Baumgartner, C., Koren, J. P., & Rothmayer, M. (2018). Automatic computer-based detection of epileptic seizures. *Frontiers in Neurology, 9*, 639. https://doi.org/10.3389/fneur.2018.00639

Beleza, P., Bilgin, O., & Noachtar, S. (2009). Interictal rhythmical midline theta differentiates frontal from temporal lobe epilepsies. *Epilepsia, 50*(3), 550–555. https://doi.org/10.1111/j.1528-1167.2008.01780.x

Benbadis, S. R. (2005). A spell in the epilepsy clinic and a history of "chronic pain" or "fibromyalgia" independently predict a diagnosis of psychogenic seizures. *Epilepsy & Behavior, 6*(2), 264–265. https://doi.org/10.1016/j.yebeh.2004.12.007

Benbadis, S. R. (2013). "Just like EKGs!" Should EEGs undergo a confirmatory interpretation by a clinical neurophysiologist? *Neurology, 80*(Suppl. 1), S47–S51. https://doi.org/10.1212/wnl.0b013e3182797539

Benbadis, S. R., & Lin, K. (2008). Errors in EEG interpretation and misdiagnosis of epilepsy: Which EEG patterns are overread? *European Neurology, 59*(5), 267–271. https://doi.org/10.1159/000115641

Benbadis, S. R., & Tatum, W. O., 4th. (2000). Prevalence of nonconvulsive status epilepticus in comatose patients. *Neurology, 55*(9), 1421–1423. https://doi.org/10.1212/wnl.55.9.1421-a

Beniczky, S., Neufeld, M., Diehl, B., Dobesberger, J., Trinka, E., Mameniskiene, R., Rheims, S., Gil-Nagel, A., Craiu, D., Pressler, R., Krysl, D., Lebedinsky, A., Tassi, L., Rubboli, G., & Ryvlin, P. (2016). Testing patients during seizures: A European consensus procedure developed by a joint taskforce of the ILAE–Commission on European Affairs and the European Epilepsy Monitoring Unit Association. *Epilepsia, 57*(9), 1363–1368. https://doi.org/10.1111/epi.13472

Berger, H. (1929). Über das Elektrenkephalogramm des Menschen: Erste Mitteilung. *Archiv für Psychiatrie und Nervenkrankheiten, 87*, 527–570.

Berger, H. (1930). Über das Elektrenkephalogramm des Menschen: Zweite Mitteilung. *Journal für Psychologie und Neurologie, 40*, 160–179.

Betting, L. E., Mory, S. B., Lopes-Cendes, I., Li, L. M., Guerreiro, M. M., Guerreiro, C. A. M., & Cendes, F. (2006). EEG features in idiopathic generalized epilepsy: Clues to diagnosis. *Epilepsia, 47*(3), 523–528. https://doi.org/10.1111/j.1528-1167.2006.00462.x

Binnie, C. D. (1999). Simple reflex epilepsy. In J. Engel & T. A. Pedley (Eds.), Epilepsy: A *comprehensive text book* (pp. 2849–2906). Lippincott Williams & Wilkins.

Blom, S., Heijbel, J., & Bergfors, P. G. (1972). Benign epilepsy of children with centro-temporal EEG foci: Prevalence and follow-up study of 40 patients. *Epilepsia, 13*(5), 609–619. https://doi.org/10.1111/j.1528-1157.1972.tb04396.x

Boulanger, J. M., Deacon, C., Lecuyer, D., Gosselin, S., & Reiher, J. (2006). Triphasic waves versus nonconvulsive status epilepticus: EEG distinction. *Canadian Journal of Neurological Sciences, 33*(2), 175–180.

Brandt, S., & Brandt, H. (1955). The electroencephalographic patterns in young healthy children from 0 to five years of age: Their practical use in daily clinical electroencephalography. *Acta Psychiatrica et Neurologica Scandinavica, 30*(1–2), 77–89. https://doi.org/10.1111/j.1600-0447.1955.tb06048.x

Brenner, R. P. (2002). Is it status? *Epilepsia, 43*(Suppl. 3), 103–113. https://doi.org/10.1046/j.1528-1157.43.s.3.9.x

Brenner, R. P., & Atkinson, R. (1982). Generalized paroxysmal fast activity: Electroencephalographic and clinical features. *Annals of Neurology, 11*(4), 386–390. https://doi.org/10.1002/ana.410110412

Brigo, F., Rossini, F., Stefani, A., Nardone, R., Tezzon, F., Fiaschi, A., Manganotti, P., & Bongiovanni, L. G. (2013). Fixation-off sensitivity. *Clinical Neurophysiology, 124*(2), 221–227. https://doi.org/10.1016/j.clinph.2012.07.017

Browne, T. R., Penry, J. K., Porter, R. J., & Dreifuss, F. E. (1974). Responsiveness before, during and after spike–wave paroxysms. *Neurology, 24*, 659–665.

Buzsáki, G. (1986). Hippocampal sharp waves: Their origin and significance. *Brain Research, 398*(2), 242–252. https://doi.org/10.1016/0006-8993(86)91483-6

Buzsáki, G. (2002). Theta oscillations in the hippocampus. *Neuron, 33*(3), 325–340. https://doi.org/10.1016/s0896-6273(02)00586-x

Carroll, W. M., & Mastaglia, F. L. (1979). Alpha and beta coma in drug intoxication uncomplicated by cerebral hypoxia. *Electroencephalography and Clinical Neurophysiology, 46*(1), 95–105. https://doi.org/10.1016/0013-4694(79)90054-3

Catarino, C. B., Vollmar, C., & Noachtar, S. (2012). Paradoxical lateralization of non-invasive electroencephalographic ictal patterns in extra-temporal epilepsies. *Epilepsy Research, 99*(1–2), 147–155. https://doi.org/10.1016/j.eplepsyres.2011.11.002

Cavazzuti, G. B. (1980). Epidemiology of different types of epilepsy in school age children of Modena, Italy. *Epilepsia, 21*(1), 57–62. https://doi.org/10.1111/j.1528-1157.1980.tb04044.x

Chatrian, G. E., Shaw, C. M., & Leffman, H. (1964). The significance of periodic lateralized epileptiform discharges in EEG: An electrographic, clinical and pathological study. *Electroencephalography and Clinical Neurophysiology, 17*, 177–193. https://doi.org/10.1016/0013-4694(64)90149-x

Cigánek, L. (1961). Theta-discharges in the middle-line—EEG symptom of temporal lobe epilepsy. *Electroencephalography and Clinical Neurophysiology, 13*(5), 669–673. https://doi.org/https://doi.org/10.1016/0013-4694(61)90099-2

Clancy, R. R., Bergqvist, A. G. C., & Dlugos, D. J. (2003). Neonatal electroencephalography. *Current Practice of Clinical Electroencephalography, 3*, 106–234.

Cobb, W. A. (1945). Rhythmic slow discharges in the electroencephalogram. *Journal of Neurology, Neurosurgery, and Psychiatry, 8*(3–4), 65–78. https://doi.org/10.1136/jnnp.8.3-4.65

Cobb, W. A., Guiloff, R. J., & Cast, J. (1979). Breach rhythm: The EEG related to skull defects. *Electroencephalography and Clinical Neurophysiology, 47*(3), 251–271. https://doi.org/10.1016/0013-4694(79)90278-5

Cooper, R. (1963). Electrodes. *American Journal of EEG Technology, 3*, 91–101.

Cruse, R., Klem, G., Lesser, R. P., & Lueders, H. (1982). Paradoxical lateralization of cortical potentials evoked by stimulation of posterior tibial nerve. *Archives of Neurology, 39*(4), 222–225. https://doi.org/10.1001/archneur.1982.00510160028005

Csercsa, R., Dombovári, B., Fabó, D., Wittner, L., Eross, L., Entz, L., Sólyom, A., Rásonyi, G., Szucs, A., Kelemen, A., Jakus, R., Juhos, V., Grand, L., Magony, A., Halász, P., Freund, T. F., Maglóczky, Z., Cash, S. S., Papp, L., ... Ulbert, I. (2010). Laminar analysis of slow wave activity in humans. *Brain, 133*(9), 2814–2829. https://doi.org/10.1093/brain/awq169

Curio, G. (2000). Linking 600-Hz "spikelike" EEG/MEG wavelets ("sigma-bursts") to cellular substrates: Concepts and caveats. *Journal of Clinical Neurophysiology, 17*(4), 377–396. https://doi.org/10.1097/00004691-200007000-00004

Dalby, M. A. (1969). Epilepsy and 3 per second spike and wave rhythms: A clinical, electroencephalographic and prognostic analysis of 346 patients. *Acta Neurologica Scandinavica*, (Suppl 40), 3+. PMID: 4979890.

Daly, D. D. (1990). Epilepsy and syncope. In D. D. Daly & T. A. Pedley (Eds.), *Current practice of clinical electroencephalography* (pp. 269–334). Raven Press.

Dan, B., & Boyd, S. G. (2006). A neurophysiological perspective on sleep and its maturation. *Developmental Medicine and Child Neurology, 48*(9), 773–779.

Das Pektezel, L., Tezer, F. I., & Saygi, S. (2023). Electroclinical presentations of fixation-off sensitivity in adults with symptomatic epilepsy. *Journal of Clinical Neurophysiology, 40*(3), 244–249. https://doi.org/10.1097/WNP.0000000000000880

Desai, B., Whitman, S., & Bouffard, D. A. (1988). The role of the EEG in epilepsy of long duration. *Epilepsia, 29*(5), 601–606. https://doi.org/10.1111/j.1528-1157.1988.tb03768.x

Desai, J., Mitchell, W. G., Rosser, T., Ramos-Platt, L., Ahsan, N., Langille, M. M., & Toczek, M. T. (2012). Clinical associations of occipital intermittent rhythmic delta activity. *Journal of Child Neurology, 27*(4), 503–506. https://doi.org/10.1177/0883073811419256

Drake, M. E. (1986). Paroxysmal hyperventilation responses in the adult electroencephalogram. *Clinical EEG (Electroencephalography), 17*(2), 61–65.

Drury, I., & Beydoun, A. (1991). Benign partial epilepsy of childhood with monomorphic sharp waves in centrotemporal and other locations. *Epilepsia, 32*(5), 662–667. https://doi.org/10.1111/j.1528-1157.1991.tb04706.x

Dumas, G., Soussignan, R., Hugueville, L., Martinerie, J., & Nadel, J. (2014). Revisiting mu suppression in autism spectrum disorder. *Brain Research, 1585*, 108–119. https://doi.org/10.1016/j.brainres.2014.08.035

Ebersole, J. S. (1994). Non-invasive localization of the epileptogenic focus by EEG dipole modeling. *Acta Neurologica Scandinavica. Supplementum, 152*, 20–28. https://doi.org/10.1111/j.1600-0404.1994.tb05179.x

Eeg-Olofsson, O. (1971a). The development of the electroencephalogram in normal children from the age of 1 through 15 years: 14 and 6 Hz positive spike phenomenon. *Neuropadiatrie, 2*(4), 405–427. https://doi.org/10.1055/s-0028-1091792

Eeg-Olofsson, O. (1971b). The development of the electroencephalogram in normal adolescents from the age of 16 through 21 years. *Neuropadiatrie, 3*(1), 11–45. https://doi.org/10.1055/s-0028-1091798

Eeg-Olofsson, O., Petersén, I., & Selldén, U. (1971). The development of the electroencephalogram in normal children from the age of 1 through 15 years: Paroxysmal activity. *Neuropadiatrie, 2*(4), 375–404. https://doi.org/10.1055/s-0028-1091791

Ellingson, R. J., & Peters, J. F. (1980). Development of EEG and daytime sleep patterns in low risk premature infants during the first year of life: Longitudinal observations. *Electroencephalography and Clinical Neurophysiology, 50*(1–2), 165–171. https://doi.org/10.1016/0013-4694(80)90333-8

Elmer, J., Rittenberger, J. C., Faro, J., Molyneaux, B. J., Popescu, A., Callaway, C. W., & Baldwin, M. (2016). Clinically distinct electroencephalographic phenotypes of early myoclonus after cardiac arrest. *Annals of Neurology, 80*(2), 175–184. https://doi.org/10.1002/ana.24697

Fattouch, J., Casciato, S., Lapenta, L., Morano, A., Fanella, M., Lombardi, L., Manfredi, M., Giallonardo, A. T., & Di Bonaventura, C. (2013). The spectrum of epileptic syndromes with fixation off sensitivity persisting in adult life. *Epilepsia, 54*(Suppl. 7), 59–65. https://doi.org/10.1111/epi.12310

Feddersen, B., & Trinka, E. (2012). Status epilepticus. *Der Nervenarzt, 83*(2), 187–194. https://doi.org/10.1007/s00115-011-3337-0

Ferrillo, F., Beelke, M., De Carli, F., Cossu, M., Munari, C., Rosadini, G., & Nobili, L. (2000). Sleep-EEG modulation of interictal epileptiform discharges in adult partial epilepsy: A spectral analysis study. *Clinical Neurophysiology, 111*(5), 916–923. https://doi.org/10.1016/s1388-2457(00)00246-7

Fisch, B., & So, E. L. (2003). Activation methods. In J. S. Ebersole & T. A. Pedley (Eds.), *Current practice of clinical electroencephalography* (pp. 246–270). Lippincott Williams & Wilkins.

Fitzpatrick, W., & Lowry, N. (2007). PLEDs: Clinical correlates. *Canadian Journal of Neurological Sciences, 34*(4), 443–450.

Foldvary-Schaefer, N., & Grigg-Damberger, M. (2009). Sleep and epilepsy. *Seminars in Neurology, 29*(4), 419–428. https://doi.org/10.1055/s-0029-1237115

Fonseca, C., Silva Cunha, J. P., Martins, R. E., Ferreira, V. M., Marques de Sá, J. P., Barbosa, M. A., & Martins da Silva, A. (2007). A novel dry active electrode for EEG recording. *IEEE Transactions on Bio-Medical Engineering, 54*(1), 162–165. https://doi.org/10.1109/TBME.2006.884649

Fountain, N. B., Kim, J. S., & Lee, S. I. (1998). Sleep deprivation activates epileptiform discharges independent of the activating effects of sleep. *Journal of Clinical Neurophysiology, 15*(1), 69–75. https://doi.org/10.1097/00004691-199801000-00009

Franco, A. C., Kremmyda, O., Rémi, J., & Noachtar, S. (2018). Positive interictal epileptiform discharges in adults: A case series of a rare phenomenon. *Clinical Neurophysiology, 129*(5), 952–955. https://doi.org/10.1016/j.clinph.2018.01.059

Gastaut, J., Roger, J., Soulayrol, R., Tassinari, C. A., Régis, H., Dravet, C., Bernard, R., Pinsard, N., & Saint-Jean, M. (1966). Childhood epileptic encephalopathy with diffuse slow spike–waves (otherwise known as "petit mal variant") or Lennnox syndrome. *Epilepsia, 7*, 139–179.

Gibbs, E. L., Gibbs, F. A., & Fuster, B. (1948). Psychomotor epilepsy. *Archives of Neurology and Psychiatry, 60*, 331–339.

Gibbs, F. A., Davis, H., & Lennox, W. G. (1935). The EEG in epilepsy and impaired states of consciousness. *Archives of Neurology and Psychiatry, 34*, 1133–1148.

Gibbs, F. A., & Gibbs, E. L. (1952). *Atlas of electroencephalography* (2nd ed.). Addison-Wesley.

Gibbs, F. A., Rich, C. L., & Giggs, E. L. (1963). Psychomotor variant of seizure discharge. *Neurology, 13*, 991–998.

Gloor, P. (1985). Neuronal generators and the problem of localization in electroencephalography: Application of volume conductor theory to electroencephalography. *Journal of Clinical Neurophysiology, 2*(4), 327–354. https://doi.org/10.1097/00004691-198510000-00002

Gloor, P., Ball, G., & Schaul, N. (1977). Brain lesions that produce delta waves in the EEG. *Neurology, 27*(4), 326–333. https://doi.org/10.1212/wnl.27.4.326

Gloor, P., Kalabay, O., & Giard, N. (1968). The electroencephalogram in diffuse encephalopathies: Electroencephalographic correlates of grey and white matter lesions. *Brain, 91*(4), 779–802. https://doi.org/10.1093/brain/91.4.779

Goldensohn, E. S. (1979). Use of EEG for evaluation of focal intracranial lesions. In D. W. Klass & D. D. Daly (Eds.), *Current practice of clinical electroencephalography* (pp. 308–340). Raven Press.

Goldensohn, E. S., & Koehle, R. (1975). *EEG interpretation: Problems of overreading and underreading*. Futura.

References

Goodin, D. S., & Aminoff, M. J. (1984). Does the interictal EEG have a role in the diagnosis of epilepsy? *Lancet, 1*(8381), 837–839. https://doi.org/10.1016/s0140-6736(84)92281-5

Goodin, D. S., Aminoff, M. J., & Laxer, K. D. (1990). Detection of epileptiform activity by different noninvasive EEG methods in complex partial epilepsy. *Annals of Neurology, 27*(3), 330–334. https://doi.org/10.1002/ana.410270317

Gotman, J., & Koffler, D. J. (1989). Interictal spiking increases after seizures but does not after decrease in medication. *Electroencephalography and Clinical Neurophysiology, 72*(1), 7–15. https://doi.org/10.1016/0013-4694(89)90026-6

Gotman, J., & Marciani, M. G. (1985). Electroencephalographic spiking activity, drug levels, and seizure occurrence in epileptic patients. *Annals of Neurology, 17*(6), 597–603. https://doi.org/10.1002/ana.410170612

Grant, A. C., Abdel-Baki, S. G., Weedon, J., Arnedo, V., Chari, G., Koziorynska, E., Lushbough, C., Maus, D., McSween, T., Mortati, K. A., Reznikov, A., & Omurtag, A. (2014). EEG interpretation reliability and interpreter confidence: A large single-center study. *Epilepsy & Behavior, 32*, 102–107. https://doi.org/10.1016/j.yebeh.2014.01.011

Gregory, R. P., Oates, T., & Merry, R. T. (1993). Electroencephalogram epileptiform abnormalities in candidates for aircrew training. *Electroencephalography and Clinical Neurophysiology, 86*(1), 75–77. https://doi.org/10.1016/0013-4694(93)90069-8

Gullapalli, D., & Fountain, N. B. (2003). Clinical correlation of occipital intermittent rhythmic delta activity. *Journal of Clinical Neurophysiology, 20*(1), 35–41.

Haglund, M. M., & Schwartzkroin, P. A. (1990). Role of Na–K pump potassium regulation and IPSPs in seizures and spreading depression in immature rabbit hippocampal slices. *Journal of Neurophysiology, 63*(2), 225–239. https://doi.org/10.1152/jn.1990.63.2.225

Halford, J. J., Sabau, D., Drislane, F. W., Tsuchida, T. N., & Sinha, S. R. (2016). American Clinical Neurophysiology Society Guideline 4: Recording clinical EEG on digital media. *Journal of Clinical Neurophysiology, 33*(4), 317–319.

Hartl, E., Rémi, J., Stoyke, C., & Noachtar, S. (2017). What is the "L" in LPDs? Localized as well as lateralized. *Acta Neurologica Scandinavica, 136*(2), 160–163. https://doi.org/10.1111/ane.12730

Hartl, E., Rémi, J., Vollmar, C., Goc, J., Loesch, A. M., Rominger, A., & Noachtar, S. (2016). PET imaging in extratemporal epilepsy requires consideration of electroclinical findings. *Epilepsy Research, 125*, 72–76. https://doi.org/10.1016/j.eplepsyres.2016.05.010

Henkel, A., Noachtar, S., Pfänder, M., & Lüders, H. O. (2002). The localizing value of the abdominal aura and its evolution: A study in focal epilepsies. *Neurology, 58*(2), 271–276. https://doi.org/10.1212/wnl.58.2.271

Hill, C. E., Blank, L. J., Thibault, D., Davis, K. A., Dahodwala, N., Litt, B., & Willis, A. W. (2019). Continuous EEG is associated with favorable hospitalization outcomes for critically ill patients. *Neurology, 92*(1), e9–e18. https://doi.org/10.1212/WNL.0000000000006689

Hirsch, L. J., Fong, M. W. K., Leitinger, M., LaRoche, S. M., Beniczky, S., Abend, N. S., Lee, J. W., Wusthoff, C. J., Hahn, C. D., Westover, M. B., Gerard, E. E., Herman, S. T., Haider, H. A., Osman, G., Rodriguez-Ruiz, A., Maciel, C. B., Gilmore, E. J., Fernandez, A., Rosenthal, E. S., ... Gaspard, N. (2021). American Clinical Neurophysiology Society's Standardized Critical Care EEG Terminology: 2021 version. *Journal of Clinical Neurophysiology, 38*(1), 1–29. https://doi.org/10.1097/WNP.0000000000000806

Hirsch, L. J., & Gaspard, N. (2013). Status epilepticus. *Continuum: Epilepsy, 19*(3), 767–794. https://doi.org/10.1212/01.CON.0000431395.16229.5a

Hockaday, J. M., Potts, F., Epstein, E., Bonazzi, A., & Schwab, R. S. (1965). Electroencephalographic changes in acute cerebral anoxia from cardiac or respiratory arrest. *Electroencephalography and Clinical Neurophysiology, 18*(6), 575–586. https://doi.org/10.1016/0013-4694(65)90075-1

Holmes, G. L., McKeever, M., & Adamson, M. (1987). Absence seizures in children: Clinical and electroencephalographic features. *Annals of Neurology, 21*(3), 268–273. https://doi.org/10.1002/ana.410210308

Hopkins, A., Garman, A., & Clarke, C. (1988). The first seizure in adult life: Value of clinical features, electroencephalography, and computerised tomographic scanning in prediction of seizure recurrence. *Lancet, 1*(8588), 721–726. https://doi.org/10.1016/s0140-6736(88)91535-8

Hrachovy, R. A. (2000). Development of the normal electroencephalogram. In K. Levin & H. O. Luders (Eds.), Comprehensive *clinical neurophysiology* (pp. 387–413). Saunders.

Hughes, J. R. (1980). Two forms of the 6/sec spike and wave complex. *Electroencephalography and Clinical Neurophysiology, 48*(5), 535–550. https://doi.org/10.1016/0013-4694(80)90289-8

Hughes, J. R. (1985). Sleep spindles revisited. *Journal of Clinical Neurophysiology, 2*(1), 37–44. https://doi.org/10.1097/00004691-198501000-00002

Hughes, J. R. (1998). The development of the vertex sharp transient. *Clinical Electroencephalography, 29*(4), 183–187. https://doi.org/10.1177/155005949802900411

Hughes, J. R., Fino, J. J., & Hart, L. A. (1987). Premature temporal theta (PT θ). *Electroencephalography and Clinical Neurophysiology, 67*(1), 7–15. https://doi.org/10.1016/0013-4694(87)90156-8

Humphrey, D. R. (1968). Re-analysis of the antidromic cortical response: II. On the contribution of cell discharge and PSPs to the evoked potentials.

Electroencephalography and Clinical Neurophysiology, 25(5), 421–442. https://doi.org/10.1016/0013-4694(68)90152-1

Husain, A. M. (2005). Review of neonatal EEG. *American Journal of Electroneurodiagnostic Technology, 45*(1), 12–35.

Husain, A. M. (2006). Electroencephalographic assessment of coma. *Journal of Clinical Neurophysiology, 23*(3), 208–220. https://doi.org/10.1097/01.wnp.0000220094.60482.b5

Ives, J. R. (1975). 4-Channel 24 hour cassette recorder for long-term EEG monitoring of ambulatory patients. *Electroencephalography and Clinical Neurophysiology, 39*(1), 88–92. https://doi.org/10.1016/0013-4694(75)90131-5

Iwasaki, M., Kellinghaus, C., Alexopoulos, A. V, Burgess, R. C., Kumar, A. N., Han, Y. H., Lüders, H. O., & Leigh, R. J. (2005). Effects of eyelid closure, blinks, and eye movements on the electroencephalogram. *Clinical Neurophysiology, 116*(4), 878–885. https://doi.org/10.1016/j.clinph.2004.11.001

Janz, D., & Christian, W. (1957). Impulsiv-Petit mal. *Deutsche Zeitschrift für Nervenheilkunde, 176*(3), 346–386. https://doi.org/10.1007/BF00242439

Jasper, H., & Van Buren, J. (1955). Interrelationship between cortex and subcortical structures: Clinical electroencephalographic studies. *Electroencephalography and Clinical Neurophysiology. Supplement* (Suppl. 4), 168–188.

Jayakar, P., & Chiappa, K. H. (1990). Clinical correlations of photoparoxysmal responses. *Electroencephalography and Clinical Neurophysiology, 75*(3), 251–254. https://doi.org/10.1016/0013-4694(90)90178-m

Jayakar, P., Duchowny, M., Resnick, T. J., & Alvarez, L. A. (1991). Localization of seizure foci: Pitfalls and caveats. *Journal of Clinical Neurophysiology, 8*(4), 414–431. https://doi.org/10.1097/00004691-199110000-00006

Jing, J., Sun, H., Kim, J. A., Herlopian, A., Karakis, I., Ng, M., Halford, J. J., Maus, D., Chan, F., Dolatshahi, M., Muniz, C., Chu, C., Sacca, V., Pathmanathan, J., Ge, W., Dauwels, J., Lam, A., Cole, A. J., Cash, S. S., & Westover, M. B. (2020). Development of expert-level automated detection of epileptiform discharges during electroencephalogram interpretation. *JAMA Neurology, 77*(1), 103–108. https://doi.org/10.1001/jamaneurol.2019.3485

Kane, N., Acharya, J., Benickzy, S., Caboclo, L., Finnigan, S., Kaplan, P. W., Shibasaki, H., Pressler, R., & van Putten, M. J. A. M. (2017). A revised glossary of terms most commonly used by clinical electroencephalographers and updated proposal for the report format of the EEG findings: Revision 2017. *Clinical Neurophysiology Practice, 2*, 170–185. https://doi.org/10.1016/j.cnp.2017.07.002

Kanner, A. M., Parra, J., Gil-Nagel, A., Soto, A., Leurgans, S., Iriarte, J., deToledo-Morrell, L., & Palac, S. (2002). The localizing yield of sphenoidal and anterior temporal electrodes in ictal recordings: A comparison study. *Epilepsia, 43*(10), 1189–1196. https://doi.org/10.1046/j.1528-1157.2002.06402.x

Kaplan, P. W., & Benbadis, S. R. (2013). How to write an EEG report: Dos and don'ts. *Neurology, 80*(1 Suppl. 1), S43–S46. https://doi.org/10.1212/WNL.0b013e3182797528

Kaplan, P. W., Gélisse, P., & Sutter, R. (2021). An EEG voyage in search of triphasic waves—The sirens and corsairs on the encephalopathy/EEG horizon: A survey of triphasic waves. *Journal of Clinical Neurophysiology, 38*(5), 348–358. https://doi.org/10.1097/WNP.0000000000000725

Kasteleijn-Nolst Trenité, D., Rubboli, G., Hirsch, E., Martins da Silva, A., Seri, S., Wilkins, A., Parra, J., Covanis, A., Elia, M., Capovilla, G., Stephani, U., & Harding, G. (2012). Methodology of photic stimulation revisited: Updated European algorithm for visual stimulation in the EEG laboratory. *Epilepsia, 53*(1), 16–24. https://doi.org/10.1111/j.1528-1167.2011.03319.x

Kasteleijn-Nolst Trenité, D. G., Binnie, C. D., Harding, G. F., & Wilkins, A. (1999). Photic stimulation: Standardization of screening methods. *Epilepsia, 40*(Suppl. 4), 75–79. https://doi.org/10.1111/j.1528-1157.1999.tb00911.x

Katz, R. I., & Horowitz, G. R. (1982). Electroencephalogram in the septuagenarian: Studies in a normal geriatric population. *Journal of the American Geriatrics Society, 30*(4), 273–275. https://doi.org/10.1111/j.1532-5415.1982.tb07101.x

Kaul, B., Shukla, G., Goyal, V., Srivastava, A., & Behari, M. (2012). Paroxysmal occipital discharges suppressed by eye opening: Spectrum of clinical and imaging features at a tertiary care center in India. *Neurology India, 60*(5), 461–464. https://doi.org/10.4103/0028-3886.103183

Kellaway, P., & Fox, B. J. (1952). Electroencephalographic diagnosis of cerebral pathology in infants during sleep: I. Rationale, technique, and the characteristics of normal sleep in infants. *Journal of Pediatrics, 41*(3), 262–287.

King, D. W., So, E. L., Marcus, R., & Gallagher, B. B. (1986). Techniques and applications of sphenoidal recording. *Journal of Clinical Neurophysiology, 3*(1), 51–65. https://doi.org/10.1097/00004691-198601000-00004

King, M. A., Newton, M. R., Jackson, G. D., Fitt, G. J., Mitchell, L. A., Silvapulle, M. J., & Berkovic, S. F. (1998). Epileptology of the first-seizure presentation: A clinical, electroencephalographic, and magnetic resonance imaging study of 300 consecutive patients. *Lancet, 352*(9133), 1007–1011. https://doi.org/10.1016/S0140-6736(98)03543-0

Kirac, L. B., Vollmar, C., Rémi, J., Loesch, A. M., & Noachtar, S. (2016). Notch filter artefact mimicking high frequency oscillation in epilepsy. *Clinical Neurophysiology, 127*(1), 979–981. https://doi.org/10.1016/j.clinph.2015.05.030

Klass, D. W., & Westmoreland, B. F. (1985). Nonepileptogenic epileptiform electroencephalographic activity. *Annals of Neurology, 18*(6), 627–635. https://doi.org/10.1002/ana.410180602

Klem, G. H., Lüders, H. O., Jasper, H. H., & Elger, C. (1999). The ten–twenty electrode system of the International Federation. The International Federation of Clinical

Neurophysiology. *Electroencephalography and Clinical Neurophysiology. Supplement, 52*, 3–6.

Kooi, K. A., Guevener, A. M., Tupper, C. J., & Bagchi, B. D. (1964). Electroencephalographic patterns of the temporal region in normal adults. *Neurology, 14*, 1029–1035. https://doi.org/10.1212/wnl.14.11.1029

Koutroumanidis, M., Tsatsou, K., Sanders, S., Michael, M., Tan, S. V, Agathonikou, A., & Panayiotopoulos, C. P. (2009). Fixation-off sensitivity in epilepsies other than the idiopathic epilepsies of childhood with occipital paroxysms: A 12-year clinical–video EEG study. *Epileptic Disorders, 11*(1), 20–36. https://doi.org/10.1684/epd.2009.0235

Kozelka, J. W., & Pedley, T. A. (1990). Beta and mu rhythms. *Journal of Clinical Neurophysiology, 7*(2), 191–207. https://doi.org/10.1097/00004691-199004000-00004

Kural, M. A., Tankisi, H., Duez, L., Sejer Hansen, V., Udupi, A., Wennberg, R., Rampp, S., Larsson, P. G., Schulz, R., & Beniczky, S. (2020). Optimized set of criteria for defining interictal epileptiform EEG discharges. *Clinical Neurophysiology, 131*, 2250–2254.

Kuratani, J., Pearl, P. L., Sullivan, L., Riel-Romero, R. M. S., Cheek, J., Stecker, M., San-Juan, D., Selioutski, O., Sinha, S. R., Drislane, F. W., & Tsuchida, T. N. (2016). American Clinical Neurophysiology Society Guideline 5: Minimum technical standards for pediatric electroencephalography. *Journal of Clinical Neurophysiology, 33*(4), 320–323.

Lacuey, N., Zonjy, B., Londono, L., & Lhatoo, S. D. (2017). Amygdala and hippocampus are symptomatogenic zones for central apneic seizures. *Neurology, 88*(7), 701–705. https://doi.org/10.1212/WNL.0000000000003613

Lieb, J. P., Walsh, G. O., Babb, T. L., Walter, R. D., Crandall, P. H., Tassinari, C. A., Portera, A., & Scheffner, D. (1976). A comparison of EEG seizure patterns recorded with surface and depth electrodes in patients with temporal lobe epilepsy. *Epilepsia, 17*(2), 137–160.

Lindsley, D. B., Bowden, J. W., & Magoun, H. W. (1949). Effect upon the EEG of acute injury to the brain stem activating system. *Electroencephalography and Clinical Neurophysiology, 1*(4), 475–486.

Llinás, R. R., & Steriade, M. (2006). Bursting of thalamic neurons and states of vigilance. *Journal of Neurophysiology, 95*(6), 3297–3308. https://doi.org/10.1152/jn.00166.2006

Lombroso, C. T. (1979). Quantified electrographic scales on 10 pre-term healthy newborns followed up to 40–43 weeks of conceptional age by serial polygraphic recordings. *Electroencephalography and Clinical Neurophysiology, 46*(4), 460–474. https://doi.org/10.1016/0013-4694(79)90147-0

Lombroso, C. T. (1997). Consistent EEG focalities detected in subjects with primary generalized epilepsies monitored for two decades. *Epilepsia, 38*(7), 797–812. https://doi.org/10.1111/j.1528-1157.1997.tb01467.x

Lombroso, C. T., Schwartz, I. H., Clark, D. M., Muench, H., Barry, P. H., & Barry, J. (1966). Ctenoids in healthy youths: Controlled study of 14- and 6-per-second positive spiking. *Neurology, 16*(12), 1152–1158. https://doi.org/10.1212/wnl.16.12.1152

Lopes da Silva, F. H., Vos, J. E., Mooibroek, J., & Van Rotterdam, A. (1980). Relative contributions of intracortical and thalamo-cortical processes in the generation of alpha rhythms, revealed by partial coherence analysis. *Electroencephalography and Clinical Neurophysiology, 50*(5–6), 449–456. https://doi.org/10.1016/0013-4694(80)90011-5

Lüders, H., Acharya, J., Baumgartner, C., Benbadis, S., Bleasel, A., Burgess, R., Dinner, D. S., Ebner, A., Foldvary, N., Geller, E., Hamer, H., Holthausen, H., Kotagal, P., Morris, H., Meencke, H. J., Noachtar, S., Rosenow, F., Sakamoto, A., Steinhoff, B. J., ... Wyllie, E. (1998). Semiological seizure classification. *Epilepsia, 39*(9), 1006–1013. http://www.ncbi.nlm.nih.gov/entrez/query.fcgi?cmd=Retrieve&db=PubMed&dopt=Citation&list_uids=9738682

Lüders, H. O., Lesser, R. P., Dinner, D. S., & Morris, H. H. (1987). Benign focal epilepsy of childhood. In H Lüders & R. P. Lesser (Eds.), *Epilepsy: Electroclinical syndromes* (pp. 303–346). Springer.

Lüders, H. O., & Noachtar, S. (2000a). *Atlas and classification of electroencephalography.* Saunders.

Lüders, H. O., & Noachtar, S. (2000b). *Epileptic seizures: Pathophysiology and clinical semiology.* Churchill Livingstone.

Lüders, H. O., & Noachtar, S. (2001). *Atlas of epileptic seizures and syndromes.* Saunders.

Lüders, H. O., Vaca, G. F.-B., Akamatsu, N., Amina, S., Arzimanoglou, A., Baumgartner, C., Benbadis, S. R., Bleasel, A., Bermeo-Ovalle, A., Bozorgi, A., Carreño, M., Devereaux, M., Francione, S., Losarcos, N. G., Hamer, H., Holthausen, H., Jamal-Omidi, S., Kalamangalam, G., Kanner, A. M., . . . Kahane, P. (2019). Classification of paroxysmal events and the four-dimensional epilepsy classification system. *Epileptic Disorders, 21*(1), 1–29.

Marshall, C. (1955). Some clinical correlates of the wave and spike phantom. *Electroencephalography and Clinical Neurophysiology, 7*(4), 633–636. https://doi.org/10.1016/0013-4694(55)90090-0

Marshall, P. J., Bar-Haim, Y., & Fox, N. A. (2002). Development of the EEG from 5 months to 4 years of age. *Clinical Neurophysiology, 113*(8), 1199–1208. https://doi.org/10.1016/s1388-2457(02)00163-3

Marshall, P. J., & Meltzoff, A. N. (2011). Neural mirroring systems: Exploring the EEG μ rhythm in human infancy. *Developmental Cognitive Neuroscience, 1*(2), 110–123. https://doi.org/10.1016/j.dcn.2010.09.001

Matsuo, F., & Knott, J. R. (1977). Focal positive spikes in electroencephalography. *Electroencephalography and Clinical Neurophysiology, 42*(1), 15–25. https://doi.org/10.1016/0013-4694(77)90147-x

Matsuo, T., Iinuma, K., & Esashi, M. (1973). A barium-titanate-ceramics capacitive-type EEG electrode. *IEEE Transactions on Bio-Medical Engineering, 20*(4), 299–300. https://doi.org/10.1109/TBME.1973.324197

Mendez, O. E., & Brenner, R. P. (2006). Increasing the yield of EEG. *Journal of Clinical Neurophysiology, 23*(4), 282–293. https://doi.org/10.1097/01.wnp.0000228514.40227.12

Metcalf, D. R., Mondale, J., & Butler, F. K. (1971). Ontogenesis of spontaneous K-complexes. *Psychophysiology, 8*(3), 340–347. https://doi.org/10.1111/j.1469-8986.1971.tb00464.x

Mizrahi, E. M. (1996). Avoiding the pitfalls of EEG interpretation in childhood epilepsy. *Epilepsia, 37*(Suppl. 1), S41–S51. https://doi.org/10.1111/j.1528-1157.1996.tb06021.x

Monod, N., Pajot, N., & Guidasci, S. (1972). The neonatal EEG: Statistical studies and prognostic value in full-term and pre-term babies. *Electroencephalography and Clinical Neurophysiology, 32*(5), 529–544. https://doi.org/10.1016/0013-4694(72)90063-6

Morris, H. H., 3rd, Luders, H., Lesser, R. P., Dinner, D. S., & Klem, G. H. (1986). The value of closely spaced scalp electrodes in the localization of epileptiform foci: A study of 26 patients with complex partial seizures. *Electroencephalography & Clinical Neurophysiology, 63*(2), 107–111.

Nakamura, Y., & Ohye, C. (1964). Delta wave production in neocortical EEG by acute lesions within thalamus and hypothalamus of the cat. *Electroencephalography and Clinical Neurophysiology, 17*(6), 671–676. https://doi.org/10.1016/0013-4694(64)90235-4

Newmark, M. E., & Penry, J. K. (1979). *Photosensitivity and epilepsy: A review.* Raven Press.

Niedermeyer, E., & da Silva, F. H. L. (2005). *Electroencephalography: Basic principles, clinical applications, and related fields.* Lippincott Williams & Wilkins.

Noachtar, S, Bilgin, O., Remi, J., Chang, N., Midi, I., Vollmar, C., & Feddersen, B. (2008). Interictal regional polyspikes in noninvasive EEG suggest cortical dysplasia as etiology of focal epilepsies. *Epilepsia, 49*(6), 1011–1017. http://www.ncbi.nlm.nih.gov/entrez/query.fcgi?cmd=Retrieve&db=PubMed&dopt=Citation&list_uids=18363706

Noachtar, S, Binnie, C., Ebersole, J., Mauguiere, F., Sakamoto, A., & Westmoreland, B. (1999). A glossary of terms most commonly used by clinical electroencephalographers and proposal for the report form for the EEG findings. The International Federation of Clinical Neurophysiology. *Electroencephalography and Clinical Neurophysiology. Supplement, 52,* 21–41. http://www.ncbi.nlm.nih.gov/entrez/query.fcgi?cmd=Retrieve&db=PubMed&dopt=Citation&list_uids=10590974

Noachtar, S., Holthausen, H., & Lüders, H. O. (1997). Epileptic negative myoclonus: Subdural EEG recordings indicate a postcentral generator. *Neurology, 49*(6), 1534–1537. http://www.ncbi.nlm.nih.gov/entrez/query.fcgi?cmd=Retrieve&db=PubMed&dopt=Citation&list_uids=9409341

Noachtar, S., & Lüders, H. O. (1999). Focal akinetic seizures as documented by electroencephalography and video recordings. *Neurology, 53*(2), 427–429. http://www.ncbi.nlm.nih.gov/entrez/query.fcgi?cmd=Retrieve&db=PubMed&dopt=Citation&list_uids=10430445

Noachtar, S., & Lüders, H. O. (2000). Akinetic seizures. In H. O. Lüders & S. Noachtar (Eds.), *Epileptic seizures. Pathophysiology and clinical semiology* (pp. 489–500). Churchill Livingstone.

Noachtar, S., & Peters, A. S. (2009). Semiology of epileptic seizures: A critical review. *Epilepsy and Behavior, 15*(1), 2–9. https://doi.org/10.1016/j.yebeh.2009.02.029

Noachtar, S., & Rémi, J. (2009). The role of EEG in epilepsy: A critical review. *Epilepsy and Behavior, 15*(1), 22–33. https://doi.org/10.1016/j.yebeh.2009.02.035

Noachtar, S., Rémi, J. (2008). Sleep and epilepsy. In S. Shorvon & T. A. Pedley (Eds.), *The epilepsies 3* (pp. 84–96). Saunders. https://doi.org/10.1016/B978-1-4160-6171-7.00007-8

Noachtar, S., Rosenow, F., & Lüders, H. O. (2004). Video analysis in the definition of the symptomatogenic zone. In J. Daube & F. Mauguiere (Eds.), *Handbook of clinical neurophysiology* (pp. 187–200). Elsevier.

Noebels, J. L., & Kellaway, P. (1989). *Problems and concepts in developmental neurophysiology.* Johns Hopkins University Press.

Nordli, D. R. J. (2012). Epileptic encephalopathies in infants and children. *Journal of Clinical Neurophysiology, 29*(5), 420–424. https://doi.org/10.1097/WNP.0b013e31826bd961

Obrist, W. D. (1954). The electroencephalogram of normal aged adults. *Electroencephalography and Clinical Neurophysiology, 6,* 235–244. https://doi.org/10.1016/0013-4694(54)90025-5

Patel, V. M., & Maulsby, R. L. (1987). How hyperventilation alters the electroencephalogram: A review of controversial viewpoints emphasizing neurophysiological mechanisms. *Journal of Clinical Neurophysiology, 4*(2), 101–120. https://doi.org/10.1097/00004691-198704000-00001

Pedley, T. A., Mendiratta, A., & Walczak, T. S. (2003). Seizures and epilepsy. *Current Practice of Clinical Electroencephalography, 3,* 506–587.

Petersén, I., & Eeg-Olofsson, O. (1971). The development of the electroencephalogram in normal children from the age of 1 through 15 years: Non-paroxysmal activity. *Neuropädiatrie, 2*(3), 247–304. https://doi.org/10.1055/s-0028-1091786

Pitt, M., & Pressler, R. (2005). Neurophysiological testing in the newborn and infant. *Early Human Development, 81*(12), 939–946. https://doi.org/10.1016/j.earlhumdev.2005.10.005

Pohlmann-Eden, B., Hoch, D. B., Cochius, J. I., & Chiappa, K. H. (1996). Periodic lateralized epileptiform discharges: A critical review. *Journal of Clinical Neurophysiology, 13*(6), 519–530. https://doi.org/10.1097/00004691-199611000-00007

Prior, P. (1973). *The EEG in acute cerebral anoxia*. Excerpta Medica.

Rechtschaffen, A., & Kales, A. (Eds.). (1968). *A manual of standardized terminology, techniques and scoring system for sleep stages of human subjects*. Brain Information Service/ Brain Research Institute.

Reiher, J., Beaudry, M., & Leduc, C. P. (1989). Temporal intermittent rhythmic delta activity (TIRDA) in the diagnosis of complex partial epilepsy: Sensitivity, specificity and predictive value. *Canadian Journal of Neurological Sciences, 16*(4), 398–401. https://doi.org/10.1017/S0317167100029450

Reiher, J, & Lebel, M. (1977). Wicket spikes: Clinical correlates of a previously undescribed EEG pattern. *Canadian Journal of Neurological Sciences, 4*(1), 39–47.

Reiher, J., Rivest, J., Maison, F. G., & Leduc, C. P. (1991). Periodic lateralized epileptiform discharges with transitional rhythmic discharges: Association with seizures. *Electroencephalography and Clinical Neurophysiology, 78*(1), 12–17. https://doi.org/10.1016/0013-4694(91)90013-T

Reilly, E. L., & Peters, J. F. (1973). Relationship of some varieties of electroencephalographic photosensitivity to clinical convulsive disorders. *Neurology, 23*(10), 1050–1057. https://doi.org/10.1212/wnl.23.10.1050

Rémi, J., & Noachtar, S. (2010). Clinical features of the postictal state: Correlation with seizure variables. *Epilepsy and Behavior, 19*(2), 114–117. https://doi.org/10.1016/j.yebeh.2010.06.039

Rémi, J., Vollmar, C., De Marinis, A., Heinlin, J., Peraud, A., & Noachtar, S. (2011a). Congruence and discrepancy of interictal and ictal EEG with MRI lesions in focal epilepsies. *Neurology, 77*(14), 1383–1390. https://doi.org/10.1212/WNL.0b013e31823152c3

Rémi, J., Vollmar, C., & Noachtar, S. (2011b). No response to acoustic stimuli: Absence or akinetic seizure? *Epilepsy and Behavior, 21*(4), 478–479. https://doi.org/10.1016/j.yebeh.2011.06.008

Rey, V., Aybek, S., Maeder-Ingvar, M., & Rossetti, A. O. (2009). Positive occipital sharp transients of sleep (POSTS): A reappraisal. *Clinical Neurophysiology, 120*(3), 472–475. https://doi.org/10.1016/j.clinph.2008.12.035

Risinger, M. W., Engel, J., Jr., Van Ness, P. C., Henry, T. R., & Crandall, P. H. (1989). Ictal localization of temporal lobe seizures with scalp/sphenoidal recordings. *Neurology, 39*(10), 1288–1293. http://www.ncbi.nlm.nih.gov/entrez/query.fcgi?cmd=Retrieve&db=PubMed&dopt=Citation&list_uids=2797451

Rona, S., Rosenow, F., Arnold, S., Carreño, M., Diehl, B., Ebner, A., Fritsch, B., Hamer, H. M., Holthausen, H., Knake, S., Kruse, B., Noachtar, S., Pieper, T., Tuxhorn, I., & Lüders, H. O. (2005). A semiological classification of status epilepticus. *Epileptic Disorders, 7*(1), 5–12.

Salanova, V., Morris, H. H., Van Ness, P., Kotagal, P., Wyllie, E., & Luders, H. (1995). Frontal lobe seizures: Electroclinical syndromes. *Epilepsia, 36*(1), 16–24.

Salinsky, M., Kanter, R., & Dasheiff, R. M. (1987). Effectiveness of multiple EEGs in supporting the diagnosis of epilepsy: An operational curve. *Epilepsia, 28*(4), 331–334.

Schaul, N. (1990). Pathogenesis and significance of abnormal nonepileptiform rhythms in the EEG. *Journal of Clinical Neurophysiology, 7*, 229–248.

Scher, M. (2005). Electroencephalography of the newborn: Normal and abnormal features. In E Niedermeyer & F. Lopes da Silva (Eds.), *Electroencephalography: Basic principles, clinical applications, and related fields* (5th ed., pp. 937–990). Lippincott Williams & Wilkins.

Scherg, M., Berg, P., Nakasato, N., & Beniczky, S. (2019). Taking the EEG back into the brain: The power of multiple discrete sources. *Frontiers in Neurology, 10*, 855. https://doi.org/10.3389/fneur.2019.00855

Scherg, M., Ille, N., Bornfleth, H., & Berg, P. (2002). Advanced tools for digital EEG review: Virtual source montages, whole-head mapping, correlation, and phase analysis. *Journal of Clinical Neurophysiology, 19*(2), 91–112. http://www.ncbi.nlm.nih.gov/entrez/query.fcgi?cmd=Retrieve&db=PubMed&dopt=Citation&list_uids=11997721

Scherg, M., Ille, N., Weckesser, D., Ebert, A., Ostendorf, A., Boppel, T., Schubert, S., Larsson, P. G., Henning, O., & Bast, T. (2012). Fast evaluation of interictal spikes in long-term EEG by hyper-clustering. *Epilepsia, 53*(7), 1196–1204. https://doi.org/10.1111/j.1528-1167.2012.03503.x

Schulz, R., Luders, H. O., Hoppe, M., Tuxhorn, I., May, T., & Ebner, A. (2000). Interictal EEG and ictal scalp EEG propagation are highly predictive of surgical outcome in mesial temporal lobe epilepsy. *Epilepsia, 41*(5), 564–570.

Schwartzkroin, P. A., & Stafstrom, C. E. (1980). Effects of EGTA on the calcium-activated afterhyperpolarization in hippocampal CA3 pyramidal cells. *Science, 210*(4474), 1125–1126. https://doi.org/10.1126/science.6777871

Selvitelli, M. F., Walker, L. M., Schomer, D. L., & Chang, B. S. (2010). The relationship of interictal epileptiform discharges to clinical epilepsy severity: A study of routine electroencephalograms and review of the literature. *Journal of Clinical Neurophysiology, 27*(2), 87–92. https://doi.org/10.1097/WNP.0b013e3181d64b1e

Sevgi, E. B., Saygi, S., & Ciger, A. (2007). Eye closure sensitivity and epileptic syndromes: A retrospective study of 26 adult cases. *Seizure, 16*(1), 17–21. https://doi.org/10.1016/j.seizure.2006.09.004

Shannon, C. E. (1998). Communication in the presence of noise. *Proceedings of the IEEE, 86*(2), 447–457. https://doi.org/10.1109/JPROC.1998.659497

Shinnar, S., Berg, A. T., Moshe, S. L., Petix, M., Maytal, J., Kang, H., Goldensohn, E. S., & Hauser, W. A. (1990). Risk of seizure recurrence following a first unprovoked seizure in childhood: A prospective study. *Pediatrics, 85*(6), 1076–1085.

Sinha, S. R., Sullivan, L., Sabau, D., San-Juan, D., Dombrowski, K. E., Halford, J. J., Hani, A. J., Drislane, F. W., & Stecker, M. M. (2016). American Clinical Neurophysiology Society Guideline 1: Minimum technical requirements for performing clinical electroencephalography. *Journal of Clinical Neurophysiology, 33*(4), 303–307.

Sofat, P., Teter, B., Kavak, K. S., Gupta, R., & Li, P. (2016). Time interval providing highest yield for initial EEG in patients with new onset seizures. *Epilepsy Research, 127*, 229–232. https://doi.org/10.1016/j.eplepsyres.2016.08.024

Speckmann, E. J., Elger, C. E., & Altrup, U. (1993). Neurophysiological basis of the EEG. In E. Wyllie (Ed.), *The treatment of epilepsy: Principles and practice* (pp. 185–201). Lea & Febiger.

Spenner, B., Krois-Neudenberger, J., Kurlemann, G., Althaus, J., Schwartz, O., & Fiedler, B. (2019). The prognostic value of sleep spindles in long-term outcome of West syndrome. *European Journal of Paediatric Neurology, 23*(6), 827–831. https://doi.org/10.1016/j.ejpn.2019.09.003

Statz, A., Dumermuth, G., Mieth, D., & Duc, G. (1982). Transient EEG patterns during sleep in healthy newborns. *Neuropediatrics, 13*(3), 115–122. https://doi.org/10.1055/s-2008-1059609

Stecker, M. M., Sabau, D., Sullivan, L., Das, R. R., Selioutski, O., Drislane, F. W., Tsuchida, T. N., & Tatum, W. O., 4th. (2016). American Clinical Neurophysiology Society Guideline 6: Minimum technical standards for EEG recording in suspected cerebral death. *Journal of Clinical Neurophysiology, 33*(4), 324–327.

Steriade, M. (2005). Sleep, epilepsy and thalamic reticular inhibitory neurons. *Trends in Neurosciences, 28*(6), 317–324. https://doi.org/10.1016/j.tins.2005.03.007

Steriade, M. (2006). Grouping of brain rhythms in corticothalamic systems. *Neuroscience, 137*(4), 1087–1106. http://www.ncbi.nlm.nih.gov/entrez/query.fcgi?cmd=Retrieve&db=PubMed&dopt=Citation&list_uids=16343791

Stockard-Pope, J. E., Werner, S. S., & Bickford, R. G. (1992). *Atlas of neonatal electroencephalography.* Raven Press.

Sundaram, M., Hogan, T., Hiscock, M., & Pillay, N. (1990). Factors affecting interictal spike discharges in adults with epilepsy. *Electroencephalography and Clinical Neurophysiology, 75*(4), 358–360. https://doi.org/10.1016/0013-4694(90)90114-Y

Sunder, T., Erwin, C., & Dubois, P. (1980). Hyperventilation induced abnormalities in the electroencephalogram of children with moyamoya disease. *Electroencephalography and Clinical Neurophysiology, 49*(3–4), 414–420. https://doi.org/10.1016/0013-4694(80)90239-4

Synek, V. M. (1988). Prognostically important EEG coma patterns in diffuse anoxic and traumatic encephalopathies in adults. *Journal of Clinical Neurophysiology, 5*(2), 161–174. https://doi.org/10.1097/00004691-198804000-00003

Synek, V. M., & Synek, B. J. L. (1987). "Theta pattern coma" occurring in younger adults. *Clinical EEG (Electroencephalography, 18*(2), 54–60.

Tatum, W. O., Selioutski, O., Ochoa, J. G., Clary, H. M., Cheek, J., Drislane, F. W., & Tsuchida, T. N. (2016). American Clinical Neurophysiology Society Guideline 7: Guidelines for EEG reporting. *The Neurodiagnostic Journal, 56*(4), 285–293. https://doi.org/10.1080/21646821.2016.1245576

Tekin Güveli, B., Baykan, B., Dörtcan, N., Bebek, N., Gürses, C., & Gökyiğit, A. (2013). Eye closure sensitivity in juvenile myoclonic epilepsy and its effect on prognosis. *Seizure, 22*(10), 867–871. https://doi.org/10.1016/j.seizure.2013.07.008

Tezer, I. F., Rémi, J., & Noachtar, S. (2009). Ictal apnea of epileptic origin. Neurology, *72*(9), 855–857.

Thomas, J. E., Reagan, T. J., & Klass, D. W. (1977). Epilepsia partialis continua: A review of 32 cases. *Archives of Neurology, 34*(5), 266–275. https://doi.org/10.1001/archneur.1977.00500170020003

Timofeev, I., Grenier, F., & Steriade, M. (2004). Contribution of intrinsic neuronal factors in the generation of cortically driven electrographic seizures. *Journal of Neurophysiology, 92*(2), 1133–1143. https://doi.org/10.1152/jn.00523.2003

Toljan, K., Pestana-Knight, E., & Nv Moosa, A. (2021). Asymmetric eye movement artifacts on EEG, secondary to unilateral retinal detachment in patients with focal epilepsy. *Epileptic Disorders, 23*(6), 961–962. https://doi.org/10.1684/epd.2021.1334

Torres, F., Faoro, A., Loewenson, R., & Johnson, E. (1983). The electroencephalogram of elderly subjects revisited. *Electroencephalography and Clinical Neurophysiology, 56*(5), 391–398. https://doi.org/10.1016/0013-4694(83)90220-1

Towne, A. R., Waterhouse, E. J., Boggs, J. G., Garnett, L. K., Brown, A. J., Smith, J. R., Jr., & DeLorenzo, R. J. (2000). Prevalence of nonconvulsive status epilepticus in comatose patients. *Neurology, 54*(2), 340–345.

Trinka, E., Cock, H., Hesdorffer, D., Rossetti, A. O., Scheffer, I. E., Shinnar, S., Shorvon, S., & Lowenstein, D. H. (2015). A definition and classification of status epilepticus: Report of the ILAE Task Force on Classification of Status Epilepticus. *Epilepsia, 56*(10), 1515–1523. https://doi.org/10.1111/epi.13121

Tükel, K., & Jasper, H. (1952). The electroencephalogram in parasagittal lesions. *Electroencephalography and Clinical Neurophysiology, 4*, 481–494.

Tveit, J., Aurlien, H., Plis, S., Calhoun, V. D., Tatum, W. O., Schomer, D. L., Arntsen, V., Cox, F., Fahoum, F., Gallentine, W. B., Gardella, E., Hahn, C. D., Husain, A. M., Kessler, S., Kural, M. A., Nascimento, F. A., Tankisi, H., Ulvin, L. B., Wennberg, R., & Beniczky, S. (2023). Automated Interpretation of Clinical Electroencephalograms Using Artificial Intelligence. *JAMA Neurology, 80*, 805–812.

Urrestarazu, E., Chander, R., Dubeau, F., & Gotman, J. (2007). Interictal high-frequency oscillations (10–500 Hz) in the intracerebral EEG of epileptic patients. *Brain, 130*(9), 2354–2366. https://doi.org/10.1093/brain/awm149

Usui, N., Kotagal, P., Matsumoto, R., Kellinghaus, C., & Lüders, H. O. (2005). Focal semiologic and electroencephalographic features in patients with juvenile myoclonic epilepsy. *Epilepsia, 46*(10), 1668–1676. https://doi.org/10.1111/j.1528-1167.2005.00262.x

Van Donselaar, C. A., Schimsheimer, R. J., Geerts, A. T., & Declerck, A. C. (1992). Value of the electroencephalogram in adult patients with untreated idiopathic first seizures. *Archives of Neurology, 49*(3), 231–237. https://doi.org/10.1001/archneur.1992.00530270045017

Verrotti, A., Trotta, D., Salladini, C., di Corcia, G., & Chiarelli, F. (2004). Photosensitivity and epilepsy. *Journal of Child Neurology, 19*(8), 571–578. https://doi.org/10.1177/088307380401900802

Vogel, F. (1958). *Über die Erblichkeit des normalen Elektroencephalogramms* [On heritability of the normal electroencephalogram]. Thieme.

Vollmar, C., Stredl, I., Heinig, M., Noachtar, S., & Rémi, J. (2018). Unilateral temporal interictal epileptiform discharges correctly predict the epileptogenic zone in lesional temporal lobe epilepsy. *Epilepsia, 59*(8), 1577–1582. https://doi.org/10.1111/epi.14514

Walter, W. G. (1936). The location of cerebral tumours by electro-encephalography. *Lancet, 228*(5893), 305–308.

Walter, W. G., Dovey, V. J., & Shipton, H. (1946). Analysis of the electrical response of the human cortex to photic stimulation. *Nature, 158*(4016), 540–541.

Watanabe, A. (1992). The neonatal electroencephalogram and sleep cycle patterns. In J. A. Eyre (Ed.), *The neurophysiological examination of the newborn infant* (pp. 11–46). Mac Keith Press.

Weber, P. (2005). Unilateral or asymmetric localization of lambda waves is not a pathologic finding. *Journal of Child Neurology, 20*(3), 250–251.

Weil, S., Arnold, S., Eisensehr, I., & Noachtar, S. (2005). Heart rate increase in otherwise subclinical seizures is different in temporal versus extratemporal seizure onset: Support for temporal lobe autonomic influence. *Epileptic Disorders, 7*(3), 199–204. http://www.ncbi.nlm.nih.gov/entrez/query.fcgi?cmd=Retrieve&db=PubMed&dopt=Citation&list_uids=16162428

Weinmann, R. L. (2007). Jack Ruby. *Neurology, 69*(9), 940–941.

Westmoreland, B. F. (1996). Epileptiform electroencephalographic patterns. *Mayo Clinic Proceedings, 71*(5), 501–511. https://doi.org/10.4065/71.5.501

Westmoreland, B. F. (2009). Electroencephalography: Electroencephalograms of infants and children. *Contemporary Neurology Series, 75*(1), 167–186.

Westmoreland, B. F., & Klass, D. W. (1981). A distinctive rhythmic EEG discharge of adults. *Electroencephalography and Clinical Neurophysiology, 51*(2), 186–191. https://doi.org/10.1016/0013-4694(81)90008-0

Westmoreland, B. F., & Klass, D. W. (1986). Midline theta rhythm. *Archives of Neurology, 43*(2), 139–141. http://www.ncbi.nlm.nih.gov/entrez/query.fcgi?cmd=Retrieve&db=PubMed&dopt=Citation&list_uids=3947252

Westmoreland, B. F., & Klass, D. W. (1990). Unusual EEG patterns. *Journal of Clinical Neurophysiology, 7*(2), 209–228. https://doi.org/10.1097/00004691-199004000-00005

Westmoreland, B. F., & Klass, D. W. (1997). Unusual variants of subclinical rhythmic electrographic discharge of adults (SREDA). *Electroencephalography and Clinical Neurophysiology, 102*(1), 1–4. https://doi.org/10.1016/S0013-4694(96)96035-6

Westmoreland, B. F., & Sharbrough, F. W. (1975). Posterior slow wave transients associated with eye blinks in children. *American Journal of EEG Technology, 15*(1), 14–19.

White, J. C., Langston, J. W., & Pedley, T. A. (1977). Benign epileptiform transients of sleep: Clarification of the small sharp spike controversy. *Neurology, 27*(11), 1061. https://doi.org/10.1212/wnl.27.11.1061

Whitehead, K., Pressler, R., & Fabrizi, L. (2017). Characteristics and clinical significance of delta brushes in the EEG of premature infants. *Clinical Neurophysiology Practice, 2*, 12–18. https://doi.org/10.1016/j.cnp.2016.11.002

Wijdicks, E. F. M. (2002). Brain death worldwide: Accepted fact but no global consensus in diagnostic criteria. *Neurology, 58*(1), 20–25. https://doi.org/10.1212/WNL.58.1.20

Wijdicks, E. F. M., & Rabinstein, A. A. (2016). Myoclonus status and prognostication of postresuscitation coma: The bigger picture. *Annals of Neurology, 80*(2), 173–174. https://doi.org/10.1002/ana.24733

Wijdicks, E. F. M., Varelas, P. N., Gronseth, G. S., & Greer, D. M. (2010). Evidence-based guideline update: Determining brain death in adults: Report of the Quality Standards Subcommittee of the American Academy of Neurology. *Neurology, 74*(23), 1911–1918. https://doi.org/10.1212/WNL.0b013e3181e242a8

Williams, G. W., Lüders, H. O., Brickner, A., Goormastic, M., & Klass, D. W. (1985). Interobserver variability in EEG interpretation. *Neurology, 35*(12), 1714–1719. https://doi.org/10.1212/wnl.35.12.1714

Wolf, P., & Goosses, R. (1986). Relation of photosensitivity to epileptic syndromes. *Journal of Neurology, Neurosurgery, and Psychiatry, 49*(12), 1386–1391.

Yang, Z. X., Cai, X., Liu, X. Y., & Qin, J. (2008). Relationship among eye condition sensitivities, photosensitivity and epileptic syndromes. *Chinese Medical Journal, 121*(17), 1633–1637. https://doi.org/10.1097/00029330-200809010-00007

Zivin, L., & Marsan, C. A. (1968). Incidence and prognostic significance of "epileptiform" activity in the EEG of non-epileptic subjects. *Brain, 91*(4), 751–778.

Index

For the benefit of digital users, indexed terms that span two pages (e.g., 52–53) may, on occasion, appear on only one of those pages.

Page references followed by *b, f,* and *t* denote boxes, figures, and tables, respectively.